The construction and principal uses of mathematical instruments. Translated from the French of M. Bion, ... To which are added, the construction and uses of such instruments as are omitted by M. Bion; ... By Edmund Stone

N. Bion

The construction and principal uses of mathematical instruments. Translated from the French of M. Bion, ... To which are added, the construction and uses of such instruments as are omitted by M. Bion; ... By Edmund Stone. The whole illustrated with twenty

Bion, N. (Nicolas)
ESTCID: T162523
Reproduction from British Library
Titlepage in red and black. The ornaments are those used by Henry Woodfall.
London : printed by H. W. [Henry Woodfall] for John Senex; and William Taylor, 1723.
vii,[1],264p.,XXVIplates ; 2°

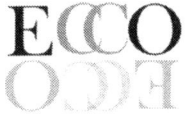

Gale ECCO Print Editions

Relive history with *Eighteenth Century Collections Online*, now available in print for the independent historian and collector. This series includes the most significant English-language and foreign-language works printed in Great Britain during the eighteenth century, and is organized in seven different subject areas including literature and language; medicine, science, and technology; and religion and philosophy. The collection also includes thousands of important works from the Americas.

The eighteenth century has been called "The Age of Enlightenment." It was a period of rapid advance in print culture and publishing, in world exploration, and in the rapid growth of science and technology – all of which had a profound impact on the political and cultural landscape. At the end of the century the American Revolution, French Revolution and Industrial Revolution, perhaps three of the most significant events in modern history, set in motion developments that eventually dominated world political, economic, and social life.

In a groundbreaking effort, Gale initiated a revolution of its own: digitization of epic proportions to preserve these invaluable works in the largest online archive of its kind. Contributions from major world libraries constitute over 175,000 original printed works. Scanned images of the actual pages, rather than transcriptions, recreate the works *as they first appeared.*

Now for the first time, these high-quality digital scans of original works are available via print-on-demand, making them readily accessible to libraries, students, independent scholars, and readers of all ages.

For our initial release we have created seven robust collections to form one the world's most comprehensive catalogs of 18th century works.

Initial Gale ECCO Print Editions collections include:

History and Geography

Rich in titles on English life and social history, this collection spans the world as it was known to eighteenth-century historians and explorers. Titles include a wealth of travel accounts and diaries, histories of nations from throughout the world, and maps and charts of a world that was still being discovered. Students of the War of American Independence will find fascinating accounts from the British side of conflict.

Social Science
Delve into what it was like to live during the eighteenth century by reading the first-hand accounts of everyday people, including city dwellers and farmers, businessmen and bankers, artisans and merchants, artists and their patrons, politicians and their constituents. Original texts make the American, French, and Industrial revolutions vividly contemporary.

Medicine, Science and Technology
Medical theory and practice of the 1700s developed rapidly, as is evidenced by the extensive collection, which includes descriptions of diseases, their conditions, and treatments. Books on science and technology, agriculture, military technology, natural philosophy, even cookbooks, are all contained here.

Literature and Language
Western literary study flows out of eighteenth-century works by Alexander Pope, Daniel Defoe, Henry Fielding, Frances Burney, Denis Diderot, Johann Gottfried Herder, Johann Wolfgang von Goethe, and others. Experience the birth of the modern novel, or compare the development of language using dictionaries and grammar discourses.

Religion and Philosophy
The Age of Enlightenment profoundly enriched religious and philosophical understanding and continues to influence present-day thinking. Works collected here include masterpieces by David Hume, Immanuel Kant, and Jean-Jacques Rousseau, as well as religious sermons and moral debates on the issues of the day, such as the slave trade. The Age of Reason saw conflict between Protestantism and Catholicism transformed into one between faith and logic -- a debate that continues in the twenty-first century.

Law and Reference
This collection reveals the history of English common law and Empire law in a vastly changing world of British expansion. Dominating the legal field is the *Commentaries of the Law of England* by Sir William Blackstone, which first appeared in 1765. Reference works such as almanacs and catalogues continue to educate us by revealing the day-to-day workings of society.

Fine Arts
The eighteenth-century fascination with Greek and Roman antiquity followed the systematic excavation of the ruins at Pompeii and Herculaneum in southern Italy; and after 1750 a neoclassical style dominated all artistic fields. The titles here trace developments in mostly English-language works on painting, sculpture, architecture, music, theater, and other disciplines. Instructional works on musical instruments, catalogs of art objects, comic operas, and more are also included.

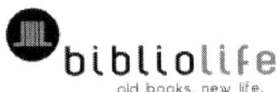

The BiblioLife Network

This project was made possible in part by the BiblioLife Network (BLN), a project aimed at addressing some of the huge challenges facing book preservationists around the world. The BLN includes libraries, library networks, archives, subject matter experts, online communities and library service providers. We believe every book ever published should be available as a high-quality print reproduction; printed on-demand anywhere in the world. This insures the ongoing accessibility of the content and helps generate sustainable revenue for the libraries and organizations that work to preserve these important materials.

The following book is in the "public domain" and represents an authentic reproduction of the text as printed by the original publisher. While we have attempted to accurately maintain the integrity of the original work, there are sometimes problems with the original work or the micro-film from which the books were digitized. This can result in minor errors in reproduction. Possible imperfections include missing and blurred pages, poor pictures, markings and other reproduction issues beyond our control. Because this work is culturally important, we have made it available as part of our commitment to protecting, preserving, and promoting the world's literature.

GUIDE TO FOLD-OUTS MAPS and OVERSIZED IMAGES

The book you are reading was digitized from microfilm captured over the past thirty to forty years. Years after the creation of the original microfilm, the book was converted to digital files and made available in an online database.

In an online database, page images do not need to conform to the size restrictions found in a printed book. When converting these images back into a printed bound book, the page sizes are standardized in ways that maintain the detail of the original. For large images, such as fold-out maps, the original page image is split into two or more pages

Guidelines used to determine how to split the page image follows:

• Some images are split vertically; large images require vertical and horizontal splits.
• For horizontal splits, the content is split left to right.
• For vertical splits, the content is split from top to bottom.
• For both vertical and horizontal splits, the image is processed from top left to bottom right.

THE
CONSTRUCTION
AND
PRINCIPAL USES
OF
Mathematical Inftruments.

Tranflated from the FRENCH of

M. BION,

Chief Inftrument-Maker to the *French* King.

To which are Added,

The *Conftruction* and *Ufes* of fuch INSTRUMENTS as
are omitted by *M. BION*; particularly of thofe
invented or improved by the ENGLISH.

By *EDMUND STONE*.

The whole Illuftrated with Twenty-fix Folio Copper-Plates, containing
the Figures, &c. of the feveral INSTRUMENTS.

*Imitetur igitur Ars Naturam, & quod ea defiderat inveniat; quod oftendit fequatur.
Nihil enim aut Natura extremum invenerit, aut Doctrina primum. fed Rerum
Principia ab Ingenio profecta funt, & Exitus Difciplina comparantur.*
Cicer. ad Heren. lib. 3.

LONDON:

Printed by *H. W.* for JOHN SENEX, at the *Globe*, over-againft
St. *Dunftan*'s Church, in *Fleetftreet*; and WILLIAM TAYLOR, at
the *Ship* and *Black-Swan* in *Pater-nofter* Row.
M.DCC.XXIII.

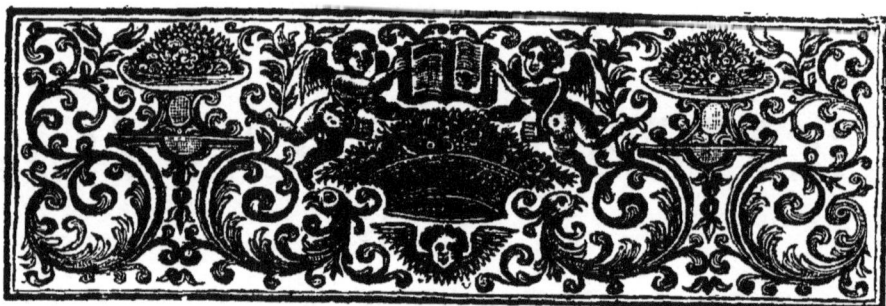

To his GRACE,

JOHN,

Duke of *Argyll* and *Greenwich*, &c.

Lord Steward of his Majefty's Houfhold.

MY LORD,

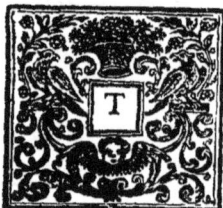

HE Subject of the following Treatife feems of Importance enough to claim Your Grace's Patronage, and of Ufe enough to deferve it. It made its firft Appearance under that of his Highnefs the Duke of *Orleans*. and, to render its fecond equally Magnificent, craves now to be introduced under that of Your Grace. Indeed, as the firft Defign of its appearing in *Englifh* was laid in Your Grace's Family, and as it was carried on and finifhed in the fame, it feems to have fome Title to Your Grace's Countenance: It naturally feeks Protection where it found its Birth, and lays claim to the Privileges of a Native of your Family, as well as thofe of a Domeftick. What I have faid of my Book, holds almoft equally good of my felf. I have been, the greateft part of my Life, an humble Retainer to Your Grace. In Your Family it was, I firft caught an Affection for MATHEMATICKS; and it was under Your Countenance, that I took occafion to Cultivate them. Your Grace therefore has a kind of Property in all I do of this kind, and it would be an Injuftice to lay it at any other Feet.

ANOTHER Perfon wou'd have here taken Occafion to expatiate on Your Grace's Character: Dedicators, Your Grace very well knows, are great Dealers in that Way, and look on it as one of the Privileges of their Place, to praife their Patrons without
Offence.

Offence. Accordingly, Your *Grace's* Lineage wou'd have been traced up to the earliest Times, and the Virtues of Your Noble Anceftors drawn out to View. Your *Grace's* perfonal Merit, fhining and confpicuous as it is, wou'd have been fet off in its full Light, and Your Heroick and Virtuous Atchievements painted in all their Colours. *Flanders, Bavaria, Spain,* and *Scotland,* wou'd have been call'd in, as Witneffes of Your Glory; of Your Prudence, as a General; and Your Bravery, as a Soldier: Nor wou'd Your Integrity, as a Minifter; Your Magnificence, as a Nobleman; or Your Love of Liberty and Your Country, as a Patriot, have been omitted. For my felf, *My Lord,* 'tis my Bufinefs rather to admire than applaud You: Panegyrick is a thing out of my Province; and Your Grace wou'd be a fufferer by the beft Things I could fay. Were I allow'd to touch on any Thing, it fhou'd be Your Private rather than Your Popular Character, rather as you're a Gentleman, than as a General, or a Hero. If You have every thing Great and Heroick in the latter; You have all that is Beautiful and Amiable in the former. To enumerate every thing of this Kind vifible in your Grace, wou'd be to give a detail of a whole Syftem of Virtues; and to draw your Picture at full, wou'd be little lefs than to collect into one Piece what is Great and Good in a thoufand: A Work fitter for a Volume than a Dedication.

MY Zeal for Your Grace had like to have driven me beyond either my Duty or Defign. It was my Refolution not to fay any thing that might look like Praife; but I find one cannot do common Juftice to Your Grace, without running into the Appearance of it. I am fenfible there is no Topick lefs inoffenfive to You, than that of Your own Merit: but the Misfortune is, there's none fo engaging or fo copious. 'Tis pity You fhould value Praife fo little; when You deferve it fo much: For hence, a Perfon, who wou'd not be Ungrateful, is under a Neceffity of becoming Troublefome. I have reafon to fear your Grace's Refentments, for having faid thus much, and yet apprehend thofe of the Publick for having faid no more. If I am Delinquent on either Side, your Grace will do me the Juftice, to believe it entirely owing to that Excefs of Devotion wherewith I am,

MY LORD,

Your Grace's moft Humble,

and moft Obedient Servant,

Edmund Stone.

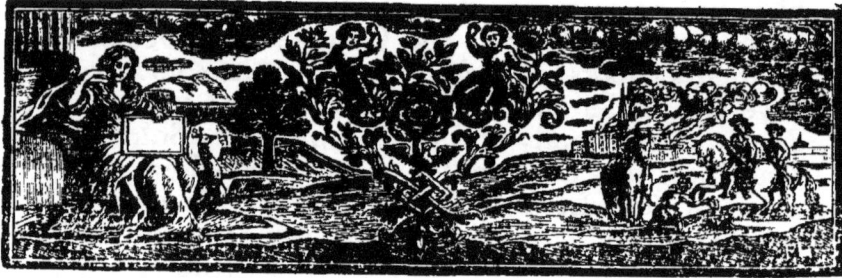

THE
TRANSLATOR's
PREFACE.

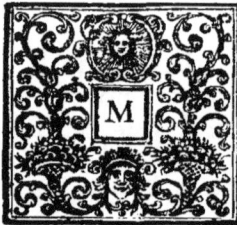

MATHEMATICKS *are now become a popular Study, and make a part of the Education of almost every Gentleman. Indeed, they are so useful, so entertaining and extensive a Branch of Knowledge, that 'tis no wonder they show'd gain Ground, and that uncommon Countenance they now find, must be esteemed as an Instance of the Felicity of the Age, and the Good Sense of the People. Mathematicks have wherewith to gratify all Tastes, and to employ all Talents. Here the greatest Genius has room to exert his utmost Faculties, and the meanest will not fail to find something on a Level with his. Their Theory, affords a noble Field for the Speculative part of Mankind; and, their Practice, an ample Province for the Men of Action and Business.*

THE Masters in Mathematicks have not been wanting in their Respect to the rest of Mankind. They have frankly communicated their Knowledge to the World, and have published Treatises on every Branch of their Art. insomuch, that a Man who has a Disposition to this Study, will find himself abundantly supplied with Helps, to what Part soever he applies himself. There seems, then, but little wanting to Mathematicks, considered as a Science. If there be any Defect, 'tis when considered as an Art. I mean, Mathematicks appears more accessible, as well as more extensive, on the Side of their Theory than on that of their Practice. Not that the latter has been less laboured by Authors than the former, but because a sufficient Regard does not seem to have been had to the Instruments, whereon it wholly depends.

MATHEMATICAL INSTRUMENTS are the Means by which those Sciences are rendered useful in the Affairs of Life. By their Assistance it is,

that

that ſubtile and abſtract Speculation is reduced into Act. They connect, as it were, the Theory to the Practice, and turn what was bare Contemplation, to the moſt ſubſtantial Uſes. The Knowledge of theſe is the Knowledge of Practical Mathematicks So that the Deſcriptions and Uſes of Mathematical Inſtruments, make, perhaps, one of the moſt ſerviceable Branches of Learning in the World. The Way then to render the Knowledge of Mathematicks general and diffuſive, is by making that of Mathematical Inſtruments ſo. With a View of which kind, our Author ſeems to have engaged in the following Treatiſe; at leaſt, 'twas from a View of this kind, that I undertook to tranſlate it.

THE Deſign of the Work, however uſeful, yet ſeems to be New among us. Particular Authors have indeed touch'd on particular Parts One, for Inſtance, having deſcribed the Globe, another the Sector, and a third the Quadiant: but for a general Courſe, or Collection of Mathematical Inſtruments, I know of none that has attempted it. 'Tis true, in Harris's Lexicon, we have the Names of moſt of them, and in Moxon's Dictionary the Figures of many. But the Accounts given of them in both are ſo ſhort, lame and deficient, that there's but little to be learn'd from either of them.

I choſe M. BION's Book for the Ground-Work of mine, as judging it better to make uſe of a good ſafe Model provided to my Hands, than run the Riſque of proceeding upon my own Bottom. The French Inſtruments deſcribed by him, are, in the main, the ſame with thoſe uſed among us. Such Engliſh Inſtruments as he has omitted, I have been careful to ſupply And throughout, have taken the Liberty not only to make up his Deficiencies, but amend his Errors.

THOSE who deſire an Inventory of the Work, have it as follows

IT is divided into Eight Books, and each of theſe ſubdivided into Chapters. To the whole are prefix'd Preliminary Definitions neceſſary for the Underſtanding of what follows.

IN the Firſt Book are laid down the Conſtruction and Principal Uſes of the moſt ſimple and common Inſtruments, as Compaſſes, Ruler, Drawing-Pen, Porte-Craion, Square, Protractor. And to theſe I have added five other Articles, of the Carpenter's Joint-Rule, the Four-foot Gauging-Rod, Everald's Sliding-Rule, Coggeſhall's Sliding-Rule, the Plotting-Scale, an Improv'd Protractor, the Plain Scale, and Gunter's Scale.

THE Second Book contains the Conſtruction and Principal Uſes of the French Sector, (or Compaſs of Proportion) thoſe of various Gauging-Rods. To this Book I have added the Conſtruction and principal Uſes of the Engliſh Sector.

THE Subject of the Third Book is very much diverſified. Under this are found the Conſtruction and Uſes of ſeveral curious and diverting as well as uſeful Inſtruments, particularly Compaſſes of various kinds, Parallel-Rules, the Parallelogram or Pentagraph, &c. Under this Head are alſo laid down ſeveral Things not eaſily to be met with elſewhere. As, the Manner of arming Load-ſtones, the Compoſition of divers Microſcopes, with ſeveral other curious Amuſements. To the firſt Chapter of this Book I have added the Deſcriptions and Uſes of the Turn-up Compaſſes and Proportional Compaſſes, with the Sector-Lines upon them, as alſo the Manner of projecting them.

IN the Fourth Book you have the Conſtruction and Uſes of the principal Inſtruments uſed in taking Plots, meaſuring or laying out Lands, taking Heights, Diſtances, acceſſible or inacceſſible; Staffs, for inſtance, Fathoms [or Toiſes] Chains, Surveying-Croſſes, Recipient-Angles, Theodolites, Semicircles,

circles, *the* Compaſs, *with their Uſes in Fortification. To this Book I have added three Articles of the* Engliſh Theodolite, Plain-Table, Circumferentor, *and* Surveying-Wheel. *What I have there added of the Uſes of thoſe Inſtruments, tho' but ſhort, yet I flatter my ſelf will be found more Inſtructive than much larger Accounts of them in the common Books of Surveying.*

THE Fifth Book contains the Conſtruction of ſeveral different kinds of Water-Levels, *with the Manner of rectifying and uſing them, for the Conveyance of Water from one Place to another. In this Book are alſo found the Conſtruction and Uſes of Inſtruments for* Gunnery *And to theſe I have added the Conſtruction and Uſe of the* Engliſh Callipers.

IN the Sixth Book are contained the Conſtruction and Uſes of Aſtronomical *Inſtruments, as the* Aſtronomical Quadrant, *and* Micrometer, *with an Inſtrument of* Mr. de la Hire's *for ſhewing the Eclipſes of the Sun and Moon, and* Mr. Huyghens's *Second* Pendulum-Clock *for Aſtronomical Obſervations. In this is alſo ſhewn the Manner of making Celeſtial Obſervations according to* Mr. de la Hire *and* Caſſini. *To this Book I have added four Chapters, containing the Deſcription and general Uſes of the Globes, with the manner of making them. The Deſcription and Uſes of the* Ptolemaick *and a* Copernican Sphere, *the* Orrery, *and a* Micrometer, *better than that deſcribed by the Author, and of* Gunter's Quadrant.

THE Seventh Book contains the Conſtruction and Uſes of the Sea-Compaſs, *the* Azimuth Compaſs, Sea-Quadrant, Fore-Staff, *and other Inſtruments for taking Altitudes at Sea, as likewiſe the Conſtruction and Uſes of the* Sinical Quadrant, *and* Mercator's Charts.

IN the Eighth Book are found the Conſtructions and Uſes of all kinds of Sun-Dials, *whether fixed or portable, with the Inſtruments uſed in drawing them, as alſo a* Moon-Dial, Nocturnal, *&c. To this is ſubjoined a ſhort Deſcription of the principal Tools uſed in making* Mathematical Inſtruments *And, laſtly, I have added, by way of Appendix, the Conſtruction of the great Eclipſe of the* Sun, *that will happen* May *the* 11th, 1724, *by the* Sector.

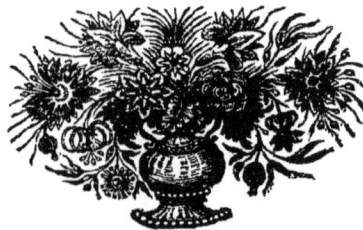

ERRATA.

ERRATA.

PAge 4 against Fig 53. should have been inserted this, *viz. an Octahedron is contained under eight equal and equilateral Triangles.* Page 8 l. 30. for *help of Division*, r *help of Addition* The Way laid down in P 10. for examining the Method of inscribing a regular *Polygon*, not being our Author's, but mine, should have been printed in *Italick* P. 15. l. 34 for *Converts*, r. *Converse.* P 60. for *Setter*, r. *Septier.* P. 156 L 60 for *Table*, r *Board.* P. 207 l 43 for *Cross Latitudes*, r. *increasing Latitudes*

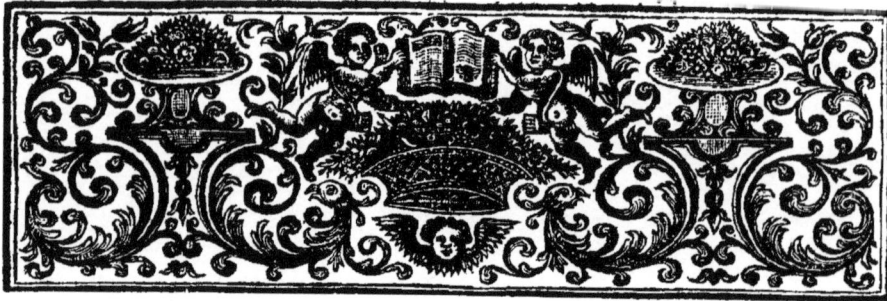

THE
CONSTRUCTION
AND
Principal Uses
OF
MATHEMATICAL INSTRUMENTS.

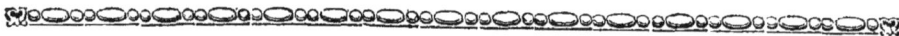

Definitions neceſſary for Underſtanding this Treatiſe.

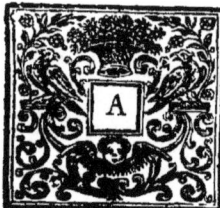

POINT is that which hath no Parts, and conſequently is indiviſible *Plate* 1. Fig 1

A Line is Length without Breadth, whoſe Original is from a Fig 2. Point

There are three kinds of Lines, *viz* Right Lines, Curve Lines, and Mix'd Lines

A Right Line is the ſhorteſt of all thoſe that can be drawn from Fig 2. one Point to another

A Curve Line is that which doth not go directly from one of its Fig. 3. Extremes to the other, but winds about

A Mix'd Line is that which hath one Part ſtrait, and the other Fig. 4. crooked

Lines compared, as to their Poſitions or Situations, are either parallel, perpendicular, or oblique

Parallel Lines are ſuch that always keep the ſame Diſtance to each other, and which, if Fig 5. both ways infinitely produced, will never meet, whether they be Right Lines, or Curves.

Perpendicular Lines are thoſe that meeting, incline no more to one ſide than to the other, Fig. 6. and therefore they make two equal Angles, which conſequently will be Right Angles

Oblique Lines are thoſe, which meeting one another, form oblique and unequal Angles, Fig. 7. that is, acute and obtuſe Angles

Moreover, Lines have other Denominations, which are as follow :

An upright, plumb, or vertical Line, is that which, if produced, would paſs thro' the Fig. 8. Center of the Earth, as the String of a ſuſpended Plummet

A horizontal Line, or Line of apparent Level, is a right Line that touches the Surface of Fig 9. the Earth in one Point, or which is parallel to a Tangent in that Point

A Line of true Level is that, whoſe Points are all equally diſtant from the Center of the Earth, as the Circumference of the ſame.

A finite Line is that whoſe Length is determined.

B

There

There are also occult Lines, drawn with the Points of Compasses, or more properly with a Pencil, because then they may be easier rubb'd out · These Lines must not be seen when the Work is finish'd, unless they are left to show how the Operation is performed, and then they are dotted, which is done with a Dotting-Wheel

Fig 10.   The Lines that must remain, and which are call'd apparent Lines, are drawn with Ink, put into a drawing Pen, as plain and small as possible, by means of the Screw belonging to it.

Fig 9.   A Tangent is a Line touching a Figure, and not cutting of it, as the Line AB.

Fig. 9.   A Subtense, or chord Line, is that which joins the Extremes of an Arc; as the Line CD

Fig. 11   An Arc is a Part of a Circumference, as the Arc DFE.

The different kinds of Curve Lines are infinite, but the simplest, most regular, and easiest to draw, is a Circle

Fig 11.   A circular Line, or the Circumference of a Circle, is a Curve, all the Parts of which are equally distant from one Point in the middle of it, which is call'd the Center of the Circle

Right Lines, drawn from the Center of a Circle to the Circumference, are call'd Radii, or Semidiameters, as NO

Those Chords that pass thro' the Center of a Circle, are call'd Diameters, as MP

The Circumference of every Circle is supposed to be divided into 360 equal Parts, call'd Degrees

The Number 360 was chosen by Geometricians for the Division of a Circle, because it may be more exactly subdivided into many equal Parts, without any Remainder, than any other[k] as for example, half of 360 is 180, $\frac{1}{3}$ is 120, $\frac{1}{4}$ is 90, $\frac{1}{5}$ is 72, $\frac{1}{6}$ is 60, and so of other of its aliquot Parts

Every Degree is divided into 60 equal Parts, call'd Minutes, every Minute into 60 Seconds, and every Second into 60 Thirds, &c which are thus distinguish'd $40^d 35^I 49^{II} 57^{III}$ signify forty Degrees, thirty five Minutes, forty nine Seconds, and fifty seven Thirds The aforesaid Division serves for measuring of Angles, but the Sub-Divisions into Seconds and Thirds are not used, unless in great Circumferences

The Opening of two different Lines cutting one another, or meeting in the same Point, is call'd an Angle

Fig 12   When two Lines cut, or meet each other in one Point on a Plan, the Angle they make with each other, is call'd a plane Angle

When the Lines that make a plain Angle, are strait Lines, the Angle is call'd a Right-lined Angle

Fig 13   If the two Lines forming an Angle, are Curves, the Angle is call'd a Curve-lined Angle

Fig 14.   If one of the Lines is a Curve, and the other a strait Line, the Angle is call'd a Mix'd-lined Angle

The two Lines that make an Angle, are call'd its Sides, the Point wherein they cut or meet each other, being the Vertex.

When an Angle is expressed by three Letters, that in the middle represents the Angle, and the other two the Sides

In producing or lessening the Sides of an Angle, the Quantity of the said Angle is not at all altered thereby, for the Magnitude of an Angle is not measured by the Magnitude of its Sides

Fig 15   The Measure of a Right-lined Angle is the Portion of a Circle comprehended between its Sides, whose Vertex is the Center of the Circle: It matters not how big the Radius of the Circle be, because whether the circular Arcs, comprehended between the Sides AB, AC, of the Angle be bigger or lesser, they still have the same Number of Degrees

If, for example, the Arc of a small Circle be 60 Degrees, which is the sixth part of the whole Circumference, the Arc of a greater Circle will likewise be 60 Degrees, or the sixth part of the Circumference of the greater Circle, and the Angle BAC will be 60 Degrees

Every Angle is either a right, acute, or obtuse Angle

Fig 16.   The Measure of a right Angle is an Arc of 90 Degrees, which is $\frac{1}{4}$ of the Circumference of a Circle

Fig 17   An acute Angle is lesser than 90 Degrees

Fig 18   An obtuse Angle is more than 90 Degrees

There can be no Angle of 180 Degrees, which is the Semi-Circumference of a Circle, for two right Lines so posited, cannot cut, but will meet each other directly, and consequently will make but one right Line, which will be the Diameter of a Circle

Fig 15   The Sine of an Angle or Arc, is half the Chord of double the same Arc as for example, to have the Sine of the Angle DAE, or of the Arc DE (which is the Measure of it) by doubling the Arc ED, you will have the Arc EDF, whose Chord is EF, whereof EH, its half, is the right Sine of the Angle DAE the Line DG is the Tangent of the same Angle, and the Line AG is its Secant

Two Arcs together making a whole Circle, have the same Chord, for it is manifest, that the Line EF is as well the Chord of the greater Arc EBCF, as of the lesser one EDF

---

* *Our Author should have said,* Lesser Number

For the same reason two Arcs, which together make a Semicircle, have but one right Sine, as the Line E H is as well the Sine of the obtuse Angle E A I, or of the Arc E B I, which is its Measure, as of the acute Angle E A D, or of the Arc E D.

The same may be said of Tangents and Secants

The Sine of 90 Degrees, which is the Radius or Semidiameter, as D A, is called the Sinus Totus

A Surface, or Superficies, is that which hath only Length and Breadth

There are two kinds of Surfaces, *viz.* Plane and Curve

A Plane Surface is that to which a right Line may be apply'd all manner of ways, as the Fig. 19. Top of a very smooth Table

A Curve Surface is that to which a right Line cannot be apply'd all manner of ways, Fig. 20 they are either Convex, or Concave, as the Outside of a Shell is Convex, and the Inside Concave

Term, or Bound, is that which limits any thing, as Points are the Bounds of Lines, Lines the Bounds of Surfaces, and Surfaces the Bounds of Solids

A Figure is that which is bounded every way.

Figures that be terminated under only one Bound, are Circles, and Ellipses, or Ovals, which are bounded by only one Curve Line

Figures terminated by several Bounds, or Lines, are the Triangle or Trigon, which hath Fig. 21 three Sides, and three Angles

The Square, or Tetragon, which hath four	Fig. 22.
The Pentagon, five.	Fig. 23
The Hexagon, six	Fig. 24
The Heptagon, seven	
The Octagon, eight.	
The Nonagon, nine	
The Decagon, ten	
The Undecagon, eleven	
And the Dodecagon, twelve	

All the aforesaid Figures, and those having a greater Number of Sides, are called by the general Name of Polygon, which signifies Figures having many Angles, and for distinguishing them, there is added the Number of Sides as a Decagon may be called a Polygon of ten Sides, likewise a Dodecagon is called a Polygon of twelve Sides, and so of others.

Figures, whose Sides and Angles are equal (as those before-named) are called regular Polygons

Those Figures, whose Sides and Angles are unequal, are called Irregular Polygons.

Triangles are distinguished by their Sides or their Angles

As to their Sides, that Triangle which hath its three Sides equal, is called an Equilateral Fig. 25. Triangle, and is also equiangular

That Triangle which hath only two equal Sides, is called an Isosceles Triangle Fig. 26.

And that which hath three unequal Sides, is called a Scalenous Triangle As to their An- Fig. 27. gles, a Triangle, which hath one right Angle, is called right-angled, and the Side op- Fig 28 posite to the right Angle, is called the Hypothenuse

That which hath one Angle obtuse, is called an obtuse angled Triangle Fig 29

That which hath all the Angles acute, is called an acute angled Triangle

Quadrilateral Figures, or Figures having four Sides, have different Appellations Fig. 30.

If the opposite Sides are parallel, the quadrilateral Figure is called by the general name of Parallelogram

If a Parallelogram hath four equal Sides, and the four Angles right ones, it is called a Fig 31 Square

If all the Sides are not equal, but the four Angles right ones, it is called an oblong, right Fig 32. angled Parallelogram, or simply a Rectangle

A right Line drawn in a Parallelogram, from one of the Angles to the opposite one, is called a Diagonal; as the Line A B

If the four Sides be equal, and also the opposite Angles, but not right ones, it is called a Fig 33. Rhombus, or Lozangé

If two opposite of the four Sides are equal, and the opposite Angles also equal, but not right ones, the quadrilateral Figure is called a Rhomboides Fig 34

Also a Square is equiangular and equilateral, an Oblong is equiangular, but not equilateral, a Rhombus is equilateral, but not equiangular ·

And a Rhomboides is neither equilateral nor equiangular

Every quadrilateral Figure, that hath neither its Opposite Sides, Parallel, or Equal, is Fig 35 called a Trapezium

A Circle is a plane Figure, comprehended under one Line, which is called its Circumfe- Fig. 36. rence, which is equally distant from a Point in the middle, called the Center.

A Semicircle is a Figure terminated by the Diameter and the Semicircumference

A Portion, or Segment of a Circle, is a Figure comprehended by a part of the Circumfe- Fig. 37 rence, and a Chord lesser than the Diameter, there is a greater and lesser Segment

A

Fig 38. A Sector of a Circle is a Figure made by a part of a Circle, terminated by two Radii, or Semidiameters, which do not make a right Line ; there is a great and small Sector

Fig. 39 An Ellipsis is a Figure longer than it is broad, comprehended but by one Curve Line, in which the * two greatest Lines that can be drawn at right Angles to one another, are called the Axes of the Ellipsis ; the greatest of which is called the great Axis, and the lesser the least Axis

The Center of an Ellipsis is that Point wherein the two Axes cut each other

Fig 40 Those Figures that have the same Center, are called Concentrick Figures

Fig. 41. Excentrick Figures are those that have not the same Center

Fig. 42 Similar Figures are those which have their Angles equal each to each , that is, which have each Angle of one Figure equal to the correspondent Angle in the other Figure, and have the Sides about the equal Angles proportional   As suppose the Side *a b* is one half, or one third of the Side A B , then all the other Sides of the lesser Figure *a b c d*, will be likewise one half, or one third of the Sides of the greater Figure A B C D

The correspondent Sides in this Figure are called homologous Sides , as the Side A B of the greater Figure, and the Side *a b* of the lesser Figure, are called homologous Sides

Equal Figures are those that equally contain an equal Number of equal Quantities

There are Figures that are similar and equal.

Others are equal, and not similar ,

And, finally, others are similar, but not equal

Fig 43. Isoperimetrical Figures are those whose Circuits are equal   As, for Example, the Triangle A B C, and the Square A B C D, are Isoperimetrical Figures, because each Side of the Triangle being 8, its Circuit is 24, and every Side of the Square being 6, its Circuit is also 24 of those equal Parts that make the Circuit of the Triangle

Body, or a Solid, is that which hath Length, Breadth, and Thickness

Fig 44. A Sphere, Globe, or Ball, is made by the entire Revolution of a Semicircle about its Diameter, which is at rest, and which is called the Sphere's Axis

Fig. 45. A Spheroid is a Solid, made by the entire Revolution of a Semi-Ellipsis about its Axis remaining at rest

Fig 46 A Pyramid is a Solid contained under several Triangular Planes meeting in one Point, and having a Polygon for its Base

Fig 47. A Cone is a Species of a Pyramid, having a circular Base. This Solid is made by the entire Revolution of a right-angled Triangle about one of the Sides, forming the right Angle, which Side is called the Axis of the Cone

Fig. 48. A Cylinder is a Solid, whose Bases are two equal Circles   This Solid is generated by the entire Revolution of a right-angled Parallelogram about one of its Sides, which is called the Cylinder's Axis.

Fig. 49 A Prism is a Solid, whose two Bases are two similar, equal, and parallel Planes, and when the parallel Planes are Triangles, the Prism is called a Triangular Prism

Fig. 50 When the two Bases of a Prism are Parallelograms, it is called a Parallelopipedon

If the Sides of the aforesaid Bodies are perpendicular to the Base, they are called right, or Isosceles Solids

If they are inclined, they are called Oblique, or Scalenous Solids

A regular Body is that which is contained under regular and equal Figures, all the solid Angles of which are likewise equal.

A solid Angle is the meeting of several Planes in one Point , as the Point of a Diamond.

There are required more than two Planes to constitute a solid Angle

There are five regular Bodies represented in the same Plate, together with the Unfoldings of their Planes, *viz.*

Fig. 51. The Tetrahedron, contained under four equal and equilateral Triangles

Fig 52. The Hexahedron, or Cube, contained under six equal Squares

Fig 53 The Dodecahedron, contained under twelve equilateral and equal Pentagons

Fig 54. The Icosahedron, contained under twenty equal and equilateral Triangles

Fig. 53. The Unfoldings nigh to each of the aforenamed regular Bodies, shew how to draw them on Brass or Pasteboard, in order to cut them out , which when done, if they are duly folded up, there will be formed the regular Bodies

All other Solids are called by the general Name of Polyhedron, which signifies a Body terminated by many Superficies

If in the following Work, Terms be used that are not here defined, they shall be defined and explained in their proper Places

---

* *Our Author should have said*, the greatest and least Lines

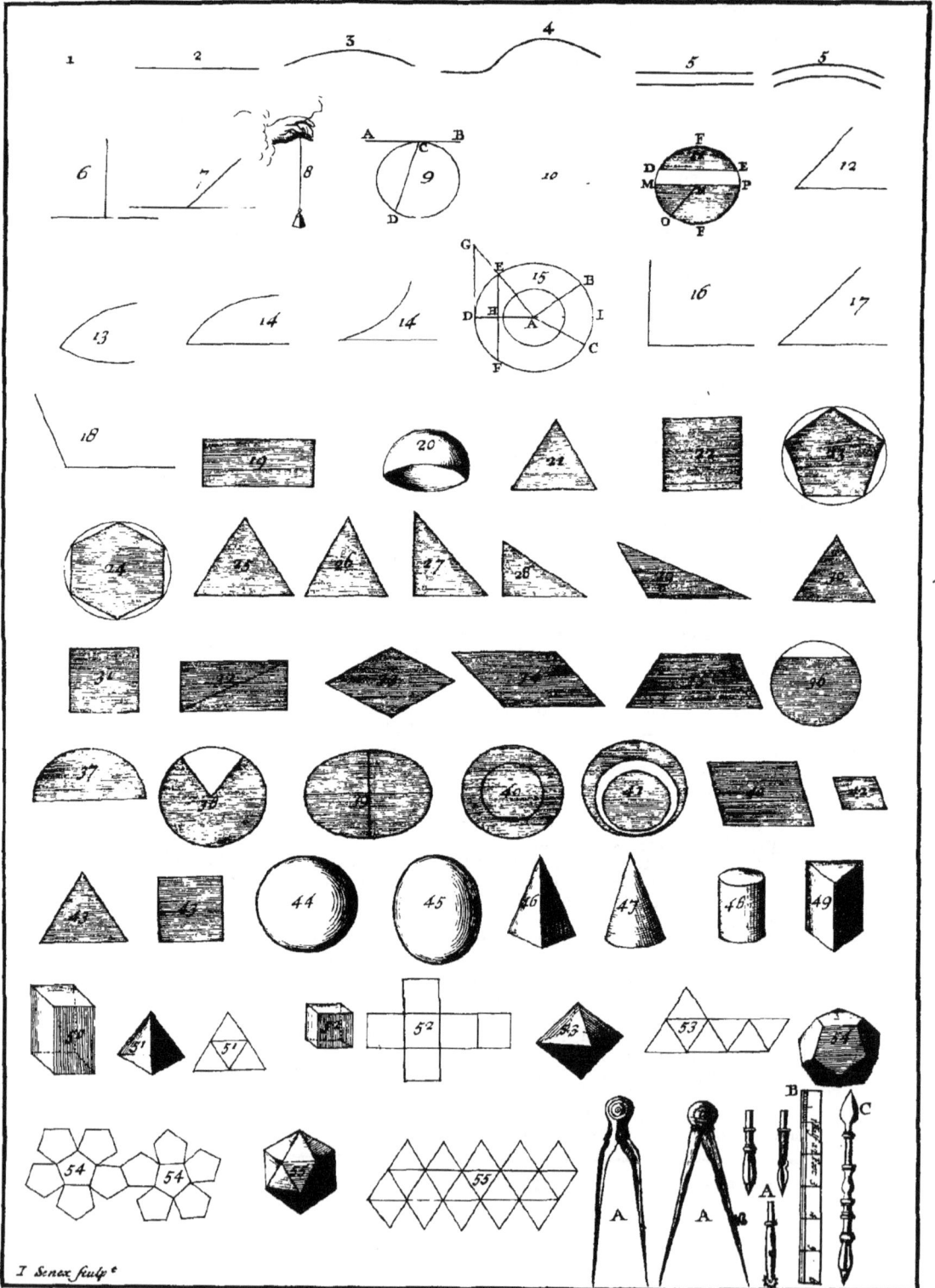

I Senex fculp.

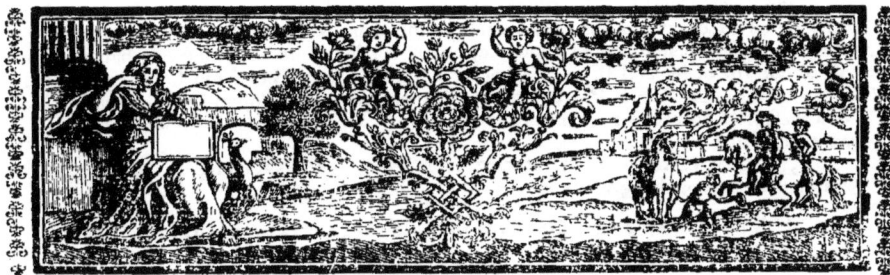

BOOK I.

Of the Construction and Use of Mathematical Instruments ; containing the common Instruments, as the Compass, *the* Ruler, *the* Drawing-Pen, *the* Porte-Craion, *the* Square, *and the* Protractor.

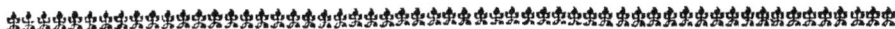

CHAP. I

Of the Construction and Use of the Compasses, *the* Ruler, *the* Drawing-Pen, *and the* Porte-Craion.

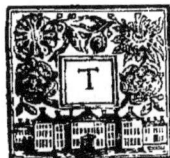

HERE are several Sorts of Compasses, of which we shall speak more fully hereafter, but that whose Uses we intend to lay down in this Chapter, is the Common Compass. Of these Compasses there are two kinds, *viz.* Simple Ones, which have their Points fixed, and others whose Points may be taken off, both kinds being of different Bigness, but they are commonly in Length from three to six Inches. To these Compasses, that shift their Points, there belongs a Drawing-Pen-Point, a Pencil-Point, and sometimes a Dotting-Wheel, to make dotted Lines.

The Goodness of Compasses consists chiefly in this, That the Motion of their Head be very equable, that so they may not leap in opening and shutting, that the Joints are well Fig. A. fitted, that they are well filed and polished, and, lastly, that the Steel-Points are well joined and equal. The Figure A sheweth these kinds of Compasses, whose Construction we shall give in the third Book.

Rulers, which are of Brass, or Wood, ought to be very strait every way, they are made Fig B. strait with Files and a Planner, whose Bottom is Steel, as also by rubbing them and another very strait Ruler together: one Side of these Rulers is sloped, to keep the Ink from blotting the Paper.

When Lines are drawn with Ink, they ought to be very fine.

To know whether a Ruler be very strait or not, draw a right Line upon a Plane, then turn the Ruler about, and apply the same Edge to the Line, and if the Edge of the Ruler exactly agrees with the right Line, it is a Sign the Ruler is very strait.

The Drawing-Pen is made of two Steel Blades joined together, and fastened to a little Fig. C. Pillar, at the other End of which is a Porte-Craion, there is a Cavity between the aforesaid Blades, in which Ink is put with a Pen. also the Blades must join each other in Points that be very equal. There is likewise a small Screw, serving more or less to open the Blades, that so Lines may be drawn fine or coarse, according to necessity.

The Porte-Craion ought to be of equal Bigness every where, and very straitly slit down the middle with a fine Saw ; also the Porte-Craion is bent towards the end, in order to fasten a Pencil in it, by means of a little Ring.

C   USE

USE I. *To divide a right Line into two equal Parts*

Plate 2
Fig. 1.

Let the given Line be A B, which is to be divided into two equal Parts · About the Point A, as a Center, or one of the Ends of the Line, deſcribe the circular Arc C D, with your Compaſſes opened to any Diſtance, but neverthelefs greater than one half of A B. Likewiſe about the other end B, as a Center, deſcribe, with the ſame Opening of your Compaſſes, the circular Arc E F, cutting the former Arc in the Points G H, then place a Ruler upon theſe two Interſections, and draw the Line G H, which will divide the Line A B into two equal Parts

Note, The two Arcs will not interſect each other, if the Opening of the Compaſſes be not greater than half of the given Line

USE II *Upon a right Line, and from a Point given in it, to raiſe a Perpendicular*

Fig 2

Let the given right Line be A B, and the Point given in it C, upon which it is required to raiſe a Perpendicular

From the given Point C, mark both ways with your Compaſſes, on the given Line, the equal Diſtances C A, C B, then about the Points A B, as Centers, and with any opening of your Compaſſes (greater than half the given Line) deſcribe the Arcs D E, F G, interſecting each other in the Point H, and draw the Line H C, which will be perpendicular to A B

Fig. 3

If the given Point C be at the End of the Line, deſcribe about the Point C, as a Centre, any Arc of a Circle, on which take twice the ſame opening of your Compaſſes, viz from B to D, and from D to E. then about the Points D, E, deſcribe two Arcs, interſecting one another in the Point F, lay a Ruler upon the Points F and C, and draw the Line F C, which will be a Perpendicular upon the End of the Line C B

If there is not room to take the Length of D E, divide the Arc B D into two equal Parts in the Point G, and make D H equal to D G, then the Line H C will be a Perpendicular

Fig 4

Or otherwife, having drawn the indefinite Line B D F, thro the Points D, F, and made D F equal to B D, F C will be a Perpendicular

Fig 5

Or again in this Manner having taken the Point P at pleaſure above the given Line, about the ſaid Point, as a Center, and with the Interval P C, deſcribe the Arc B C D, then draw the Line B P, and produce it till it cuts the aforeſaid Arc in the Point D, and from the Point D to the Point C, draw the Perpendicular D C

USE III *From a Point given without a Line, to let fall a Perpendicular to the ſaid Line*

Let the given Point be C, from which, to the given Line A B, it is required to draw a Perpendicular

Fig 6.

About the Point C, as a Center, deſcribe an Arc of a Circle cutting the Line A B in the two Points D E, then from the Points D E, make the Interſection F, lay a Ruler upon the Points C and F, and draw the Perpendicular C G

Note, The Interſection F may be made above or below the given Line, but it is beſt to have it below it, becauſe when the Points C F are at a good Diſtance, the Perpendicular may be drawn truer than when they are nigh

When the Portion of the Circle deſcribed about the Point C, does not cut the Line A B in two Points, the Line muſt be continued if it can, if it cannot, Recourſe muſt be had to the Method of *Fig 5* for raiſing a Perpendicular on the End of a Line as ſuppoſe a Perpendicular is to be let fall from the Point D, on the Line C D, draw, at pleaſure, the Line D B, which biſect in the Point P, then about this Point, as a Centre, and with the Diſtance P D, deſcribe the Arc D C B, cutting the Line A B in the Point C Laſtly, lay a Ruler upon the Points C and D, and draw the Line C D, which will be the Perpendicular required

Fig. 7.

Otherwiſe, let A B be the given Line, and C the Point without it, take two Points 1 and 2 at pleaſure, on the ſaid Line A B, then about the Points 1 and 2, and with the Diſtances 1 C, 2 C, deſcribe Arcs of Circles, interſecting each other in two Points, as in C and D, then lay a Ruler on the two Interſections, and draw a Line, which will be the Perpendicular required

USE IV *To cut a right-lined Angle into two equal Parts.*

Let A C B be the Angle to be cut into two equal Parts

Fig. 8.

About the Point C, as a Center, deſcribe the Arc D E at pleaſure, then about the Points D and E, deſcribe two other Arcs, cutting each other in the Point F, and draw the Line F C thro the Points F, C, which will cut the given Angle into two equal Parts

If it be required to divide the Angle A C B into three equal Parts, the Arc D E muſt tentatively be divided by your Compaſſes into three equal Parts; becauſe the Triſection of an Angle by right Lines, hath not yet been geometrically found

USE V *To raiſe a right Line on a given Line, that may incline no more on one Side than the other*

Make the ſame Operation as before, and produce the Line F C G   Fig 8

USE VI *Upon a given right Line, and from a Point given in it, to make an Angle equal to a given Angle*

Let A B be the given Line, and A the given Point upon which it is required to make an Angle equal to the given Angle E F G

About the Point F, as a Center, deſcribe the Portion of a Circle, and with the ſame Fig 9 opening of your Compaſſes, deſcribe about the Point A another Portion, then take the Big-neſs of the Arc E G between your Compaſſes, which Diſtance lay off on the Arc B C now thro the Points A, C, draw the Line A C, and the Angle B A C will be equal to the Angle E F G

USE VII *To draw a Line from a given Point, parallel to a given Line*

Let A B be the given Line, and C the Point thro which it is required to draw a Line parallel to A B

About the Point C, as a Center, and with any opening of your Compaſſes, taken at pleaſure, deſcribe the Arc D B cutting the given Line in the Point B, alſo about the ſame Fig 10. Point B, as a Center, and with the ſame opening of your Compaſſes, deſcribe the Arc C A, then take the Diſtance of the Points C, A, and lay it off from B to D, and thro the Points C and D, draw the Line C D, which will be parallel to A B

Otherwiſe, about the Point C, as a Center, deſcribe an Arc touching the given Line, and about another Point, taken at pleaſure in the Line A B, deſcribe, with the ſame opening Fig 11 of your Compaſſes, the Arc D then thro the Point C, draw a Line touching the Arc D, and the Line C D will be parallel to A B

But as it is difficult to find whereabouts the Point of Contact will be, there is another way which is better, and is thus ·

About the Point C, as a Center, and with any Diſtance, deſcribe an Arc cutting the Line Fig 12. A B in A

And about another Point in the ſame Line, as B, deſcribe another Arc, with the ſame opening of your Compaſſes, then open the Compaſſes to the Diſtance A B, and about the Point C, as a Center, deſcribe an Arc cutting the former one in the Point D, and thro the Points C and D draw a Line, which will be parallel to A B

USE VIII *To divide a given Line into any number of equal Parts*

Let the Line given be A B, which is required to be divided into eight equal Parts · firſt, Fig 13 draw the Line B C, at pleaſure, making any Angle with the Line A B Likewiſe draw the Line A D parallel to B C, then divide B C into eight equal Parts, taken at pleaſure, and make the ſame Parts on the Line A D, and thro the Diviſions of them, draw Lines, which will divide the Line A B into eight equal Parts

Or otherwiſe, draw the Line *a b* parallel to A B, which is propoſed to be divided, then Fig 14 take 8 equal Parts on the Line *a b* Now thro the Ends of the two Parallels draw two Lines, which form Triangles with the Parallels, and interſect each other in the Point C; then from the Point C, draw Lines to the Diviſions made on the Line *a b*, which will cut the Line A B in the Number of equal Parts required

This Diviſion of Lines ſerves to make Diagonal Scales, as ſuppoſe the Line A B is to make a Scale of eighty Parts, or eighty Fathom, each Part of this Line, divided into eight, Fig 15. contains ten Fathom · but ſince it is difficult to divide each of the aforeſaid Parts into ten others, you muſt raiſe from the Ends of the Line A B, the Perpendiculars A D and B C, on which take ten Parts at pleaſure, from every of which, you muſt draw Parallels to the Line A B, then the ſame Diviſions muſt be made on the Line D C, as on A B, and the tranſ-verſal Lines A E, 10 F, 20 G, &c muſt be drawn

Now it is eaſy to take off any Number of Fathoms from this Scale. as, for Example, to take off 23 Fathoms; Take the Concourſe of the Tranſverſal 20 G, with the Parallel 3, that is at the Point Z, and Z 3 will be 23 Fathom Moreover, if 58 Fathom is required, take the Concourſe of the Tranſverſal 50 H, with the Parallel 8, which is Y, and Y 8 will repre-ſent 58 Fathom, and ſo of others Feet might be put upon this Scale, by making a greater Diſtance between the Parallels; and by ſub-dividing them into 12 equal Parts, there would be obtained Inches

But now to divide a very ſhort Line into a great Number of equal Parts, as into 100 or 1000 For Example, Suppoſe the Line A D is to be divided into 1000 equal Parts, firſt, Fig 16 from the Ends A D, raiſe the Perpendiculars A B, D C, and divide each of theſe Perpendi-culars into 10 equal Parts, and draw thro the Diviſions the like Number of Parallels to A D, then divide each of the Lines A D, B C, into 10 equal Parts, which join by the like Num-

ber

ber of Perpendiculars   Again, ſubdivide the firſt Space A E, and its Parallel, into 10 more Parts, which join by tranſverſal or oblique Lines, as the Line E 1, &c

By this Means the firſt Interval A E, will be divided into 100 equal Parts, for which Reaſon, the Numbers 200, 300, 400, 500, &c. to 1000, are placed on this Scale, as may be ſeen in *Fig* 16

The Manner of taking off any Number of equal Parts from the aforeſaid Scale, is the ſame as that which hath been already ſhewn in the precedent Figure   We ſhall again mention this Scale in the Chapter of the Sector   There are alſo Sines, Tangents, and Secants, projected upon Scales, in the following Manner . If from each Degree of the Quadrant I F, beginning from the Point I, Perpendiculars are let fall to the Radius A I, theſe will be the Sines of each Degree, the greateſt of which is the Radius of the Circle, or Sinus Totus A F, and the Lengths of all theſe Sines may be projected upon the Radius, in order to make a Scale, beginning from the Point A, as the Sine D K is lay'd off from A towards G, &c

And if the Tangent I E, be indefinitely produced towards E, and from the Center A, Lines, as A F, be drawn thro each Degree of the Quadrant, to the Tangent I E produced, theſe will be the Secants of each Degree of the Quadrant   Whence it is manifeſt, that any one of the Secants is greater than the Radius A I   It is likewiſe plain, that every Tangent I E, is terminated by its Secant A E, in the Line I E, which will be a Scale of Tangents . and it is in this manner, that the ſimple Scales of Sines, Tangents, and Secants, are made in taking between your Compaſſes each of thoſe Diſtances, and laying them off upon a Ruler The Tables of Sines, Tangents, and Secants, are likewiſe made on this Principle : for the Radius of a Circle, or Sine of a right Angle, is ſuppoſed to be divided into 10000, and then there is found how many of theſe Parts every right Sine contains, as alſo the Tangents and Secants from one Minute to 90 Degrees, which, when put in order, are called the Tables of Sines, Tangents, and Secants

Logarithms are Numbers in an Arithmetical Progreſſion, to which anſwer other Numbers in a Geometrical Progreſſion, as the two following Progreſſions

Prog Geom Numb 1, 2, 4, 8, 16, 32, 64, 128, 256, &c.

Prog Arith Log   0, 1, 2, 3, 4, 5, 6, 7, 8, &c   Logarithms were invented to perform Multiplication by only the help of Diviſion, and Diviſion by Subſtraction, by which Operations are infinitely ſhortened, and ſo they are of excellent Uſe in Aſtronomical Calculations

Note, The Uſe of theſe Tables is explained in Books of the Tables of Sines, Tangents, and Secants

USE IX. *To cut off from a given Line any Part aſſigned*

Let the Line A B be the given Line from which it is required to cut off the fourth Part

Draw the indefinite Line A C, making any Angle with the Line A B, which divide into four equal Parts at pleaſure, then from the laſt Diviſion, draw the Line B 4, and afterwards the Line D I, parallel to B 4, which will be a fourth Part of A B

USE X *To draw a right Line thro a given Point, that ſhall touch a Circle*

If the given Point be in the Circumference, draw the Radius A B, and on the Point B raiſe the Perpendicular B C, which will be a Tangent in the Point B   But if the given Point B be without the Circle, draw a right Line from the Center A, to the Point B, which biſect in the Point D. then about the ſaid D, as a Center, and with the Diſtance B D, deſcribe a Semi-Circle cutting the Circle in the Point E, and draw B E, which will be a Tangent

If a Circle be given with its Tangent, and the Point of Contact be required, let fall the Perpendicular A B from the Center of the Circle, and the Interſection of the Tangent with the ſaid Perpendicular, will be in the Point of Contact

USE XI *Upon a given Line to deſcribe a Spiral, making any Number of Revolutions*

Let the given Line be A B, upon which it is required to deſcribe a Spiral of 3 Revolutions Firſt, biſect that Line in the Point C, about which Point, as a Center, deſcribe a Semi-Circle, whoſe Diameter may be equal to the given Line A B, then trifect the Semi-Diameter in the Points D E, and about the ſame Center deſcribe, on the ſame Side the Line A B, two other Semi-Circles paſſing thro the Points D E · again, ſubdivide the Space C E, into two equal Parts in the Point F, about which, as a Center, deſcribe on the other Side of the given Line, three other Semi-Circles, and a Spiral of three Revolutions will be had   If the Spiral is required to make four Revolutions, you muſt divide the Semi-Diameter A C into 4 equal Parts

USE XII *Upon a given right Line, to deſcribe an equilateral Triangle*

Let A B be the given Line on which it is required to deſcribe an equilateral Triangle

About the Point A, and with the Diſtance A B, deſcribe an Arc of a Circle, and about the Point B, as a Center, with the Diſtance B A, deſcribe another Arc cutting the precedent one in the Point C; then draw the Lines C A, C B, and the Triangle A B C, will be an equilateral Triangle.

USE

Fig 17

Fig 18

Fig. 19 & 20

Fig. 21.

Fig 22.

USE XIII *Upon a given right Line, to make a Triangle equal and ſimilar to a given one*

Let the given Triangle be A B C, to which it is required to make another ſimilar, as Fig 24 and 25 D E F

Make the Line D E equal to A B, then about the Point D, as a Center, and with the Radius A C deſcribe an Arc, alſo about the Point E, as a Center, and with the Radius B C deſcribe another Arc, cutting the former one in the Point F, then draw the Lines D F, E F, and there will be a Triangle made equal and ſimilar to the given one

USE XIV *Upon a given right Line to make a Triangle ſimilar to a given one*

Let the given Line be H I, upon which it is required to make a Triangle ſimilar (but Fig 26. not equal) to the Triangle A B C and 27

Make the Angle H equal to the Angle A, and the Angle I equal to the Angle B, then draw the Lines H G, I G, till they meet each other, and the Triangle H I G will be that required.

USE XV *To make a Triangle of three right Lines given, but any two of them muſt be longer than the third*

Let the three given Lines be A, B, C, firſt make the Line D E equal to the Line A, and Fig 28 about the Point E as a Center, with an Interval, equal to the Line B, deſcribe the Portion of a Circle, alſo about D, as a Center, with an Interval equal to C, deſcribe another Portion of a Circle, cutting the former one in the Point F, then draw the right Lines F D, F E, and the Triangle D F E will be that required ●

USE XVI *Upon a given right Line to make a Square*

Let the given Line be A B, on which it is required to deſcribe a Square, whoſe Side Fig 29 may be equal to the given Line, firſt about the Point A, as a Center, and with the Diſtance A B, deſcribe the Arc B D, and about the Point B the Arc A E, interſecting it in the Point C, and divide the Arc C A, or C B, into two equal Parts in the Point F now make the Intervals C E, and C D, equal to C F, and draw the Lines A D, B E, D E, and the Square will be made.

Or, otherwiſe, upon the End of the Line A B, raiſe the Perpendicular A D equal to A B, and about the Point D, as a Center, with the Diſtance A D, deſcribe an Arc, likewiſe, Fig 30. with the ſame opening of your Compaſſes about the Point B, deſcribe another Arc, and 31. cutting the firſt in the Point E, and draw the Lines A D, D E, E B, and the Square will be made

I ſhall ſhew, in the Uſes of the Protractor and Sector, how to make any regular Polygon upon a given Line, but, by the way, I ſhall give one general Method for conſtructing them, by means only of a Ruler and Compaſſes

USE XVII *To inſcribe any regular Polygon in a Circle*

Suppoſe, for Example, a Pentagon is to be made   Now if the Circle be given, divide its Diameter into five equal Parts (by *Uſe* VIII) but if it be not given, draw with your Pencil an indefinite Line for a Diameter, which being divided into five equal Parts, open your Compaſſes the whole Extent of the Diameter, and ſetting one Foot of them upon the Ends Fig. 32. of the Diameter, deſcribe two Arcs interſecting each other in the Point C, that thereby an equilateral Triangle may be formed, then having drawn a Circle about the Diameter, lay a Ruler upon the ſaid Point C, and upon the ſecond Diviſion of the Diameter, and draw a Line, cutting the concave Part of the Circumference in the Point D, then the Arc A D will be nighly a fifth part of the Circumference   therefore the Extent A D will divide the Circle into five equal Parts, and drawing five Lines, the propoſed Polygon will be made

This is a general Method to make all regular Polygons   As, to make a Heptagon, there is no more to do but divide the Diameter A B into ſeven equal Parts (that is, into as many Parts as the Figure hath Sides) and always drawing a Line from the Point C, thro' the ſecond Diviſion of the Diameter

The Conſtruction of a Hexagon is ſimpler, becauſe, without any Preparation, the Radius, or Semidiameter of the Circle will divide the Circumference into ſix equal Parts

And the Dodecagon is made in only biſecting each Arc of the Hexagon; therefore to make a Decagon, every Arc of the Pentagon muſt be biſected

This Problem is almoſt the ſame as that deſcribed in *cap* 17 *lib* 1 of the Chevalier *de Ville*'s Fortification, except, that for dividing the Circle, he draws a Line from the exterior Angle of the equilateral Triangle, thro' the firſt Point of Diviſion of the Diameter, and afterwards he doubles the Arc of the Circle, but his Method is far from being exact · for, in the Deſcription of a Pentagon, the Angle at the Center is too great by forty four Minutes; in the Heptagon it is too great one Degree and five Minutes, and ſo the Error will be augmented in Polygons of a greater number of Sides   But by making the Line paſs thro' the ſecond Point of Diviſion of the Diameter, the Angle at the Center of the Pentagon will be but

D   about

about fix Minutes too little, and in the Heptagon it is too great by about fix Minutes, which are much lefs Errors, and almoft infenfible in the Defcription of the Polygons

' The Truth of the aforefaid Method of infcribing any regular Polygon in a Circle, which
' is mentioned in *Sturmy's Mathefis Juvenilis*, may, by the help of Trigonometry, be eafily
' examined For, fuppofe A C G to be a Circle, D the Center, A C the Diameter, A B C an
' equilateral Triangle, E the fecond Point of Divifion of the Diameter divided into any Num-
' ber of equal Parts, B F drawn thro' the Points B, E, D B, perpendicular to A C, and the
' Points D, F, joined Now becaufe the Semidiameter DC, and the whole Diameter BC are
' given, the Perpendicular D B (*per Prop* 47 *hb* 1 *Eucl*) will be had

' Again, becaufe the Number of equal Parts the Diameter is divided into, is given, the
' Line C E, which is two of thofe equal Parts, will be given, and confequently the Part D E,
' then in the right-angled Triangle B D E, the Sides B D, D E being given, the Angle DB E
' may be found, by faying, as D B is to D E, fo is Radius to the Tangent of the Angle
' D B E.

' Moreover, becaufe in the Triangle B D F, the Sides D B, and D F (equal to D C) are
' given, and the Angle F B D (which is now found), the Angle B F D may be found, by fay-
' ing, as D F is to D B, fo is the Sine of the Angle D B F, to the Sine of the Angle D F B
' which being found, add it to the Angle D B F, and fubftract the Sum from 180 Degrees,
' then the Remainder will be the Angle B D F, from which take the right Angle B D C,
' and the Remainder will be the Angle F D C of the Center of the Polygon

' I have calculated, according to the aforefaid Directions, the Quantity of the Angle F DC
' for a Pentagon, which I find to want about 14 Minutes of 72 Degrees, the Angle of the
' Center for a Pentagon, (tho' our Author fays it wants but fix) likewife the Hexagon wants
' 12 Minutes of 60 Degrees, the Angle at the Center, that of the Octagon is one Degree too
' great, and that of the Dodecagon 29 Minutes too great therefore this Method is very er-
' roneous, and not to be ufed, it being only true for infcribing a Square '

USE XVIII *To draw a Circle thro' three given Points, provided they be not in a right Line.*

Let the given Points be A B C firft draw a Line from the Point A to the Point B, and another from the Point B to the Point C, both of which divide into two equal Parts by the Lines D E, F G, drawn at right Angles to them, and meeting each other in the Point H, which will be the Center of the Circle: Now about the Point H as a Center, and with the Diftance H A, H B, or H C, defcribe a Circle, and what was required will be done

By this means the Circumference of a Circle begun, may be finifhed, in taking three Points in it, and proceeding as before.

USE XIX *To find the Center of a Circle.*

Let A B D be the given Circle, whofe Center is required to be found, draw the Line A B, which bifect by the Line C D at right Angles likewife bifect the Line C D by the Line E F, cutting the Line C D in the Point G, which will be the Center of the Circle

USE XX *To draw a right Line equal to the Circumference of a Circle, and, contrariwife, to make the Circumference of a Circle equal to a given Line*

Let the given Circle A B C D be that whofe Circumference it is required to make a right Line equal to Firft draw a right Line, and lay off upon it three times and ⅐ of the Dia-meter, as from G to H, then this right Line G H will be almoft equal to the Circumference of the Circle I fay almoft, for if it could be exactly had equal to the Circumference, the Quadrature of the Circle would alfo be had, which hath not yet been Geometrically found

USE XXI *To defcribe an Oval upon a given right Line.*

Let A B be the given Line, upon which it is required to defcribe an Oval, trifect it in the Points C and D, then upon the Part C D defcribe two equilateral Triangles, whofe Sides produce; and about the Points C, D, with the Diftance C A, or D B, defcribe Portions of a Circle to the Sides of the Triangles, produced to the Points E, F, G, H, then about the Points I, K, as Centers, and with the Radius I E, or I G, defcribe the Arc E G on one Side, and the Arc F H on the other, and the Oval will be made

USE XXII *To defcribe an Ellipfis, having the two Axes given*

Let the great Axis be A B, and the fmall one C D, interfecting each other at right Angles in the Point G

First take with your Compaffes, or a String, half the Length of the great Axis, that is, A G, or G B, and with this Length fetting one foot of your Compaffes in the Point C, de-fcribe a Circle cutting the great Axis in the Points E, F, which will be the Foci of the Ellip-fis. This being done, place Pins in thefe Foci; or if the Ellipfis to be defcribed be re-quired large, and to be on the Ground, as in a Garden, drive Pegs into them: Then take a Thread, or String, equal in Length to the great Axis A B, and after having doubled it, put it about the two Pins or Pegs placed in the Foci E, F, fo that the two Ends which you hold in your Hand may be in the End C of the fmall Axis: then holding a Pencil, or fome-thing

thing elſe propei to make a Mark, in your Hand at C, move it round, keeping the String always tight, till it, together with the Ends of the Thread or String, come again to the Point C, and the Elliplis A D B C will be deſcribed by the Pencil

Note, This Method of deſcribing an Elliplis is the beſt of any ; as alſo if the Thread, or String, be in Length augmented or diminiſhed, without changing the Diſtance of the Foci, theie will be had Elliplies of another kind   Moreover, if without changing the Length of the Thread, or String, the Diſtance of the Foci be diminiſhed, there will ſtill be had another Species of Elliplies , and when the Foci's Diſtance is infinitely diminiſhed, a Circle will be deſcribed · But it the Length of the great Axis be augmented or diminiſhed, together with the String (which is equal to it) in the ſame Proportion as the Diſtance of the Foci, all the Elliplies will be of the ſame kind, but of different Magnitudes

To draw an Elliplis another way

The two Foci L, F, being found (as in the precedent Figure) any Number of Points, thro' which the Elliplis muſt paſs, may in this manner be found   Open your Compaſſes at pleaſure to any Diſtance greater than A F, as to the Diſtance A I, then ſet one of their Points in the Focus F, and with the other deſcribe the Arc O R , afterwards open the Com-   Fig 39 paſſes the Diſtance I B, which is the remaining part of the great Axis, and ſetting one of its Points in the other Focus L, with the Diſtance I B deſcribe the Arc S T, and the Point P of Interſection will be in the Periphery of the Elliplis   In like manner, the Diſtances A L, L B, deſcribed about the Foci, will interſect each other in the Point H   and, finally, by opening your Compaſſes to different Diſtances, any Number of Points may be found , which being joined, an Elliplis will be had

Note, Every Opening of your Compaſſes ſerves to find four Points equally diſtant from the Axes, as alſo if, from any Point taken at pleaſure in the Periphery of an Elliplis, two right Lines, as P F, P E, are drawn to the Foci, theſe will be both together equal to the great Axis.

USE XXIII *To make one Figure equal and ſimilar to another Figure*

Let the propoſed Figure be A B C D E, to which another is to be made ſimilar and equal

Firſt divide it into Triangles by the Lines A C, A D, then draw the Line *a b* equal to A B, and about the Point *b*, with the Diſtance B C, deſcribe an Arc   alſo about the Point *a*, Fig 40 and with the Diſtance A C, deſcribe another Arc, cutting the former one in the Point *c*, and draw the Line *b c*   In like manner proceed for the other Sides, and the Figure *a b c d e* will &c be ſimilar to the propoſed Figure A B C D E

USE XXIV. *To reduce great Figures to leſſer ones, and contrariwiſe.*

Becauſe the Reduction of Figures is uſeful, there is here three ways given to reduce them

Firſt, a Figure may be reduced in taking a Point within it, and drawing of Lines to all Fig 41. the Angles   for Example, let the Figure A B C D E be propoſed to be reduced to a leſſer

Take the Point F, about the middle of the Figure, and draw Lines to all the Angles A B C D E , then draw the Line *a b* parallel to the Line A B, the Line *b c* parallel to B C, and the Figure *a b c d e* will be ſimilar to the Figure A B C D E

It a greater Figure be required, there is no more to do but produce the Lines drawn from the Center of the Figure, and then drawing Parallels to its Sides

To reduce a Figure by the Scale

Meaſure all the Sides of the propoſed Figure A B C D E, with the Scale G H , then take another leſſer Scale K L, containing as many equal Parts as the greater   Now make the Side Fig. 42. *a b* as many Parts of the leſſer Scale, as the Side A B contains of the greater one's Parts , alſo make *b c* as many Parts as B C, and *a c* as many as A C, &c   by which means the Fi-gure will be reduced to a leſſer one

To reduce a leſſer Figure to a greater one, a greater Scale muſt be had, and proceed as before

To reduce Figures by the Angle of Proportion

Let the propoſed Figure A B C D E be that which is to be diminiſhed in the proportion of the Line A B, to the Line *a b*

Firſt draw the indefinite Line G H, and take the Length A B, and lay off from G to H , Fig 43. then about the Point G, deſcribe the Arc H I   Again, take the Length of the given Side *a b*, as a Chord of the Arc H I, draw the Line G I, and the Angle I G H will give all the Sides of the Figure to be reduced

As to have the Point *c*, take the Interval B C, and about the Point G deſcribe the Arc K L , alſo about the Point *b*, with the Diſtance L K, deſcribe a ſmall Arc   Now take the Diſtance A C, and about the Point G deſcribe the Arc M N , likewiſe about the Point *a*, with the Diſtance M N, deſcribe an Arc, cutting the precedent one in the Point *c*, which will be that which muſt be had to draw the Side *b c* · in like manner proceed for all the other Sides and Angles of the Figure

It by this means a ſmall Figure is to be reduced to a greater, the ſame manner of pro-ceeding will do it , but the Side of the Figure to be augmented muſt be leſſer than double

of

On or next the other Edge of the Rule, you have the Line of Board-Measure; and when the Figures stand upright, you see it numbered 7, 8, 9, &c to 36 which is just 4 Inches from the right Hand   It is thus divided, suppose the Division 7 is to be marked, divide 144, which is the Number of Inches in a square Foot, by 7, and the Quotient will be $20\frac{4}{7}$ Inches, whence the Division 7 must be against $20\frac{4}{7}$ Inches on the other Side of the Rule   Again, to mark the Division 8, divide 144 by 8, and the Quotient, which is 18 Inches, must be placed on the Line of Board-Measure against 18 Inches on the other Side   proceed thus for the other Divisions of the said Line   But because the Side of a long Square, that is either 1, 2, 3, 4, 5 Inches, requires the other Side to be more than 24 Inches, which is the whole Length of the Rule, therefore there is a Table placed at the other end of the Rule, made in dividing 144 Inches by each of the Numbers in the upper Row, and then each of the Quotients by 12, to bring them into Feet

USE *of the Carpenter's Joint-Rule*

The Inches on this Rule are to measure the Length or Breadth of any given Superficies or Solid, and the manner of doing it is superfluous to mention, it being not only easy, but even natural to any Man, for holding the Rule in the left Hand, and applying it to the Board, or any thing to be measured, you have your Desire   But now for the Use of the other Side, I shall shew in two or three Examples in each Measure, that is, Superficial and Solid

Example I   *The Breadth of any Superficies, as Board, Glass, or the like, being given: to find how much in Length makes a Square Foot*

To do which, look for the Number of Inches your Superficies is broad, in the Line of Board Measure, and keep your Finger there, and right against it, on the Inches Side, you have the Number of Inches that makes up a Foot of Board, Glass, or any other Superficies   Suppose you have a Piece 8 Inches broad, how many Inches make a Foot?   Look for 8 on the Board Measure, and just against your Finger (being set to 8) on the Inch-Side, you will find 18, and so many Inches long, at that Breadth, goes to make a superficial Foot

Again, suppose a Superficies is 18 Inches broad, then you will find that 8 Inches in Length will make a superficial Foot, and if a Superficies is 36 Inches broad, then 4 Inches in Length makes a Foot

Or you may do it more easy thus   Take your Rule, holding it in your left Hand, and apply it to the Breadth of the Board or Glass, making the End, which is next 36, even with one Edge of the Board or Glass, and the other Edge of the Board will shew how many Inches, or Quarters of an Inch, go to make a square Foot of Board or Glass   This is but the Converts of the former, and needs no Example, for laying the Rule to it, and looking on the Board-Measure, you have your Desire

Or else you may do it thus, in all narrow Pieces under 6 Inches broad   As suppose $3\frac{1}{4}$ Inches, double $3\frac{1}{4}$, it makes $6\frac{1}{2}$, then twice the Length from $6\frac{1}{2}$ to the End of the Rule, will make a superficial Foot, or so much in Length makes a Foot

Example II   *A Superficies of any Length or Breadth being given, to find the Content*

Having found the Breadth, and how much makes one Foot, turn that over as many times as you can upon the Length of the Superficies, for so many Feet are in that Superficies   But if it is a great Breadth, you may turn it over two or three times, and then take that together, and so say 2, 4, 6, 8, 10, &c or 3, 6, 9, 12, 15, 18, 21, till you come to the End of the Superficies

The USE *of the Table at the End of the Board-Measure*

If a Superficies is 1 Inch broad, how many Inches in Length must there go to make a superficial Foot?   Look in the upper Row of Figures for 1 Inch, and under it, in the second Row, you will find 12 Feet, which shews that 12 Feet in Length, and 1 Inch in Breadth, will make a superficial Foot

Again, a Superficies 5 Inches broad, will be found, in the said Table, to have 2 Feet and about 5 Inches in Length to make a superficial Foot, and a Piece 8 Inches broad, will have a Length of 1 Foot 6 Inches to make a superficial Foot

USE *of the Line of Timber-Measure*

The Use of this Line is much like the former   for first you must learn how much your Piece is square, and then look for the same Number on the Line of Timber-Measure, and the Space from thence to the End of the Rule, is the true Length at that Squareness to make a Foot of Timber

Example. There is a Piece that is 9 Inches square, look for 9 on the Line of Timber-Measure, and then the Space from 9, to the End of the Rule, is the true Length to make a solid Foot of Timber, and it is $21\frac{1}{3}$ Inches

Again, suppose a Piece of Timber is 24 Inches square, then 3 Inches in Length will make a Foot, for you will find three Inches on the other Side against 24   But if it is small Timber, as under 9 Inches square, you must seek the Square in the upper Rank in the Table, and

and right under you have the Feet and Inches that go to make a ſolid Foot, as was in the Table of Board Meaſure : As ſuppoſe a Piece of Timber is 7 Inches ſquare, look in the Table for 7, in the upper Row of Numbers, and you will find directly under 2 Feet, 11 Inches, which is the Length of the Piece of Timber that goes to make a ſolid Foot But if a Piece be not exactly ſquare, *viz.* is broader at one Side than the other, then the uſual way is to add them both together, and take half the Sum for the Side of the Square , but if they differ much, this way is very erroneous for that half is always too great, which from hence will eaſily be manifeſt

Fig 3. Let A C be the longeſt Side, C D the ſhorteſt, and B D, or A B, half their Sum, which is taken for the Side of the Square, that is, for the Side of a Square whoſe Area is equal to the Product of the two Sides A C, and C D, into one another, or the Rectangle under them · Now with the Diſtance B D, and on the Center B, deſcribe a Semicircle , draw the Diameter E B, at right Angles, to A D, and from the Point C raiſe the Perpendicular F C, then it is manifeſt, *per Prop* 13 *lib* 6 *Eucl* that F C is a mean Proportional between the Sides A C, C D , that is, F C is the true Side of the Square, which, *per Prop* 15 *lib* 3 *Eucl.* is much leſs than E B, or its Equal A B, or B D

The uſual way likewiſe for round Timber, is to take a String, and girt it about, and the fourth part of it is commonly allowed for the Side of the Square, that is, for the Side of a Square equal to the circular Baſe, and then you deal with it as if it was juſt Square But this way is alſo erroneous , for by this Method you loſe above ⅟ of the true Solidity But for maintaining this ill Cuſtom, they plead, The Overplus Meaſure may well be allowed, becauſe the Chips cut off are of little Value, and will not near countervail the Labour of bringing the Timber to a Square, to which Form it muſt be brought before it be fit to uſe

The Deſcription of Gunter's Line, or the Line of Numbers

The Line of Numbers is only the Logarithms transferred on a Ruler from the Tables, by means of a Scale divided into a great Number of equal Parts , and whereas in the Logarithms, by adding or ſubſtracting them from one another, the *Quæſita* is produced , ſo here, by turning a Pair of Compaſſes forwards or backwards, according to due Order on this Line, the *Quæſita* will in like manner be produced The Conſtruction of this Line I ſhall give in ſpeaking of *Gunter*'s Scale

As to the Length of the Line of Numbers, the longer it is, the better it is , whence it hath been contrived ſeveral ways As firſt upon a Rule of two Foot, and a Rule of three Foot long, by *Gunter*, which (as I ſuppoſe) is the Reaſon why it is called *Gunter*'s Line ; then that Line was doubled, or laid ſo together, that you might work either right on, or croſs from one to another, by Mr *Windgate* , afterwards projected in a Circle, by Mr *Oughtred*, and alſo to ſlide one by another, by the ſame Author , and laſt of all projected into a kind of Spiral, of 5, 10, or 20 Turns, more or leſs, by Mr *Brown*, the Uſes being in all of them in a manner the ſame, only ſome with Compaſſes, as Mr *Gunter*'s and Mr *Windgate*'s, and ſome with flat Compaſſes, or an opening Index, as Mr *Oughtred*'s and Mr *Brown*'s, and ſome without either, as the Sliding-Rules

The Order of the Diviſions on this Line of Numbers, and commonly on moſt others, is thus , it begins with 1, and ſo proceeds with 2, 3, 4, 5, 6, 7, 8, 9 , and then 1, 2, 3, 4, 5, 6, 7, 8, 9, 10, whoſe Order of Numeration is thus The firſt 1 ſignifies one Tenth of any whole Number or Integer, and conſequently the next 2 is two Tenths, 3, three Tenths , and all the ſmall intermediate Diviſions are 100 Parts of an Integer, or a Tenth of one of the former Tenths , ſo that 1 in the middle is one whole Integer , the next 2, two Integers, and 10 at the end, 10 Integers Thus the Line is in its moſt proper Acceptation, or natural Diviſion.

But if you are to deal with a Number greater than 10, then 1 at the beginning muſt ſignify 1 Integer, and 1 in the middle 10 Integers, and 10 at the end 100 Integers But if you would have it to a Figure more, then the firſt 1 is 10, the ſecond 100, and the laſt 10 a 1000 If you proceed further, then the firſt 1 is 100, the middle 1 a 1000, and the 10 at the end 10000, which is as great a Number as can well be diſcovered, on this or moſt ordinary Lines of Numbers , and ſo far, with convenient Care, you may reſolve a Queſtion tolerably exact

Numeration on the Line of Numbers.

Any whole Number being given under four Figures, to find the Point on the Line of Numbers that repreſents the ſame

Firſt look for the firſt Figure of your Number amongſt the long Diviſions that are figured, and that leads you to the firſt Figure of your Number , then for the ſecond Figure, count ſo many Tenths from that long Diviſion forwards, as that ſecond Figure amounts to , then for the third Figure, count from the laſt Tenth ſo many Centeſmes as the third Figure contains, and ſo for the fourth Figure, count, from the laſt Centeſme, ſo many Millions as that fourth Figure has Units, or is in Value, and that will be the Point where the Number propounded is on the Line of Numbers Two or three Examples will make this manifeſt

Firſt, 'to find the Point upon the Line of Numbers repreſenting the Number 12 Now becauſe the firſt Figure of this Number is 1, you muſt take the 1 in the middle for the firſt Figure ,

Figure, then the next Figure being 2, count two Tenths from that 1, and there will be the Point reprefenting 12

Secondly, To find the Point reprefenting 144   Firft, as before, take for 1 the firft Figure of the Number 144, the middle Figure 1, then for the fecond (*viz* 4) count four Tenths forwards, laftly, for the other 4, count four Centefms further, and that is the Point for 144

Thirdly, To find the Point reprefenting 1728   Firft, as before, for 1000 take the middle 1 on the Line   Secondly, for 7 reckon feven Tenths forwards, and that is 700,   Thirdly, for 2, reckon two Centefms, from that 7th Tenth, for 20   And, Laftly, for 8 you muft reafonably eftimate that following Centefm to be divided into 10 Parts (if it be not ex-preffed, which in Lines of ordinary Length cannot be done) and 8 of that fuppofed 10 Parts is the precife Point for 1728, the Number propounded to be found, and the like of any other Number

But if you was to find a Fraction, you muft confider, that properly, or abfolutely, the Line only expreffes Decimal Fractions, as thus, $\frac{1}{10}$, or $\frac{1}{100}$, or $\frac{1}{1000}$, and more near the Rule in common Acceptation cannot exprefs, as one Inch, one Tenth, one Hundredth, or one Thoufandth Part of an Inch, it being capable to be applied to any thing in a decimal way. (But if you would ufe other Fractions, as Quarters, Half-Quarters, &c. you muft reafonably read them, or elfe reduce them into Decimals)

The fundamental Ufes of the Line of Numbers.

USE I   *Two Numbers being given, to find a third Geometrically proportional to them, and to three a fourth, and to four a fifth, &c*

Extend your Compaffes upon the Line of Numbers, from one Number to another; which done, if that Extent is applied (upwards or downwards, as you would either increafe or di-minifh the Number) from either of the Numbers, the moveable Point will fall upon the third proportional Number required   Alfo the fame Extent, applied the fame way from the third, will give you a fourth, and from the fourth a fifth, &c   For Example, let the Numbers 2 and 4 be propofed, to find a third Proportional, &c to them   Extend the Com-paffes upon the firft Part of the Line of Numbers, from 2 to 4, which done, if the fame Extent is applied upwards from 4, the moveable Point will fall upon 8, the third Proportio-nal required, and then from 8 it will reach to 16, the fourth Proportional, and from 16 to 32 the fifth, &c   Contrariwife, if you would diminifh, as from 4 to 2, the moveable Point will fall on 1, and from 1 to $\frac{1}{10}$, or 5, and from 5 to .25, &c as is manifeft from the Na-ture of the Logarithms, and *Prop* 20 *lib* 7 *Eucl*

But generally in this, and moft other Work, make ufe of the fmall Divifions in the middle of the Line, that you may the better eftimate the Fractions of the Numbers you make ufe of, for how much you mifs in fetting the Compaffes to the firft and fecond Term, fo much the more you will err in the fourth, therefore the middle Part will be moft ufeful: As for Example, as 8 to 11, fo is 12 to 16 50, if you imagine one Integer to be divided but in-to 10 Parts, as they are on the Line on a two-foot Rule

USE II   *One Number being given to be multiplied by another given Number, to find the Product.*

Extend your Compaffes from 1 to the Multiplicator, and the fame Extent, applied the fame way from the Multiplicand, will caufe the moveable Point to fall upon the Product, as is manifeft from the Nature of the Logarithms, and *Defin* 15 *lib* 7 *Eucl*

Example   Let 6 be given to be multiplied by 5, extend your Compaffes from 1 to 5, and the fame Extent will reach from 6 to 30, the Product fought   Again, fuppofe 125 is to be multiplied by 144, extend your Compaffes from 1 to 125, and the moveable Point will fall from 144 on 18000 the Product

USE III   *One Number being given to be divided by another, to find the Quotient*

Extend your Compaffes from the Divifor to 1, and the fame Extent will reach from the Dividend to the Quotient; or, extend the Compaffes from the Divifor to the Dividend, the fame Extent will reach the fame way from 1 to the Quotient, as is manifeft from the Nature of the Logarithms, and this Property, that as the Divifor is to Unity, fo is the Dividend to the Quotient

Example   Let 750 be a Number given, to be divided by 25, (the Divifor) extend your Compaffes downwards from 25 to 1, then applying that Extent the fame way from 750, and the other Point of the Compaffes will fall upon 30, the Quotient fought   Again, let 1728 be given to be divided by 12, extend your Compaffes from 12 to 1, and the fame Extent will reach the fame way from 1728 to 144

If the Number is a Decimal Fraction, then you muft work as if it was an abfolute whole Number, but if it is a whole Number joined to a decimal Fraction, it is worked here as properly as a whole Number   As fuppofe 1114 is to be divided by 1.728, extend your Com-paffes from 1.728 to 1, the fame Extent, applied from 1114, will reach to 645   So again, 564 being to be divided by 8 75, and the Quotient will be found to be 6 45.

Now to know of how many Figures any Quotient ought to confift, it is neceffary to write down the Dividend, and the Divifor under it, and fee how often it may be written under

F

it, for fo many Figures muft there be in the Quotient · As in dividing this Number 12231 by 27, according to the Rules of Division, 27 may be written 3 times under the Dividend; therefore there muft be 3 Figures in the Quotient for if you extend the Compaffes from 27 to 1, it will reach from 12231 to 453, the Quotient fought.

Note, That in this Ufe, or any other, it is beft to order it fo, that your Compaffes may be at the clofeft Extent, for you may take a clofe Extent more eafy and exact than a large Extent, as by Experience you will find

USE IV. *Three Numbers being given, to find a fourth in a direct Proportion.*

Extend your Compaffes from the firft Number to the fecond, that done, the fame Extent apply'd the fame way from the third, will reach to the fourth Proportional fought, as is manifeft from the Nature of the Logarithms, and *Prop*. 19 *lib* 7 *Eucl* from whence it may be gathered, that the third Number multiply'd by the fecond, divided by the firft, will give the fourth fought

Example If 7 give 22, what will 14 give? Extend your Compaffes upwards from 7 to 14, and that Extent apply'd the fame way, will reach from 22 to 44, the fourth Proportional required Again, if 38 gives 76, what will 96 give? Extend your Compaffes from 38 to 96, and the fame Extent will reach from 76 to 192, the fourth Proportional fought.

USE V *Three Numbers being given, to find a fourth in an Inverfe Proportion*

Extend your Compaffes from the firft of the given Numbers to the fecond of the fame Denomination, if that Diftance be apply'd from the third Number backwards, it will reach to the fourth Number fought

Example If 60 give 5, what will 30 give? Extend your Compaffes from 60 to 30, and that Extent apply'd the contrary way from 5, will give 25 the Anfwer Again, If 60 give 48, what will 40 give? Extend your Compaffes from 60 to 40, that Extent apply'd the contrary way from 48, will reach to 32, the fourth Number fought

USE VI *Three Numbers being given, to find a fourth in a duplicate Proportion*

This Ufe concerns Queftions of Proportions between Lines and Superficies, now if the Denominations of the firft and fecond Terms are Lines, then extend your Compaffes from the firft Term to the fecond (of the fame kind of Denomination ·) this done, that Extent apply'd twice the fame way from the third Term, and the moveable Point will fall upon the fourth Term required, which is manifeft from the nature of the Logarithms, and from hence, *viz.* Becaufe the fourth Number to be found is only a fourth Proportional to the Square of the firft, the Square of the fecond, and the third, it is plain that the third, multiply'd by the Square of the fecond, divided by the third, will be the fourth Number fought

Example If the Area of a Circle, whofe Diameter is 14, be 154, what will the Content of a Circle be, whofe Diameter is 28? Here 14 and 28 having the fame Denomination, *viz* both Lines, extend the Compaffes from 14 to 28, then applying that Extent the fame way from 154 twice, the moveable Point will fall upon 616, the fourth Proportional or Area fought: Becaufe Circles are to each other as the Squares of their Diameters, *per Prop* 2 *lib.* 12 *Eucl*

USE VII *Three Numbers being given, to find a fourth in a triplicate Proportion*

This Ufe is to find the Proportion between the Powers of Lines and Solids, that is, two Lines being given and a Solid, to find a fourth Solid, that has the fame Proportion to the given Solid, as the given Lines have to one another Therefore extend the Compaffes from the firft Line to the fecond, and that Extent, apply'd three times from the given Solid or third Number, will give the fourth fought Becaufe the third multiply'd by the Cube of the fecond, divided by the Cube of the firft, will give the fourth

Example. If an Iron Bullet, whofe Diameter is 4 Inches, weighs 9 Pounds, what will another Iron Bullet weigh, whofe Diameter is 8 Inches? Extend your Compaffes from 4 to 8, that Extent apply'd the fame way three times from 9, will give 72, the Weight of the Bullet fought Becaufe the Weight of homogeneal Bodies are as their Magnitudes, and Spheres are to one another as the Cubes of their Diameters, *per Prop* 16 *lib.* 12 *Eucl.*

USE VIII. *To find a mean Proportional between two given Numbers*

Bifect the Diftance between the given Numbers, which Point of Bifection will fall on the mean Proportional fought · Becaufe the fquare Root of the Quotient of the two Extremes divided by one another, multiply'd by the leffer, is equal to the Mean.

Example The Extremes being 8 and 32, the middle Point between them will be found to be 16.

USE IX *To find two mean Proportionals between two given Lines*

Trifect the Space between the two given Extremes, and the two Points of Trifection will give the two Means Becaufe the Cube Root of the Quotient of the Extremes divided by one another, multiply'd by the leffer Extreme, will give the firft of the Mean Proportionals fought, and that firft Mean multiply'd by the aforefaid Cube Root, will give the fecond

Example.

ing of Divifions at every Place in the Face of the Rod, to which the Water arifes, until the Hogfhead be full, and then the Scale for a Hogfhead, on the third Face, will be divided. Proceed, in the fame manner, in making the Divifions for the other Scales of Lines ufed in finding the Wants in the feveral Veffels aforementioned lying down   And taking off the Head of a Butt that is ftanding, and pouring of Water in the fame manner as in the Hogfhead, putting the Rod downright into the Butt, and making Divifions on the Rod, as was done for the Hogfhead, the Line will be finifhed, when figured.

Note, The Divifions for Half-Gallons, marked by long Dots on the fourth Face, are made by pouring in of Half-Gallons fucceffively, &c.

USE *of the Diagonal Lines on the Gauging-Rod.*
To find the Content of a Veffel in Beer or Wine-Gallons

Put the brafed End of the Gauging-Rod into the Bung-hole of the Cask, with the Diagonal Lines upwards, and thruft the brafed End to the meeting of the Head and Staves

Then with Chalk make a Mark on the middle of the Bung-hole of the Veffel, and alfo on the Diagonal Lines of the Rod, right againft, or over one another, when the brafed End is thruft home to the Head and Staves

Then turn the Gauging-Rod to the other End of the Veffel, and thruft the brafed End home to the End as before

And fee if the Mark made on the Gauging-Rod come even with the Mark made on the Bung-Hole, when the Rod was thruft to the other End, which if it be, the Mark made on the Diagonal Lines, will, on the fame Lines, fhew the whole Content of the Cask in Beer or Wine-Gallons

But if the Mark firft made on the Bung-hole be not right againft that made on the Rod, when put the other way, then right againft the Mark made on the Bung-hole, make another on the Diagonal Lines. then the Divifion on the Diagonal Line, between the two Chalks, will fhew the Veffel's whole Content in Beer or Wine-Gallons   As for Example, if the Diagonal Line of a Veffel be 28 Inches 4 Tenths, its Content in Beer-Gallons will be near 51, and in Wine-Gallons 62.

But if a Veffel be open, as a Half-Barrel, Tun, or Copper, and the Meafure from the middle on one Side, to the Head and Staves, be 38 Inches, the Diagonal Line gives 122 Beer-Gallons, half of which, *viz.* 61, is the Content of the open Half-Tub

But if you have a large Veffel, as a Tun, or Copper, and the Diagonal Line, taken by a long Rule, prove 70 Inches, then the Content of that Veffel may be found thus:

Every Inch, at the Beginning-End of the Diagonal Line, call 10 Inches, then 10 Inches becomes 100 Inches

And every Tenth of a Gallon call 100 Gallons, and every whole Gallon, with a Figure, call 1000 Gallons   Example, at 44 8 Inches, on the Diagonal Beer-Line, is 200 Gallons, fo alfo at 4 Inches 48 Parts, now called 44 Inches 8 Tenths, is juft two Tenths of a Gallon, now called 200 Gallons

Alfo if the Diagonal Line be 76 Inches and 7 Tenths, a clofe Cask, of fo great a Diagonal, will hold 1000 Beer-Gallons   but an open Cask but half fo much, *viz.* 500 Beer-Gallons

For reducing of Wine-Gallons to Beer-Gallons, or, *vice verfa,* by Infpection, this may be done

Thus 30 Wine-Gallons, is 24 ½ Beer-Gallons, &c.

USE *of the Gauge-Line.*
USE I *To find the Content of any Cylindrical Veffel in Ale-Gallons*

Seek the Diameter of the Veffel in the Inches, and juft againft it, on the Gauge-Line, is the Quantity of Ale-Gallons contained in one Inch deep   then this multiplied by the Length of the Cylinder, will give its Content in Ale-Gallons   For Example, fuppofe the Length of the Veffel be 32 06, and the Diameter of its Bafe 25 Inches, what is the Content in Ale-Gallons?   Right againft 25 Inches, on the Gauge-Line, is 1 Gallon, and 745 of a Gallon, which multiplied by 32 06, the Length, gives 55 9447 Gallons for the Content of the Veffel

USE II *The Bung-Diameter of a Hogfhead is 25 Inches, the Head-Diameter 22 Inches, and the Length 32 06 Inches, to find the Quantity of Ale-Gallons contained in it*

Seek 25, the Bung-Diameter, on the Line of Inches, and right againft it, on the Gauge-Line, you will find 1 745, take ⅓ of it, which is 580, and fet it down twice   Seek 22 Inches, the Head-Diameter, and againft it you will find, on the Gauge-Line, 1 356, ⅓ of which added to twice 580, gives 1 6096, which multiplied by the Length 32 06, the Product will be 51 603776, the Content in Ale-Gallons   This Operation fuppofes, that the aforefaid Hogfhead is in the Figure of the middle Fruftum of a Spheroid

The Ufe of the Lines on the two other Faces of the Rod, is very eafy, for you need but put it downright into the Bung-hole (if the Veffel you defire to know the Quantity of Ale-Gallons contained therein be lying) to the oppofite Staves; and then where the Surface of the Liquor cuts any one of the Lines appropriated for that Veffel, will be the Number of Gallons contained in that Veffel   G   CHAP

C H A P. III.

Of the Construction and Use of Everard's *Sliding-Rule for Gauging.*

THIS Instrument is commonly made of Box, exactly a Foot long, one Inch broad, and about six Tenths of an Inch thick. It consists of three Parts, *viz.* A Rule, and two small Scales or Sliding-Pieces to slide in it ; one on one Side, and the other on the other. So that when both the Sliding-Pieces are drawn out to their full Extent, the whole will be three Foot long.

On the first broad Face of this Instrument are four Lines of Numbers, the first Line of Numbers consists of two Radius's, and is numbered 1, 2, 3, 4, 5, 6, 7, 8, 9, 1 and then 2, 3, 4, 5, &c. to 10. On this Line are placed four Brass Center Pins, the first in the first Radius, at 2150 42, and the third likewise at the same Number taken in the second Radius, having M B set to them, signifying, that the aforesaid Number represents the Cubic Inches in a Malt Bushel. the second and fourth Center Pins are set at the Numbers 282 on each Radius, they have the Letter A set to them, signifying that the aforesaid Number 282 is the Cubic Inches in an Ale-Gallon. *Note,* The little long black Dots, over the Center Pins, are put directly over the proper Numbers. This Line of Numbers hath A placed at the End thereof, and is called A for Distinction-sake.

The second and third Lines of Numbers which are on the Sliding-Piece (and which may be called but one Line) are exactly the same with the first Line of Numbers : They are both, for Distinction, called B. The little black Dot, that is hard by the Division 7, on the first Radius, having S*i* set after it, is put directly over 707, which is the Side of a Square inscribed in a Circle, whose Diameter is Unity. The black Dot hard by 9, after which is writ S *e*, is set directly over 886, which is the Side of a Square equal to the Area of a Circle, whose Diameter is Unity. The black Dot that is nigh W, is set directly over 231, which is the Number of Cubic Inches in a Wine-Gallon. Lastly, the black Dot by C, is set directly over 3.14. which is the Circumference of a Circle, whose Diameter is Unity.

The fourth Line, on the first Face, is a broken Line of Numbers of two Radius's, numbered 2, 10, 9, 8, 7, 6, 5, 4, 3, 2, 1, 9, 8, 7, 6, 5, 4, 3, the Number 1 is set against M B on the first Radius. This Line of Numbers hath M D set to it, signifying *Malt Depth.*

On the second broad Face of this Rule, are,

I. A Line of Numbers of but one Radius, which is numbered 1, 2, 3, &c. to 10, and hath D set at the End thereof for distinguishing it. There are upon it four Brass Center Pins the first, to which is set W G, is the Gauge-Point for a Wine-Gallon, that is, the Diameter of a Cylinder, whose Height is an Inch, and Content 231 Cubic Inches, or a Wine-Gallon, which is 17 15 Inches. The second Center-Pin A G stands at the Gauge-Point for an Ale-Gallon, which is 18 95 Inches. The third Center-Pin M S stands at 46 3, which is the Side of a Square, whose Content is equal to the Inches in a solid Bushel. The fourth Center-Pin M R is the Gauge-Point for a Malt Bushel, which is 52 32 Inches.

II. Two Lines of Numbers on the Sliding-Piece, which are exactly the same as on the Sliding-Piece on the other Side the Rule, they are called C. The first black Dot something on this Side the Division of the Number 8, to which is set ⊙ *c*, is set to 795, which is the Area of a Circle whose Circumference is Unity, and the second, to which is set ⊙ *d*, stands at 785, the Area of a Circle, whose Diameter is Unity.

III. Two Lines of Segments, each numbered 1, 2, 3 to 100, the first is for finding the Ulage of a Cask, taken as the middle Frustum of a Spheroid, lying with its Axis parallel to the Horizon, and the other for finding the Ulage of a Cask standing.

Again, on one of the narrow Faces of this Rule, is, (1) A Line of Inches, numbered 1, 2, 3, 4, &c. to 12. each of which is subdivided into ten equal Parts. (2) A Line, by means of which, and the Line of Inches, is found a mean Diameter for a Cask in the Figure of the middle Frustum of a Spheroid, it is figured 1, 2, 3, &c. to 7 at the End thereof is writ *Spheroid.* (3.) A Line for finding the mean Diameter of a Cask in the Figure of the middle Frustum of a parabolic Spindle, which by Gaugers is called, *the second Variety of Casks ;* it is numbered 1, 2, 3, 4, 5, 6, and at its End is writ, 2 *Variety* (4) A Line, by means of which may be found the mean Diameter of a Cask of the third Variety ; that is, a Cask in the Figure of two parabolic Conoids abutting upon a common Base. it is numbered 1, 2, 3, 4, 5, at the End thereof is writ 3 *Variety*

And on the other narrow Face, is, (1) A Foot divided into 100 equal Parts, every ten of which are numbered, F M stands at the beginning of it, signifying Foot-Measure. (2) A Line of Inches, like that before spoken of, having I M set to the beginning thereof, signifying Inch-Measure. (3) A Line for finding the mean Diameter for the fourth Variety of Casks, which is the middle Frustum of two Cones, abutting upon one common Base, it is numbered 1, 2, 3, 4, 5, 6. and at the beginning thereof is writ F C, signifying Frustum of a Cone.

These

USE II *To meaſure Round Timber the true way*

The manner of meaſuring Round-Timber in the laſt Uſe, being the common way, but not the true one, as I have already ſaid in ſpeaking of the Carpenter's Rule. I ſhall now give you a Point on the Girt-Line D, which muſt be uſed inſtead of 12, which is 10 635, at which there ought to be placed a little Braſs Center-Pin: this 10 635 is the Side of a Square, equal to a Circle, whoſe Diameter is 12 Inches.

Example. Let a Length be (as in the ſecond Example of the laſt Uſe) 15 Feet, and the ¼ of the Girt 42 Inches: ſet the ſaid Point 10 635, to 15 the Length, then againſt 42, at the beginning of the Girt-Line, is 233 Feet for the Content ſought · but by the common way, there ariſes only 184 Feet

Note, As the Area, or Content of a Circle (in Inches) whoſe Diameter is 12 Inches, is to the Length of any Cylinder in Feet, ſo is the Square of ¼ of the Circumference of the Baſe of the Cylinder, in Inches, to the ſolid Content of the Cylinder in Feet

Alſo the common Meaſure is to the true Meaſure, as 11 is to 14; that is, as the Area, or Content of a Circle, to the Square of its Diameter, which, from hence, will be eaſily mani-feſt. Call the Diameter of any Circle D, and ¼ the Circumference C, then the Content of the ſaid Circle will be equal to D×C, therefore D×C is to D×D, as 11 is to 14. But the common Meaſure (becauſe the Length of the Piece is the ſame) will be to the true Meaſure, as C×C, the Square of ¼ the Circumference, to D×C the Content of the ſaid Circle, whence D×C muſt be to D², as C² is to D×C, and by comparing the Rectangles under the Means and Extremes, they will be found equal, therefore what I propoſed is true

If the Girt of a Piece of Timber be taken in Feet, the Point for true Meaſure is 886, or 89, which is the Side of a Square, equal to the Content of a Circle, whoſe Diameter is Unity. And then, for the foregoing Example, the Length being 15 Feet, and ¼ of the Girt 42 Inches, ſet the aforeſaid Point 89 on the Girt-Line, to the Length 15 Feet on the Line C, (in the firſt Radius) then againſt 3 5 Feet (which is 35) on the Girt-Line D, is 233 Feet on the Line C, the true Content required.

USE III *To meaſure a Cube.*

Let there be a Cube whoſe Sides are 6 Feet, to find the Content: ſet 12 on the Girt-Line D, to 6 on the Line C, then againſt 72 Inches (the Inches in 6 Feet) on the Girt-Line D, is 216 Feet on the Line C, which is the Content required.

USE IV *To meaſure unequal ſquared Timber; that is, if the Breadth and Depth are not equal.*

Meaſure the Length of the Piece, and the Breadth and Depth (at the End) in Inches, then find a mean Proportional between the Breadth and Depth of the Piece, which mean Propor-tional is the Side of a Square equal to the End of the Piece. which being found, the Piece may be meaſured as ſquare Timber

Example I. Let there be a Piece of Timber whoſe Length is 13 Feet, the Breadth 23 In-ches, and the Depth 13 Inches: ſet 23 on the Girt-Line D, to 23 on the Line C; then a-gainſt 13 on the Line C, is 17 35 on the Girt-Line D for the mean Proportional. Now again, ſetting 12 on the Girt-Line D, to 13 Feet, the Length, on the Line C, then againſt 17 35 on the Girt-Line D, is 27 Feet the Content required

Example II. Let there be a Piece of Stone 7 4 Feet in Length, 30 Inches in Breadth, and 23 5 Deep. ſet 30 Inches on the Girt-Line D, to 30 on the Line C, then againſt 23 5, on the Line C, is 26 5 on the Girt-Line D, then ſet 12 on the Girt-Line D, to 7 4 on the Line C, and againſt 26 5, on the Girt-Line, is 36 Feet the Content ſought

USE V *To find the Content of a Piece of Timber in Form of a triangular Priſm*

You muſt firſt find a mean Proportional between the Baſe, and half the Perpendicular of the triangular End, or between the Perpendicular and half the Baſe, both meaſured in Inches, and that mean Proportional will be the Side of a Square equal to the Triangle

Then to find the Content, ſet 12 on the Girt-Line D, to the Length in Feet on the Line of Numbers C, and againſt the mean Proportional on the Girt-Line D, is the Content on the Line of Numbers C

But the Dimenſions being all taken in Foot Meaſure, and the mean Proportional found in the ſame; then ſet 1 on the Girt-Line, to the Length on the Line C, and againſt the mean Proportional in the Girt-Line, is the Content in the Line C

Example There is a Piece of Timber 19 Feet 6 Inches in Length, the Baſe of the Trian-gle at each End 21 Inches, and the Perpendicular 16 Inches · to find the Content

Set 21 Inches on the Girt-Line D, to 21 on the Line C, then againſt 8 on the Line C, is 12 95 on the Line D, the mean Proportional, then ſet 12 on the Line D, to 19 5 Feet the Length, on the Line C; and againſt 12 95 (the mean Proportional) on the Girt-Line D, is 22 8 Feet the Content on the Line C. Or thus, take all the Dimenſions in Foot-Meaſure, and then the Length 19 Feet 6 Inches, is 19 5, the Baſe 21 Inches, is 1 75, and the Perpen-dicular 16 Inches, is 1 33. Now ſet 1 on the Girt-Line D, to the Length 19.5 on the dou-

I ble

ble Line C, and againſt 1 08 on the Girt-Line D, is 22 8 Feet on the Line C, for the Content.

USE VI   *To meaſure Taper Timber*

The Length being meaſured in Feet, note one third of it, which may be found thus · ſet 3 on the Line A, to the Length on the Line B, then againſt 1 on the Line A, is the third Part on the Line B: then if the Solid be round, meaſure the Diameter at each End in Inches, and ſubſtract the leſſer Diameter from the greater, and add half the Difference to the leſſer Diameter, the Sum is the Diameter in the middle of the Piece, then ſet 13 54 on the Girt-Line D, to the Length on the Line C, and againſt the Diameter in the middle, on the Girt-Line, is a fourth Number on the Line C   Again, ſet 13 54 on the Girt-Line, to the third part of the Length on the Line C   then againſt half the Difference on the Girt-Line, is another fourth Number on the Line C, theſe two fourth Numbers added together, will give the Content

Example Let the Length be 27 Feet, (one third of which will be 9) the greater Diameter 22 Inches, and the leſſer 18, the Sum of the greater and leſſer Diameters will be 40, their Difference 4, half their Difference 2, which added to the leſſer Diameter, gives 20 Inches for the Diameter in the middle of the Piece   Now ſet 13 54 on the Girt-Line D, to 27 on the Line C, and againſt 20 on the Line D, is 58 9 Feet   Again, ſet 13 54 of the Girt-Line, to 9 on the Line C, then againſt 2 on the Girt-Line, (repreſented by 20) is 196 Parts therefore, by adding 58 9 Feet, to 196 Feet, the Sum is 59 096 Feet the Content. If all the Dimenſions are taken in Foot-Meaſure, then you muſt add the greater and leſſer Diameters together, which in this Example make 3 33 Feet, half of which is the Diameter in the middle of the Piece, *viz* 1 67 Feet, the difference of the Diameters is 0 33 Feet, half of which Difference is 0 17 Feet

Then ſet 1 13 on the Girt-Line, to the Length 27 Feet on the Line C, and againſt 1 67 on the Line D, is 58 9 Feet : then again, ſet 1 13 on the Line D, to 9 Feet on the Line C ; and then againſt 0 17 on the Line D, is 196 Parts of a Foot, and both added together is the Content, that is, 58 9 and 196 added, makes 59 096 Feet as before

If the Solid is ſquare, and has the ſame Dimenſions, that is, the Length 27 Feet, the Side of the greater End 22 Inches, and the Side of the leſſer End 18 Inches, to find the Content in Inch-Meaſure · ſet 12 on the Girt-Line, to 27 the Length of the Solid, on the Line C ; and againſt 20 Inches, the Side of the mean Square on the Girt-Line, is 75 4 Feet   Again ; ſet 12 on the Girt-Line, to 9 Feet, one third of the Length, on the Line C, and againſt 2 Inches, half the difference of the Sides of the Squares of the Ends, on the Girt-Line, is 25 Parts of a Foot, both together is 75 65 Feet the Content of the Solid   or thus, When all the Dimenſions are the 1 Foot Meaſure ſet 1 on the Girt-Line, to the Length 27 Feet on the Line C, then againſt 1 67 Feet, the Side of the middle Square on the Girt-Line, ſtands 75 4 Feet, and ſetting 1 on the Girt-Line to 9 Feet, one third of the Length on the Line C, againſt 0 167, half the Difference of the Sides of the Squares of the Ends on the Girt-Line, is on the Line C, 25 Parts of a Foot, which added to the other, makes 75 65 Feet, as before, for the Content

Note, The fixed Numbers 13 54, and 1 13 are, the firſt, the Diameter of a Circle whoſe Area, or Content is 144, that is, the Number of ſquare Inches in a ſuperficial Foot, and the other, the Diameter of a Circle whoſe Area is Unity.

USE VII   *To find how many Inches in Length will make a Foot-Solid, at any Girt, being the Side of a Square not exceeding 40 Inches*

Let the Girt, or Side of the Square, taken upon the Girt-Line, be ſet to 1 on the Line C   then againſt 41 57 of the Girt-Line, is the Number of Inches on the Line C, that will make a Solid-Foot

Example. Let the Side of a Square be 8 Inches   ſet 8 on the Girt-Line D, to 1 on the Line C, then againſt 41 57 on the Girt-Line D, is 27 Inches for the Length of one ſolid Foot   To do this in Foot Meaſure, the Side of the Square 8 Inches, in Foot-Meaſure, is .66 Parts, which taken on the Girt-Line, and being ſet to 1 on the Line C, againſt 1 on the Girt-Line, is 2 25 Feet, for the Length to make one Foot of Timber.

Note, 41 57 is the Square-Root of 1728, the Number of Cubic Inches in a ſolid Foot.

USE VIII   *The Diameter of a Circle, or round Piece of Timber, being given to find the Side of a Square within the Circle, or to know how many Inches the Side of the Square will be, when the round Timber is ſquared.*

Rule Set 8 5 on the Line A, to 6 on the Line B, then againſt the Diameter on the Line A, is the Side of the Square on the Line B.

Example Let the Diameter be 18 Inches · ſet 8 5 on A, to 6 on B, then againſt 18 on A, is 12 ¼ on the Line B, for the Side of a Square within the Circle   The ſame done in Foot-Meaſure   the Diameter being 18 Inches, is in Foot-Meaſure 1 5, then ſet 1 on the Line A, to 707 on the Line B, and againſt the Diameter 1 5 on the Line A, is 1 7 on the Line B, that is, 1 7 Foot is the Side of an inſcribed Square in a Circle, whoſe Diameter is 1 5 Foot

Note,

Note, the given Numbers 8 5 and 6, or more exacter, 1 and 707, are, the one the Diameter of a Circle, and the other the Side of a Square inſcribed in that Circle

USE IX.   *The Girt of a Tree, or round Piece of Timber being given , to find the Side of a Square within.*

Rule Set 10 to 9 on the Lines A and B , then againſt the Girt on the Line A, are the Inches for the Side of the Square on the Line B

Let the Girt be 12 Inches, ſet 10 on the Line A, to 9 on the Line B , then againſt 12 on the Line A, is 10 8 on the Line B, for the Side of the Square   By Foot-Meaſure it is thus , the Girt 12 Inches is one Foot , then ſet 10 on the Line A, to 9 on the Line B , and againſt the Girt 1 Foot, on the Line A, is 89 Parts of a Foot for the Side of the Square within

Note, The Numbers 10 and 9, or 1 and 9, ſhew when the Square within the Circle is 1, the fourth Part of the Circumference is 9 Parts of the ſame   Alſo, by this and the laſt Uſe, you may know, before a Piece of Timber be hewn, how many Boards or Planks of any Thickneſs it will make

USE X   *The fourth Part of the Girt of a round Piece of Timber being given , to find the Side of a Square equal to it*

Rule Set 1 on the Line A, to 1 128, on the Line B , then againſt the one fourth of the Girt, on the Line A, is on the Line B, the Side of the Square equal to it

Example Let the Girt, (that is, one fourth of the whole Girt) be 16 Inches ; what is the Side of a Square equal to it ? Set 1 to 1 13, on the Lines A and B , then againſt 16 on the Line A, is 18 on the Line B , which ſhews, that a Square, whoſe Side is 18 Inches, is equal to a Circle, whoſe Girt is 64 Inches, and ¼ of its Girt 16 Inches

USE XI   *To find the Solidity of a Cone*

Let the Diameter of the Baſe of a Cone be 12 Feet, and its Altitude or Height, 24, to find the Content

This Uſe may be ſolved at one Operation, thus , ſet 1 95 on the Girt Line, to the Height of the Cone 24, on the Line C, then againſt the Diameter of the Baſe of the Cone 12, on the Girt Line, ſtands on the Line C, 904 8 Feet, for the Content

Note, 1 95 is the Square Root of the Quotient of 42 divided by 11 ∙ and as the Quotient of 42 divided by 11, is to the Height of any Cone, ſo is the Square of the Diameter of its Baſe to the ſolid Content

USE XII   *To find the Solidity of a Square Pyramid*

Suppoſe the Side of the Baſe is 8 Inches, and the Height 30, ſet 7 on the Girt Line, to ⅐ of the Length, *viz* 10, on the Line C, then againſt the Side of the Baſe 8, on the Girt Line, is 640 Inches, on the Line C, for the Solidity

USE XIII   *To find the Solidity of a Sphere, by having the Circumference given*

Let the Circumference of a Sphere be 22 Inches, to find the Content   As 2904 is to 49, ſo is the Cube of the Circumference of a Sphere to its ſolid Content   therefore ſet 53 8 (the Square Root of 2904) on the Girt Line, to 49 on the Line C, then againſt the Circumference 22 Inches on the Girt Line, is a fourth Number, *viz* 8 09   Again, ſet 1, on the Line B, to 22 on the Line A , then againſt 8 09, on the Line C, ſtands 1796 on the Line A, for the Content of the ſaid Sphere in ſolid Inches   If the Diameter had been given, you muſt have uſed the fixed Numbers 4 57 and 11, inſtead of 53 8 and 49, and then have proceeded as before   becauſe as 21 is to 11, ſo is the Cube of the Diameter of a Sphere to the ſolid Content thereof

This Uſe may be otherwiſe ſolved at one Operation, thus   ſet 7 69 on the Girt Line D, to the Circumference of the Sphere 22 Inches, on the Line C, then againſt 22 Inches, on the Girt Line D, ſtands, on the Line C, the ſolid Content 1796 Inches   If the Diameter be given to find the Solidity at one Operation, you muſt ſet 1 38, on the Girt Line to the Diameter on the Line C, then againſt the ſame Diameter, on the Girt Line, ſtands, on the Line C, the Content.

Note, 7 69, and 1 38 are, the one, the Square Root of the Quotient of 2904 divided by 49 , and the other, the Square Root of the Quotient of 21, divided by 11

USE XIV   *The Circumference of a Sphere being given, to find its Superficies*

Suppoſe the Circumference of a Sphere be 20 Inches, what is the Area of its Superficies ? Set 4 69 (the Square Root of 22) on the Girt Line D, to 7 on the Line C, then againſt 20 Inches on the Girt Line, ſtands upon the Line C 136 5, the Area of the Superficies of the Sphere

The reaſon of this is, becauſe as 22 is to 7 , ſo is the Square of the Circumference of a Sphere to the ſuperficial Area thereof

USE

USE XV   *To find the Solidity of the Segment of a Sphere*

Say, as 21 is to the Sine, so is 11 times the Square of the said Sine, added to 33 times the Square of half the Chord, to the solid Content of the Segment. As suppose the Sine be 10 Inches, and half the Chord 16 Inches; to find the Content. Say, as 21 is to 10, so is 9548, the Sum of 11 times the Square of 10, added to 33 times the Square of 16, to the Content 4546 6 Inches.

USE XVI   *To find the Area of the Convex Superficies of the Segment of a Sphere*

Say, as 14 is to 44 times the Diameter of a Sphere, so is the Length of the Sine of any Segment thereof, to the convex Superficies of the said Segment. Suppose the Sine be 12 Inches, and the Diameter 30, say, as 14 is to 1320, so is 12 to 1131 4 Inches, the Content sought.

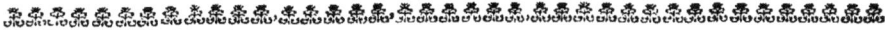

CHAP. V.

Of the Construction and Uses of the Plotting-Scale, and an improv'd Protractor.

THE Plotting-Scale is generally made of Box-Wood, and sometimes of Brass, Ivory, or Silver, exactly a Foot, or half a Foot in Length, about an Inch and a half broad, and of a convenient Thickness: Those that are but half a Foot long, have that Length given them, that thereby they may be put into Cases of Instruments.

Plate 4.
Fig. 1

On one Side of this Scale is placed seven several Scales of Lines, five of which are divided into as many equal Parts as the Length of the Plotting-Scale will permit. The other two are likewise equal Parts, but have two Lines of Chords of different Lengths joined to them. The first of the equal Divisions, on the first Scale of Lines, is subdivided into 10 equal Parts, at the beginning of which is set the Number 10, signifying, that ten of those Subdivisions make an Inch; that is, in this Case, every of the Divisions on the first Scale, is exactly an Inch, at the End of the first of which, is set o, at the End of the second 1; at the End of the third 2, and so on to the End of the Scale. The first of the equal Divisions, on the second Scale of Lines, which are lesser than the Divisions on the first Scale, is likewise subdivided into 10 equal Parts, and hath the Number 16 set at the beginning of it, signifying, that 16 of those Subdivisions make an Inch, or one of the Divisions $\frac{1}{16}$ of an Inch, at the End of the first of which is placed o, at the End of the second 1, at the End of the third 2 and so on to the End of the Scale. The first of the equal Divisions on the third Scale of Lines, which are lesser than the Divisions of the precedent Scale's, is also subdivided into 10 equal Parts, at the beginning of which is set the Number 20, signifying, that 20 of those Subdivisions go to make an Inch, or that one of the Divisions is $\frac{1}{20}$ or of an Inch, which Divisions are marked, o, 1, 2, 3, and so on to the End of the Scale. Understand the same for the other four Scales, at the beginnings of which are writ, 24, 32, 40, 48, only the Divisions of the two last Scales of Lines are not continued to the End of the Scale, because of two Lines of Chords of different Lengths, the Beginnings of which are marked by the Letters C, C, signifying Chords. The Construction of which see in the next Chapter.

Note, Each of the aforesaid Scales of Lines are aptly distinguish'd from one another, by being call'd Scales of 10, 16, 20, 24, 32, or 48, in an Inch, as the first Scale, is a Scale of 10 in an Inch, the second, 16 in an Inch, the third, 20 in an Inch, the fourth, 24, and so on.

Fig 2

On the back Side of this Scale, is placed a Diagonal Scale, the first of whose Divisions, which is half an Inch, if the Scale is a Foot long, and one fourth, if the Scale is but half a Foot long, is diagonally subdivided into 100 equal Parts. Also at the other End of the Scale is another Diagonal Subdivision of an Inch into 100 equal Parts, if the Scale is a Foot long, but if it is half a Foot, the Subdivision is of half an Inch into 100 equal Parts. The Figure of this Diagonal Scale, and what our Author has already said of it, in Use 8, is sufficient to shew its Construction and Use.

There is also next to the Diagonal Scale, a Foot divided into 100 equal Parts, if the Scale is a Foot long, every 10 of which are numbered 10, 20, 30, &c. There is likewise next to that the Divisions of Inches, numbered 1, 2, 3, &c. each of which is subdivided into ten equal Parts.

Use of the Plotting-Scale

This Scale's principal Use is to lay down Chains and Links taken in surveying Land

USE

Plate III

fronting page 36

Fig 1

A

Fig 3

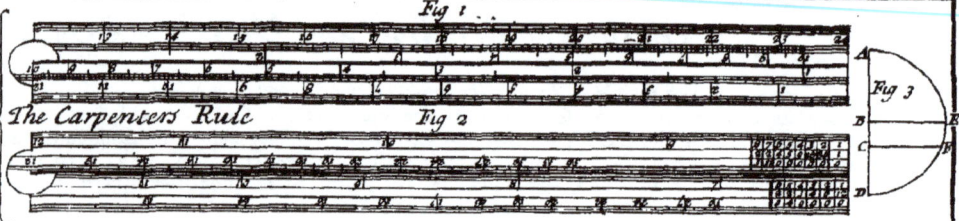

The Carpenters Rule

Fig 2

B

C

D

E

Four foot Gauging Rod

Everards Slyding Rule

Cogeshals Rule

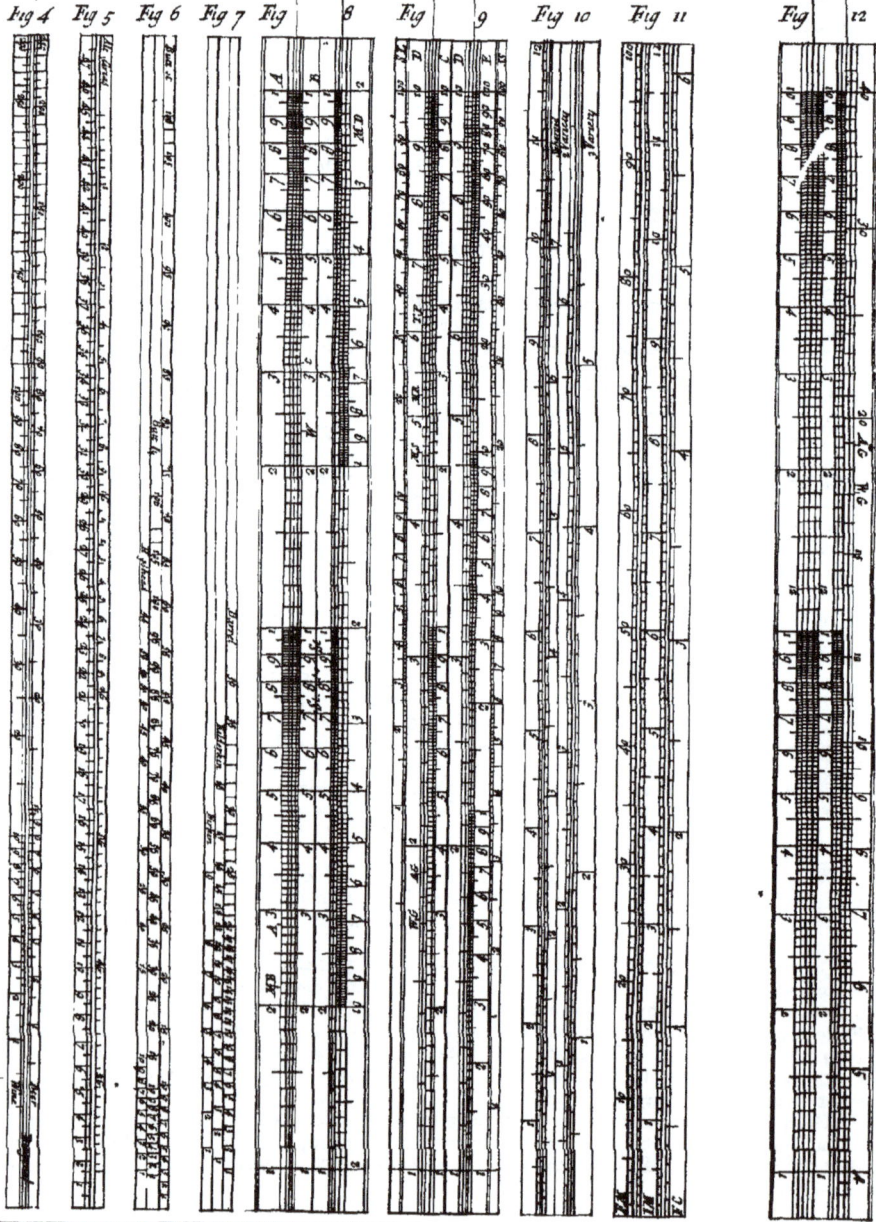

Fig 4   Fig 5   Fig 6   Fig 7   Fig 8   Fig 9   Fig 10   Fig 11   Fig 12

USE I *Any Diſtance being meaſured by your Chain, to lay it down upon Paper*

Suppoſe, that meaſuring along a Hedge, or the D ſtance between any two Marks, or Pla-Fig 3. ces, with your Chain, you find the Length thereof to contain 6 Chains, 50 Links Now to take this D ſtance from your Scale, and lay it down upon Paper, do thus

Firſt draw the Line A B, then place one Foot of your Compaſſes upon your Scale at the Figure 6, for the 6 Chains, and extend the other Foot to 5 of the Subdiviſions, (which repreſents the 50 Links) then ſet this Diſtance upon the Line drawn from A to B, and the Line A B will contain 6 Chains, 50 Links, if you take the Diſtance from the Scale of 10 in an Inch

But if you wou'd have the Line ſhorter, and yet to contain 6 Chains 50 Links, then take your Diſtance from a ſmaller Scale, as of 16, 20, 24, &c in an Inch, and then the 6 Chains, 50 Links, will end at C if taken from the Scale of 16 in an Inch, or at ,D, if taken from the Scale of 20 in an Inch, &c either of which Lines will contain 6 Chains, 50 Links, and be proportional one to another, as the Scales from which they were taken And in this manner any Number of Chains and Links may be taken from any of the Scales

USE II *A right Line being given, to find how many Chains and Links are therein contain'd, according to any aſſigned Scale*

Suppoſe A B was a given Line, and it is required to find how many Chains and Links are Fig. 3. contained therein, according to the Scale of 10 in an Inch Take in your Compaſſes the Length of the Line A B, and applying it to the Scale of 10 in an Inch, you will find that the Extent of your Compaſſes will reach from 6 of the great Diviſions, to 5 of the ſmall ones, whence the Line A B, contains 6 Chains, 50 Links The like muſt be done for any Line, and alſo by any of the other Scales

But note, that in laying down the Lengths of Lines by your Scales, whatſoever Scale you begin your Work with, with the ſame Scale you muſt continue it to the End, not laying down one Line by one Scale, and another by another, but if you would have a large Work in a little room, then uſe a ſmall Scale, as of 32, 40, or 48 in an Inch But contrariwiſe, if you would expreſs every ſmall Particular, then it is beſt to uſe the Scales of 10, or 16 in an Inch.

The Uſe of the Lines of Chords on the Plotting-Scale, is to protract or lay down Angles, when a Protractor is wanting, which is much more convenient in laying off Angles *vide* Uſes of the Plain-Scale To take off Parts from the Diagonal Scale, ſee Uſe VIII of our Author's.

Of the Conſtruction and Uſe of an improved Protractor.

This Protractor is made of Braſs, as the others commonly are, and has likewiſe its Semi- Fig. 4. circular Limb divided into 180 Degrees, there is an Index adjuſted in the Center of this Protractor, by means of which, an Angle of any Number of Degrees and Minutes, may be protracted there is a Circle cut out in the Piece, whoſe Edge, next to the Limb, ſerves for the Diameter of the Semicircle, the Center of this Circle is in the Center of the Limb, and it is cut ſloping, ſo that it makes the Fruſtum of a Cone, the greateſt Baſe being underneath In this Circle is adjuſted a Ring, to which the Ring of the end of the Index is rivetted, by which means the Index will move freely about the Limb There is a little Steel Point fixed to the Ring, adjuſted in the aforeſaid Circle, the End of which terminates in the Center of the Circle, the End of this Point muſt be laid to the angular Point to be protracted

The Index conſiſts of two Pieces, one End of that which comes out beyond the Limb of the Protractor is cut ſlopewiſe, ſo as exactly to fit the Edge of the Limb of the Protractor, which is likewiſe ſloped underneath, and is faſtened to the other Piece, by which means the Index is kept down cloſe to the Limb.

The Diviſions on both Edges of that Part of the Index beyond the Limb, are 60 equal Parts of the Portions of Circles (paſſing thro the Center of the Protractor, and two Points aſſumed in the outward Edge of the Limb of that Piece of the Index nigheſt the Center) intercepted by two other right Lines drawn from the Center, ſo that they each make, with Lines drawn to the aſſumed Points from the Center, Angles of one Degree

To lay off any Number of Degrees and Minutes by this Protractor, you muſt move the Index, ſo that one of the Lines drawn upon the Limb, from one of the aforementioned Points, may be upon the Number of Degrees ſought, and then pricking off as many of the equal Parts on the proper Edge of the Index, as there are Minutes given, and drawing a Line from the Center, to that Point ſo prick'd off, you will have an Angle, with the Diameter of the Protractor, of the propoſed Number of Degrees or Minutes The reaſon of this Contrivance is from *Prop* 27 *Lib* 3 *Eucl* where it is proved that Angles inſiſting upon the ſame Arcs, in equal Circles, or in the ſame Circle, (for it is the ſame thing) are equal

K   CHAP.

CHAP. VI.

The Projection of the Plain-Scale.

Fig. 5, 6. FIRST, draw a Circle A B D C, which crofs at right Angles with the Diameters A D, C B; then continue out A D to G, and upon the Point B, raife B F perpendicular to C B Now draw the Chord A B, and divide the Quadrant A B into 9 equal Parts, fetting the Figures 10, 20, 30, &c to 90 to them, each of which 9 Parts again fubdivide into 10 more equal Parts, and then the Quadrant will be divided into 90 Degrees Now fetting one Foot of your Compaffes in the Point A, transfer the faid Divifions to the Chord Line A B, and fet thereto the Figures 10, 20, 30, &c and the Line of Chords A B, will be divided, and then may be put upon your Scale, reprefented in *Fig 6* Now to project the Sines, divide the Arc B D into 90 Degrees, as before you did A B, from every of which Degrees, let fall Perpendiculars on the Semidiameter E B, which Perpendiculars will divide E B into a Line of Sines, to which you muft fet 10, 20, 30, &c beginning from the Center, and then you may transfer the Line of Sines to your Scale

Again, to project the Line of Tangents, from the Center E, and thro every Divifion of the Arc B D, draw right Lines cutting B F, which will divide it into a Line of Tangents, fetting thereto the Numbers 10, 20, 30, &c. which you muft transfer to your Scale

To project the Line of Secants, transfer the Diftances E 10, E 20, E 30, &c that is, the Diftance from E to 10, 20, 30, &c. on the Tangent Line, upon the Line E G, and fetting thereto the Numbers 10, 20, 30, &c the Line E G will be divided into a Line of Secants, which muft be transfer'd on the Scale

To project the Semi-tangents, draw Lines from the Point C, thro every Degree of the Quadrant A B, and they will divide the Diameter A E into a Line of Semi-tangents · but becaufe the Semitangents, or Plane-Scales of a Foot in Length, run to 160 Degrees, continue out the Line A E, and draw Lines from the Point C, thro the Degrees of the Quadrant C A, cutting the faid continued Portion of A E, and you will have a Line of Half-tangents to 160 Degrees, or further, if you pleafe.

Note, The Semitangent of any Arc, is but the Tangent of half that Arc, as will eafily appear from its manner of Projection, and *Prop 20 Lib 3. Eucl.* where it is proved, that an Angle at the Center, is double to one at the Circumference

Moreover, to draw the Rhumb Line, from every 8th part of the Quadrant A C, fetting one Foot of your Compaffes in A, defcribe Arcs cutting the Chord A C, which will divide A C into a Line of whole Rhumbs, and in the fame Manner may the Subdivifions of half and quarter Rhumbs be made

Laftly, to project the Line of Longitude, draw the Line H D, equal and parallel to the Radius C E, which divide into 60 equal Parts, (becaufe 60 Miles make a Degree of Longitude under the Equator) every 10 of which Number fet Figures to. Now from every of thofe Parts, let fall Perpendiculars to C E, cutting the Arc C D, and having drawn the Chord C D, with one Foot of your Compaffes in D, transfer the Diftances from D, to each of the Points in the Arc C D, on the Chord C D, and fet thereto the Numbers 10, 20, &c and the Line of Longitude will be divided.

The Reafon of this Conftruction is, that as Radius is to the Sine Complement of any Latitude, fo is the Length of a Degree of Longitude under the Equator, which is 60 Miles, to the Length of a Degree of Longitude in that Latitude

Thefe being all the Lines commonly put upon the Rulers, call'd Plain-Scales, excepting equal Parts, therefore I fhall proceed to fhew their manner of ufing in Trigonometry, and Spherical Geometry.

But by the way, note, That Plain-Scales are commonly of thefe two Lengths, *viz* fome one foot long, and others, which are put into Cafes of Inftruments, but half a foot in Length; and on one Side is a Diagonal Scale they are generally made of Box, and fometimes of Brafs or Ivory.

USE I. *To make an Angle in the Point A, at the End of the Line A B, of any Number of Degrees, fuppofe 40*

Fig 7. Take in your Compaffes 60 Degrees from the Line of Chords, and fetting one Foot in the Point A, defcribe the Arc C B, then take 40 Degrees, which is the Number propofed, from the fame Line of Chords, and lay them off on the Arc from B to E, draw the Line A E, and the Angle B A E will be 40 Degrees, as is manifeft from the Conftruction of the Line of Chords, and *Prop 15 Lib 4 Eucl* which fhews that the Semidiameter of any Circle, is equal to the Side of a Hexagon infcribed in the fame Circle, that is, to the Chord of 60 Degrees. USE

U S E II *The Angle E A B being given, to find the Quantity of Degrees it contains*

Take in your Compasses 60 Degrees from the Line of Chords, and describe the Arc BC , Fig 7. then take the Extent from B to E in the Compasses ; which Extent apply on the Line of Chords, and the Quantity of the Angle will be shewn   This Use, which is only the Reverse of the former, may be likewise done by the Lines of Sines and Tangents, the Method of doing which is enough manifest from Use I

U S E III *The Base of a Triangle being given 40 Leagues, the Angle A B C 36 Degrees, and the Angle B A C 41 Degrees; to make the Triangle, find the Lengths of the Sides A C, C B, and also the other Angle*

Draw the indefinite right Line A D, and take the Extent of 40 Leagues, from the Line Fig 8 of Leagues, between your Compasses, which lay off upon the said Line from A to B for the Base of the Triangle ; at the Points A and B make, by Use I the Angles A B C, B C A , the first 36 Degrees, and the last 41 Degrees, and the Triangle A C B will be formed , then take in your Compasses the Length of the Side A C, and apply it to the same Scale of Leagues, and you will find its Length to be 24 Leagues   Do thus for the other Side B C, and you will find it 27 Leagues and a half ; and, by Use II. the Angle A C B will be found 103 Degrees

By this Use the following Problem in Navigation may be solved, *viz* Two Ports, both lying under the same Meridian, being any Number of Miles distant from each other, suppose 30, and the Pilot of a Ship, out at Sea on a certain time, finds the Bearing of one of the Ports is S W by S, and the Bearing of the other N W   the Ship's Distance from each of the Ports at that time is required ?

To solve this Problem , draw the right Line A B equal to 3 Inches, or 3 of the largest equal Parts on the Diagonal Scale, which is to represent the 30 Miles, or the Distance from one of the Ports, as A to the other B ; at the Point B make an Angle, equal to the bearing Fig 9. of the Port B from the Ship, which must be 33 Degrees, 45 Minutes , likewise make another Angle at the Point A, equal to the bearing of the Port A from the Ship, which must be 45 Degrees, then the Point C will be the Place the Ship was in at the time of Observation.

Now to find the Distance of the Ship from the Port A, take the Length of the Side A C in your Compasses, and applying it to the Diagonal Scale, you will find it to be 17 $\frac{7}{10}$ Miles. In the same manner the Distance of the Ship, from the Port B, will be found 21 $\frac{1}{4}$ Miles.

Note, The Reason why the Angles A and B are equal to the bearing of the Ship from each of those Ports, depends on *Prop. 29. lib. 1 Eucl*

U S E IV *The Base A B of a Triangle being given 60 Leagues, the opposite Angle A C B 108 Fig 10. Degrees, and the Side C B 40 Leagues , to make the said Triangle, and find the Length of the other Side A C*

Draw the Line *a b* equal to A B, the given Base ; and because in any Triangle the Sines Fig 11. of the Sides are proportionable to the Sines of the opposite Angles (as is demonstrated by Trigonometrical Writers) it follows, that as A B is to the Sine of the given Angle C, which is of 72 Degrees, *viz* the Complement of 108 Degrees to 180 , so is the given Side B C, to the Sine of the Angle C A B   therefore make *b c* equal to the given Side B C of 40 Leagues Take in your Compasses, upon the Line of Sines, the Sine of 72 Degrees, to which Length make *b e* equal, and draw the Line *a c*, likewise draw *e d* parallel to *a c*, and (by *Prop* 4. *lib. 6 Eucl*) *b d* will be the Sine of the Angle C A B, which will be found, by applying it to the Line of Sines, about 39 Degrees   therefore make an Angle at the Point A of 39 Degrees, then take in your Compasses the Length 40 Leagues, and setting one foot in the Point B, with the other describe an Arc, which will cut the Side A C in the Point C, and consequently the Triangle A B C will be made, and the Length of the Side A C will be found 34 Leagues.

U S E V. *Concerning the Line of Rhumbs*

The Use of the Line of Rhumbs is only to lay off, or measure, the Angles of a Ship's Course in Navigation, more expeditiously than can be done by the Line of Chords : As suppose a Ship's Course is N N E, it is required to lay it down

Draw the Line A B, representing the Meridian ; take 60 Degrees from the Line of Fig 12. Chords, and about the Point A describe the Arc B C.   Now because N N E is the third Rhumb from the North, therefore take the third Rhumb in your Compasses, on the Line of Rhumbs, and lay it off upon the Arc from B to C ; draw the Line A C, and the Angle B A C will be the Course

U S E VI *Of the Line of Longitude.*

The Use of this Line is to find in what Degrees of Latitude a Degree of Longitude is 1, 2, 3, 4, *&c* Miles, which is easily done by means of the Line of Chords next to it . for it is only seeing what Degree of the Line of Chords answers to a proposed Number of Miles, and that Degree will be the Latitude, in which a Degree of Longitude is equal to that proposed

poſed Number of Miles As for Example , againſt 10 Miles, on the Line of Longitude, ſtand 80 Degrees, and ſomething more , whence, in the Latitude of about 80 Degrees, a Degree of Longitude is 10 Miles. Again, 30 Miles on the Line of Longitude, anſwers to 60 Degrees on the Line of Chords , therefore in the Latitude of 60 Degrees, a Degree of Longitude is 30 Miles. Moreover, againſt 58 Miles, on the Line of Longitude, ſtands 15 Degrees of the Line of Chords, which ſhews that a Degree of Longitude, in the Latitude of 15 Deg is 58 Miles , and ſo for others

USE of the Plain-Scale in Spherical Geometry.

USE I. To find the Pole of any Great Circle.

If the Pole of the Primitive Circle be required, it is its Center

If the Pole of a right or perpendicular Circle be ſought, it is 90 Degrees diſtant, reckoned upon the Limb from the Points, where this Circle, which is a Diameter, cuts it

If the Pole of an oblique Circle be required,

(1) Conſider that this Circle muſt cut the primitive in two Points, that will be diſtant from each other juſt a Diameter, as is the Caſe of the Interſection of all great Circles

(2) The Pole of this Circle muſt be in a right Line perpendicular to its Plane

(3) This Circle's Pole cannot but lie between the Center of the primitive one, and its own

Fig 13   *Example* Let the Pole of the oblique Circle A B C be required

1 Draw the Diameter A C, and then another, as D E, perpendicular to it

2 Lay the Edge of your Scale from A to B, it will cut the Limb in F , then take the Chord of 90 Degrees, and ſet it from F to *h*

3 Lay the Edge of your Scale from *h* to A, it will cut D E in *g*, which Point *g* is the Pole required

Note, To find the Points F and *h*, is called reducing B to the primitive Circle, and to the Diameter Alſo, *Note*, that every of the primitive Circles in this Uſe, and the following ones, are ſuppoſed to be deſcribed from 60 Degrees, taken off from the leſſer Line of Chords on the Scale

USE II To deſcribe a Spherical Angle of any Number of given Degrees.

1. If the angular Point be at the Center of the primitive Circle, then it is at any plane Angle, numbring the Degrees in the Limb from the Line of Chords , for all Circles paſſing thro the Center, and which are at right Angles with the Limb, muſt be projected into right Lines

2 If the Angle given is to be deſcribed at the Periphery of the primitive Circle, draw a Diameter, as A C , then take the Secant of the Angle given in your Compaſſes, and ſetting one Foot in A, croſs the Diameter in *e* or if no Diameter be drawn, placing one Foot in C, and croſſing the former Arc, you will find the ſame Point *e*, which is the Center of the Circle A *a* C, which, with the Primitive, makes the Angle D A *a* required.

Note, If the Angle given be obtuſe, take the Secant of its Supplement to 180 Degrees.

3 If a Point, as *a*, were aſſigned, thro which the Arc of the Circle conſtituting the Angle muſt paſs, draw the Diameter A C (as before) then take the Secant of the given Angle, and ſetting one Foot in A or C, ſtrike an Arc as at *e* , and then with the Secant of the given Angle, ſetting one Foot in *a*, croſs the other Arc in *e* ; which will be the Center of the oblique Circle required

USE III To draw a great Circle thro any two Points given, as a and b, within the primitive one

Fig. 14.   Draw a Diameter thro that Point which is furtheſt from the Center, as D R, producing it beyond the Limb if there be Occaſion , ſet 90 Degrees of Chords from D or R, to O, and draw O *a*

Then erect O H perpendicular to *a* O, and produce it till it cuts the Diameter prolonged in H , that Interſection H is a third Point, thro which, as alſo *a* and *b*, if a Circle be drawn, it will be a great Circle, as *e a b g*

Which is eaſily proved, by drawing the Lines *e* C *g*, for that Line is a Diameter, becauſe its Parts, multiplied into one another, are equal to *a c* × C H, equal to O C ſquared. *Per Prop* 35. *lib* 3 *& Coroll.* 8 *lib* 6 *Eucl*

USE IV To draw a great Circle perpendicular to, or at right Angles with another

Let it paſs through its Poles, and it is done

Of which there will be four Caſes ·

1. To draw a Circle perpendicular to the Primitive, which is done by any ſtrait Line paſſing thro' the Center

2. To draw a Circle perpendicular to a right Circle, is only to draw a Diameter at right Angles with that right Circle

3 To draw an oblique Circle perpendicular to a right one, only draw a right Circle that ſhall paſs thro both the Poles of ſuch a right Circle

                                           Thus

Thus the oblique Circle **D C R** is perpendicular to the right one **O Q**, becaufe it paffes thro its Poles **D** and **R**.

4 To draw an oblique Circle perpendicular to another . *Plate 5*

First find **P**, the Pole of the given oblique Circle **C *e* B**, and then draw any-how the Diameter **D R**. fo a Circle, drawn thro the three Points **D, P,** and **R**, will be the Circle required ; for paffing thro the Poles of the oblique Circle **C *e* B**, it muft be perpendicular to it

USE V *To meafure the Quantity of the Degrees of any Arc of a great Circle*

1 If the Arc be part of the Primitive, it is meafured on the Line of Chords

2 If the Arc be any part of a right Circle, the Degrees of it are meafured on the Scale of Semi-Tangents, fuppofing the Center of the primitive Circle to be in the beginning of the Scale, fo that if the Degrees are to be reckoned from the Center, you muft account according to the Order of the Scale of Half-Tangents

But if the Degrees are to be accounted from the Periphery of the Primitive, as will often happen, then you muft begin to account from the end of the Scale of Half-Tangents, calling 80, 10, 70, 20, &c

3 To meafure any part of an oblique Circle, first find its Pole, and there laying the Ruler, reduce the two Extremities of the Arc required to the primitive Circle, and then meafure the Diftance between thofe Points on the Line of Chords

Thus, in the laft Figure, if the Quantity of *e* B, an Arc of the oblique Circle **C *e* B** be required, lay a Ruler to **P** the Pole, and reduce the Points *e* B to the primitive Circle, fo *Fig 1.* fhall the Diftance between **O** and **B**, meafured on the Line or Chords, be the Quantity of Degrees contained in the Arc *e* B

USE VI *To meafure any Spherical Angle*

1 If the angular Point be at the Center of the primitive Circle, then the Diftance between the Legs taken from the Limb, and meafured on the Chords, is the Quantity of the Angle fought

2 If the angular Point be at the Periphery, as **A C B**, here the Poles of both Circles being in the fame Diameter, find the Pole of the oblique Circle **C B O**, which let be **P** ; then the Diftance of **B P**, meafured on the Scale of Half-Tangents, is the Meafure of the Angle **A C B**

For the Poles of all Circles muft be as far diftant from each other, as are the Angles of the Inclinations of their Planes

But if the two Poles are not in the fame Diameter, being both found in their proper Diameter, reduce thofe Points to the primitive Circle, and then the Diftance between them there, accounted on the Line of Chords, is the Quantity of the Angle fought

When the angular Point is fomewhere within the primitive Circle, and yet not at the *Fig 3.* Center, proceed thus Suppofe the Angle *a b* C be fought, find the Pole **P** of the Circle *a b d*, and then the Pole of the Circle *e b c*, after which lay a Ruler to the angular Point, and the two Poles **P** and **Q**, and reduce them to the primitive Circle by the Points *x* and *z*, fo is the Arc *x z*, meafured on the Line of Chords, the Meafure of the Angle *a b* C required

USE VII *To draw a Parallel-Circle*

1. If it be to be drawn parallel to the primitive Circle, at any given Diftance, draw it from the Center of the Primitive, with the Complement of that Diftance taken from the Scale of Half-Tangents

2 If it be to be drawn parallel to a right Circle, as fuppofe *a b*, parallel to **A B**, was to *Fig. 4* be drawn at 23 Deg 30 Min. Diftance from it, from the Line of Chords take 23 Deg 30 Min and fet it both-ways on the Limb from **A** to *a*, and **B** to *b* (or fet its Complement 66 Deg 30 Min both-ways from **P** the Pole of **A B**) to the Points *a* and *b*

Then take the Tangent of the Parallel's Diftance from the Pole of the right Circle **A B**, which is here 66 Deg 30 Min and fetting one foot in *a* and *b*, with the other ftrike two little Arcs, to interfect each other fomewhere above **P**, which will give **C**, the Center of the parallel Circle *a b d* required.

3 If it be drawn parallel to an oblique Circle, and at the Diftance fuppofe of 40 Degrees . *Fig. 5.*

First find **P**, the Pole of the oblique Circle **A B C**, and then meafure, on the Scale of Half-Tangents, the Diftance *g* **P**, which fuppofe to be 34 Degrees, then add to it 50 Degrees, the Complement of the Circle's Diftance, it will make 84 Degrees ; and alfo fubftracting 50 from it, or it from 50, it will make 16 Degrees : Then this Sum and Difference taken from the Scale of Half-Tangents, and fet each way from **P** the Pole of the oblique Circle, will give the two Extremes *a b* of the Diameter, or the Points of the Interfection of the Parallel, and then the middle Diftance between *a* and *b*, is the Center of the true parallel Circle **P** *a b*, which is parallel to the given oblique Circle **A B C**, and at the given Diftance of 40 Degrees . or the Half-Tangent of 84, fet from *g*, will give *b*, and the Half-Tangent of 16 Degrees, fet alfo from *g*, and the Points *a* and *b*, the two Ends of the parallel Circle's Diameter will be had.

L   USE

USE VIII. *To meaſure any projected Arc of a parallel Circle*

1. If it be parallel to the Primitive, then a Ruler, laid thro the Center and the Diviſion of the Limb, will divide the Parallel into the ſame Degrees, or determine, in the Limb, the Quantity of any Arc parallel to it.

2 If the Circle be parallel to a right one, as *a d b* is, in caſe the ſecond of the laſt Uſe, and it were required to meaſure that Arc *a b*, or to divide it into proper Degrees Since that parallel Circle is 66 Deg 30 Min. diſtant from P, the nearer Pole of the right Circle A B, and conſequently 113 Deg 30 Min diſtant from its other Pole, take the Half-Tangent of 113 Deg 30 Min or the Tangent of its half, 56 Deg 45 Min and with that Diſtance, and on the Center of the Primitive, draw a Circle parallel to the Limb, and divide that half of it, which lies towards the oppoſite Pole of A B, into its Degrees Then a Ruler laid from P, and the equal Diviſions of that Semicircle, will divide *a b*, or meaſure any part thereof

3. To meaſure or divide the Arc of a Circle which is projected, parallel to an oblique one.

As ſuppoſe the Circle *a b*, which is parallel to the oblique one A B C, *Fg Caſe 3* of the precedent Uſe, and at the Diſtance of 40 Degrees, this parallel Circle being 40 Degrees diſtant from the Plane of the Circle A B C, muſt be 50 Degrees diſtant from its Pole, and conſequently 130 Degrees from its oppoſite Pole : therefore take the Semi-Tangent of 130 Degrees, or the Tangent of its half, 65 Degrees, and with that, as a Radius, draw a Circle parallel to the Limb of the Primitive, which Circle divide into proper Degrees, then ſhall a Ruler laid thro P, and the equal Diviſion of that Circle, cut the little Circle *a b* into its proper Degrees, or truly give the Meaſure of any part thereof

Theſe being moſt of the general Uſes of the Scales of Lines commonly put upon Plain-Scales, their particular Applications in Navigation, Spherical Trigonometry, and Aſtronomy, would take up too much room, therefore I proceed to *Gunter*'s Scale.

As for its Uſe in the Projection of the Sphere, ſee *Uſes of the* Engliſh *Sector.*

CHAP. VII.

Of the Conſtruction and Uſes of Gunter's-Scale.

Fig 6.

THIS Scale is commonly made of Box, and ſometimes of Braſs, exactly two Foot long (tho there are others but a Foot long, which are not ſo exact) about an Inch and ½ broad, and of a convenient Thickneſs

The Lines that are put on one Side of it are the Line of Numbers, marked on the Scale *Numbers*, the Line of artificial Sines, marked *Sines*, the Line of artificial Tangents, marked *Tangents* ; the Line of artificial verſed Sines, marked V S ſignifying Verſed Sines, the artificial Sines of the Rhumbs, marked S R ſignifying the Sines of the Rhumbs, the artificial Tangents of the Rhumbs, marked T. R ſignifying Tangents of the Rhumbs ; the Meridian-Line in *Mercator's* Chart, marked *Merid* ſignifying Meridian-Line, and equal Parts, marked E P. ſignifying equal Parts

There are commonly placed on theſe Scales, that are but a Foot long, the Lines of Latitudes, Hours, and Inclinations of Meridians.

On the Back-ſide of this Scale are placed all the Lines that are put upon a Plain-Scale

The Lines of artificial Sines, Tangents, and Numbers are ſo fitted on this Scale, that, by means of a Pair of Compaſſes, any Problem, whether in right-lined, or ſpherical Trigonometry, may be ſolved by them very expeditiouſly, with tolerable Exactneſs, and therefore the Contrivance of theſe Lines on a Scale is extremely uſeful in all Parts of Mathematicks that Trigonometry hath to do with, as Navigation, Dialling, Aſtronomy, &c.

Conſtruction of the Line of Numbers.

The Conſtruction of the Line of Numbers is thus · Having pitched upon its Length, which, on *Gunter's* Scale, let be 23 Inches, take exactly half that Length, which will be the Length of either of the Radius's, then take that half Length, and divide into 10 equal Parts, one of which diagonally ſubdivide into 100 equal Parts, that is, make a Diagonal Scale of 1000 equal Parts of the aforeſaid Half-Length, which may eaſily be done from our Author's 8th Uſe.

Now having drawn, on *Gunter's* Scale, three Parallels, for better diſtinguiſhing the Diviſions of the Line of Numbers, and made a Mark for the beginning of it, half an Inch from the beginning-end of the Scale, look in the Table of Logarithms for the Number 200, and againſt it you will find 2 301030 ; and rejecting the Characteriſtick 2, and alſo the three laſt Figures 030, becauſe the Length of the Radius is divided but into 1000 equal Parts, take 301 of thoſe 1000 Parts in your Compaſſes, and lay off that Diſtance from the beginning of
the

Plate IV

Fig 2   Fig 1
The Ploting Scale

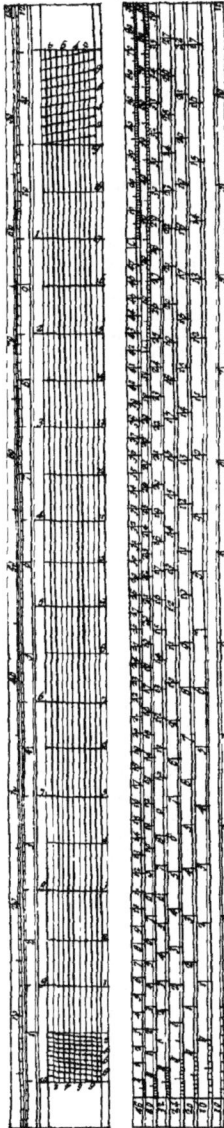

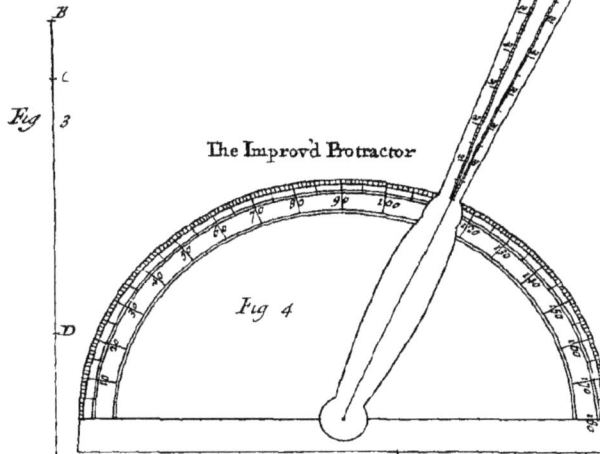

The Improv'd Protractor

Fig 6
Plain Scale

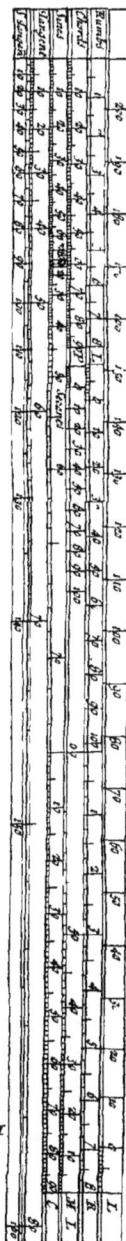

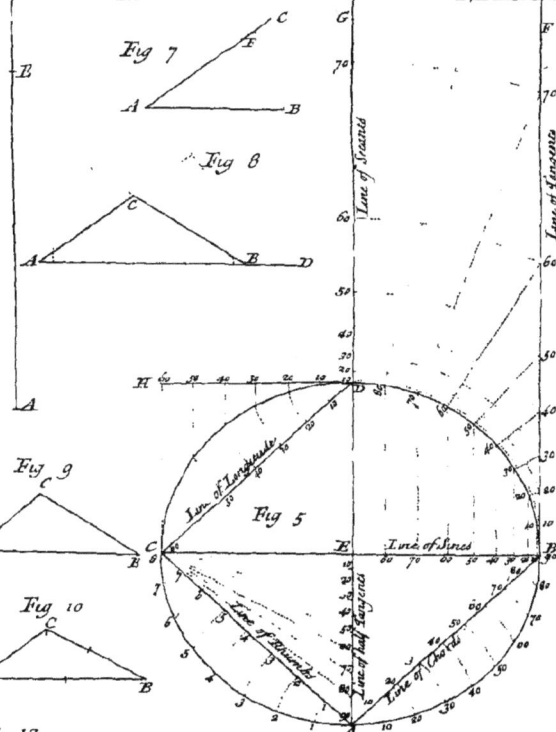

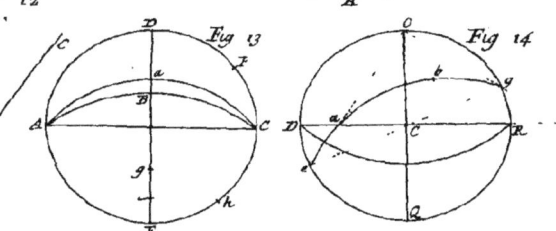

Fig 4

Fig 7

Fig 8

Fig 9

Fig 5

Fig 10

Fig 11

Fig 12

Fig 13

Fig 14

Line of Sines

Line of Tangents

Line of Longitude

Line of Sines

Line of half Tangents

Line of Rhumbs

Line of Chords

I Senex sculp

the Line, at the end of which write 2 for the first Prime.   Again, to find the Division for the second Prime, look in the Table of Logarithms for the Number 300, and against it you will find 2 477121, and rejecting the Characteristick 2, and the three last Figures 121, as before, take 477 from your Diagonal Scale, and lay off that Distance from 1 at the beginning, at the end of which write 3 for the second Prime In this manner proceed for all the Primes of the first Radius to 1, which will be the whole Length of your Diagonal Scale, or 1000 equal Parts   And because each of the Primes of the second Radius are at the same Distance from 1, at the end of the first Radius, as the same Primes, on the first Radius, are distant from 1 at the beginning, the Primes on the second Radius are easily found.

The Divisions of the Tenths, between each of the Primes in both Radius's, are found thus   Look in the Table of Logarithms for 110, and against it you will find 2 041393, and rejecting the Characteristick 2, and the three last Figures, there will remain 41, which taken from the aforesaid Diagonal Scale of 1000, will give the first Tenth in the first Prime. Again, look in the Table for 120, and against it you will find 2 079181, and by rejecting the Characteristick, and the three last Figures, there will remain 79, which taken from the Diagonal Scale, will give the second Tenth in the first Prime   Proceed thus for all the Tenths in the first Primes of both Radius's.   And to find the Tenths in the second Primes of both Radius's, look in the Table for the Number 210, and against it you will find 2 322210, whence rejecting as before, you will have 322, which laid off from the beginning of the first Prime, will give the first Tenth in the second Prime   Again, to find the second Tenth in the second Prime, look for the Number 220, and against it you will find 2 342423, whence by rejecting, as before, you will have 342 for the second Tenth, in the second Prime   In like manner may the Tenths in all the Primes of both Radius's be found

To find every two Centesms in the first Prime of the second Radius, look for the Number 102 in the Table of Logarithms, and against it you will find 2 008600, and by rejecting, as at first, you will have 8 for the second Centesm   Again, look in the Table for 104, and proceed as before, and you will have 17 for the third Centesm   In like manner you may have every second Centesm in the first, and also the Second Primes of the second Radius

Note, In bisecting every of the two Centesms in the first Prime, Centesms will be had. Note also, that the third, fourth, and fifth Primes, cannot be divided into every two Centesms, but only into every five, because of the Smallness of the Divisions.

Construction of the Line of artificial Sines and Tangents

The Line of artificial Sines on *Gunter's* Scale, is nothing but the Logarithms of the natural Sines, translated from the Tables of artificial Sines and Tangents, almost in the same Manner as the Logarithms of the natural Numbers was, the Method of doing which is thus:

Having drawn three Parallels under the Line of Numbers for distinguishing the Divisions of the Line, and marked a Point exactly half an Inch from the beginning-end of the Scale, representing the beginning of the Line of Sines, look in the Tables of artificial Sines and Tangents, for the Sine of 40 Minutes, which is the first Subdivision of the Line, and it will be found 8 065776: then rejecting the Characteristick 8, and the three last Figures 776, as in the Construction of the Line of Numbers, the 65 remaining, must be taken on the same Scale of 1000 Parts, as served before for the Line of Numbers, this 65 laid off from the beginning of the Line of Sines, will give the Division on the Line of Sines for 40 Minutes. Again, to make the next Division which is for 50 Minutes, seek in the Table for the Sine of 50 Minutes, which will be found 8 162681, then rejecting the Characteristick 8, and the three last Figures 681, take the Remainder 162, from your Scale of 1000 Parts, and lay it off from the beginning of the Line, and that will give the Division for 50 Minutes   Moreover, to make the Division for 1 Degree, seek the Sine of 1 Degree, which is 8 241855, and rejecting as before, take the Remainder 241 from the Scale of 1000, and lay it off from the beginning on the Line of Sines, which will give the Division for 1 Degree   Proceed thus for the other Degrees and Minutes to 90, only take notice, that when you come to 5 Degrees, 50 Minutes, the Parts to be taken off the Scale are more than 1000, and consequently longer than the Scale itself   In that Case you must make a Mark in the Middle of the Line of Sines, from which lay off all the Parts found above 1000, for the Degrees and Minutes: As, to make the Division for 6 Degrees, the Sine of which is 9.019235, the Parts to be taken off the Scale will be 1019, therefore lay off 19 from the middle Point, representing 1000, and the Division for 6 Degrees will be had   Proceed in the same manner for the Line of artificial Tangents, till you come to 45 Degrees, whose Length is equal to Radius; and the Divisions for the Degrees and Minutes above 45, which should go beyond 45, are set down by their Complements to 90   For Example, the Division of 40 Degrees hath its Complement 50 set to it, because the proper equal Parts taken off the Scale of 1000 to make the Division, for the Tangent of 50 Deg will be as much above 1000 (which are the equal Parts for the Tangent of 45 Degrees, to be laid off from the middle of the Line of Tangents) as the equal Parts for the Division of the Tangent of 40 Degrees wants of 1000, an Example of which will make it manifest   The Tangent of 40 Degrees is 9 924813, and by rejecting the Characteristick, and the three last Figures, the Parts of 1000, *viz.* 924 taken from 1000, and there remains 76, which are the Parts that the Tangent of 40 Degrees is distant from the

Tangent

Tangent of 45 Degrees   Again, the Tangent of 50 Degrees is 10076186, and by rejecting the Characteriſtick, and the three laſt Figures, the Parts 76 above 1000, for the Diviſion of the Tangent of 50 Degrees, which muſt fall beyond 45 Degrees, are equal to the Parts that the Diviſion of 40 Degrees wants of 1000   Underſtand the ſame for the Tangent of any other Degree, or Minute, and its Complement. the Reaſon of this is, becauſe Radius is a mean Proportional between any Tangent and its Complement

The Conſtruction of the artificial Sines of the Rhumbs, and quarter Rhumbs, is deduced from a Conſideration that the firſt Rhumb makes an Angle of 11 Deg 15 Min with the Meridian, the ſecond, 22 Deg. 30 Min the third, 33 Deg. 45 Min the fourth, 45 Deg &c. therefore to make the Diviſion on *Gunter's* Scale, for the firſt Rhumb, take the Extent of the artificial Sine of 11 Deg 15 Min. on the Scale, and lay it off upon the Line drawn to contain the Diviſions of the Line of Rhumbs, and that will give the Diviſion for the firſt Rhumb   Again, take the Extent, on the Line of artificial Sines, of the Sine of 22 30 Min. and lay it off in the ſame manner as before, and you will have the ſecond Rhumb ∙ proceed thus for all the other Rhumbs. The Diviſions for the half Rhumbs, and quarter Rhumbs, are alſo made in the ſame manner the Diviſions of the artificial Tangents of the Rhumbs, are made in the ſame manner as the Diviſions of the artificial Sines of the Rhumbs, by taking the artificial Tangents of the ſeveral Angles that the Rhumbs and quarter Rhumbs make with the Meridian.

The Conſtruction of the Line of artificial vers'd Sines

This Line, which begins at about 11 Deg 45 Min and runs to 180 Deg. which is exactly under 90 of the Line of Sines (tho on the Scale they are numbered backwards; that is, to the vers'd Sine of each 10 Degrees above 20, are ſet the Numbers of their Complements to 182, for a Reaſon hereafter ſhewn) may be thus made, by means of the Table of Sines, and the aforeſaid equal Parts   Suppoſe the Diviſion for the verſed Sine of 15 Degrees be to be made   Take half 15 Degrees, which will be 7^d. 30^m, the Sine of which doubled will be 18231396, and by ſubſtracting the Radius therefrom, you will have 8231396, and rejecting the three laſt Figures, and the Characteriſtick, there will remain 231, this 231 taken from your Scale of 1000, and laid off from a Point directly under the beginning of the Line of Sines, will give the Diviſion for the verſed Sine of 15 Degrees, at which is ſet 165, *viz.* the Complement of 15^d to 180^d Again, to make the Diviſion for 20 Degrees, twice the Sine of 10 Degrees, (its half) will be 18479340, from which, ſubſtracting Radius, and rejecting the Characteriſtick, and the three laſt Figures, you will have 479, which taken from your Scale, and laid off from the beginning of the Line, will give the Diviſion for the verſed Sine of 20 Degrees   And in this manner may the Line of verſed Sines be divided to 180 Degrees, by obſerving what I have ſaid in the Conſtruction of the Line of Sines

The Manner of projecting the Lines of Numbers, artificial Sines and Tangents, in Circles, and Spirals of any Number of Revolutions

Fig. 7.

Suppoſe the Circle B C is to be divided into a Line of Numbers of but one Radius, firſt, divide the Limb into 1000 equal Parts, beginning from the Point G, then take 301 of thoſe Parts, which ſuppoſe to be at *p*, and lay a Ruler from the Center A, on the ſaid Point *p*, and that will cut the Periphery of the Circle B C in the Point for the Log. of 2   Again; take 477 Parts upon the Limb, and a Ruler laid from the Center upon the ſaid Diviſion, will cut the Circle B C in the Point for the Log of the Number 3   and thus by taking the proper Parts upon the Limb, from the Point G, which were before directed to be uſed in dividing this Line upon the Scale, and laying a Ruler from the Center, may the Line of Numbers be projected upon the Circle B C   And in the ſame manner may the Lines of artificial Sines and Tangents be projected, from the Sine of 5^d 45^m, and Tangent of 5^d 42^m to the Sine of 90^d, and the Tangent of 45^d, by taking (as before directed in the Conſtruction of the ſtraight Lines of Sines and Tangents) the Parts of 1000 for the Degrees and Minutes, and laying them off upon the Limb from the Point G, and then laying a Ruler from the Center, which will divide the Circles into Lines of Sines and Tangents

Fig. 8.

Now to project a Line of Numbers upon the Spiral of *Fig* 8 having four Revolutions, or Turns, firſt, divide the Limb into 1000 equal Parts, beginning from the Point G; then take 301, which is the Log of the Number 2 (when the Characteriſtick, and the three laſt Figures are rejected) and multiply it by 4, becauſe the Spiral hath four Revolutions, and the Product is 1204   then if 204 of the Parts of 1000, be taken upon the Limb from G to *p*, and a Ruler be laid from the Center A to *p*, it will cut the ſecond Revolution of the Spiral in the Point for the Number 2   Again, having multiply'd 477, the Log of the Number 3, by 4, the Product will be 1908, whence, taking 908 Parts from the Point G on the Limb, to the Point *q*, lay a Ruler from A to *q* and that will cut the ſecond Revolution of the Spiral, in the Point for the Number 3   Moreover, multiply 602 by 4, and the Product will be 2408; whence take 408 Parts upon the Limb from G, and laying a Ruler from A, it will cut the third Revolution of the Spiral in the Point, for the Number 4   and in thus proceeding may the Spiral be divided into a Line of Numbers, whoſe beginning is at the Point C, and

end

End at the Point B   This being underſtood, it will be no difficult Matter to projeſt the Sines and Tangents in a Spiral of any Number of Revolutions.

In uſing either the Circular or Spiral Lines of Numbers, Sines, and Tangents, there is an opening Index placed in the Center A, conſiſting of two Arms, the one called the antecedent Arm, and the other the conſequent Arm ; then three Numbers, Sines, or Tangents being given, to find a fourth   If you move the antecedent Arm to the firſt, and open the other Arm to the ſecond (the two Arms keeping the ſame Opening) and afterwards the antecedent Arm be moved to the third, the conſequent Arm will fall upon the fourth required

But, *Note,* that as many Revolutions of the Spiral as the ſecond Term is diſtant from the firſt, ſo many Revolutions will the fourth Term be diſtant from the third

Of the Meridian Line

The Meridian Line, on *Gunter's* Scale, is nothing but the Table of Meridional Parts in *Mercator's* Projection transferred on a Line, which may be done in the following manner, by help of the Line of equal Parts ſet under it, and a Table of Meridional Parts

Take any one of the large Diviſions of the aforeſaid Line of equal Parts, whoſe Length Fig. 9. let be A B, and divide it into ſix equal Parts up on ſome Plane, at the Points A B raiſe the Perpendiculars A C, B D, equal to A B, and compleat the Parallelogram A B D C, divide the Sides A C, B D, into ten equal Parts, and the Side D C into ſix, draw the Diagonals A F, 10 20, *&c* as per Figure, and you will have a Diagonal Scale, by which any part of the aforeſaid Diviſion under 60 may readily be taken

Now to make the Diviſions of the Meridian Line, look in the Table of meridional Parts for 1 Degree, and againſt it you will find 60   and rejecting the laſt Figure, which in this Caſe is 0, take ſix equal Parts from the aforementioned Diagonal Scale, and lay it off on the Meridian Line, which will give the Diviſion for one Degree   Again, to find the Diviſion for 2 Degrees, ſeek in the Table of Meridional Parts, for the Parts againſt 2 Degrees, and they will be found 120: whence rejecting the laſt Figure (which always muſt be done) take 12 from your Scale, and lay it off from the beginning of the Meridian Line, and the Diviſion for 2 Degrees will be had   Moreover, to find the Diviſion for 11 Degrees, you will find anſwering to it 664, and rejecting the laſt Figure, the remainder will be 66, which muſt be laid off from the beginning of the Meridian Line to have the Diviſion for 11 Degrees. But becauſe 66 cannot be taken from the Diagonal Scale, you muſt take only 6 from it, and for the 60, take its whole Length, or elſe lay off the 6 from the End of the firſt Diviſion of the Line of equal Parts, and the Diviſion for 11 Degrees will be had   In this manner may the Meridian Line be divided into Degrees and every thirty Minutes, as it is upon the Scale

There are ſeveral other ways of dividing this Meridian Line, but let this ſuffice.
The Uſe of this Line is to project a *Mercator's* Chart

Projection of the Line of Latitudes and Hours.

Upon the end A, of the Diameter of the Circle, erect a Line of Sines at right Angles, of Fig. 10. the Length of the Diameter ; then from the Point B, the other end of the Diameter, draw right Lines to each Degree of that Line of Sines, cutting the Quadrant A C   Now having drawn the Chord-Line A C, which is to be the Line of Latitudes, ſet one foot of your Compaſſes upon the Point A, and with the other transfer the Interſections made by the Lines drawn from B, on the Quadrant, to the Chord-Line A C, by means of which it will be divided into a Line of Latitudes   Or the Line of Latitudes may be made by this Canon, viz. As Radius is to the Chord of 90 Deg ſo is the Tangent of any Degree, to another Tangent, the natural Sine of whoſe Arc, taken from a Diagonal Scale of equal Parts, will give the Diviſion, for that Degree, on the Line of Latitudes, and ſo for any other Degree

Again, to graduate the Line of Hours, draw the Tangent G H equal to the Diameter A B, and parallel thereto, then divide each of the Arcs of half the Quadrants A K, K B, into three Parts, for the Degrees of every Hour from 12 to 6, which muſt again be each ſubdivided into Halfs, Quarters, *&c* then if thro' each of the aforeſaid Diviſions and Subdiviſions, Lines be drawn from the Center, cutting the Tangent Line G H, they will divide the ſaid Line into a Line of Hours

As for the Line of Inclination of Meridians, uſually put upon Scales, it is nothing but the Line of Hours numbered with Degrees inſtead of Time, and the Lines of the Style's Height, and Angle of 12 and 6, ſometimes put upon Scales, are made from Tables of the Style's Height, *&c* and no otherwiſe uſed

Whence the Line of Hours is but two Lines of natural Tangents to 45 Degrees, each ſet together at the Center, and from thence beginning and continued to each End of the Diameter, and from one End thereof, numbered with 90 Deg to the other End, and may otherwiſe be thus divided: Let A B be the Radius of a Line of Tangents, C D another Radius Fig. 11. equal and parallel thereto, and C B the Diameter to either of the ſaid Radius's, which is to be divided into a Line of Hours.   Now if right Lines are drawn from the Point D, to every Degree of the Tangent-Line A B, thoſe Lines will divide G B, half of the Line of

M   Hours,

Hours, as required , and Lines drawn from the Point A, to every Degree of the Tangent C D, will divide the other half of C B: therefore from the ſimilar Triangles C D F, E F B, it will be as the Radius C D is to the Tangent E B of any Arc under 45 · ſo is C F to F B, that is, as Radius is to the Tangent of any Arc under 45 Degrees, ſo is Radius *plus* the Cotangent of the ſaid Arc to 45 Degrees, to Radius *leſs* the ſaid Cotangent, as in *Fig* 12.

Fig. 12.

As the Radius A B, to the Tangent B C of any Arc, ſo is A B + E G, to A B — E G : for call A B, *r* , and B C, *b* , and from the Point C, draw C F parallel to E G, and make B D equal to A B Then D F (= F C) = $\sqrt{rr - 2rb + bb}$, and A F = $\sqrt{rr + 2rb + bb}$:

Whence as A F $\left(\frac{\sqrt{rr + 2rb + bb}}{2}\right)$ F C $\left(\frac{\sqrt{rr - 2rb + bb}}{2}\right)$. A B (*r*) : E G $\left(\frac{rr - rb}{r + b}\right)$ therefore it will be A B   (*r*)   B C (*b*) ·   A B + E G $\left(\frac{2rr}{r+b}\right)$. A B — E G $\left(\frac{2rb}{r+b}\right)$

Thus having given the Conſtruction of the Lines on *Gunter's* Scale, I now proceed to ſhew their manner of uſing , but, *Note*, theſe Lines are alſo put upon Rulers to ſlide by each other, and are therefore called *Sliding-Gunters*, ſo that you may uſe them without Compaſſes , but any Perſon that underſtands how to uſe them with Compaſſes, may alſo, by what I have ſaid of *Everard's* and *Coggeſhall's* Sliding-Rules, uſe them without.

USE *of the Lines of Numbers, Sines, and Tangents.*

U S E I. *The Baſe of a right-angled right-lined Triangle being given* 30 *Miles, and the oppoſite Angle to it* 26 *Degrees, to find the Length of the Hypotenuſe.*

As the Sine of the Angle, 26 Degrees, is to the Baſe, 30 Miles, ſo is Radius to the Length of the Hypothenuſe Set one Foot of your Compaſſes upon the 26th Degree of the Line of Sines, and extend the other to 30 on the Line of Numbers . the Compaſſes remaining thus opened, ſet one Foot on 90 Degrees, or the End of the Line of Sines, and cauſe the other to fall on the Line of Numbers, which will give 68 Miles and about a half, for the Length of the Hypotaenuſe ſought.

U S E II *The Baſe of a right-angled Triangle being given* 25 *Miles, and the Perpendicular* 15, *to find the Angle oppoſite to the Perpendicular*

As the Baſe 25 Miles is to the Perpendicular 15 Miles, ſo is Radius to the Tangent of the Angle ſought , becauſe if the Baſe is made Radius, the Perpendicular will be the Tangent of the Angle oppoſite to the Perpendicular Extend your Compaſſes on the Line of Numbers, from 15, the Perpendicular given, to 25, the Baſe given, and the ſame Extent will reach the contrary way, on the Line of Tangents, from 45 Degrees to 31 Degrees, the Angle ſought.

U S E III *The Baſe of a right-angled Triangle being given,* ſuppoſe 20 *Miles, and the Angle oppoſite to the Perpendicular* 50 *Degrees, to find the Perpendicular.*

As Radius is to the Tangent of the given Angle 50 Degrees, ſo is the Baſe 20 Miles to the Perpendicular ſought. Extend your Compaſſes on the Line of Tangents, from the Tangent of 45 Degrees to the Tangent of 50 Degrees, and the ſame Extent will reach on the Line of Numbers the contrary way, from the given Baſe 20 Miles, to the required Perpendicular, about 23 ¾ Miles

Note, The Reaſon why the Extent on the Line of Numbers was taken from 20 to 23 ¾ forwards, is, becauſe the Tangent of 50 Degrees (as I have already mentioned in the Conſtruction of the Line of Tangents) ſhould be as far beyond the Tangent of 45 Degrees, as its Complement 40 Degrees wants of 45 Degrees.

U S E IV. *The Baſe of a right-angled Triangle being given,* ſuppoſe 35 *Miles, and the Perpendicular* 48 *Miles, to find the Angle oppoſite to the Perpendicular*

As the Baſe 35 Miles is to the Perpendicular 48 Miles, ſo is Radius to the Tangent of the Angle ſought Extend your Compaſſes from 35, on the Line of Numbers, to 48 , the ſame Extent will reach the contrary way on the Line of Tangents, from the Tangent of 45 Degrees, to the Tangent of 36 Degrees 5 Minutes, or 53 Degrees 55 Minutes , and to know which of thoſe Angles the Angle ſought is equal to, conſider that the Perpendicular of the Triangle is greater than the Baſe , therefore (becauſe both the Angles oppoſite to the Perpendicular and Baſe together make 90 Degrees) the Angle oppoſite to the Perpendicular will be greater than the Angle oppoſite to the Baſe, and conſequently the Angle 53 Degrees 55 Minutes, will be the Angle ſought.

USE V *The Hypothenuse of a right-angled Spherical Triangle being given, suppose 60 Degrees, and one of the Sides 20 Degrees, to find the Angle opposite to that Side*

As the Sine of the Hypothenuse 60 Degrees is to Radius, so is the Sine of the given Side 20 Degrees, to the Sine of the Angle sought. Extend your Compasses, on the Line of Sines, from 60 Degrees to Radius or 90 Degrees, and the same Extent will reach on the Line of Sines the same way, from 20 Degrees, the given Side, to 23 Degrees 10 Minutes, the Quantity of the Angle sought

USE VI. *The Course and Distance of a Ship given, to find the Difference of Latitude and Departure*

Suppose a Ship sails from the Latitude of 50 Deg 10 Min North, S. S W 48 5 Miles: As Radius is to the Distance sailed 48 5 Miles, so is the Sine of the Course, which is two Points, or the second Rhumb, from the Meridian, to the Departure Extend your Compasses from 8, on the artificial Sine Rhumb-Line, to 48 5 on the Line of Numbers, the same Extent will reach the same way from the second Rhumb, on the Line of artificial Sines of the Rhumbs, to the Departure Westing 18 6 Miles Again, as Radius is to the Distance sailed 48 5 Miles, so is the Co-Sine of the Course 67 Deg 30 Min to the Difference of Latitude Extend your Compasses from Radius, on the Line of Sines, to 48 5 Miles on the Line of Numbers, the same Extent will reach the same way, from 67 Deg 30 Min on the Line of Sines, to 44 8 on the Line of Numbers; which converted into Degrees, by allowing 60 Miles to a Degree, and substracted from the given North-Latitude 50 Deg 10 Min. leaves the Remainder 49 Deg 25 Min the present Latitude

USE VII *The Difference of Latitude and Departure from the Meridian being given, to find the Course and Distance*

A Ship, from the Latitude of 59 Deg North, sails North-Eastward till she has altered her Latitude 1 Deg 10 Min or 70 Miles, and is departed from the Meridian 57 5 Miles, to find the Course and Distance

As the Difference of Latitude 70 Miles is to Radius, so is the Departure 57 5 Miles to the Tangent of the Course 39 Deg 20 Min or three Points and a half from the Meridian Extend your Compasses from the fourth Rhumb, on the Line of artificial Tangents of the Rhumbs, to 70 Miles on the Line of Numbers the same Extent will reach from 57 5 on the Line of Numbers, to the third Rhumb and a half on the Line of artificial Tangents of the Rhumbs Again, as the Sine of the Course 39 Deg 20 Min is to the Departure 57 5 Miles, so is Radius to the Distance 90 6 Miles Extend your Compasses from the third Rhumb and a half, on the artificial Sines of the Rhumbs, to 57 5 Miles on the Line of Numbers, and that Extent will reach from the Sine of the eighth Rhumb, on the Sines of the Rhumbs, to 90 6 Miles on the Line of Numbers

USE *of the Line of Versed Sines.*

The three Sides of an oblique Spherical Triangle being given, to find the Angle opposite to the greatest Side

Suppose the Side A B be 40 Degrees, the Side B C 60 Degrees, and the Side A C 96 Degrees, to find the Angle A B C. First add the three Sides together, and from half the Sum substract the greater Side A C, and note the Remainder, the Sum will be 196 Degrees, half of which is 98 Degrees, from which substracting 96 Degrees, the Remainder will be two Degrees Fig. 13.

This done, extend your Compasses from the Sine of 90 Degrees, to the Sine of the Side A B 40 Degrees, and applying this Extent to the Sine of the other Side B C 60 Degrees, you will find it to reach to a fourth Sine about 34 Degrees Again, from this fourth Sine extend your Compasses to the Sine of half the Sum, that is, to the Sine of 72 Degrees, the Complement of 98 Degrees to 180, and this second Extent will reach from the Sine of the Difference 2 Degrees, to the Sine of 3 Deg 24 Min against which, on the Versed Sines, stands 151 Deg 50 Min which is the Quantity of the Angle sought

That the Reason of this Operation may appear, it is demonstrated in most Books of Trigonometry, that as Radius is to the Sine of A B, so is the Sine of B C to a fourth Sine, then as this fourth Sine is to Radius, so is the Difference of the versed Sines of A C and A B + B C to the Versed Sine of the Complement of the Angle A B C to 180 Degrees It is also demonstrated, that as Radius is to the Sine of half the Sum of any two Arcs, so is the Sine of half their Difference to half the Difference of the Versed Sines of these two Arcs. whence, if the Sine of A B be called a, the Sine of B C, b, and the Sine of A C, c, the

fourth Sine in the first Analogy will be had; in saying, as $:: a - b \dfrac{ab}{r}$ Now to get the

Difference of Versed Sines of A C, and A B + B C, let us call the Sine of $\dfrac{AB + BC + AC}{2}$ p,

and

and the Sine of $\frac{A B + B C - A C}{2}$ q, then as r p q . $\frac{p\,q}{r}$, which laſt Term will be half

the Difference of the verſed Sines of A C, and A B + B C therefore if we again ſay, as

$\frac{a\,b}{r}$ r : . $\frac{2\,p\,q}{r}$ $\frac{2\,r\,p\,q}{a\,b}$ this laſt Term will be the verſed Sine of the Complement of the

Angle A B C : To find which at two Operations, you muſt ſay, As r a · : b · $\frac{a\,b}{r}$, then as

$\frac{a\,b}{r}$ · p : q : $\frac{p\,q}{a\,b}$, which laſt Term, multiplied by 2, will be the verſed Sine Complement
ſought But to avoid multiplying by 2, the verſed Sines on Scales are fitted from this Pro-
portion, *viz.* As Radius is to half the Sine of an Arc, ſo is half the Sine of the ſame Arc,
to half the verſed Sine of that Arc

USE *of the Line of Latitudes and Hours*

Theſe Lines are conjointly uſed, in readily pricking down the Hour-Lines from the Subſtyle, in an Iſoſceles Triangle, on any kind of upright Dials, having Centers in any given
Latitude , that is, by means of them there will be this Proportion worked, *viz.* As Radius
is to the Sine of the Style's Height, ſo is the Tangent of the Angle at the Pole, to the
Tangent of the Hour-Lines Diſtance from the Subſtyle

Now ſuppoſe the Hour-Lines are to be pricked down upon an upright Declining-Plane,
declining 25 Deg Eaſtwards : Firſt draw C 12 the Meridian, perpendicular to the Horizontal Line of the Plane, and make the Angle F C 12 equal to the Subſtyle's Diſtance from the
Meridian, and draw the Line F C for the Subſtyle This being done, draw the Line B A
perpendicular to the ſaid Subſtyle, paſſing thro the Center C, then out of your Line of
Latitudes ſet off C A, C B, each equal to the Style's Height, and fit in the Hour-Scale,
ſo that one End being at A, the other may meet with the Subſtyle Line at F

Now get the Difference between 30 Deg 47 Min the Inclination of Meridians, and 30
Degrees, the next Hour's Diſtance leſſer than the ſaid 30 Deg 47 Min and the Difference is
47 Minutes, that is, 3 Minutes in time ; then count upon the Line of Hours,

Hours	Min			
0	3	} from F to	10	{ And make Points at the Ter-
1	3		11	minations, to which draw-
2	3		12	ing Lines from the Center
3	3		11	C, they ſhall be the Hour-
4	3		2	Lines on one Side
5	3		3	

Again, fitting in the Hour-Scale from B to F, count from that End at B, the former Arcs
of Time

Hours	Min			
00	03	} from B to	4	{ And make Points at the Ter-
1	3		5	minations, thro which draw
2	3		6	Lines from the Center C, and
3	3		7	they will be the Hour-Lines
4	3		8	on the other Side the Sub-
5	3		9	ſtyle

You muſt proceed thus for the Halfs and Quarters, in getting the Difference between the
Half-Hour next leſſer (in this Example 22 Deg 30 Min) under the Arc of Inclination of
Meridians , the Difference is 1 Deg 17 Min which in time is 33 Minutes, to be continu-
ally augmented an Hour at a time, and ſo be pricked off, as before was done for the whole
Hours

If the Hour-Scale reach above the Plane, as at B, ſo that B C cannot be pricked down,
then may an Angle be made on the upper Side of the Subſtyle, equal to the Angle F C A
on the under Side, and thereby the Hour-Scale laid in its due Poſition, having firſt found
the Point F on the Subſtyle.

That the Reaſon of the conjoint Uſe of theſe Lines, in pricking off the Hour-Lines from
the Subſtylar-Line may appear , let us ſuppoſe A C to be the Subſtylar-Line, A the Center
of a Dial, B A a Portion of the Line of Latitudes, at right Angles to A C, and B C the
Line of Hours fitted thereto. Now if C D be the Quantity of any Arc taken on the Line of
Hours, and a right Line be drawn from the Center A thro the Point D, the Angle F A C
will be the ſame, as that found by ſaying, As Radius is to the Sine of the Number of
Degrees pricked off upon the Line of Latitudes (that is, to the Sine of the Style's Height)
from A to B , ſo is the Tangent of that Number of Degrees pricked off from C to D on
the Line of Hours (that is, the Tangent of the Angle at the Pole) to another Tangent,
whoſe

Fig. 14

Fig 15.

whofe Arc will be equal to F A C (that is, to the Tangent of the Diftance of the Hour-Line A F from the Subftyle)

Now to prove this, it is evident, from the Conftruction of the Line of Latitudes, that as the Radius B C is to the Sine B G of an Arc, fo is A C to A B whence if A C be fuppofed Radius, B A is the Sine of the Arc pricked down from the Line of Latitudes

Again, from the Nature of the Line of Hours; if C D be taken for the Tangent of an Arc, B D will be the Radius thereto This being evident, let C E be the Tangent of the Angle F A C, then the Triangles B A D, D E C, will be fimilar, whence as the Radius B D is to B A, the Sine of an Arc, fo is C D, the Tangent of an Arc, to E C, the Tangent of the Angle F A C.

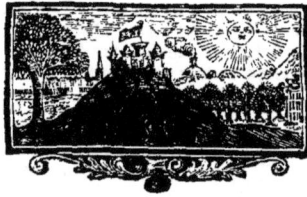

N   B O O K

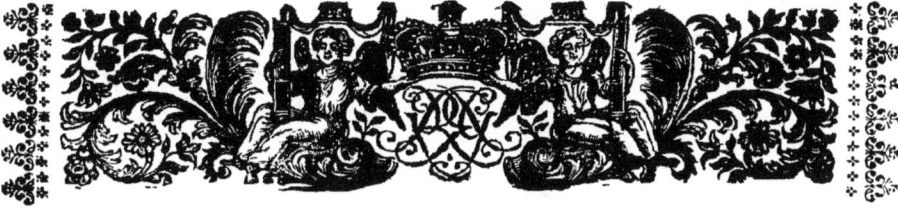

BOOK II.

Of the Conſtruction and Uſes of the SECTOR.

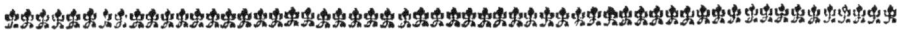

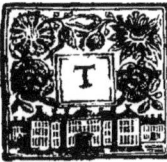

CHAP. I.

Of the Conſtruction of the Sector.

T H E Sector is a Mathematical Inſtrument, whoſe Uſe is to find the Proportion between Quantities of the ſame kind, as between one Line and another, between one Superficies and another, between one Solid and another, &c

This Inſtrument is made of two equal Rules, or Legs, of Silver, Braſs, Ivory, or Wood, joined to each other by a Rivet, ſo worked, as to render its Motion regular and uniform   To do which, firſt make two Slits with a Saw, about an Inch deep, at one End of one of the Rules, in order to fit therein the Head-Pieces, which muſt be well rivetted. Afterwards the Head muſt be rounded, by filing off the Superfluities, in ſuch manner, that the Middle-Piece and Head-Pieces may be even with each other   Then to find the Center of the Rivet, ſet one Foot of your Compaſſes at the bottom of the Middle-Piece, and mark with the other Foot four Sections in the middle of the Rivet, by opening the Middle-Piece of the Joint to four or more different Angles, and the Middle-Point of thoſe Sections will be the Center of the Rivet, and conſequently alſo the Center of the Sector   This being done, a Line muſt be drawn upon the Rule from the Center, near the inward Edge, by which Line the inward Edge of the Rule muſt be filed ſtrait, the inward Edge of the other Rule being alſo made ſtrait, and ſlit, to receive the Middle-Piece, you muſt cut away its Corner in an Arc, ſo as it may well fit the Joint, and then rivet, with three or four little Rivets, the Rule to the Middle-Piece, by which means the two Legs may eaſily open and ſhut, and keep at any Opening required   But Care muſt be taken that the Legs are filed very flat, and do not twiſt, Care muſt alſo be taken that the Sector be well center'd, that is, that being entirely opened, both Inſide and Outſide, may make a right Line, and that the Legs be very equal in Length and Breadth; in a word, that it be very ſtrait every way.   *Note,* The Length and Breadth of the aforeſaid Rules are not determinate, but they are commonly ſix Inches long, three quarters of an Inch broad, and about one quarter in Thickneſs

There are commonly drawn upon the Faces of this Inſtrument ſix kind of Lines, *viz* the Line of equal Parts, the Line of Planes, and the Line of Polygons on one Side, the Line of Chords, the Line of Solids, and the Line of Metals on the other

There is generally placed, near the Edge of the Sector, on one Side, a divided Line, whoſe Uſe is to find the Bores of Cannons, and on the other Side, a Line ſhewing the Diameters and Weights of Iron-Bullets, from one Quarter to 64 Pounds, whoſe Conſtruction and Uſes we ſhall give, in ſpeaking of the Inſtruments belonging to the Artillery

SECTION

Plate V.   fronting page 46

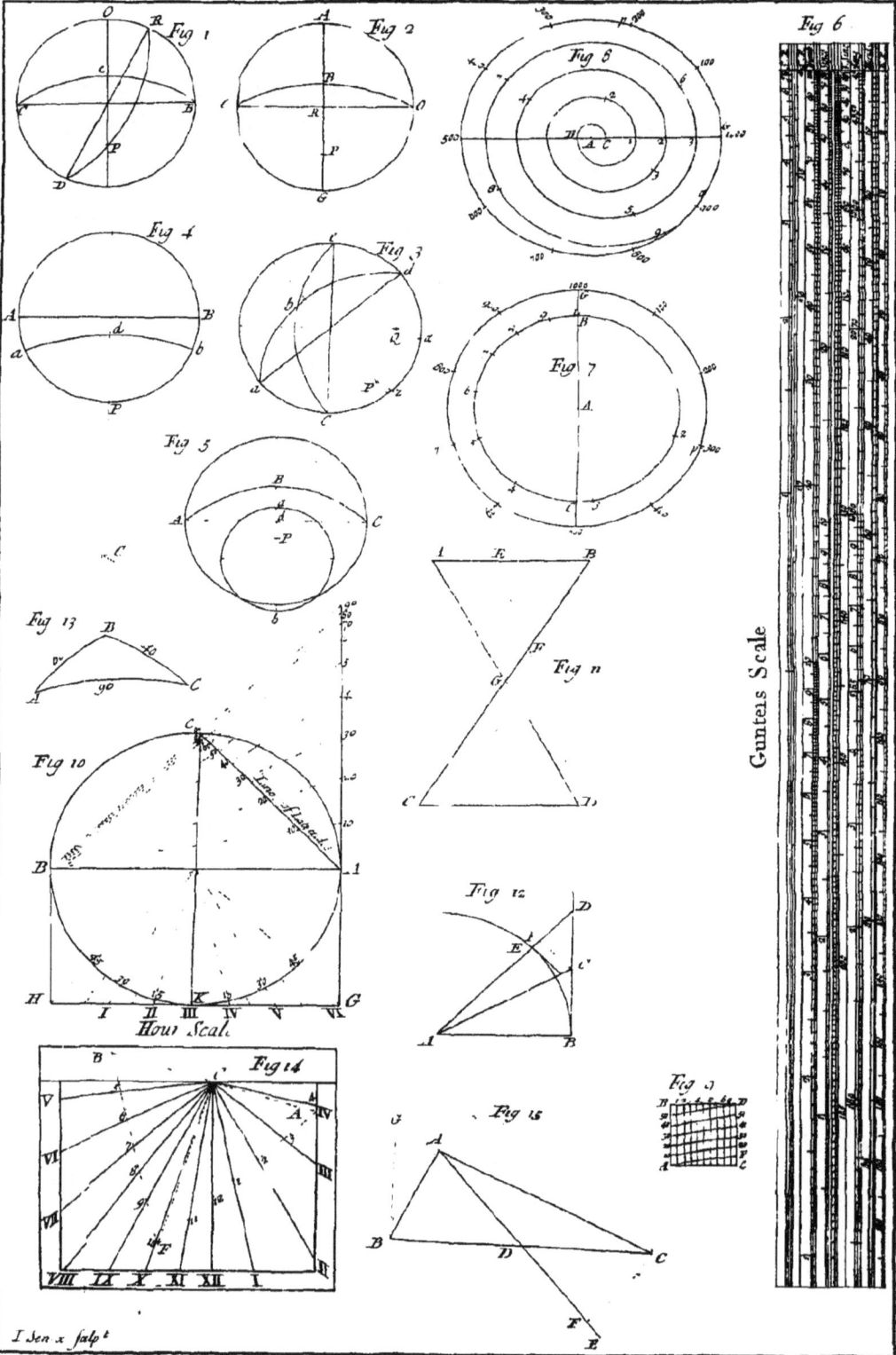

Fig 1

Fig 2

Fig 8

Fig 6

Fig 4

Fig 3

Fig 7

Guntels Scale

Fig 5

Fig n

Fig 13

Fig 10

Fig 12

Fig 9

Hour Scale

Fig 14

Fig 15

I Sen x sculpt

SECTION I.

Of the Line of Equal Parts.

THIS Line is so called, because it is divided into equal Parts, whose Number is com- *Plate 6.* monly 200, when the Sector is six Inches long *Fig 1.*

Having drawn upon one of the Faces of each Leg the equal Lines A B, A B, from the Center of the Joint A First, divide them into two equal Parts, each of which will consequently be 100, then each of those Parts being again divided into two equal Parts, and each Part arising will be 50; then divide each of these last Parts into five others, and each Part produced will be 10, and finally dividing each of these new Parts into 2, and each of these last into five equal Parts, and by this means the Lines A B, A B, will be each divided into 200 equal Parts, every 5 of which must be distinguished by short Strokes, and every 10 numbered from the Center A to 200, at the other End

Now because the two other Lines, drawn upon the same Faces of each Leg, must terminate in the Center A, the Extremity B of the Line of equal Parts must be drawn as near as possible to the outward Edges of each Leg, that so there may be Space enough left to draw the Line of Planes in the middle of the Breadth of the said Legs, and the Line of Polygons near their inward Edges, but Care must be taken, in drawing of these Lines, that each one, and its Fellow, be equally distant from the interior Edges of each Leg, as may be seen in the Figure

SECTION II.

Of the Line of Planes.

THIS Line is so called, because it contains the homologous Sides of a certain Number of similar Planes, Multiples of a small one, beginning from the Center A, that is, whose Surfaces are double, triple, quadruple, &c that small Plane, from Unity, according to the natural Order of Numbers, to 64, which is commonly the greatest Term of the Divisions, denoted upon the Line A C

This Line may be divided two ways, both of which are founded upon *Prop 20 lib. 6. Eucl* which demonstrates, That similar Plane Figures are to each other, as the Squares of their homologous Sides The first way of dividing this Line is by Numbers, and the second without Numbers, as follows:

Having drawn the Line A C, from the Center A, upon each Leg of the Sector; first divide it into eight equal Parts, the first of which, next to the Center A, which represents the Side of the least Plane, hath no need of being drawn The second Division from the Center, which is double the first, is the Side of a similar Plane quadruple the least Plane, (whose Side is supposed one of the eight Parts the Line A C is divided into) because the Square of 2 is 4 The third Division, which is three times the first, is the Side of a similar Plane, nine times greater than the first, because the Square of 3 is 9 The fourth Division, which is four times the first, and consequently half of the whole Scale, is the Side of a similar Plane, sixteen times greater than the first, because the Square of 4 is 16 Lastly, the eighth Division, which is eight times the first, is the Side of a similar Plane, sixty four times greater, because the Square of 8 is 64

There is something more to do to find the homologous Sides of Planes that are double, triple, quadruple, &c of the first For you must have a Scale divided into 1000 equal Parts, *Fig. 2.* (as that whose Construction we have already given in Book I) whose Length must be equal to the Line A C, and because the Side of the least Plane is ⅛ of the Line A C, it will consequently be ⅛ of 1000, which is 125 Again, to have in Numbers the Side of a Plane double the least, the square Root of a Number twice the Square of 125 must be found. This Square is 15625, which doubled is 31250, the Square Root of which is about 177, the Side of a similar Plane double the least, whose Side is supposed to be 125. Moreover, to have the Side of a Plane three times the first, the square Root of a Number three times the Square of the first must be found The Number is 46875, and its Root, which is about 216, is the Side of a similar Plane three times the least, and so of others, therefore by laying off from the Center A, upon the Line of Plans, 177 Parts of the aforesaid Scale, you will have the Length of the Side of a similar Plane double the least Plane Again, laying off 216 Parts of the same Scale from the Center A, the Length of the Side of a similar Plane will be had, which is three times the least Plane.

According to the aforesaid Directions the following Table is calculated, that shews the Number of equal Parts which are contained in the homologous Sides of all the similar Planes that are double, triple, quadruple, &c of a Plane whose Side is 125, to the Plane 64, that is, which contains it 64 times, and whose Side is 1000

A

A TABLE *for dividing the Line of Planes.*

1	125	17	515	33	718	49	875	
2	177	18	530	34	729	50	884	
3	216	19	545	35	739	51	892	
4	250	20	559	36	750	52	901	
5	279	21	573	37	760	53	910	
6	306	22	586	38	770	54	918	
7	330	23	599	39	780	55	927	
8	353	24	612	40	790	56	935	
9	375	25	625	41	800	57	944	
10	395	26	637	42	810	58	952	
11	414	27	650	43	819	59	960	
12	433	28	661	44	829	60	968	
13	450	29	673	45	839	61	976	
14	467	30	684	46	848	62	984	
15	484	31	696	47	857	63	992	
16	500	32	707	48	866	64	1000	

Fig. 2

Each of the ten Diviſions which the Scale of 1000 Parts contains, is 100 ; and each of the Subdiviſions of the Line A B is 10   therefore if it is to be uſed for dividing any of the Lines of the Sector ; as, for Example, the Line of Planes , take on the Scale a Line denoting the Hundreds, and the Exceſs above muſt be taken in the Space between the Points A B : As to denote the firſt Plane, to which the Number 125 anſwers, place your Compaſſes on the fifth Line of the Space marked 100, and open them to the Diſtance O P , in the ſame manner, if the Plane 50 is to be denoted, to which the Number 884 anſwers, for 800 take the 8th Space of the Scale, and for 84 take in the Space A B, the Interſection of the 8th Tranſverſal, with the fourth Parallel, which will be the Diſtance N L

5.

The Line of Planes may otherwiſe be divided in the following manner without Calculation, founded on *Prop 47 lib 1. Eucl.* Make the right-angled Iſoſceles Triangle K M N, whoſe Side K M, or K N, let be equal to the Side of the leaſt Plane, and then the Hypothenuſe M N will be the Side of a ſimilar Plane double to it , therefore having laid off with your Compaſſes the Diſtance M N, on the Side K L produced, from K to 2, the Length K 2 will be the Side of a Plane double the leaſt Plane   In like manner lay off the Diſtance M 2, from K to 3, the Line K 3 will be the Side of a Plane triple the firſt. Again, lay off the Diſtance M 3, from K to 4, the Line K 4 (twice K M) will be the Side of a Plane four times greater, that is, which will contain the leaſt Plane four times , and ſo of others, as may be ſeen in the Figure

SECTION III.

Of the Line of Polygons.

This Line is ſo called, becauſe it contains the homologous Sides of the firſt twelve regular Polygons inſcribed in the ſame Circle, that is, from an equilateral Triangle to a Dodecagon.

The Side of the Triangle being the greateſt of all, muſt be the whole Length of each of the Legs of the Sector , and becauſe the Sides of the other regular Polygons, inſcribed in the ſame Circle, ſtill diminiſh as the Number of Sides increaſe, the Side of the Dodecagon is leaſt, and conſequently muſt be nigheſt the Center of the Sector.

Now ſuppoſing the Side of a Triangle to be a thouſand Parts, the Length of the Sides of every of the other Polygons muſt be found , and becauſe the Sides of regular Polygons, inſcribed in the ſame Circle, are in the ſame Proportion as the Chords of the Angles of the Center of each of the Polygons, it is neceſſary to ſhew here how to find the ſaid Angles.

To do which, divide 360 Deg by the Number of the Sides of any Polygon, and the Quotient will give the Angle of the Center

If, for Example, the Angle of the Center of a Hexagon is required, divide 360 Deg by 6, and the Quotient will be 60 ; which ſhews that the Angle of the Center of a Hexagon is 60 Deg   If likewiſe the Angle of the Center of a Pentagon be required, divide 360 Deg by 5, the Number of Sides, and the Quotient will be 72 , which ſhews that the Angle of the Center of a Pentagon is 72 Deg and ſo of others

The Angle of the Center being known, if it be ſubſtracted from 180 Degrees, the Remainder will be the Angle of the Polygon : As, for Example, the Angle of the Center of a

Pentagon

Pentagon being 72 Degrees, the Angle of the Circumference will be 108 Degrees, and so of others, as may be seen in the following Table.

Regular Polygons		Angles of the Center		Angles at the Circumference	
		Degrees		Degrees	
Triangle.	————	—120		60	
Square	————	90		90.	
Pentagon.	————	72		108.	
Hexagon	————	60	Min	120	Min
Heptagon.	————	51	26	128.	34
Octogon	————	45		135	
Nonagon	————	40		140.	
Decagon	————	36		144	
Undecagon.	————	32	44	147.	16.
Dodecagon.	————	30		150	

Now to find in Numbers the Sides of the regular Polygons inscribed in the same Circle Having supposed that the Side of the equilateral Triangle is 1000 equal Parts, instead of the Chords of the Angles of the Center, take their Halves, which are the Sines of half the Angles at their Centers, and make the following Analogy

For Example, to find the Side of the Square, say, As the Sine of 60 Degrees, half the Angle of the Center of the equilateral Triangle, is to the Side of the same Triangle, supposed 1000 , so is the Sine of 45 Degrees half the Angle of the Center of the Square, to the Side of the same Square, which, by calculating, will be found 816

And in this manner are the following Tables of Polygons constructed.

The Side of an equilateral Triangle, denoted on the				*Equal Parts*
Sector by the Number	———	3.		1000.
Of a Square by the Number	———	4	————	816.
Of the Pentagon by the Numb		5	————	678
Of the Hexagon by the Numb.		6.	————	577.
Of the Heptagon by the Numb		7	————	501.
Of the Octagon by the Numb		8.	————	442.
Of the Nonagon by the Numb		9	————	395.
Of the Decagon by the Numb.		10.	————	357.
Of the Undecagon by the Numb.		11.	————	325.
Of the Dodecagon by the Numb.		12	————	299.

We have neglected the Fractions remaining after the Calculation in this Table, as in all others , as being but thousandth Parts, which are not considerable

Those that will not denote an equilateral Triangle upon the Sector, because of the Facility of describing it, and which consequently begin at the Square, use the following Table, wherein the Side of the Square is supposed 1000 Parts

Another Table of Polygons				*Parts*
Square.	————		————	1000
Pentagon	————		—	831
Hexagon	————		—	707
Heptagon	————		—	613
Octagon	————			540
Nonagon.	————		—	484
Decagon.	————		————	437.
Undecagon.	————		—	398
Dodecagon.	————		—	366.

To make the Line of Polygons upon the Sector (the same Scale of 1000 equal Parts being used, as that for making the Line of Planes) you must lay off from the Center A, upon both the Lines A D, the Number of Parts expressed in the Table, that thereby the Numbers 3, 4, 5, &c. may be graved upon the Sector, signifying the Numbers of the Sides of the regular Polygons

SECTION IV.

Of the Line of Chords.

THIS Line is fo named, becaufe it contains the Chords of all the Degrees of a Semi-circle, whofe Diameter is the Length of that Line, which is denoted upon the other Sur-face of each Leg of the Sector, from the Point A, which is the Center of the Joint, to the end F of each Leg, fo that the two Lines A F are exactly equal, and equidiftant from the interior Edges of the Sector

Note, The Line of Chords muft be drawn directly under the Line of equal Parts, becaufe of fome Operations that require a Correfpondence between thofe two Lines

It is alfo proper for the Line of Solids to be drawn under the Line of Planes, and the Line of Metals under the Line of Polygons

For the Divifion of the aforefaid Line A F, defcribe a Semicircle, whofe Diameter let be equal to it, which divide into 180 Degrees, afterwards lay off the Lengths of the Chords of all thofe Degrees upon the Diameter of the Semicircle, then lay the Diameter of the Se-micircle upon the Legs of the Sector, and mark upon them Points that reprefent the Degrees of the Semicircle, every fifth of which, diftinguifh by fhort Strokes, and every tenth by Numbers, beginning from the Point A, and going on to F

The fame Degrees may otherwife be denoted, upon the Line of Chords, by help of Num-bers, in fuppofing the Semidiameter of a Circle, or the Chord of 180 Degrees, to be 1000 equal Parts, all of which Numbers may be found ready calculated in the common Tables of Sines for inftead of the Chords, there is no more to do but to take their halves, which are the Sines of half their Arcs. As for Example, inftead of the Chord of 10 Degrees, the Sine of 5 muft be taken, and becaufe the Calculation in Tables is made for a Radius of 100000 Parts, the two laft Numbers muft be taken away, as may be feen in the following Table, where the Chords of all the Degrees to 180 are denoted

Note, This Divifion is made with a Scale of 1000 Parts.

A TABLE *for the Line of Chords.*

D	Ch	D	Ch.	D	Ch	D	Ch.	D.	Ch	D.	Ch
1	8	31	267	61	507	91	713	121	870	151	968
2	17	32	275	62	515	92	719	122	874	152	970
3	26	33	284	63	522	93	725	123	879	153	972
4	35	34	292	64	530	94	731	124	883	154	974
5	43	35	300	65	537	95	737	125	887	155	976
6	52	36	309	66	544	96	743	126	891	156	978
7	61	37	317	67	552	97	749	127	895	157	980
8	70	38	325	68	559	98	754	128	899	158	981
9	78	39	334	69	566	99	760	129	902	159	983
10	87	40	342	70	573	100	766	130	906	160	985
11	96	41	350	71	580	101	771	131	910	161	986
12	104	42	358	72	588	102	777	132	913	162	987
13	113	43	366	73	595	103	782	133	917	163	989
14	122	44	374	74	602	104	788	134	920	164	990
15	130	45	382	75	609	105	793	135	924	165	991
16	139	46	390	76	615	106	798	136	927	166	992
17	145	47	399	77	622	107	804	137	930	167	993
18	156	48	406	78	629	108	809	138	933	168	994
19	165	49	414	79	636	109	814	139	936	169	995
20	173	50	422	80	643	110	819	140	939	170	996
21	182	51	430	81	649	111	824	141	941	171	997
22	191	52	438	82	656	112	829	142	945	172	997
23	199	53	446	83	662	113	834	143	948	173	998
24	208	54	454	84	669	114	838	144	951	174	998
25	216	55	462	85	675	115	843	145	954	175	999
26	225	56	469	86	682	116	848	146	956	176	999
27	233	57	477	87	688	117	852	147	959	177	999
28	242	58	485	88	694	118	857	148	961	178	1000
29	250	59	492	89	701	119	861	149	963	179	1000
30	259	60	500	90	707	120	866	150	966	180	1000

SECTION V.

Of the Line of Solids.

THIS Line is so called, because it contains the homologous Sides of a certain Number of similar Solids, Multiples of a lesser from Unity, according to the natural Order of Numbers, to 64, which is commonly the greatest of the Divisions of this Line, which is marked Fig. 4. A H, next to the Line of Chords.

To make the Divisions upon it, the Scale of 1000 Parts must be used, and the Side of the 64th and greatest Solid must be supposed 1000 equal Parts, then because the Cube-Root of 64 is 4, and the Cube-Root of 1 is 1, it follows that the Side of the 64th Solid is quadruple the Side of the first and least Solid, which consequently will be 250, because (*per Prop* 33. *lib.* 11 *Eucl.*) similar Solids are to each other, as the Cubes of their homologous Sides.

The Number 500 (twice 250) is the Side of the eighth Solid, that is, of a Solid eight times as great as the first: because the Cube of 2, which is 8, is eight times the Cube of Unity

Likewise the Number 750, which is three times 250, is the Side of the 27th Solid, because the Cube of 3, which is 27, is 27 times the Cube of Unity

There are more Calculations required to find the Sides of Solids double, triple, quadruple, &c the first, which cannot exactly be expressed in Numbers, because their Roots are incommensurable, nevertheless they may be sufficiently approached for Use, by the following Method.

For Example, to find the Number expressing the Side of a Solid, twice the first and least: its Side 250 must be cubed, which is 15625000, then this Number must be doubled, and the Cube-Root of it extracted, which will be almost 315, for the Side of a Solid double the first. To have the Side of a Solid triple the first, the said Cube must be tripled, and its Cube-Root, which is 360, will be the Side of a Solid triple the first; and so of others, as may be seen in the following Table.

A TABLE *for the Line of Solids.*

1	250	17	643	33	802	49	914
2	315	18	655	34	810	50	921
3	360	19	667	35	818	51	927
4	397	20	678	36	825	52	933
5	427	21	689	37	833	53	939
6	454	22	700	38	840	54	945
7	478	23	711	39	848	55	951
8	500	24	721	40	855	56	956
9	520	25	731	41	862	57	962
10	538	26	740	42	869	58	967
11	556	27	750	43	876	59	973
12	572	28	759	44	882	60	978
13	588	29	768	45	889	61	984
14	602	30	777	46	896	62	989
15	616	31	785	47	902	63	995
16	630	32	794	48	908	64	1000

The Sides of all these Solids being thus found in Numbers, they are denoted on the Line of Solids, by laying off from the Center A the Parts which they contain, taken upon the Scale.

SECTION VI.

Of the Line of Metals.

THIS Line is so named, because it is used to find the Proportion between the six Metals, of which Solids may be made

It is placed upon the Legs of the Sector, hard by the Line of Solids, and the Metals are Fig. 4. figured thereon by the Characters, which have been appropriated to them by Chymists and Naturalists

The Division of this Line is founded upon Experiments that have been made of the different Weights of equal Masses of each of these Metals, from whence their Proportions are calculated, as in the following Table.

A

A TABLE *for the Line of Metals.*

Gold	☉	730.
Lead	♄	863
Silver	☽	895
Brafs	♀	937.
Iron	♂	974.
Tin	♃	1000.

Advertifement.

That of all the fix Metals which has the leaft Weight, which is Tin, is marked at the End of each Leg (as A G) at a Diftance from the Center, equal to the Length of the Scale of 1000 Parts, and the other Metals nigher the faid Center (each according to the Numbers which correfpond with them) taken upon the fame Scale.

Becaufe moft of the aforementioned Lines, marked on the Sector, are divided by means of the Scale of 1000 equal Parts, it is requifite that they be exactly equal between themfelves and to the faid Scale, therefore becaufe they all center in one Point (which is the Center of the Joint) they muft all be terminated at the other End by an Arc, made upon the Surface of each of the Legs

It is not always neceffary to divide the Sector by the Methods we have given, for, to make them fooner, prepare a Ruler of the fame Length, Breadth, and Thicknefs as the Sector, and draw upon it the fame Lines we have already prefcribed · then with a Beam-Compafs transfer the fame Divifions upon the Sector, having firft drawn upon it the Lines to contain them

SECTION VII.

Containing the Proofs of the Six Lines commonly put upon the Sector.

The Proof of the Line of equal Parts.

The Divifion of this Line is fo eafy, that there is no need of any other Proof, but to examine, with your Compaffes, whether the two correfpondent Lines, drawn upon the Legs of the Sector, are very equal, and equally divided, which may be known by taking between your Compaffes (whofe Points let be very fharp) any Number at pleafure of thofe equal Parts, beginning any where : for if the Line of equal Parts be well divided, by carrying that fame Opening of your Compaffes on the faid Line, the two Points will always contain between them the fame Number of equal Parts upon either of the Legs, reckoning from the Center, or from any other Point of Divifion.

The Proof of the Line of Chords.

The Method before explained will not ferve to know whether the Line of Chords be well divided, becaufe the Divifions are not equal : the Chord of 10 Degrees, for Example, is greater than half that of 20, likewife the Chord of 20 Degrees is greater than the half of that of 40 Degrees, and fo on · fo that the Divifions are greater towards the Center of the Sector, than towards the Ends of its Legs, as is manifeft from the Nature of the Circle But becaufe we have given two Methods for dividing the Line of Chords, one by help of Numbers, and the other by means of the Chords of Arcs, one of thefe Methods will ferve to prove the other

But there is ftill another Method, which is this : Take at pleafure, on the Line of Chords, two Numbers equally diftant from 120 Degrees, as for Example, 110 and 130, which are each 10 Degrees diftant from it, the firft in Defect, and the laft in Excefs Then take in your Compaffes the Diftance of the two Numbers 110 and 130, which muft be equal to the Chord of 10 Degrees, or to the Diftance of the Point 10, upon the Line of Chords, from the Center of the Sector

You will find, by the fame means, that the Diftance between 100 and 140 Degrees, is equal to the Chord of 20 Degrees; as likewife the Diftance between 90 and 150 is equal to the Chord of 30 Degrees, which is the Number by which 120 exceeds 90, and by which 150 exceeds 120, and fo of others, as may eafily be noted by the aforegoing Table of Chords, where you may fee (for Example) the Number 44, which is the Chord of 5 Degrees, is the Difference between 843, which is the Chord of 115 Degrees, and 887, which is the Chord of 125, as likewife 87, the Chord of 10 Degrees, is the Difference between the Chord of 110 Degrees and 130, &c. which are equally diftant from 120 Degrees

Proof of the Line of Polygons

You may know whether this Line be well divided, by help of the Line of Chords, in the following manner

Take in your Compaffes, upon the Line of Polygons, the Diftance of the Number 6, denoting a Hexagon, from the Center of the Joint, then carry this Diftance upon the Line of Chords, putting each Point of your Compaffes upon the correfpondent Points, from 60 to 60, denoting the Angle of the Center of an Hexagon

The

The Sector being thus opened, take upon each Line of Chords the Distance of the two Points, marked 72 from the Center, and lay it off upon the Line of Polygons, placing one Foot in the Center of the Joint, then the other Foot must reach to the Point 5, which appertains to a Pentagon, whose Angle at the Center is 72 Degrees

Likewise in taking upon the Line of Chords the Distance of the two Points, denoting 90, and laying it off upon the Line of Polygons, the Foot of your Compasses must meet the Point 4, appertaining to a Square, whose Angle of the Center is 90 Deg and so of others.

Proof of the Line of Planes

Because we have given two Methods for dividing the Line of Planes, one may serve to prove the other, but still you may easier know whether the Divisions be well made, in the following manner Take between your Compasses the Distance of any Point upon this Line from the Center of the Joint, and lay it off from the same Point on the other Side of the same Line of Planes, then the Foot of your Compasses will fall upon the Number of a Plane four times greater than that which was taken towards the Center and if again your Compasses thus opened should be once more turned over, towards the End of the said Line, the Point would fall upon the Number of a Plane nine times greater As, for Example, if you take the Distance from the Center to the Plane 2, in placing one Point of your Compasses on 2, the other ought to fall upon 8, and by turning the Compasses once more, one of its Points must fall upon 18, which contains 9 times 2. Moreover, in turning the Compasses once more over, the other Point ought to fall upon the Number 32, containing 2, 16 times If, lastly, you turn over the Compasses again, it must fall upon 50, and so of other similar Planes, because they are to each other as the Squares of their homologous Sides It is this that facilitates the Division of the Line of Planes, for having the first, these are likewise had, viz. the 4th, the 9th, the 16th, the 20th, the 25th, the 36th, the 49th, and the 64th Having found the 2d, the 8th, the 18th, the 32d, and the 50th will be had likewise having found the 3d, the 12th, the 27th and the 48th will be had, and so of others

Proof of the Line of Solids

You may know whether this Line be well divided, in the following manner Take between your Compasses the Distance of some Point on this Line from the Center of the Joint, then place one of its Points, thus opened, upon this Point of Division, and turn the other Point over towards the End of the Line Now this Point must fall upon the Number of a Solid 8 times greater than that which was taken. Again, if the Compasses be once more turned over, it will fall upon a Solid 27 times greater than that which was first taken. As, for Example, the Distance of the first Solid from the Center, will be equal to the Distance from 8 to 27, and from 27 to 64 Likewise, twice the Distance from the Center to 3, will be equal to the Distance from 3 to 24. By the 4th Solid, the 32d will be had Moreover, the 5th Solid will give the 40th, by the 6th the 48th Solid will be had, and, in a word, by help of the 7th, the 56th Solid will be had, because similar Solids are to each other, as the Cubes of their homologous Sides, which facilitates the Division of the Line of Solids

Proof of the Line of Metals

We have already mentioned, that the Division of this Line is founded upon Experiments made of the different Weights of a Cubic Foot of each of the six Metals, as they are here denoted

Metals		Weights of a Cubic Foot	
Gold	———	1326 Pounds,	4 Ounces
Lead	———	802	2
Silver	——	720	12
Brass	———	627	12
Iron	————	558.	00
Tin	———	516	2

From these different Weights of the six Metals the beforementioned Table was calculated, by means of which the Line of Metals was divided

Now because Tin is the lightest of the said six Metals, it is manifest that if, for Example, a Ball of Tin is to be made of the same Weight as a Ball of Iron, or Brass, the Ball of Tin must be greater than either of them, as also the Ball of Iron ought to be greater than that of Brass, and so on to that which will be the least Therefore supposing the Diameter of a Ball of Tin to be 1000, the Question is to find the Lengths of the Diameters of Iron and Brass-Balls, that may be of the same Weight as the Ball of Tin

Now to do this, you must make a Rule of Three, whose first Term let always be the heaviest of the two Metals to be compared; the second Term must be the Weight of the Tin, and the third must be the Number 64, which is the greatest Solid of the Table of Solids, to which the Number 1000 answers As, for Example, to compare Iron, a Cubic Foot of which weighs 558 Pounds, with Tin, a Cubic Foot of which weighs 516 Pounds, 2

Ounces

Ounces Having reduced them all into Ounces, the 558 Pounds make 8928 Ounces, and the 516 Pounds, 2 Ounces, make 8258 Ounces then fay, if 8928 gives 8258, what will 64 give ? The Rule being finifhed, the fourth Term will be 59 and a fmall Remainder, then look for the Number 59 in the Table of Solids, and the Number anfwering thereto is 973, inftead of which take 974, becaufe of the remaining Fraction therefore, I fay, that the Diameter of the Ball of Iron muft be 974. In the fame manner, by making four other Rules of Proportion, you may know whether the Numbers, marked againft the four other Metals, are well calculated, and confequently whether the Line of Metals be well divided

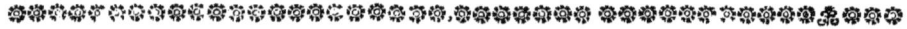

CHAP. II.

Of the Ufe of the Sector.

THE Ufes we fhall here lay down, are only thofe that moft appertain to the Sector, and which by it can be better performed, than by any other Inftrument

SECTION I

Of the USE of the Line of equal Parts.

USE I *To divide a given Line into any Number of equal Parts, for Example, into feven*

Plate 7
Fig 1

TAKE between your Compaffes the propofed Line, as A B, and carry it, upon the Line of equal Parts, to a Number on both Sides, that may eafily be divided by 7, as 70, whofe 7th Part is 10, or elfe the Number 140, whofe 7th Part is 20 Then keeping the Sector thus opened, fhut the Feet of your Compaffes, fo that they may fall on the Numbers 10 on each Leg of the Sector, if the Number 70 be ufed, or upon the Numbers 20, if 140 be taken for the Length of the propofed Line, and this opening of your Compaffes will be the 7th Part of the propofed Line

Note, If the Line to be divided be too long to be applied to the Legs of the Sector, only divide one half, or one fourth of it by 7, and the double, or quadruple, of this 7th Part, will be the 7th Part of the whole Line

USE II *Several right Lines, conftituting the Perimeter of a Polygon, being given, one of which is fuppofed to contain any Number of equal Parts to find how many of thefe Parts are contained in each of the other Lines*

Take that Line's Length, whofe Meafure is known, between your Compaffes, and fet it over, upon the Line of equal Parts, to the Number on each Side, expreffing its Length. The Sector remaining thus opened, carry upon it the Lengths of each of the other Lines, parallel to the beforementioned Line, and the Numbers that each of them falls on will fhew their different Lengths: But if any one of the faid Lines doth not exactly fall upon the fame Number of the Lines of equal Parts, upon both Legs of the Sector, but, for Inftance, one of the Points of the Compaffes falls upon 29, and the other upon 30, the Length of the faid Line will be 29 and a half

USE III. *A right Line being given, and the Number of equal Parts it contains, to take from it a leffer Line, containing any Number of its Parts*

Let, for Example, the propofed Line be 120 equal Parts, from which it is required to take a Line of 25 Firft take the propofed Line between your Compaffes, and then open the Sector, fo that the Feet of your Compaffes may fall upon 120, on the Line of equal Parts, upon each Leg of the Sector: The Sector remaining thus opened, take the Diftance from 25 to 25, and that will give the Line defired It is manifeft, from the three aforementioned Ufes, that the Line of equal Parts, upon the Legs of the Sector, may very fitly ferve as a Scale for all kinds of plane Figures, provided that one of their Sides be known, and that, by means of this Line, they may be augmented or diminifhed.

USE IV *Two right Lines being given, to find a third Proportional and three being given, to find a fourth*

If there be but two Lines propofed, then take the Length of the firft between your Compaffes, and lay it off upon the Line of equal Parts from the Center, in order to know the Number whereon it terminates; then open the Sector, fo that the Length of the fecond Line may be terminated by the Length of the firft. The Sector remaining thus opened, lay off the Length of the fecond Line upon one of the Legs from the Center, and, *Note,* the Number whereon it terminates, and the Diftance between that Number, on both Legs of the Sector, will give the third Proportional required

Let,

Let, for Example, the first Line proposed be A B, 40 equal Parts, and the second C D, 20 First take the Length of 20 between your Compasses, and opening the Sector, set over this Distance upon 40, and 40 on each Leg of the Sector The Sector remaining thus opened, take the Distance from 20 to 20, which will be the Length of the third Proportional sought; which being measured, on the Line of equal Parts, from the Center, you will find it 10, for as 40 is to 20, so is 20 to 10

But if three Lines be given, and a fourth Proportional to them required, take the second Line between your Compasses, and, opening the Sector, apply this Extent to the Ends of the first, laid off from the Center, on both Legs of the Sector The Sector being thus opened, lay off the third Line from the Center, and the Extent between the Number, whereon it terminates on both Legs of the Sector, will be the fourth Proportional required

Let the first of the three Lines be 60, the second 30, and the third 50, carry the Length of 30 to the Extent from 60 to 60, and the Sector remaining thus opened, take the Distance from 50 to 50, which is 25, and this will be the fourth Proportional sought for 60 is to 30 as 50 to 25

USE V *To divide a Line into any given Proportion*

As for Example, to divide a Line into two Parts, which may be to each other as 40 is to 70 First add the two Numbers together, and their Sum will be 110, then take between your Compasses the Length of the Line proposed, which suppose 165, and carry this Length to the Distance, from 110 to 110, on both Legs of the Sector The Sector remaining thus opened, take the Extent from 40 to 40, and also from 70 to 70, the first of the two will give 60, and the latter 105, which will be the Parts of the Line proposed, for 40 is to 70, as 60 is to 105

USE VI *To open the Sector, so that the two Lines of equal Parts may make a right Angle*

Find three Numbers, that may express the Sides of a right-angled Triangle, as 3, 4, or 5, or their Equimultiples, but since it is better to have greater Numbers, let us take 60, 80, and 100. Now having taken, between your Compasses, the Distance from the Center of the Sector to 100, open the Sector, so that one Point of your Compasses, set upon 80 on one Leg, may fall upon 60, of the Line of equal Parts, upon the other Leg, and then the Sector will be so opened, that the two Lines of equal Parts make a right Angle.

USE VII. *To find a right Line equal to the Circumference of a given Circle*

The Diameter of a Circle is to the Circumference almost as 50 to 157, therefore take, between your Compasses, the Diameter of the Circle, and set it over, upon the Legs of the Sector, from 50 to 50, on both Lines of equal Parts The Sector remaining thus opened, take the Distance from 157 to 157, between your Compasses, and that will be almost equal to the Circumference of the proposed Circle, I say almost, for the exact Proportion of the Diameter of a Circle to its Circumference hath not yet been Geometrically found

SECTION II.

Of the USE of the Line of Planes

USE I *To augment or diminish any Plane Figures in a given Ratio*

LET, for Example, the Triangle A B C be given, and it is required to make another Triangle similar, and triple to it Fig. 4,

Take the Length of the Side A B between your Compasses, and open the Sector, so that the Points of your Compasses fall upon 1 and 1, on each Line of Planes, the Sector remaining thus opened, take the Distance from the third Plane to the third, on each Leg of the Sector, which will be the Length of the homologous Side to the Side A B After the same manner may the homologous Sides to the other two Sides of the given Triangle be found, and of these three Sides may be formed a Triangle triple to the proposed one *Note,* If the proposed Plane Figure hath more than three Sides, it must be reduced into Triangles, by drawing of Diagonals

If a Circle is to be augmented or diminished, you must proceed in the same manner with its Diameter

USE II *Two similar Plane Figures being given, to find the Ratio between them*

Take either of the Sides of one of the Figures, and open the Sector, so that it may fall upon the same Number or Division, on the Line of Planes, on both Legs of the Sector. Then take the homologous Side of the other Figure, and apply that to some Number or Division on both Legs of the Sector, and then the two Numbers, on which the homologous Sides fall, will express the Ratio of the two Figures As suppose the Side *a b*, of the lesser Fig. 5. Figure, falls upon the fourth Plane, and the homologous Side A B, of the greater, falls upon the sixth Plane, the two Planes are to each other as 4 to 6 But if the Side of a Figure is applied to the Extent of some Plane, on both Legs of the Sector, and the homologous Side cannot
not

not be adjusted parallel to it, so as it may fall on a whole Number on both Legs of the Sector, then you must place the Side of the first Figure upon some other Number, on each Leg, till a whole Number is found on both Legs of the Sector, whose Extent is equal to the Length of the homologous Side of the other Figure, to avoid Fractions

If the proposed Figures are so great, that their Sides cannot be applied to the opening of the Legs of the Sector, take the half, third, or fourth Parts of any of the two homologous Sides of the said Figures, and compare them together, as before, and you will have the Proportion of the said Figures

USE III *To open the Sector, so that the two Lines of Planes may make a right Angle.*

Take between your Compasses the Extent of any Plane from the Center of the Sector, as, for Example, the 40th then apply this opening of your Compasses, upon the Line of Planes, on both Sides, to a Number equal to half the precedent one, which, in this Example, is 20, then the two Lines of Planes will be at right Angles because, by the Construction of the Line of Planes, the Number 40, which may represent the longest Side of a Triangle, signifies a Plane equal to two other similar Planes, denoted by the Number 20 upon the Legs of the Sector Whence, from *Prop* 48 *lib* 1 *Eucl* the aforenamed Angle is a right one

USE IV *To make a plane Figure similar and equal to two other given similar plane Figures*

Open the Sector (by the precedent Use) so that the Lines of Planes be at right Angles, and carry any two homologous Sides, of the two proposed Figures, upon the Line of Planes, from the Center, the one upon one Leg, and the other upon the other Leg, and then the Distance of the two Numbers found will give the homologous Side of a plane Figure similar and equal to the two given ones

As, for Example, the Side of the lesser Figure being laid off from the Center, will reach to the fourth Plane, and the homologous Side of the greater Figure, likewise laid off upon the other Leg, will extend to the ninth Plane then the Distance from 4 to 9 is the homologous Side of a Figure equal to the two proposed ones, by means of which it will be easy to make a Figure similar to them

By means of this Use may be added together any Number of similar plane Figures, viz in adding together the two first, and then adding their Sum to the third, and so on

USE V *Two similar unequal plane Figures being given, to find a third equal to their Difference*

Open the Sector, so that the two Lines of Planes may make a right Angle, then lay off one Side of the lesser Figure from the Center of the Sector This being done, take the homologous Side of the greater Figure, and set one Foot of your Compasses upon the Number whereon the first Side terminates, and the other Point will fall on the other Leg, upon the Number required

As, for Example, having laid off the Side of the lesser Figure from the Center, which falls upon the Number 9, take the Length of the homologous Side of the greater Figure, and setting one Foot of your Compasses upon the Number 9, the other will fall on the Number 4 of the other Leg, therefore taking the Distance of the Number 4 from the Center of the Sector, that will be the homologous Side of a Figure similar and equal to the Difference of the two given Figures, whose Ratio is as 9 to 13

USE VI *To find a mean Proportional between two given Lines*

Lay off both the given Lines upon the Line of equal Parts, in order to have their Lengths expressed in Numbers, the lesser of which suppose 20, and the greater 45 Then open the Sector, so that the Distance from 45 to 45, of the Lines of Planes, be equal in Length to the greater Line The Sector remaining thus opened, take the Distance from 20 to 20 of the Line of Planes, which will be the mean Proportional sought, and having measured it upon the Line of equal Parts from the Center, you will find it to be 30 : for as 20 is to 30, so is 30 to 45

But because the greatest Number on the Line of Planes is 64, if any one of the Lines proposed be greater than 64, the Operation must be made with their half, third, or fourth Parts, in the following manner Suppose the lesser Number be 32, and the greater 72, open the Sector, so that half of the greater Number, viz 36, may be equal to the Distance from 36 to 36, of the Line of Planes, upon both Legs of the Sector, and then the Distance from 16 to 16 doubled, will be the mean Proportional sought

SECTION III.

Of the USES of the Line of Polygons.

USE I *To inscribe a regular Polygon in a given Circle*

Fig. 6.

TAKE the Semidiameter A C, of the given Circle, between your Compasses, and adjust it to the Number 6, upon the Line of Polygons, on each Leg of the Sector ; and the Sector remaining thus opened, take the Distance of the two equal Numbers, expressing the Number

ber of Sides the Polygon is to have for Example, take the Diftance from 5 to 5, to infcribe a Pentagon, from 7 to 7 for a Heptagon, and fo of others : either of thefe Diftances, carried about the Circumference of the Circle, will divide it into fo many equal Parts And thus you may eafily defcribe any regular Polygon, from the equilateral Triangle to the Dodecagon

USE II. *To defcribe a regular Polygon upon a given right Line*

If, for Example, the Pentagon of *Fig 6* is to be defcribed upon the Line A B Take the Length of the faid Line between your Compaffes, and apply it to the Extent of the Numbers 5, 5, on the Line of Polygons : The Sector remaining thus opened, take, upon the fame Lines, the Extent from 6 to 6, which will be the Semidiameter of the Circle the Polygon is to be infcribed in, therefore if, with this Diftance, you defcribe, from the Ends of the given Line A B, two Arcs of a Circle, their Interfection will be the Center of the Circle.

If an Heptagon was propofed, apply the Length of the given Line to the Extent of the Numbers 7 and 7, on both Legs of the Sector, and always take the Extent from 6 to 6, to find the Center of the Circle, in which it will be eafy to infcribe an Heptagon, each Side of which will be equal to the given Line

USE III *To cut a given Line, as D E, into extreme and mean Proportion*

Apply the Length of the given Line to the Extent of the Numbers 6 and 6, on both Sides, upon the Line of Polygons, and the Sector remaining thus opened, take the Extent of the Numbers 10 and 10, on both Legs of the Sector, which are thofe for a Decagon This Extent will give D F, the greateft Segment of the propofed Line, becaufe the greateft Segment of the Radius of a Circle, cut into mean and extreme Proportion, is the Chord of 36 Degrees, which is the 10th Part of the Circumference

If the greater Segment is added to the Radius of the Circle, fo as to make but one Line, the Radius will be the greater Segment, and the Chord of 36 Degrees will be the leffer Segment.

USE IV *Upon a given Line D F, to defcribe an Ifofceles Triangle, having the Angles at the Bafe double to that at the Vertex*

Open the Sector, fo that the Ends of the given Line may fall upon 10 and 10, of the Line of Polygons, upon each Leg of the Sector The Sector remaining thus opened, take the Diftance from 6 to 6, and this will be the Length of the two equal Sides of the Triangle to be made

It is manifeft that the Angle, at the Vertex of this Triangle, is 36 Degrees, and that each of the Angles at the Bafe is 72 Degrees, but the Angle of 36 Degrees, is the Angle of the Center of a Decagon.

USE V *To open the Sector fo, that the two Lines of Polygons may make a right Angle*

Take between your Compaffes the Diftance of the Number 5, from the Center, on the Line of Polygons, then open the Sector, fo that this Diftance may be applied to the Number 6 on one Side, and to the Number 10 on the other, and then the two Lines of Polygons will make a right Angle, becaufe the Square of the Side of a Pentagon is equal to the Square of the Side of a Hexagon, together with the Square of the Side of a Decagon

SECTION IV
Of the USES of the Line of Chords.

USE I *To open the Sector, fo that the two Lines of Chords may make an Angle of any Number of Degrees.*

FIRST take the Diftance, upon the Line of Chords, from the Center of the Joint, to the Number of Degrees propofed, then open the Sector, fo that the Diftance, from 60 to 60 on each Leg, be equal to the aforefaid Diftance, and then the Lines of Chords will make the Angle required

As, to make an Angle of 40 Degrees, take the Diftance of the Number 40 from the Center, then open the Sector, till the Diftance from 60 to 60, be equal to the faid Diftance of 40 Degrees If a right Angle be required, take the Diftance of 90 Degrees from the Center, and then let the Diftance from 60 to 60 be equal to that, and fo of others.

USE II *The Sector being opened, to find the Degrees of its Opening.*

Take the Extent from 60 Degrees to 60 Degrees, and lay it off upon the Line of Chords from the Center, then the Number, whereon it terminates, fheweth the Degrees of its Opening

Sights are fometimes placed upon the Line of Chords, by means of which Angles are taken, in adding to the Sector a Ball and Socket, and placing it upon a Foot, to elevate it to the height of the Eye, but thefe Operations are better performed with other Inftruments

Q   USE

USE III *To make a right-lined Angle, upon a given Line, of any Number of Degrees.*

Describe, upon the given Line, a circular Arc, whose Center let be the Point whereon the Angle is to be made ; then set off the Radius, from 60 to 60, on the Lines of Chords The Sector remaining thus opened, take the Distance of the two Numbers upon each Leg, expressing the proposed Degrees, and lay it from the Line upon the Arc described Lastly, draw a right Line from the Center, thro the End of the Arc, and it will make the Angle proposed

Fig. 10,

Suppose, for Example, an Angle of 40 Degrees is to be made at the End B, of the Line A B, having described any Arc about the Point B, always lay off the said Radius from 60 to 60 on the Line of Chords, (because the Radius of a Circle is always equal to the Chord of 60 Degrees) and lay off the Distance of 40 Deg and 40 Deg from C to D Lastly, drawing a Line thro the Points B and D, the Angle of 40 Degrees will be had   *Vid. Fig* 10.

By this Use a Figure, whose Sides and Angles are known, may be drawn

USE IV *A right-lined Angle being given, to find the Number of Degrees it contains*

About the Vertex of the given Angle describe the Arc of a Circle, and open the Sector, so that the Distance from 60 to 60, on each Leg, be equal to the Radius of the Circle Then take the Chord of the Arc between your Compasses, and carrying it upon the Legs of the Sector, see what equal Number, on each Leg, the Points of your Compasses fall on, and that will be the Quantity of Degrees the given Angle contains.

USE V *To take the Quantity of an Arc, of any Number of Degrees, upon the Circumference of a given Circle*

Open the Sector, so that the Distance from 60 to 60, on each Line of Chords, be equal to the Radius of the given Circle The Sector remaining thus opened, take the Extent of the Chord of the Number of Degrees upon each Leg of the Sector, and lay it off upon the Circumference of the given Circle

By this Use may any regular Polygon be inscribed in a given Circle, as well as by the Line of Polygons, *viz* in knowing the Angle of the Center, by the Method and Table before expressed, in the Construction of the Line of Polygons

Fig 11,

For Example, to make a Pentagon by means of the Line of Chords : Having found the Angle of the Center, which is 72 Degrees, open the Sector, so that the Distance from 60 to 60, on each Leg of the Sector, be equal to the Radius of the given Circle, and then take the Extent from 72 to 72, on each Leg, between your Compasses, which carried round the Circumference, will divide it into five equal Parts, and the five Chords being drawn, the Polygon will be made

USE VI *To describe a regular Polygon upon the given right Line* F G

As, for Example, to make a Pentagon, whose Angle of the Center is 72 Degrees, open the Sector, so that the Distance from 72 Degrees to 72 Degrees, on each Line of Polygons, be equal to the Length of the given Line The Sector remaining thus opened, take the Distance from 60 to 60, on each Leg, between your Compasses, with this Distance, about the Ends of the given Line, as Centers, describe two Arcs intersecting each other in D, and this D will be the Center of a Circle, whose Circumference will be divided, by the given Line, into five equal Parts

SECTION V

Of the USES of the Line of Solids

USE I *To augment or diminish any similar Solids in a given Ratio*

Fig. 12

LET, for Example, a Cube be given, and it is required to make another double to it Carry the Side of the given Cube to the Distance of some equal Number, on both Lines of Solids, at pleasure, as, for Example, to 20 and 20 The Sector being thus opened, take the Extent, on both Legs of the Sector, of a Number double to it, that is, of 40 and 40, and this is the Side of a Cube double the proposed one

If a Ball or Globe be proposed, and it is required to make another thrice as big, carry the Diameter of the Ball to the Distance of some equal Number, on both Lines of Solids, at pleasure, as to 20 and 20, then take the Distance from 60 to 60, (because 60 is thrice 20) and that will be the Diameter of a Ball three times greater than the proposed one, because Balls are to each other as the Cubes of their Diameters

If, again, a Chest, in figure of a right-angled Parallelopipedon, contains three Measures of Grain, and it be required to make another similar Chest to contain five Measures, open the Sector, so that the Distance from 30 to 30, on each Line of Solids, be equal to the Length of the Base of the Chest ; then the Distance from 50 to 50, on each Leg, will be the homologous Side of that Solid to be made. Again, apply the Breadth of the Base to the Distance of the said Numbers 30 and 30, and then the Distance from 50 to 50 will be the homologous

mologous Side to the said Breadth Now having made a Parallelogram with these two Lengths, your next thing will be to find the Depth To do which, open the Sector, so that the Distance from 30 to 30 be equal to the Depth of the given Chest, then the Distance from 50 to 50 will be the Depth of the Chest to be made This being done, it will be easy to make the Parallelopipedon, containing the five proposed Measures

It the Lines are so long, that they cannot be applied to the Legs of the Sector, take any of their Parts, and with them proceed as before, then the respective Parts of the required Dimensions will be had

USE II *Two similar Bodies being given, to find their Ratio*

Take either of the Sides of one of the proposed Bodies between your Compasses, and having carried it to the Distance of some equal Number, on each Line of Solids, take the homologous Side of the other Solid, and note the Number on each Leg it falls upon, and then the said Numbers will shew the Ratio of the two similar Solids

But if the Side of the first Solid be so applied to some Number on each Leg of the Sector, that the homologous Side of the other cannot be applied to the Extent of some Number on each Leg, then you must apply the Side of the first Solid to such a Number on each Line, that the Length of the Side of the second Solid may fall upon some whole Number on each Line of Solids, to avoid Fractions

USE III *To construct and divide a Line, whose Use is to find the Diameters of Cannon-Balls.*

It is found, by Experience, that an Iron Ball, three Inches in Diameter, weighs 40 Pounds, whence it will be easy to find the Diameters of other Balls of different Weights, and the same Metal, in the following manner : Open the Sector, so that the Distance from the 4th Solid to the 4th Solid, on each Line of Solids, be equal to three Inches The Sector remaining thus opened, take upon the Lines of Solids the Distances of all the Numbers, from 1 to 64, on one Leg, to the same Numbers on the other Leg, then lay off all these Lengths upon a right Line drawn on a Ruler, or upon one of the Legs of the Sector, and where the Diameters terminate, denote the Weights of the Balls

But now to mark the Fractions of a Pound, as $\frac{1}{4}, \frac{1}{2}, \frac{3}{4}$, open the Sector, so that the Distance of the 4th Solid, on each Leg of the Sector, be equal to the Diameter of a Ball of one Pound The Sector remaining thus opened, the Distance from the 1st Solid to the 1st on each Leg of the Sector, will give the Diameter for $\frac{1}{4}$ of a Pound, from the 2d to the 2d, for $\frac{1}{2}$ of a Pound, and from the 3d to the 3d, for $\frac{3}{4}$ of a Pound, and so of others When the Diameters of Balls are known, the Diameters or Bores of Cannon, to which they are proper, will likewise be known : but there are commonly two or three Lines given for the Vent of great Balls, and for lesser ones in proportion The Diameters of Balls are measured with spherick Compasses, as will be more fully explained among the Instruments for Artillery

USE IV *To make a Solid similar and equal to the Sum of any Number of similar given Solids*

Open the Sector, and apply either of the Sides of either of the Bodies to the same Number on each Line of Solids ; then note on what equal Numbers, on both Legs of the Sector, the homologous Sides of the other Solids fall This being done, add together the said Numbers, and take the Extent, on both Lines of Solids, of the Number arising from that Addition, and this Extent will be the homologous Side of a Body, equal and similar to the Sum of the given Bodies

Example, Suppose the Side chosen of the first Solid be applied to the fifth Solid, on each Leg of the Sector, and the homologous Sides of the others fall, the one on the 7th, and the other on the 8th Solid, on each Line of Solids, add the three Numbers 5, 7, and 8 together, and their Sum is 20, therefore the Distance from 20 to 20, on each Line of Solids, will be the homologous Side of a Body, equal and similar to the three others

USE V *Two similar and unequal Bodies being given, to find a third similar and equal to their Difference*

Open the Sector, and apply either of the Sides of either of the Bodies to some equal Number on each Leg of the Sector, and see what equal Numbers, on both Legs, the homologous Sides of the other Solids fall upon, then substract the lesser Number from the greater, and take the Distance from the remaining Number, on one Line of Solids, to the same on the other, and this will be the homologous Side of a Body, equal to the Difference of the two given ones

As, for Example, the Side of the greatest being set over, upon the Line of Solids, from 15 to 15, the homologous Side of the lesser will be equal to the Distance from 9 to 9, then taking 9 from 15, there remains 6 · therefore the Distance from 6 to 6 will be the homologous Side of the Solid sought.

USE VI *To find two mean Proportionals between two given Lines*

For Example, suppose there are two Lines, one of which is 54, and the other 16: open the Sector, so that the Distance from 54 to 54, on each Leg of the Sector, be equal to the Length

Length of the longeſt Line. The Sector remaining thus opened, the Diſtance from 16 to 16, on each Leg, will be equal to the greater of the mean Proportionals, and will be found to be 36. Again, ſhutting the Legs of the Sector cloſer, till the Diſtance between 54 and 54, on each Leg, be equal to 36, then the Diſtance from 16 to 16 will be the leſſer of the mean Proportionals, and will be found to be 24. Whence theſe four Lines will be in continual Proportion, 54, 36, 24, 16.

It the Lines be too long, or the Numbers of their equal Parts too great, you muſt take their halfs, thirds, or fourths, &c. and proceed as before. For Example, to find two mean Proportionals between two Lines, one of which is 32, and the other 256, take the fourth Parts of both the Lines, which are 8 and 64. This being done, open the Sector, ſo that the Diſtance from 8 to 8, on each Line of Solids, be equal to 8, then take the Diſtance from 64 to 64, and that gives 16, for ¼ of the firſt of the two mean Proportionals. Again, open the Sector, ſo that the Diſtance from 8 to 8 be equal to 16, the Sector being thus opened, the Diſtance from 64 to 64 will give 16, for ¼ of the ſecond of the mean Proportionals ſought: whence the mean Proportionals are 64 and 128, for 32, 64, 128, 256, are proportional.

USE VII. *To find the Side of a Cube equal to the Side of a given Parallelopipedon.*

Firſt, find a mean Proportional between the two Sides of the Baſe of the Parallelopipedon; then between the Number found, and the Height of the Parallelopipedon, find the firſt of two mean Proportionals, which will be the Side of the Cube ſought.

For Example, let the two Sides of the Parallelopipedon be 24 and 54, and its Height 63, the Side of a Cube equal to it is ſought.

Open the Sector, ſo that the Diſtance between 54 and 54, on the Line of Planes, be equal to the Side of 54, then take the Diſtance from 24 to 24 on the ſame Line, which, meaſured upon the Line of equal Parts, will give 36 for a mean Proportional. This being done, take 36 between your Compaſſes, and open the Sector, ſo that the Points of the Compaſſes may fall upon 36 and 36, on each Line of Solids, then take the Diſtance from 63 to 63 on the Lines of Solids, which will be found almoſt 44 ½, for the Side of a Cube equal to the given Parallelopipedon.

USE VIII. *To conſtruct and divide a Gauging-Rod to meaſure Casks, and other the like Veſſels, proper to hold Liquors.*

Fig 13.

The Gauging-Rod, of which we are now going to ſpeak, is a Ruler made of Metal, divided into certain Parts, whereby the Number of Pints contained in a Veſſel may be found, in putting it in at the Bung-hole, till its End touches the Angle, made by the Bottom, with that part of the Side oppoſite to the Bung-hole, as the Line A C diagonally ſituated.

The Gauging-Rod being thus poſited, the Diviſion, anſwering to the middle of the Bung-hole, ſhews the Quantity of Liquor, or Number of Pints the Veſſel, when full, holds.

But it is neceſſary to change the Poſition of the aforeſaid Rod, ſo that its End C may touch the Angle of the other Bottom B, in order to ſee whether the middle of the Bung-hole be in the middle of the Veſſel, for if there is any Difference, half of it muſt be taken.

The Uſe of this Gauging-Rod is very eaſy ; for, without any Calculation by it, the Dimenſions of Casks may immediately be taken, all the Difficulty conſiſts only in well dividing it.

Now, in order to divide it, a little Cask, holding a *Setter*, or eight Pints, muſt be made ſimilar to the Veſſels that are commonly uſed, for this Rod will not exactly give the Dimenſions of diſſimilar Veſſels, that is, ſuch that have the Diameters of the Heads, thoſe of the Bungs, and the Lengths not proportional to the Diameters of the Head, Bung, and Length of that which the Diviſions of the Rod are made by.

Now ſuppoſe the Diameter, at the Head of a Cask, be 20 Inches, the Diameter of the Bung 22, and the interior Length 30 Inches, this Veſſel will hold 27 *Setters* of *Paris* Meaſure, and its Diagonal Length, anſwering to the middle of the Bung-hole, will be 25 Inches, 9 Lines and a half, as is eaſy to find by Calculation: becauſe in the right-angled Triangle A D C, the Side C D being 15 Inches, and D A 21, by adding their Squares together, you will have (*per Prop* 47 *lib.* 1 *Eucl.*) the Square of the Hypothenuſe A C, and by extracting the Square Root, A C will be had.

According to the ſame Proportions a Cask, whoſe Dimenſions are one Third of the former ones, will contain one *Setter*, or eight Pints, that is, if the Diameter of the Head be 6 Inches, and 8 Lines, that of the Bung 7 Inches, 8 Lines, the Length 8 Inches, 8 Lines, and its Diagonal 8 Inches, 7 Lines.

Another Cask, whoſe Dimenſions are half of that before-mentioned, will contain one Pint, that is, if the Diameter of the Head be 3 Inches, 4 Lines; that of the Bung 3 Inches, 8 Lines, the interior Length of the Cask 5 Inches, and the Diagonal, anſwering to the middle of the Bung-hole, 4 Inches, 3 Lines and a half.

Now take a Rod about 3 or 4 Feet long, and chuſe either of the three Meaſures, which you judge moſt proper. As, for Example, if you will make Diviſions for *Setters* upon the Rod, make a Point, in the middle of its Breadth, diſtant from one of its Ends, 8 Inches, 7 Lines, and there make the Diviſion for one *Setter* upon it, double that Extent, and there make a Mark for 8 *Setters*, triple the ſame Extent, and there make a Mark for 27 *Setters*,

quadruple

quadruple it, and there make a Mark for 64 Setiers, becaufe fimilar Solids are to each other, as the Cubes of their homologous Sides

Again, to make Divifions upon it for the other Setiers, take between your Compaffes the Length of 8 Inches, 7 Lines, fet over this Diftance, upon each Line of Solids of your Sector, from the firft Solid to the firft The Sector remaining thus opened, take the Diftance from the fecond Solid to the fecond, which mark upon the Rod for the Divifion of two Setiers

Again, take the Diftance from the third Solid to the third, which mark upon the Rod for the Length of the Diagonal, agreeing to three Setiers, and fo on, by which means the Rod will be divided, for taking the Dimenfions of Veffels in Setiers With the fame facility may the Divifions for Pints be made upon the Rod, for half of the Diftance of the Divifion of two Setiers, will give the Divifion for two Pints; half of the Diftance of the Divifion for three Setiers, will give the Divifion for three Pints, half of the Diftance of the Divifion for four Setiers, will give the Divifion for four Pints, and fo on

If the Sector be not long enough to take the Diagonal Length anfwerable to one Setier, from the firft Solid to the firft, take the Diagonal Length anfwerable to one Pint, and having divided the Rod for any Number of Pints, the Diagonal Lengths of the fame Number of Setiers may be had, by doubling the Diagonal Lengths of the Pints As, for Example, if the Diagonal Length for 6 Pints be doubled, that Diftance will be the Diagonal Length of a Veffel holding 6 Setiers Alfo if the Diagonal Length of 7 Pints be doubled, the Length of the Diagonal of a Veffel, holding 7 Setiers, will be had, and fo of other Diagonal Lengths

If the Diagonal Length is yet too long to be applied to the Diftance of the Divifion for the firft Solid, on each Leg of the Sector, its half muft be applied to the fame, and the Sector remaining thus opened, take the Diftance of the Divifions for the fecond Solid on both Lines of Solids, and double it, then you will have the Diagonal Length of a Veffel holding two Pints. Having again taken the Diftance of the Divifion for the third Solid upon each Leg of the Sector, which Diftance being double, the Diagonal Length of a Veffel holding three Pints will be had, and may be marked upon your Rod, and fo of others

The Divifions for Setiers go acrofs the whole Breadth of the Rod, upon which are their refpective Numbers graved, and the Divifions for Pints are fhorter than the others, for their better Diftinction

In order for this Gauging-Rod to ferve to take the Quantity of Liquor contained in different diffimilar Veffels, other Divifions may be made upon its Faces, according to the different Proportions of their Lengths and Diameters, and at the bottom of the Faces muft be writ the Diameters and Lengths by which the Divifions were made For Example, at the bottom of the Face, upon which the precedent Divifions were made, there is wrote, the Diameter of the Head 20, the Diameter of the Bung 22, and the Length 30

If, for dividing another Face, you ufe a Veffel, whofe Diameter of the Head is 21 Inches, that of the Bung 23, and the interior Length 27 ½ Inches, this Veffel is fhorter than that before-named, but contains almoft the fame Quantity of Liquor, when full, *viz* 27 Setiers, and the Length of its Diagonal will be 26 Inches

If another Veffel hath all its Dimenfions ⅔ of the precedent ones, this Veffel will hold one Setier, and its Diagonal A C will be 8 Inches and 8 Lines in Length Now by means of this Veffel, and its Diagonal Length, you may divide the aforefaid Face in the manner directed for dividing the firft Face, and at the bottom of this Face you muft write, *Diameter reduced 22, Length 27 ½*

If the four Faces of the Rod are divided, as before-named, you will have four different Gauges for gauging four different kinds of Veffels, and by examining the Proportions of the Diameters of the Heads and Lengths, you muft make ufe of fuch a Face accordingly

Inftead of ufing the Sector in dividing the before-mentioned Gauging-Rod, it is better ufing the Table of Solids

For having found, by Calculation, that the Length of the Diagonal of a Veffel, holding 27 Setiers, is 6 Inches, it will be eafy to find the Diagonals of Veffels of any propofed Bigneffes, having the fame Proportions to the Diameters reduced, as 22 to 27 ½, or as 4 to 5

As, for Example, it is required to find the Diameter of a *Quarteau*, which holds 9 Setiers, feek, in the Table of Solids, the Number anfwering to the 9th Solid, which will be found 520, at the fame time find the correfpondent Number to the 27th Solid, which will be found 750 then ftate a Rule of Three, in the following manner; 750 520 26 18, whence 18 Inches will be the Length of the Diagonal of a Veffel holding 9 Setiers The Coopers about *Paris* make their Veffels almoft in the Proportion of 4 to 5, as is, for Example, a half *Mud*, having 19 Inches 2 Lines in Diameter reduced, and 24 Inches in Length, in which Cafe the Diagonal will be 22 Inches, 8 ½ Lines, as you will eafily find by Calculation

But, in general, as foon as the Proportions ufed in making Veffels are known, the Diagonal of fome one of thofe Veffels, holding a known quantity of Setiers being firft found (*per Prop 47 lib 3 Eucl*) you may afterwards find the Lengths of the Diagonals of all Veffels made in the fame proportion, by means of the aforefaid Table of Solids

R   SECTION

SECTION VI.

Of the Conſtruction and Uſe of other kinds of Gauging-Rods.

THE Gauging-Rod, of which we have already ſpoken, ſerves only to find the Quantity of Liquor contained in ſimilar Veſſels, but that which we are now going to mention, may be uſed in taking the Dimenſions of diſſimilar Veſſels.

In order to conſtruct the firſt Gauge of this kind, the Meaſure which you uſe muſt be determined, by comparing it with ſome regular Veſſel, as a Concave Cylinder, in which a Quart or a Gallon of Water being poured, you muſt exactly note the Depth occupied by the Water

As, for Example, if a Gauge is to be made for *Paris*, where a Pint is 48 Cubic Inches, or 61 Cylindrick Inches, you will find, by Calculation, that a Concave Cylinder, 3 Inches, 11 ½ Lines in Diameter, and the like Number in Depth, contains one Pint of *Paris*, and a Cylinder, whoſe Dimenſions are double the aforeſaid ones, that is, 7 Inches, 10 ⅔ Lines, will hold one Setier · for ſimilar Solids are to each other, as the Cubes of their like Sides

Fig. 14
This being ſuppoſed, lay off that Length of 3 Inches 11 ½ Lines, upon one Face of the Rod, as often as the Length of the Rod will admit, and mark Points, whereon ſet 1, 2, 3, 4, 5, &c each of theſe Parts may be ſubdivided into 4 or more This Face, thus divided, is called the Face of equal Parts, and is uſed in meaſuring the Lengths of Veſſels

You muſt likewiſe mark, upon another Face of the Rod, the Diameter of the Cylinder of 3 Inches, 11 ½ Lines, and then the Diameters of Circles double, triple, quadruple, &c. by any of the Methods before explained for dividing the Line of Planes on the Sector, the eaſieſt
Fig. 15
and ſhorteſt of which is to make a right-angled Iſoſceles Triangle A B C, each of the Legs about the right Angle of which being 3 Inches, 11 ½ Lines, the Hypothenuſe B C will be the Diameter of a Circle double to that, whoſe Diameter is 3 Inches, 11 ½ Lines therefore having produced one of the Legs A B towards D, lay off the ſaid Hypothenuſe from A towards D, and at the Point whereon it terminates mark the Number 2, then take the Diſtance C 2, and having laid it off upon the Line A D, mark the Number 3 at the Point whereon it terminates Again, take the Diſtance C 3, and having laid it off upon the Line A D, there mark the Number 4, &c

Note, A 4, which is the Diameter of a Circle quadruple the firſt, is double A C, or A B, becauſe Circles are to each other as the Squares of their Diameters whence ſince A B is 1, its Square is alſo 1, and the Line A 4 being 2, its Square muſt conſequently be 4.

To uſe this Gauge, you muſt firſt apply the Face of equal Parts to the exterior Length of the Veſſel, from which you muſt take the Depth of the two Croes, that thereby the true interior Length may be had

This being done, apply the Face of Diameters to the Diameters of the Heads of the Veſſel, and note the Number anſwering to them, and whether they are equal, for if there be any Difference between the Diameters of the Heads, you muſt add them together, and take half their Sum for the mean Head-Diameter

Again, put the Rod downright in at the Bung-hole, in order to have the Diameter of the Bung, which add to the Head-Diameter, and take half the Sum for an arithmetical Mean, this being multiplied by the Length of the Veſſel, will give the Number of Pints the Veſſel holds

As ſuppoſe the interior Length of a Veſſel is 4 ¾ of the equal Parts of the Rod, the Diameter at the Head 15, and the Bung-Diameter 17, add 15 to 17, and their Sum is 32, half of which is 16, which multiplied by the Length 4 ¾, and the Product 76 will give the Number of Pints the Veſſel holds

Now to conſtruct the ſecond kind of Rods, it is found, by Experience, that a Cylinder, whoſe Height and Diameter is 3 Foot, 3 Inches, and 6 Lines, holds 1000 *Paris* Pints

Then take upon a Ruler a Length of 3 Feet, 3 Inches, and 6 Lines, which divide into 10 Parts, each of which will be the Height and Diameter of a Cylinder holding one Pint, (becauſe ſimilar Cylinders are to each other as the Cubes of their Diameters.) Again, divide each of theſe Parts into 10 more, which may eaſily be done by help of the Line of Lines on the Sector, then each of theſe laſt Parts will be the Height and Diameter of a Cylinder holding the 1000th part of a Pint · Every five of theſe ſmall Parts being numbered, your
Fig. 16
Rod will be made One of theſe Rods, of 4 or 5 Feet in Length, will ſerve to gauge great Veſſels, as Pipes, &c

To uſe this Rod, you muſt note how many of the ſmall Diviſions of the Rod the Diameters of the Head and Bung, as alſo the Length, contains

But, *Note,* by the Length of a Veſſel is underſtood the interior Length, which is the Diſtance between the Head and the Bottom, and by the Diameters is underſtood the interiour Diameters included between the Staves

Note alſo, if the Diameters at Top and Bottom are unequal, compare one of them with the Bung-Diameter, and the middle between theſe two is called the mean Diameter of the Veſſel

But

But if the Diameters at Top and Bottom are unequal, add them together, and take half of the Sum, which is called the mean Diameter of the Head and Botton, then compute this mean Diameter with the Diameter at the Bung, add them together, and take half their Sum for the mean Diameter of the Vessel

Then square the mean Diameter of the Vessel, and multiply the said Square by the Length of the Vessel, then the Product will give you the Quantity of Liquor in 10000 Parts the Vessel holds, and by casting away the last three Figures, you will have the Number of Pints contained in the Vessel, when full

Let, for Example, the Diameter at the Head be 58 Parts of the Gauging Rod, and the Bung-Diameter 62, add these two Numbers together, and their Sum will be 120, whose half 60 is the mean Diameter of the Vessel then the Square of this mean Diameter will be 3600, and if this Square be multiplied by the Length of the Vessel, which suppose 80, the Product will be 288000, and by taking away the three last Figures, the Number of *Paris* Pints the Vessel holds will be 288

This way of Gauging is exact enough for Practice, when there is but a small Difference between the Bung and Head-Diameters, as are the Diameters of *Paris-Muids*, but when the Difference between the Bung and Head-Diameters is considerable, as in the Pipes of *Anjou*, whose Bung-Diameters are much greater than the Head-Diameters, Dimensions taken in the before-directed manner will not give the Quantity of Liquor exact enough But to render the Method more exact, divide the Difference of the Bung and Head-Diameters into 7 Parts, and add 4 of them to the Head-Diameter, and that will give you the mean Diameter for Example, if the Diameter of the Head is 50, and the Bung-Diameter 57, the mean Diameter of the Vessel will be 54, with which mean Diameter proceed as before

Having found by the Rod how many *Paris* Pints a Vessel holds, you may find how many other Measures the same Vessel holds, in the following manner

A *Paris* Pint of fresh Water weighs 1 Pound, 15 Ounces, therefore you need but weigh the sought Measure full of Water, and by the Rule of Three you may have your Desire

As, for Example, a certain Measure of Water weighs 50 Ounces, and it is required to find how many of the same Measures is contained in a *Paris-Muid*, which holds 288 Pints : Say, by the Rule of Three, As 50 is to 31, so is 288 Pints to a fourth Number, which will be 178, of the said Measures

There may be marked Feet and Inches upon the vacant Faces of the aforesaid Gauging-Rod, each of which Inches may be subdivided into four equal Parts, which will be a second means to gauge Vessels, the Feet are marked with Roman Characters, and the Inches with others

We have already said, that a *Paris* Pint contains 61 Cylindrick Inches, therefore having the Solidity of a Vessel in Cylindrick Inches, it must be divided by 61, to have the Number of Pints the Vessel holds An Example or two will make this manifest

Let the Length of a Vessel be 36 Inches, the Head-Diameter 23, and the Bung-Diameter 25, add the two Diameters together, and their Sum will be 48, half of which is 24 for the mean Diameter This Number 24 being squared, will be 576, and this Square being multiplied by the Length 36, gives 20736 Cylindrick Inches which being divided by 61, the Quotient will give 339 Pints, and about ½

If the Diameters and Lengths of Vessels are taken in fourth Parts of Inches, the last Product must be divided by 3904, to have the Number of Pints contained in a Vessel, when full

Let, for Example, the Length of a Vessel be 35 ¼ Inches, the Head-Diameter 23 Inches, and the Diameter at the Bung 25 ¼ Inches, add the two Diameters together, and their Sum will be 48 ¼, half of which will be 24 ¼, which, for ease of Calculation, reduce to 4ths 97 is the Number to be squared, which will be 9409, which multiply by 141, and that Product again by 35 ¼, reduced to 4ths of Inches, will give this Product 1326669, which being divided by 3904, the Quotient will (as before) be 339 Pints, and about ½

The Construction and USE of a new Gauging-Rod

Mr *Sauveur*, of the Academy of Sciences, has communicated to us a new Gauging-Rod of his Invention, by means of which may be found, by Addition only, the Quantity of Liquor that any Vessel holds, when full, whereas hitherto Multiplication and Division has been used in Gauging

To make this Gauging-Rod, you must first chuse a Piece of very dry Wood, as Sorbaple Fig 17. or Pear-tree, without Knots, about 5 Foot long, in Figure of a Parallelopipedon, and 6 or 7 Lines in Breadth, *Fig* 17 shews its four Faces

Now upon the first of the four Faces are made Divisions for taking the Diameters of Vessels

The Divisions of the second Face serves to measure the Lengths of the Diameters

The Divisions upon the third Face are for finding the Contents of Vessels

And, Lastly, upon the fourth Face, the Numbers of Setiers and Pints, which the Vessel holds, are marked

The aforesaid Divisions are made in the following manner

First, divide the fourth Face into Inches, and each Inch into 10 equal Parts, those Divisions denote Pints, and are numbered 1, 2, 3, 4, 5, 6, &c every 8 being Setiers, because

I Se-

1 Setier is 8 Pints   On the end of this fourth Face is written *Pints* and *Setiers*.

The Divisions of the other three Faces are made by help of Logarithms, in manner following.

Note, The Divisions of the fourth Face serve as a Scale to the third, and ought to be contiguous to it.

To divide the third Face of the Rod

If you have a mind to place any Number upon the third Face of your Rod, for Example, 240 seek in the Table of Logarithms for 240, or the nighest Number to it, which will be found against 251 in your Table, then place 240 upon the third Face, over against 251 Pints on the fourth Face, and, proceeding in this manner, you may divide the third Face.

But because, in the Table of Logarithms, 240 doth not stand against 251, but instead thereof there stands 2 39996, which nighly approaches it, therefore to make the Divisions as exact as possible, you must add 1 to the first Number of the Logarithm 2 40, and then seek for 3.40, over against which stands 25 12, which shews, that the Logar. 240 must be placed not over against 25 1 of the Divisions of Pints, but against 251 and two Parts of the Division of a Pint, supposed to be divided into 10 Parts more. You must write *Contents* at one End of this third Face.

The Manner of dividing the second Face

A Cylindrical Vessel, whose Length and Diameter is 3 Inches, 11½ Lines, holds one *Paris Pint*; therefore the first part of the second Face, which is without Divisions, must be of that Length. This said Length must be laid off ten times, and more, if possible, upon the said Face, upon which make occult Marks, then one of these Parts must be divided into 100 more, upon a separate Ruler, serving as a Scale.

This being done, suppose any Number is to be placed upon the second Face, as, for Example, 60. Seek in the Table of Logarithms for 60, which will be found against 39 and 40, or rather against 3981, without having regard to the Numbers 1, 2, 3, that precede it, and which are called Characteristicks · therefore I take 98, or 981, by esteeming one Part divided into 10, upon the small Scale divided into 100, and I place this Distance next to the third occult Point, which denotes three Centesms, or three Thousandths. You must thus mark Divisions from 5 to 5, and every of these 5ths must again be subdivided into 5 equal Parts. Finally, upon the End of this Face, you must write *Lengths*.

The Manner of dividing the first Face.

The first Part of this Face, which is not divided, represents the Diameter of a Cylindrical Vessel holding one *Paris Pint*; therefore its Length must be 3 Inches, 11½ Lines.

And for dividing this Face, lay off upon it the Divisions of the second Face, but instead of writing 5, 10, 15, 20, 25, &c write their Doubles, 10, 20, 30, 40, 50, &c and subdivide the Intervals into 10 Parts, and at the End of this Face write *Diameters*.

The USE of the New Gauging-Rod

Measure the Length of the mean Diameter of the Vessel with the Face of *Diameters* of your Rod, which suppose to be 153 00. Likewise take the Length of the Vessel with the second Face of your Rod, which suppose to be 92 85, add these two Numbers together, then seek their Sum 245 85 upon the third Face, and over against it, on the fourth Face, you will have 36 Setiers, or 288 Pints.

153 00
92 85
————
245 85

But to make the Use of this Rod general, suppose the Weight of a Pint of fresh Water of some Country be 50 Ounces Avoirdupoise, then seek 31, the Number of Ounces Avoirdupoise a *Paris* Pint of fresh Water weighs, upon the fourth Face of *Setiers* of the Rod, which will be found against 239 4 on the third Face.

Likewise, against 50 on the fourth Face, answers 260 2 on the third Face.

Then from 260.2   Again from 245 85 before found
Take 239   Take 20 80
—————   —————
And there remains 20 8   And there remains 225 05

Now against this Number 225 05, on the third Face, you will find, on the fourth Face, 22 Setiers 2 Pints, or 178 Pints, which is the Number of Pints of that Country a Vessel of the aforesaid Dimensions holds.

SECTION VII.

Of the USE of the Line of Metals.

USE I   *The Diameter of a Ball, of any one of the six Metals, being given, to find the Diameter of another Ball of any one of them, which shall have the same Weight.*

OPEN the Sector, and taking the given Diameter of the Ball between your Compasses, apply its Extremes to the Characters upon each Line of Metals, expressing the Metal the Ball is made of. The Sector remaining thus opened, take the Distance of the Characters of the Metal, the sought Diameter is to be of, upon each Line of Metals, and this will be the Diameter sought As, for Example, let A B be the Diameter of a Ball of Lead, and it is required to find the Diameter of a Ball of Iron, having the same Weight Open the Sector, so that the Distance between the Points ♄ and ♄ be equal to the Line A B The Sector remaining thus opened, take the Distance of the Points of ♂ on each Line of Metals, and that will give C D, the Length of the Diameter sought If, instead of Balls, similar Solids of several Sides had been proposed, make the same Operation, as before, for finding each of their homologous Sides, in order to have the Lengths, Breadths, and Thicknesses of the Bodies to be made Fig. 18.

USE II *To find the Proportion that each of the six Metals have to one another, as to their Weight*

For Example, it is required to find what Proportion two similar and equal Bodies, but of different Weights, have to one another

Having taken the Distance from the Center of the Joint of your Sector, to the Point of the Character of that Metal of the two proposed Bodies which is least, (and which is always more distant from the Center) apply the said Distance across to any two equal *Divisions* on both the Lines of Solids The Sector remaining thus opened, take the Distance on the Line of Metals, from the Center of the Joint to the Point, denoting the other Metal · and applying it to both Lines of Solids, see if it will fall upon some equal Number on each Line; if it will, that Number, and the other before, will, by permuting them, shew the Proportions of the Metals proposed

As, for Example · to find the Proportion of the Weight of a Wedge of Gold, to the Weight of a similar and equal Wedge of Silver.

Now because Silver weighs less than Gold, open the Sector, and having taken the Distance from the Center of the Joint to the Point ☽, apply it to the Numbers 50 and 50 on each Line of Solids The Sector remaining thus opened, take the Distance from the Center to the Point ☉, and applying it on each Line of Solids, and you will find it to fall nearly upon the 27th Solid on each Line Whence I conclude, the Weight of the Gold to the Weight of the Silver, is as 50 to 27 $\frac{3}{8}$, or as 100 to 54 $\frac{3}{4}$, that is, if the Wedge of Gold weighs 100 Pounds, the Wedge of Silver will weigh 54 $\frac{3}{4}$ Pounds, and so of other Metals, whose Proportions are more exactly laid down by the Numbers of Pounds and Ounces that a cubick Foot of each of the Metals weighs, as is expressed in the Table adjoining to the Proof of the Line of Metals If nevertheless their Proportions are required in lesser Numbers, you will find, that if a Wedge of Gold weighs 100 Marks, a Wedge of Lead, of the same Bigness, will weigh about 60 $\frac{1}{2}$, one of Silver 54 $\frac{3}{4}$, one of Brass 47 $\frac{1}{4}$, one of Iron 42 $\frac{1}{10}$, and one of Tin 39 Marks.

USE III *Any Body of one of the six Metals being given, to find the Weight of any one of the five others, which is to be made similar and equal to the proposed one*

For Example, let a Cistern of Tin be proposed, and it is required to make another of Silver equal and similar to it. First weigh the Tin-Cistern, which suppose 36 Pounds This being done, open the Sector, and having taken the Distance from the Center of the Sector to the Point ☽, (which is the Metal the new Cistern is to be made of) apply that Distance to 36 and 36 on each Line of Solids Then take the Distance, upon the Line of Metals, of the Point ♃, from the Center, and applying that Distance cross-wise on each of the Lines of Solids, you will find it nearly fall upon 50 and 50 on each Line Whence the Weight of a Silver Cistern must be 50 $\frac{1}{4}$ Pounds, to be equal in Bigness to the Tin-Cistern The Proof of this Operation may be had by Calculation, *viz* in multiplying the different Weights reciprocally by those of a Cubick Foot of each of the Metals As, in this Example, multiplying 720 *lib* 12 Ounces, which is the Weight of a Cubick Foot of Silver, by 36 *lib* which is the Weight of the Tin-Cistern, and again, multiplying 516 *lib* 2 Ounces, which is the Weight of a Cubick Foot of Tin, by 50 $\frac{1}{4}$ Pounds, which is the Weight of the Silver Cistern, the two Products ought to be equal

USE IV. *The Diameters, or Sides, of two similar Bodies of different Metals, being given, to find the Ratio of their Weights*

Let, for Example, the Diameter of a Ball of Tin be the right Line E F, and the Line G H the Diameter of a Ball of Silver, it is required to find the Ratio of the Weights of these two Balls Open the Sector, and taking the Diameter E F between your Compasses, apply it to the Points ♃ on each Line of Metals The Sector remaining thus opened, take the Distance of the Points ☽ on each Leg of the Sector, which compare with the Diameter G H, in order to see whether it is equal to it for if it be, the two Balls must be of the same Weight But if the Diameter of the Ball of Silver be lesser than the Distance of the Points ☽, on each Leg of the Sector, as here K L is, it is manifest that the Ball of Silver weighs less than the Ball of Tin, and to know how much, the Diameters G H and G L must be compared together. Wherefore apply the Distance of the Points ☽, which is G H, on each Leg of the Sector, to some equal Number on both the Lines of Solids, as, for Example, Fig. 19.

ple, to the Numbers 60 and 60, then note upon what equal Number, on both Lines of Solids, the Diameter K L falls, which fuppofe 20. whence the Ball of Silver, whofe Diameter is K L, weighs but ⅟ of the Weight of the Ball of Tin, whofe Diameter is E F.

USE V. *The Weight and Diameter of a Ball, or the Side of any other Body, of one of the fix Metals, being given to find the Diameter or homologous Side of another fimilar Body of one of the other five Metals, which fhall have a given Weight.*

Fig 20.

Let, for Example, the right Line M N be the Diameter of a Ball of Brafs, weighing 10 Pounds, and the Diameter of a Ball of Gold is required weighing 15 Pounds You muft firft find the Diameter of a Ball of Gold, weighing as much as that of Silver, and then augment it by means of the Line of Solids To do which, open the Sector, fo that the Diftance between the Points ♀, on each Line of Metals, be equal to M N The Sector remaining thus opened, take the Diftance of the Points ☉ and ☉ on each Line of Metals, which fuppofe to be the Diameter of the Ball of Gold O P, then open the Sector again, and apply this Diftance to 10 and 10 of the Line of Solids, on each Leg of the Sector The Sector remaining thus opened, take the Diftance from 15 to 15, on each Line of Solids, and this laft Extent Q R will be the Diameter of a Ball of Gold weighing 15 Pounds

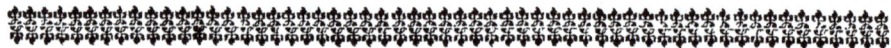

Of the Confiruction and Ufes of the ENGLISH
SECTOR.

Plate 6

T H E principal Lines that are now generally put upon this Inftrument, to be ufed Sector-wife, are the Line of Equal Parts, the Line of Chords, the Line of Sines, the Line of Tangents, the Line of Secants, and the Line of Polygons

The Line of equal Parts, called alfo the Line of Lines, is a Line divided into 100 equal Parts, and if the Length of the Legs of the Sector is fufficient, it is again fubdivided into Halfs and Quarters : they are placed on each Leg of the Sector, on the fame Side, and are numbered by 1, 2, 3, &c to 10, which is very near the End of each Leg Thefe Lines are denoted by the Letter L, it is divided into the fame Number of equal Parts, as the fame Line on the Sector defcribed by our Author And here note, that this 1 may be taken for 10, or for 100, 1000, 10000, &c as Occafion requires, and then 2 will fignify 20, 200, 2000, 20000, &c and fo of the reft

The Line of Chords is a Line divided after the ufual way of the Line of Chords, from a Circle, whofe Radius is nearly equal in Length to the Legs of the Sector, beginning at the Center, and running towards the End thereof. It is numbered with 10, 20, &c to 60, and to this Line, on each Leg, is placed the Letter C

The Line of Sines is a Line of natural Sines, divided from a Circle of the fame Radius, as the Line of Chords on the Sector was, thefe are alfo placed upon each Leg of the Sector, and numbered with the Figures 10, 20, 30, &c to 90 ; at the end of which, on each Leg, is fet the Letter S

The Line of Tangents, is a Line of natural Tangents, divided from a Circle, and is placed upon each Leg of the Sector, and runs to 45 Degrees It has the Numbers 10, 20, &c to 45 placed upon it, with the Letter T for Tangent.

There is likewife another fmall Line of Tangents, divided from a Radius, of about two Inches, and is placed upon each Leg of the Sector, it begins at 45, which ftands at the Length of the Radius from the Center, and runs to about 75 Degrees or farther, having the Numbers 45, 50, &c to 75 with the Letter t fet thereto The Ufe of this Line (as hereafter fhall be fhewn) is to fupply the Defect in the great Line

The Line of Secants is only a Line of natural Secants, divided from a Circle of about two Inches Radius. Thefe are placed upon each Leg of the Sector, beginning, not from the Center, but at two Inches Diftance therefrom, and run to 75 Degrees To thefe are fet the Numbers 10, 20, &c to 75, with the Letter S at the End thereof for Secants

Finally, the Line of Polygons, denoted by the Letter P on each Leg of the Sector, is divided in the fame manner as the Line of Polygons on the *French* Sector, only there the Number 3, for an equilateral Triangle, is the firft Polygon, and here the Number 4 for a Square.

Thefe are the principal Lines that are now put upon this Sector, to be ufed Sector-wife.

The other Lines, that are placed near and parallel to the outward Edges of the Sector, on both Faces thereof, and which are to be ufed, as on *Gunter*'s Scale, are,

1ft, The Line of artificial Sines, numbered (as *per Fig*) with 1, 2, 3, 4, 5, on one of the Legs, and with 6, 7, 8, &c to 90, on the other Leg, which laft Numbers, as they appear in the Figure, muft be fet backwards, to the end, that when the Sector is quite opened, they may become forwards This Line is denoted by the Letter S, fignifying Sines

2dly, The

2dly, The Line of artificial Tangents, placed next below the Line of artificial Sines, is numbered, on one Leg, 1, 2, 3, 4, 5, and on the other 6, 7, 8, &c to 45 which last are likewife set backwards ; but the Numbers 80, 70, 60, 50, placed at the Divifions 10, 20, 30, 40, which fignify their Complements, are set forwards

3dly, Near the Edges, on the other Face of the Sector, is a Foot divided into 12 Inches, numbered 1, 2, 3, &c and each Inch into 20 equal Parts   There is set to it *In* fignifying Inches

4thly, and *Laftly,* Next to that is placed *Gunter*'s Line of Numbers, denoted by the Letter N, as *per* Figure

There are also fome other Lines placed fometimes upon the vacant Spaces of the Sector, as the Lines of Hours, Latitudes, and Inclinations of Meridians, which are no otherwife ufed than if they were placed upon common Scales.

All the aforefaid Lines, except the fmall Lines of Tangents, Secants, and the Line of Polygons, are furnifhed with Parallels, and the Divifions marked by unequal Lines, that the Eye may the better diftinguifh them

SECTION I.

Of the general USE *and Foundation of the Sector.*

The Excellency of this Inftrument above the common Scales, or Rules, is, that it may be made to fit all Scales and Radius's, for by the Sector you may divide a Line, not exceeding its Length when quite opened, into any Number of equal Parts ; also from the Line of Chords, Sines, Tangents, &c placed on the Sector, as before directed, you may have a Line of Chords, Sines, Tangents, &c to any Radius, betwixt the Breadth and Length of the Sector when opened, by which Contrivance a Sector is made almoft a univerfal Inftrument   The Invention and Contrivance of this Inftrument arofe from a premeditate Confideration of *Prop* IV *Lib* 6 *Eucl* where it is demonftrated that fimilar Triangles have their Homologous Sides proportional

For let the Lines A B, A C, reprefent the Legs of the Sector, and A D, A E, two equal *Plate* 7. Sections from the Center . then, I fay, if the Points C, B, also D, E, are joined, the Lines C B, Fig 21. D E, *per Prop.* II *Lib* 6 *Eucl* will be parallel, therefore becaufe the Lines D E, C B, are parallel, the Triangles A D E, A C B, *per Schol Prop* IV *Lib* 6 *Eucl* will be fimilar, and confequently from the faid *Prop* IV the Sides A D, D E, A B, B C, are proportional that is, as A D to D E, fo is A B to B C, whence if A D is the half, or a third part of the Side A B, D E will be a half, or a third part of the Parallel C B, the like Reafon holds of all other Sections   whence you fee that if A D is the Chord, Sine, or Tangent of any Number of Degrees, to the Radius A B, D E will be the Chord, Sine, or Tangent of the fame Number of Degrees to the Radius B C.

Now the Lines found out by the Sector, are of two Sorts, *viz* Lateral or Parallel   Lateral are fuch as are found upon the Sides of the Sector, as A B, A C   Parallel are the Lines that run from one Leg of the Sector to the other, in equal Divifions from the Center, as D E, C B

And here note, that the innermoft of the Parallels, is the true divided Line, and therefore in ufing the Compaffes, you muft set them upon the innermoft Line, both in lateral and parallel Entrance

And further note, that the Lines are placed upon this Sector, different from thofe that are placed upon Sectors formerly made, for inftead of putting the fame Lines at equal Diftances from the inward Edges of both the Legs of the Sector, they are put at unequal Diftances, as may be feen in the Figure : where, upon one Leg the Line of Chords is innermoft, upon the other the Line of Tangents is innermoft, that is, the innermoft Line of Chords and Tangents are equally diftant from the inward Edge, and fo are the outermoft Line of Chords and Tangents   The Benefit of the Contrivance is this, When you have fet the Sector to a Radius for the Chords, it ferves also for the Sines and Tangents without ftirring it, for the Parallel betwixt 60 and 60 of the Chords, 90 and 90 of the Sines, also 45 and 45 of the Tangents, are all equal, which is the Reafon that the Chords run but to 60 Degrees

SECTION II.

Of the general USE *of the Lines of Chords, Sines, Tangents, and Secants, on the Sector.*

By difpofing and placing thefe Lines, as before directed, on this Inftrument, we have Scales to feveral Radius's, that is, having a Length, or Radius given, (not exceeding the Length of the Sector when opened) we can by the Sector find the Chord, Sine, &c thereto, for which Property, this Inftrument is often of great Ufe

For Example, Suppofe the Chord, Sine, or Tangent of 10 Degrees, to a Radius of three Inches, is required . take that three Inches, and make it a Parallel between 60 and 60 on the
Line

Line of Chords, then, as I have already said, the same Extent will reach from 45 to 45, on the Line of Tangents, also on the other Side of the Sector, the same Distance of three Inches, will reach from 90 to 90 on the Line of Sines so that if the Lines of Chords be set to any Radius, the Lines of Sines and Tangents are also set to the same Now the Sector being thus opened, if you take the parallel Distance between 10 and 10 on the Line of Chords, it will give the Chord of 10 Degrees Also if you take the parallel Distance on the Line of Sines between 10 and 10, you will have the Sine of 10 Degrees. Lastly, if you take the parallel Extent on the Line of Tangents, between 10 and 10, it will give you the Tangent of 10 Degrees.

If the Chord, or Tangent of 70 Degrees, had been required, then for the Chord you must take the parallel Distance of half the Arc proposed, that is, the Chord of 35 Degrees, and repeat that Distance twice on the Arc you lay it down on, and you will have the Chord of 70 Degrees, and for finding the Tangent of 70 Degrees to the aforesaid Radius, you must make use of the small Line of Tangents for the great one running but to 45 Degrees, the Parallel of 70 cannot be taken on that, therefore take the Radius of three Inches, and make it a Parallel between 45 and 45 on the small Line of Tangents, and then the parallel Extent of 70 Degrees on the said Line, is the Tangent of 70 Degrees to 3 Inches Radius

If you would have the Secant of any Arc, then take the given Radius, and make it a Parallel between the beginning of the Line of Secants, that is 0 and 0, so the parallel Distance between 10 and 10, or 70 and 70, on the said secant Line, will give you the Secant of 10, or 70 Degrees, to the Radius of three Inches

After this manner may the Chord, Sine, or Tangent of any Arc be found, provided the Radius can be made a Parallel between 60 and 60 on the Line of Chords, or between the small Tangent of 45, or Secant of 0 Degrees But if the Radius be so large, that it cannot be made a Parallel between 45 and 45 on the small Line of Tangents, then there cannot be found a Tangent of any Arc above 45 Degrees, nor the Secant of no Arc at all to such a Radius, because all Secants are greater than the Radius, or Semi-diameter of a Circle.

If the Converse of any of these things be required, that is, if the Radius is sought, to which a given Line is the Chord, Sine, Tangent, or Secant of any Arc, suppose of 10 Degrees, then it is but making that Line (if it be a Chord) a Parallel on the Line of Chords between 10 and 10, and the Sector will stand at the Radius required, that is, the parallel Extent between 60 and 60, on the said Chord-Line, is the Radius.

And so if it be a Sine, Tangent, or Secant, it is but making it a Parallel between the Sine, Tangent, or Secant of 10 Degrees, according as it is given, then will the Distance of 90 and 90 on the Sines, if it be a Tangent, the Extent from 45 to 45 on the Tangents, and if it be a Secant, the Extent or Distance between 0 and 0, be the Radius

Hence, you see, it is very easy to find the Chord, Sine, Tangent, or Secant to any Radius.

SECTION III.
Of the USE of the Sector in Trigonometry.

USE I. *The Base A C of the right-lined right-angled Triangle A B C being given 40 Miles, and the Perpendicular A B 30 : to find the Hypothenuse B C.*

Fig 22

Open the Sector, so that the two Lines of Lines may make a right Angle (by Use VI of our Author's) then take, for the Base, A C, 40 equal Parts upon the Line of Lines on one Leg of the Sector ; and for the Perpendicular A B, 30 equal Parts on the Line of Lines upon the other Leg of the Sector Then the Extent from 40 on one Line, to 30 on the other, taken with your Compasses, will be the Length of the Hypothenuse B C, and applying it on the Line of Lines, you will find it to be 50 Miles

USE II *The Perpendicular A B of the right-angled Triangle A B C being given 30 Miles, and the Angle B C A 37 Degrees, to find the Hypothenuse B C*

Fig. 22.

Take the given Side A B, and set it over, as a Parallel, on the Sine of the given Angle A C B, then the parallel Radius will be the Length of the Hypothenuse B C, which will be found 50 Miles, by applying it on the Line of Lines.

USE III. *The Hypothenuse B C being given, and the Base A C, to find the Perpendicular A B*

Fig. 22.

Open the Sector, so that the two Lines of Lines may be at right Angles ; then lay off the given Base A C on one of these Lines from the Center, take the Hypothenuse B C in your Compasses, and setting one Foot in the Term of the given Base A C, cause the other to fall on the Line of Lines on the other Leg of the Sector, and the Distance from the Center to where the Point of the Compasses falls, will be the Length of the Perpendicular A B

USE IV. *The Hypothenuse B C being given, and the Angle A C B ; to find the Perpendicular A B*

Take the given Hypothenuse B C, and make it a parallel Radius, and the parallel Sine of the Angle A C B will be the Length of the Side A B.

USE

The French Sector　　Plate VI

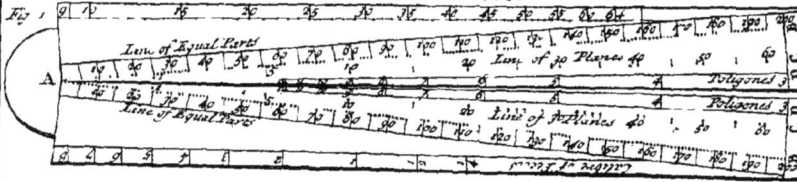

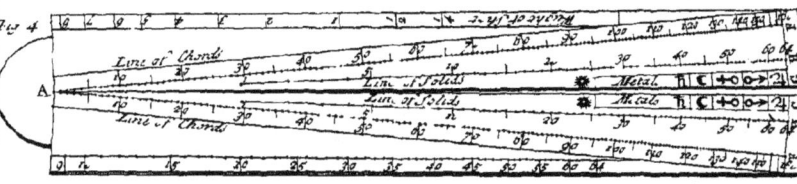

fronting page 66

Fig 1

Line of Equal Parts

Line of 30 Planes

Polygones

Polygones

Line of Equal Parts

Fig 4

Line of Chords

Line of Solids　Metal

Line of Solids　Metals

Line of Chords

Fig 3

English Cases of Instruments

Chords

Fig 3

Chords

French Cases of Instruments

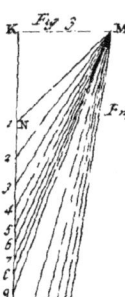

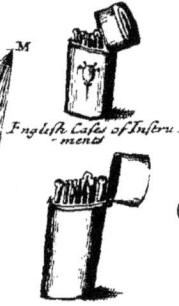

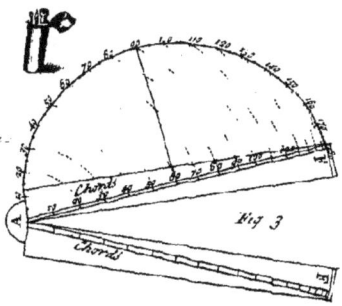

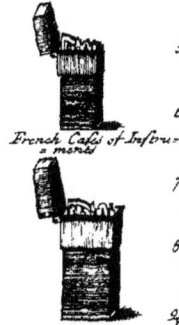

The English Sector

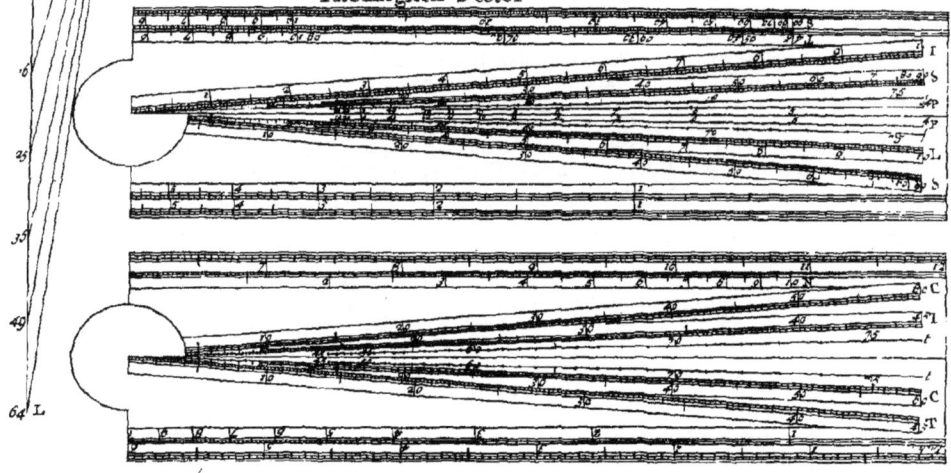

I Senex sculpt.

USE V *The Bafe* A C, *and Perpendicular* A B, *being given, to find the Angle* B C A

Lay off the Bafe A C on both Sides of the Sector from the Center, and note its Extent, then take the Perpendicular A B, and to it open the Sector in the Terms of the Bafe A C fo the Parallel Radius will be the Tangent of B C A

USE VI *In any right-lined Triangle, as* A B C, *the Sides* A C, *and* B C, *being given, one* 20 *Miles, and the other* 30, *and the included Angle* A C B 110 *Degrees, to find the Bafe* A B

Open the Sector, fo that the two Lines of Lines may make an Angle equal to the given An- Fig. 23 gle A C B of 110 Degrees, then take out the Sides A C, C B, of the Triangle, and lay them off from the Center of the Sector on each of the Lines of Lines, and take in your Compaffes the Extent between their Terms, or Ends, and that will be the Length of the fought Side A B, which will be found 41 ½ Miles

USE VII *The Angles* C A B, *and* A C B, *being given, and the Side* C B. *to find the Bafe* A B

Take the given Side C B, and turn it into the parallel Sine of its oppofite Angle C A B, Fig. 23. and the parallel Sine of the Angle A C B, will be the Length of the Bafe A B.

USE VIII *The three Angles of a Triangle, as* A B C, *being given, to find the Proportion of the Sides* A B, A C, B C

Take the lateral Sines of the Angles A C B, C B A, C A B, and meafure them in the Line Fig. 23. of Lines, for the Numbers belonging to thofe Lines will give the Proportions of the Sides.

USE IX *The three Sides* A C, A B, C B, *being given, to find the Angle* A C B

Lay the Sides A C, C B, on the Lines of Lines of the Sector from the Center, and let the Fig. 23 Side A B be fitted over in their Terms, fo fhall the Sector be opened in thofe Lines, to the Quantity of the Angle A C B

USE X *The Hypotheanfe* A C, *of the right-angled Spherical Triangle* A B C, *being given, fup-pofe* 43 *Degrees, and the Angle* C A B, 20 *Degrees, to find the Side* C B

As Radius is to the Sine of the given Hypothenufe 43 Degrees, fo is the Sine of the given Fig. 24. Angle C A B 20 Degrees, to the Sine of the Perpendicular C B

Take either the lateral Sine of the given Angle C A B, 20 Degrees, and make it a parallel Radius, that is, take 20 Degrees from the Center on the Line of Sines, in your Compaffes, and fet that Extent from 90 to 90, then the parallel Sine of 43 Degrees, the given Hypothenufe, will, when meafured from the Center on the Line of Sines, give 13 Deg. 30 Min. Or take the Sine of the given Hypothenufe A C, 43 Degrees, and make it a parallel Radius; and the parallel Sine of the given Angle C A B, taken and meafured laterally on the Line of Sines, will give the Length of the Perpendicular C B, 13 Deg 30 Min as before

USE XI *The Perpendicular* B C *given, and the Hypothenufe* A C, *to find the Bafe* A B

As the Sine Complement of the Perpendicular B C, is to Radius, fo is the Sine Comple- Fig. 24. ment of the Hypothenufe A C, to the Sine Complement of the Bafe required

Make the Radius a parallel Sine of the given Perpendicular B C, viz 76 Deg 30 Min and then the parallel Sine of the Complement of the given Hypothenufe, viz 47 Degrees, meafured laterally on the Line of Sines, will be found 49 Degrees, 25 Minutes therefore the Complement of the required Bafe, will be 49 Degrees, 25 Minutes, and confequently the Bafe will be 40 Degrees, 35 Minutes

The Ufe of the Sector in the Solution of the before-mentioned Cafes of Trigonometry, being underftood, its Ufe in folving the other Cafes, which I have omitted, will not be difficult

Note, The feveral Ufes of the Line of Lines, and Line of Polygons, on this Sector, are the fame as the Ufes of thefe Lines upon the French Sector, which fee.

I now proceed to give fome of the particular Ufes of the Sector in Geometry, Projection of the Sphere, and Dialling

SECTION IV.

USE I *To make any regular Polygon, whofe Area fhall be of a given Magnitude*

LET it be required to find the Length of one of the Sides of a regular Pentagon, whofe fuperficial Area fhall be 125 Feet, and from thence to make the Polygon

Having extracted the fquare Root of ⅕ Part of 125 (becaufe the Figure is to have 5 Sides) which Root will be 5, make the Square A B, whofe Side let be 5 Feet then by means of the Line of Polygons (as directed by our Author in *U S E* I of the Line of Polygons) upon any Fig. 25. right Line, as C D, make the Ifofceles Triangle C G D fo, that C G, being the Semi-diameter of a Circle, C D may be the Side of a regular Pentagon infcribed in it, and let fall the
T
Perpendicular

Perpendicular G E   Now continuing the Lines E G, and E C, make E F equal to the Si of
the Square A B, and from the Point F, draw the right Line F H parallel to G C, then a mean
Proportional between G E, and E F, will be equal to half the Side of the Polygon fought,
which doubled, will give the whole Side   Now having found the Length of the whole Side,
you must, upon the Line expressing its Length, make a Pentagon, (as directed by our Author
in USE II of the Line of Polygons) which will have the required Magnitude

Fig 26

USE II   *A Circle being given, to find the Side of a Square equal to it*

Let E F be the Diameter of the given Circle, which divide into 14 equal Parts, by means of
the Line of Lines (as directed by our Author in the Use of the Line of equal Parts) then E P,
which is 12 4 of those Parts, will be the Side of the Square fought.

Note, 12 4 is the square Root of 11 × 14

Fig. 27.

USE III   *A Square being given, to find the Diameter of a Circle equal to it*

Let A B be one Side of the given Square, which divide into 11 equal Parts, by means of
the Line of Lines on the Sector, then continue the said Side, so that A G may be 12 4, that
is, 14 of those Parts more, and the Line A G, will be the Diameter of a Circle, equal to the
Square whose Side is A B

Fig. 28.

USE IV   *The transverse and conjugate Diameters of an Ellipsis being given, to find the Side of a Square equal to it*

Let A B, and C D, be the transverse and conjugate Diameters of an Ellipsis first, find a
mean Proportional between the transverse and conjugate Diameters, which let be the Line
E F, then divide the said Line E F, into 14 equal Parts, 12 and $\frac{2}{8}$ of which, will be E G,
the Side of the Square equal to the aforesaid Ellipsis

Fig. 29.

USE V.   *To find the Magnitude of two right Lines which shall be in a given Ratio, about which, an Ellipsis being described, in taking them for the transverse and conjugate Diameters, the Area of the said Ellipsis, may be equal to a given Square*

Let the given Proportion that the transverse and conjugate Diameters are to have, be as
2 to 1 ; then divide the Side A B of the given Square, into 11 equal Parts   Now as 2 is to
1, (the Terms of the given Proportion) so is 11 × 14 = 154 to a fourth Number, the square
Root of which being extracted, will be a Number to which, if the Line A G is taken equal,
(supposing one of those 11 Parts the Side of the Square is divided into, to be Unity) the said
Line A G, will be the conjugate Diameter fought.   Then to find the transverse Diameter,
fay, as 1 is to 2, so is the conjugate Diameter A G, to the transverse Diameter fought.
To work the first of the said Proportions by the Line of Lines on the Sector, set 1 over as a
Parallel on 2, then the parallel Extent of 154 taken, and laterally measured on the Line of
Lines, will give 77, the fourth Proportional fought   In the same manner may the latter
Proportion be worked

Fig. 30.

USE VI   *To describe an Ellipsis, by having the transverse and conjugate Diameters given.*

Let A B, and E D, be the given Diameters   take the Extent A C, or C B, between your
Compasses, and to that Extent, open the Legs of the Sector so, that the Distance between
90 and 90 of the Line of Sines, may be equal to it.   then may the Line A C be divided into
a Line of Sines, by taking the parallel Extents of the Sine of each Degree, on the Legs of the
Sector, between your Compasses, and laying them off from the Center C, the Line A C being divided into a Line of Sines (I have only divided it into the Sine of every 10 Degrees)
from every of them raise Perpendiculars both ways   Now to find Points in the said Perpendiculars, thro which the Ellipsis must pass, take the Extent of the semi-conjugate Diameter
C E, between your Compasses, and then open the Sector so, that the Points of 90 and 90,
on the Lines of Sines of the Sector, may be at that Distance from each other   This being
done, take the parallel Sines of each Degree, of the Lines of Sines of the Sector, and lay
them off, on those Perpendiculars drawn thro their Complements, in the Line of Sines A C,
both ways from the said Line A C, and you will have two Points in each of the Perpendiculars thro which the Ellipsis must pass

As for Example, the Sector always remaining at the same Opening, take the Distance from
80 to 80, on the Lines of Sines, between your Compasses, and setting one Foot in the Point
10, on the Line A C, with the other make the Points a and b, in the Perpendicular passing
thro that Point   then the Points a and b, will be the two Points in the said Perpendicular,
thro which the Ellipsis must pass   All the other Points, in this manner, being found, if they
are joined by an even Hand, there will be described the Semi-Ellipsis D A E   In the same
manner may the other half of the Ellipsis be described

Fig. 31.

USE VII   *The Bearings of three Towers, standing at A B C, to each other being given, that is, the Angles A B C, B C A, and C A B, and also the Distances of each of them from a fourth Tower standing between them, as at D, being given, that is, B D, D C, and A D being given.*

to find the Distances of the Towers at A B C from each other, that is, to find the Length of the Sides A B, B C, A C, of the Triangle A B C.

Having drawn the Triangle E F G similar to A B C, divide the Side E G in the Point H, F so that E H may be to H G, as A D is to D C, which may be done by taking the Sum of the Lines A D and D C between your Compasses, and setting that Extent over as a Parallel on the Line of Lines of the Sector, upon the Side E G of the Triangle, laterally taken on the Line of Lines, for then the parallel Extent of A D will give the Length of E H, and consequently the Point H will be had.

In like manner must the Side E F (or F G) be divided so in I, that E I may be to I F, as A D is to D B (or F G must be so divided, that the Segments must be as B D to D C.)

Again, having continued out the Sides E G, E F, say, As E H — H G is to H G, so is E H + H G to G K, and as E I — I F is to I F, so let E I + I F be to F M, which Proportions may easily be worked by the Line of Lines on the Sector. This being done, bisect H K and I M, in the Points L N, and about the said Points, as Centers, and with the Distances L H and I N describe two Circles intersecting each other in the Point O, to which, from the Angles E F G, draw the right Lines E O, F O, and O G, which will have the same Proportion to each other, as the Lines A D, B D, D C. Now if the Lines E O, F O, and G O are equal to the given Lines A D, B D, D C, the Distances E F, F G, and E G, will be the Distances of the Towers sought. But if E O, O F, O G are lesser than A D, D B, D C, continue them out so, that P O, O R, and O Q be equal to them, then the Points P, Q, R being joined, the Distances P R, R Q, and P Q will be the Distances of the Towers sought. Lastly, if the Lines E O, O F, O G, are greater than A D, D B, D C, cut off from them Lines equal to A D, B D, D C, and join the Points of Section by three right Lines, then the Distances of the said three right Lines, will be the sought Distances of the three Towers.

Note, If E H be equal to H G, or E I to I F, the Centers L and N, of the Circles, will be infinitely distant from H and I, that is, in the Points H and I there must be two Perpendiculars raised to the Sides E F, E G, instead of two Circles, till they intersect each other. But if E H be lesser than H G, the Center L will fall on the other Side of the Base E G continued, understand the same of E I, I F.

USE VIII. *To project the Sphere Orthographically upon the Plane of the Meridian.*

Let the Radius of the Meridian Circle, upon which the Sphere is to be projected, be A E; *Plate 8* then divide the Circumference of the said Circle into four equal Parts in E, P, Æ, S, and *Fig. 1.* draw the Diameters E Æ, P S, the former of which will represent the Equator, and the latter P S, the Hour-Circle of 6, as also the Axis of the World, P being the North-Pole, and S the South Pole. Then must each Quarter of the Meridian be divided into 90 Degrees, by making the Extent from 60 to 60 of the Lines of Chords, on the Sector, equal to the Radius of the Meridian Circle, and taking the parallel Extent of every Degree, and laying them off from the Equator towards the Poles, in which if 23 Deg. 30 Min. be numbered, (*viz.* the Sun's greatest Declination) from E to ♋ Northwards, and from Æ to ♑ Southwards, the Line drawn from ♋ to ♑ will be the Ecliptick, and the Lines drawn Parallel to the Equator, thro ♋ and ♑, will be the Tropicks.

Now if each Semidiameter of the Ecliptick be divided into Lines of Sines (by making the Distance of the Points of 90 and 90, on the Lines of Sines of the Sector, equal to either of the Semidiameters, and taking out the parallel Extent of each Degree, and laying them off both ways from the Center A) the first 30 Degrees, from A towards ♋, will stand for the Sign *Aries*, the 30 Degrees next following for *Taurus*, the rest for ♊, ♌, ♍, &c in their Order.

If, again, A P, A S, are divided into Lines of Sines, and have the Numbers 10, 20, 30, &c. to 90 set to them, the Lines drawn thro each of these Degrees, parallel to the Equator, will represent the Parallels of Latitude, and shew the Sun's Declination.

If, moreover, A E, A Æ, are divided into Lines of Sines, and also the Parallels, and then there is a Line carefully drawn thro each 15 Degrees, the Lines so drawn will be *Elliptical,* and will represent the Hour-Circles, the Meridian P E S the Hour of 12 at Noon, that next to it, drawn thro 75 Degrees from the Center, the Hours of 11 and 1, that which is drawn thro 60 Degrees from the Center, the Hours of 10 and 2, &c.

Then with respect to the Latitude, you may number it from E, Northwards, towards Z, and there place the Zenith, (that is, make the Arc E Z 51 Deg. 32 Min for *London,*) thro which, and the Center, the Line Z A N being drawn, will represent the vertical Circle passing thro the Zenith and Nadir East and West, and the Line M A H, crossing it at right Angles, will represent the Horizon. These two being divided, like the Ecliptick and Equator, the Lines drawn thro each Degree of the Radius A Z, parallel to the Horizon, will represent the Circles of Altitude, and the Divisions in the Horizon, and its Parallels will give the Azimuths, which will be Ellipses.

Lastly, If thro 18 Degrees in A N, be drawn a right Line I K, parallel to the Horizon, it will show the Time of Day-breaking, and the End of Twilight. For an Example of this Projection, let the Place of the Sun be the last Degree of ♉, the Parallel passing thro this Place is L D, and therefore the Meridian Altitude will be M L, the Depression below the

Horizon

Horizon at Midnight H D, the femidiurnal Arc L C, the feminoćturnal Arc C D, the Declination A b, the afcenfional Difference b C, the Amplitude of Afcenfion A C. The Difference between the End of Twilight, and the Break of Day, is very fmall, for the Sun's Parallel hardly croffes the Line of Twilight

If the Sun's Altitude be given, let a Line be drawn for it parallel to the Horizon, fo it fhall crofs the Parallel of the Sun, and there fhew both the Azimuth and the Hour of the Day As fuppofe the Place of the Sun being given, as before, the Altitude in the Morning was found, 25 Degrees, the Line F G, drawn parallel to the Horizon thro 20 Degrees in A Z, would crofs the Parallel of the Sun in ☉, wherefore F ☉ fhews the Azimuth, and L ☉ the Quantity of the Hour from the Meridian, which is about half an Hour paft 6 in the Morning, and about half a Point from the Eaft. The Diftance of two Places may be alfo fhewn by this Projection, in having their Latitudes and Difference of Longitude given

For fuppofe a Place in the Eaft of *Arabia* hath 20 Degrees of North Latitude, whofe Difference of Longitude from *London*, by an Eclipfe, is found to be five Hours and an half : Let Z be the Zenith of *London*, and the Parallel of Latitude for that other Place be L D, in which the Difference of Longitude is L ☉, wherefore ☉ reprefenting the Pofition of that Place, draw thro ☉ a Parallel to the Horizon M H, croffing the vertical A Z about 70 Degrees from the Zenith › which multiplied by 69, the Number of Miles in a Degree, gives 4830 Miles, the Diftance of that Place from *London*

USE IX *To project the Sphere Stereographically upon the Plane of the Horizon, fuppofe for the Latitude of 51 Degrees, 32 Minutes*

Fig 2

Draw a Circle of any Magnitude at pleafure, as N E, S W, reprefenting the Horizon, in which draw the two Diameters, W E, N S, croffing one another at right Angles, which will be the Reprefentations of two great Circles of the Sphere croffing each other at right Angles in the Zenith   Let N reprefent the North, E the Eaft, S the South, and W the Weft Part of the Horizon

Note, In all thefe Projections, the Eye is commonly fuppofed to be in the Under-pole of the primitive Circle, projecting that Hemifphere which is oppofed to the Eye, which will all fall within the primitive Circle, but that Hemifphere in which the Eye is, will all fall without the primitive Circle, and will run out in an infinite annular Plane, in the Plane of the Projection, and confequently cannot all of it be projected by Scale and Compafs

I. But now let us begin with projecting the Equinoctial   And here we muft firft determine the Line of Meafures, in which the Center of this Circle will be, and this will be done by determining in what Points a Plane, perpendicular to the primitive Circle, will cut the Horizon, whether in the North and South, Eaft and Weft, or in what other intermediate Points fuch a Plane fhall cut it   The Pole of the World, in this Projection, is elevated 51 Deg 32 Min and confequently the Equinoctial, on the Northern Part of the Horizon, will fall below the Horizon, and it is the Southern Part which here muft be projected, or which will fall within the primitive Circle, that Plane, whofe Interfection with the Horizon fhall produce the Line of Meafures, will be the Plane of a Meridian paffing thro the North and South Parts of the Horizon   wherefore N S will be the Line of Meafures, in which the Center of the projected Equinoctial muft fall, and fince it is the Southern Part of the Equinoctial which we are to project, its Center will be towards the North

To find whereabouts in the Line of Meafures the faid Center will fall, you muft firft open the Legs of the Sector, fo that the Diftance from 45 Degrees to 45 Degrees, on the Lines of Tangents, is equal to the Radius of the primitive Circle, then take the parallel Extent of the Tangents of 38 Deg 28 Min the Height of the Equinoctial above the Plane of the Horizon, and lay it off from Z to n, and n will be the Center of the projected Equinoctial, and the Secant of the fame, 38 Deg 30 Min will give its Radius, with which the Circle W Q E muft be defcribed, which is the Reprefentation of that part of the Equinoctial which is above our Horizon, for the Latitude of 51 Deg 32 Min

II We will next project the Ecliptick, which being a great Circle of the Sphere, muft cut the Equinoctial at a Diameter's Diftance, that is, in E, W, the Eaft and Weft Points of the Horizon, and confequently will have the fame Line of Meafures with that of the Equinoctial, *viz* N S Now let us confider whether the Center of the Ecliptick falls towards the North, or towards the South of the Horizon, and this will eafily be determined, by confidering that the Equinoctial is elevated above the Southern Part of the Horizon 38 Deg 28 Min. and the Northern Part of the Ecliptick, or the Northern Signs, are elevated above the Equinoctial 23 Deg 30 Min which in all, make 62 Degrees, which is leffer than 90 Deg So that it muft fall towards the South, and confequently the Center muft be Northwards, and will be found, (the Sector remaining open as before) by fetting off the Tangent of 62 Deg from z to b, and the Secant of 62 Deg will give its Radius, with which the Circle W C E, the Reprefentation of the Northern half of the Ecliptick, muft be defcribed

The Southern Part of the Ecliptick is likewife, for the moft part, projected on the horizontal Projection, and made to fall within the primitive Circle, but this cannot be, the Globe remaining fixed for that part of the Ecliptick, which is below the Horizon, will be thrown out of the primitive Circle, fo that it cannot be projected, unlefs the Globe be fuppofed to be

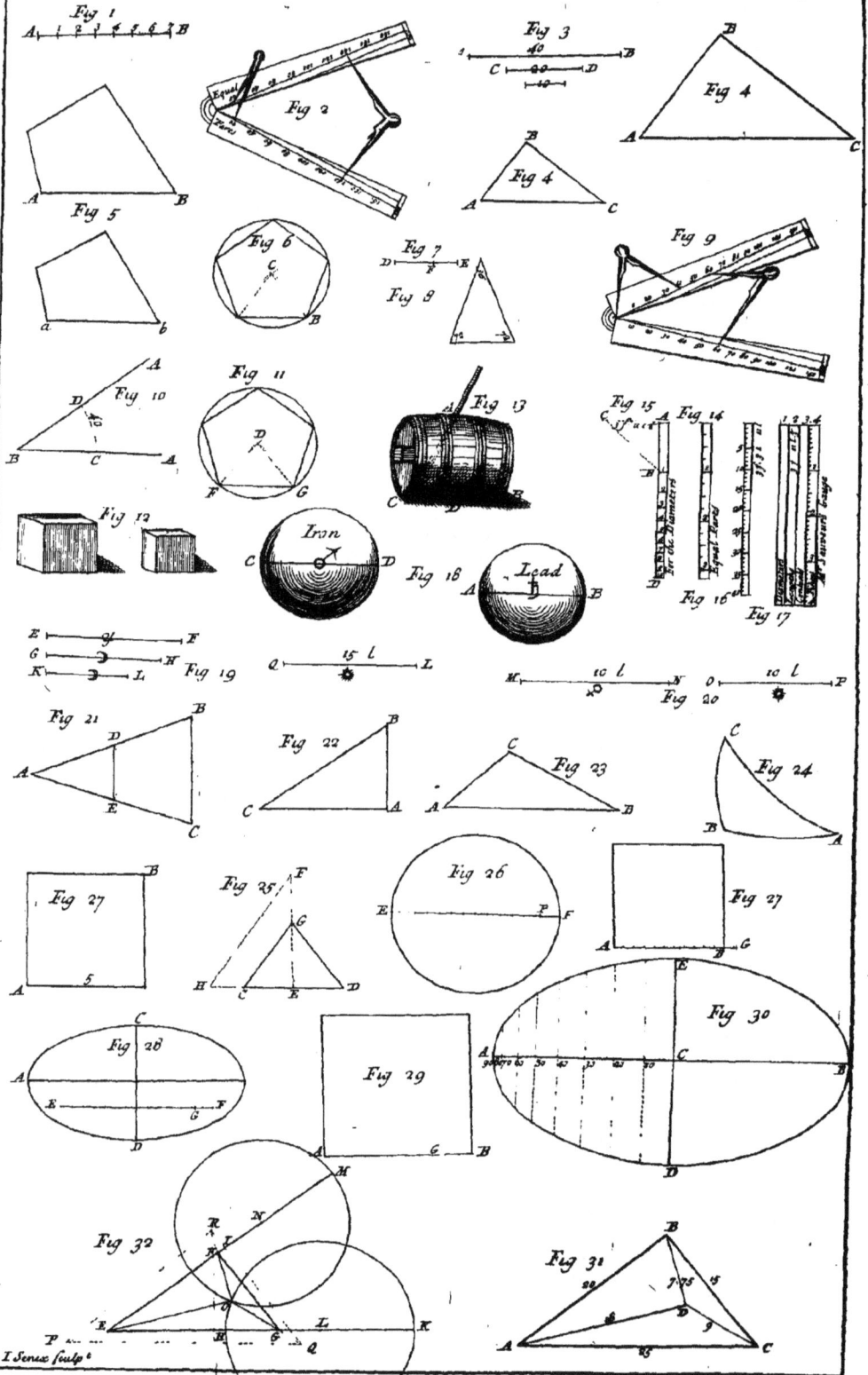

Plate VII

Fig 1

A · 1 2 3 4 5 6 · B

Fig 2

Fig 3
40
1 ———————————————————— B
C ——— 60 ——— D
—— 40 ——

Fig 4
B
A C

Fig 5
A B

Fig 6
C

Fig 7
D ——— E

Fig 8
B
A C

Fig 9

Fig 5
a b

Fig 10
A
D
B C A

Fig 11
D
F G

Fig 13
A
C B

Fig 15
G if act A
D

Fig 14
E

Fig 16

Fig 17
1 2 3 4

Fig 12

Iron
C D
Fig 18

Lead
A B

Fig 19
E ——— F
G ——— H
K ——— L

Q ——— 15 l ——— L

Fig 20
M ——— 10 l ——— N O ——— 10 l ——— P

Fig 21
D B
A
E
C

Fig 22
B
C A

Fig 23
C
A B

Fig 24
C
B A

Fig 27
B
A 5

Fig 25
F
G
H C E D

Fig 26
E F

Fig 27
C
A G

Fig 28
C
A
E F
D

Fig 29
B
G

Fig 30
E
A C B
D

Fig 32
M
N
R
L
P E H G Q L K

Fig 31
B
A C

I Senex Sculpt

be turned round, and by that means the Southern Part of the Ecliptick to be brought above the Horizon, but fuch a Revolution of the Sphere, where it makes any Alteration, is fcarce allowable however, I fhall fhew how it is ufually projected

The fame Line of Meafures N S remains ftill, and the Circle muft fall to the South, and confequently its Center to the North of the Horizon, therefore nothing remains but to find its Elevation above the Horizon. The Northern Part of the Eclyptick falls 23 Deg. 30 Min. nearer the Zenith than the Equinoctial does, therefore the Southern Part, being brought above the Horizon, muft be 23 Deg. 30 Min. nearer the Horizon than the Equinoctial fo that 23 Deg. 30 Min. being taken from 38 Deg. 28 Min. there remains 15 Deg. for the Diftance of that part of the Eclyptick above the Horizon. It will be reprefented by W e E, which is defcribed by fetting off the Tangent of 15 Degrees for the Center, and taking the Secant of the fame for the Radius

III. N S produced will alfo be the Line of Meafures for all Parallels of Declination, and Parallels of Latitude for the Poles of leffer Circles being the fame as thofe of the great Circles, to which they are parallel, it is manifeft that the fame Plane, which is at right Angles to the Equinoctial and Horizon, will alfo be at right Angles to all leffer Circles parallel to the Equinoctial, and the fame will hold as to Circles parallel to the Eclyptick. But N S is the Line of Meafures of the Equinoctial and Eclyptick, and confequently muft be the Line of Meafures of all Circles parallel to either of them, therefore the Centers of fuch leffer Circles will be in N S produced, if there be Occafion. Now to project them, for Inftance, the Tropick of Cancer, confider, in this Pofition of the Sphere, what will be its neareft and greateft Diftance from the Zenith, or the Pole of the primitive Circle, which you will find to be 28 Degrees, for the Equinoctial being elevated 38 Deg. 28 Min. above the Horizon, and the Tropick of *Cancer* being 23 Deg. 30 Min. from the Equinoctial, which, being added together, gives 62 Deg. which fubftracted from 90 Deg. leaves 28 Deg. its Diftance from the Zenith on the South-fide of the Horizon, therefore the Half-Tangent of 28 Deg. or the Tangent of 14 Deg. fet from Z to C, will give one Extremity of its projected Diameter. Then the Diftance from the Zenith to the Pole, being 38 Deg. 28 Min. and from the Pole to the Tropick of *Cancer* 66 Deg. 30 Min. the Sum of thefe, viz. 104 Deg. 58 Min. will be its greateft Diftance from the Zenith, the Half-Tangent of which, fet from Z to a, will give the other Extremity of its projected Diameter. therefore having got C a the Diameter, bifect it, and defcribe the Circle ♋ C ♋

The Tropick of *Capricorn* may be defcribed in the fame manner. for the Diftance of the Equinoctial and the Zenith being 51 Deg. 32 Min. if to this be added 23 Deg. 30 Min. you will have 55 Deg. 2 Min. equal to the neareft Diftance of the Tropick of *Capricorn*, on the South-fide of the Horizon, the Half-Tangent of which being fet from Z to e, will give one Extremity of its Diameter. Then the Diftance between the Zenith and the Pole, viz. 38 Deg. 28 Min. and the Diftance between the Pole and the Equinoctial, which is 90 Deg. and the Diftance between the Equinoctial and the Tropick of *Capricorn*, which is 23 Deg. 30 Min. being all added together, will give the greateft Diftance of the Tropick of *Capricorn*, from the Zenith, viz. 152 Deg. 2 Min. the Semi-tangent of which being fet from Z towards the North, will give the other Extremity of the Diameter. Bifect the Diameter found in e, and defcribe the Circle ♑ C ♑, which is the Reprefentation of fo much of the Tropick of *Capricorn*, as falls within the primitive Circle

IV. The Polar Circle is 23 Deg. 30 Min. from the Pole, but the Pole being elevated, on the North-fide the Horizon, 51 Deg. 32 Min. and 51 Deg. 32 Min. added to 23 Deg. 30 Min. whofe Sum is 75 Deg. 2 Min. is leffer than 90 Deg. fo that it does not pafs beyond the Zenith, therefore 75 Deg. 2 Min. taken from 90 Deg. leaves 15 Deg. which is the neareft Diftance of the Polar Circle from the Zenith. And the Half-Tangent of 15 Deg. fet from Z to v, will give one Extremity of its projected Diameter, and then 15 Deg. added to 47 Deg. equal to 62 Deg. will be its greateft Diftance from the Zenith. the Half-Tangent of which Diftance, fet from Z to P, will give the other Extremity of its projected Diameter, fo that its Diameter v p being found, it is but bifecting it, and the Circle may be defcribed

V. I fhall now fhew how to project the Hour-Circles. And, Firft, a Line of Meafures muft be determined, in which their Centers fhall be, if poffible, but you may eafily difcover it impoffible for one Line of Meafures to ferve them all. for they are differently inclined to the Horizon, and fo the Plane of no one great Circle can be at right Angles to the Horizon and all the Hour-Circles, therefore the Plane of a great Circle at right Angles to the Horizon, and one of them, muft be found which is poffible, becaufe the Hour-Circles being all at right Angles to the Plane of the Equinoctial, their Poles will be all found in this Circle, but the Poles of all great Circles, being 90 Degrees diftant from their Planes, the Hour-Circle of 12, and the Hour-Circle of 6, muft of neceffity pafs thro each other's Poles, and fo will be at right Angles to one another · But the Hour-Circle of 12 is at right Angles to the Horizon, and interfects it in N S, therefore the Line N S will be the Line of Meafures, in which the Center of the Hour-Circle of 6 will be, and its Center will be towards the South-Parts of the Horizon, becaufe all the Hour-Circles pafs thro the Pole which falls towards the North, the Elevation of this Circle above the Horizon being the fame with that

U   of of the Pole, *viz* 51 Deg 32 Min. then take the Tangent of 51 Deg 32 Min and set it from Z to K , and upon the Center K, and with the Secant of the fame Elevation, defcribe W P E, which is the Circle required

The Point P, where N S, W E, interfect one another, is the Reprefentation of the Pole of the World ; for N S being the Reprefentation of the Hour-Circle of 12, the projected Pole muft be fomewhere in this Line , but it muft be fomewhere in W E, which is likewife the Projection of an Hour-Circle : therefore it muft be in that Point where thefe two projected Circles interfect one another, that is, in the Point P , P is the Point thro which all the Hour-Circles muft pafs in the Projection

In order to draw the reft of the Hour-Circles, we muft have recourfe to a *Secondary* Line of Meafures, which may thus be determined : To P K, at the Point K, erect D B at right Angles, and produce the Circle W P E, till it meet the Line D B, in the Points D and B, and the Line D B will be the fecondary Line of Meafures in which the Centers of all the Hour-Circles will be found , for let the Hour-Circle of 6, D P B, be confidered as the primitive Circle, in whofe Under-Pole (which will be in the Equinoctial) K, let the Eye be placed , then D B will be the Reprefentation of the Equinoctial, for it paffing thro the Eye will be projected into a right Line . but the Equinoctial is at right Angles to the Hour-Circles, both the primitive and all the reft ; therefore it will be the fecondary Line of Meafures, upon this Suppofition, upon which will be all their Centers In order to find which, fet the Sector to the Radius P K, then take off parallel-wife the Tangents of 15 Deg 30 Deg 45 Deg the Elevations of the Hour-Circles above the Hour-Circle at 6, and fet them both ways, from K to *r*, from K to *s*, from K to *t*, &c. then upon thofe Centers, and with the Secants of the fame Elevations, defcribe the Circles P P, P Q, and P T, which will be the Hour-Circles , for they are all great Circles of the Sphere, paffing thro the Pole P, and make Angles with one another of 15 Deg or are 15 Deg diftant from each other and the Portions of thofe Circles which fall within the primitive Circle N E S W, as H P *h*, are the Reprefentations of thofe Halves of the Hour-Circle, which are above our Horizon in our Latitude

VI. In like manner the Circles of Longitude may be drawn, by determining the fecondary Line of Meafures R S, in which all their Centers will be , and this Line will be determined after the fame manner with D B above, and the Circles of Longitude drawn as before the Meridians were drawn · for the Line N S will be the Line of Meafures, with refpect to one of them paffing thro E and W, the Eaft and Weft Points of the Horizon In order to draw this Circle, confider its Elevation above the Horizon, which will be found by confidering the Diftance of the Pole of the Ecliptick, from the Pole of the World, which will be 28 Deg. 2 Min the Elevation of this Circle above the Horizon Set the Tangent of 28 Deg 2 Min. from Z to Q, and with the Secant of the fame Diftance, defcribe the Circle W *p* E, to *p* Q, at the Point Q, erect R S at right Angles, which will be the fecondary Line of Meafures. In this Line from Q (the Sector being fet to *p* Q) fet off the Tangents of 24 Deg. 40 Deg according to the Number of Circles you have a Defire to draw, from Q to *x*, from Q to *y*, &c. and with the Secants of 20 Deg. 40 Deg. &c defcribe the Circles of Longitude, M P *m*, &c

VII The Reprefentations of Azimuths, in this Projection, will be all right Lines, and any Number of them may be drawn, making any affigned Angles with one another, if the Limb be divided into its Degrees by help of the Sector, and thro thefe Degrees be drawn Diameters to the primitive Circle

VIII. All Parallels of Altitude, in this Projection, will be Circles parallel to the primitive Circle, and may be eafily drawn, by dividing a Radius of the primitive Circle, into Half-Tangents, and defcribing upon the Center Z, thro the Points of Divifion, concentrick Circles I fhall omit drawing of them, left the Scheme be too much perplexed

USE X *To project the Sphere Stereographically upon the Plane of the Solftitial Colure for the Horizon of 51 Deg 32 Min.*

Fig 3.

Draw the Circle H B O C, reprefenting the primitive Circle ; and the Diameter H O, reprefenting the Horizon · Set off the Chord of 51 Deg. 32 Min. from O to P, having firft fet the Sector to the Radius of the Circle, which will give the Polar Point, and draw the Diameter P *p*, reprefenting the Hour-Circle of 6

I. The Equinoctial may be reprefented, by drawing the Diameter E Q at right Angles to the Diameter P *p*.

II Set off 23 Deg. 30 Min from the Chords, from E to ♋, and from Q to ♑, which will reprefent the Ecliptick

III. The Tropicks of *Cancer* and *Capricorn* may be drawn thus : Take the Secant of 66 Deg. 30 Min the Diftance of each of them from their refpective Poles, and fet it both ways, from the Center A in P *p* produced, which will give the two Points *e e* the Centers of the two Circles, and their Radii will be the Tangents of the fame, 66 Deg 30 Min.

IV. The Polar Circles, as alfo all other Parallels of Declination, may be drawn in the fame manner

V The Line of Meafures for the Azimuths will be H O, and the Line of Meafures for the Almacanters will be B C

VI

VI. ♋, ♑, or the Ecliptick, will be the Line of Measures for the Circles of Longitude, and the Line of Measures for the Circles of Latitude will be N S, all of which may be easily drawn from what is said in the precedent Use

VII The Ecliptick may be divided into its proper Signs in this Projection, by setting off the Tangents of 15 Deg. 30 Deg. 45 Deg both ways from A.

USE XI   *To draw the Hour-Lines upon an erect direct South Plane, as also on an Horizontal Plane*

First, draw the indefinite right Line C C, for the Horizon and Equator, and cross it at right Angles in the Point A, about the middle of the Line, with the indefinite right Line A B, serving for the Meridian, and the Hour Line of 12 then take out 15 Deg from the Line of Tangents, on the Sector (the Sector being set to a parallel Radius lesser than the Extent from 45 Deg. to 45 Deg of the lesser Lines of Tangents, when the Sector is quite opened) and lay them off in the Equator on both Sides from A, and one Point will serve for the Hour of 11, and the other for the Hour of 1.   Again, take out the Tangent of 30 Deg (the Sector being opened to the same Radius) and lay it off on both Sides the Point A in the Equator, and one of these Points will serve one for the Hour of 10, and the other for the Hour of 2 In the same manner, lay off the Tangent of 45 Deg for the Hours of 9 and 3, the Tangent of 60 Deg for the Hours of 8 and 4, and the Tangent of 75 Deg for the Hours of 7 and 5. But note, because the greater Tangents on the Sector run but to 45 Deg therefore you must set the parallel Radius of the lesser Tangents, when you come above 45 Deg to the Extent of the Radii of the greater Tangents

Now if you have a mind to set down the Parts of an Hour, you must allow 7 Deg 30 Min for every half Hour, and 3 Deg 45 Min. for one quarter This done, you must consider the Latitude of the Place in which the Plane is, which suppose 51 Deg. 30 Min. then if you take the Secant of 51 Deg 32 Min off from the Sector, it remaining opened to the parallel Radius of the lesser Tangents, and set it off from A to V, this Point V will be the Center of the Plane, and if you draw from V, right Lines to 11, 10, 9, &c. and the rest of the Hour Points, they will be the required Hour Lines.

But if it happen, that some of these Hour Points fall out of the Plane, you may thus remedy yourself, by means of the larger Tangents

At the Hour Points of 3 and 9, draw occult Lines parallel to the Meridian ; then the Distances D C, between the Hour-Line of 6, and the Hour Points of 3 and 9, will be equal to the Semi-diameter A V ; and if they be divided in the same manner as the Line A C is divided, you will have the Points of 4, 5, 7, and 8, with their Halves and Quarters.

For take out the Semi-diameter A V, and make it a parallel Radius, by fitting it over in the Tangents of 45 and 45 , then take the parallel Tangent of 15 Deg and it will give the Distance from 6 to 5, and from 6 to 7 The Sector remaining thus opened, take out the parallel Tangent of 30 Deg. and it will give the Distance from 6 to 4, and from 6 to 8 : the like may be done for Halves and Quarters of Hours

The Hour Points may be otherwise denoted thus : Having drawn a right Line for the Equator, as before, and assumed the Point A for the Hour of 12, cut off two equal Lines A 10, and A 2 then upon the Distance between 10 and 2, make an equilateral Triangle, and you will have B for the Center of the Equator, and the Line A B, will give the Distance from A to 9, and from A to 3 This done, take out the Distance between 9 and 3, and this will give the Distance from B to 8, and from 8 to 7, and from 8 to 1 and again, from B to 4, and from 4 to 5, and from 4 to 11, so have you the Hour Points and if you take out the Distances B 1, B 3, B 5, &c the Points may be found not only for the Half-Hours, but for the Quarters

In the same manner are the Hour Lines drawn on a Horizontal Plane, only with this Difference, that A H is the Secant of the Complement of the Latitude, and the Hour Lines of 4, 5, 7, 8, are continued thro the Center

USE XII   *To draw the Hour Lines upon a Polar Plane, as also on a Meridional Plane.*

In a Polar Plane, the Equator may be also the same with the Horizonal Plane, and the Hour Points may be denoted as before, in the last Use but the Hour Lines must be drawn parallel to the Meridian

In a Meridional Plane, the Equator will make an Angle with the Horizontal Line, equal to the Complement of the Latitude of the Place, then may you assume the Point A, and there cross the Equator with a right Line, which will serve for the Hour Line of 6 : then the Tangent of 15 Deg. being laid off in the Equator on both Sides from 6, will give the Hour Points of 5 and 7 , and the Tangent of 30 Deg. the Hour Points of 8 and 4 , the Tangent of 45 Deg the Hour Points of 3 and 9 , the Tangent of 60 Deg the Hour Points of 2 and 10 . and lastly, the Tangent of 75 Deg will give the Hour Points of 1 and 11 ; and if right Lines are drawn thro these Hour Points, crossing the Equator at right Angles, these shall be the Hour Lines required.

USE

USE XIII. *To draw the Hour Lines upon a vertical declining Plane.*

Fig. 6

Firſt draw A V the Meridian, and A E the Horizontal Line, croſſing one another in the Point A, then take out A V, the Secant of the Latitude of the Place, which ſuppoſe 51 De 32 Min and prick it down on the Meridian from A to V. Now becauſe the Plane declines, which ſuppoſe 40 Deg Eaſtward, you muſt make an Angle of the Declination upon the Cen ter A, below the Horizontal Line, on the left Side of the Meridian, becauſe the Plane declines Eaſtwards, for if it had declined Weſtward, the ſaid Angle muſt have been made on the right Side of the Meridian. This being done, take A H, the ſecant Complement of the Latitude, out of the Sector, and prick it down in the Line of Declination from A to H, as was done for the Semi-diameter in the Horizontal Plane · then draw an indefinite right Line thro the Point A, perpendicular to A H, which will make an Angle, with the Horizontal Line, equal to the Plane's Declination, and will be as the Equator in the Horizontal Plane. Again, take the Hour Points out of the Tangents, as in the laſt Problem, and prick them down in this Equator on both Sides, from the Hour of 12 at A, then lay your Ruler, and draw right Lines thro the Center H, and each of theſe Hour Points, and you will have all the Hour Lines of an Horizontal Plane, except the Hour of 6, which is drawn thro H perpendicular to H A. Laſtly, you muſt note the Interſections that theſe Hour Lines make with A E, the Ho rizontal Line of the Plane, and then if right Lines are drawn thro the Center V, and each of theſe Interſections, they will be the Hour Lines required.

The Hour Points may be pricked down otherwiſe, thus. Take out the Secant of the Plane's Declination, and prick it down in the Horizontal Line from A to E, and thro E draw right Lines parallel to the Meridian, which will cut the former Hour Lines of 3 or 9, in the Point C; then take out the Semi-diameter A V, and prick it down in thoſe Parallels from C to D, and draw right Lines from A to C, and from V to D, the Line V D will be the Hour of 6 and if you divide thoſe Lines A C, D C, in the ſame manner as D C is divided in the Horizontal Plane, the Hour Points required will be had.

Or you may find the Point D, in the Hour of 6, without knowing either H or C, for ha ving pricked down A V in the Meridian Line, and A E in the Horizontal Line, and drawn Parallels to the Meridian thro the Points at E, take the Tangent of the Latitude out of the Sector, and fit it over in the Sines of 90 Deg. and 90 Deg and the parallel Sine of the Plane's Declination, meaſured in the ſame Tangent Line, will there ſhew the Complement of the Angle D V A, which the Hour Line of 6 makes with the Meridian then having the Point D, take out the Semi-diameter V A, and prick it down in thoſe Parallels from D to C, ſo ſhall you have the Lines D C, A C, to be divided, as before.

Thus have you the Uſe of the Sector apply'd in reſolving ſeveral uſeful Problems. I might have laid down many more Problems in all the practical Parts of Mathematicks, wherein this Inſtrument is uſeful, but what I, and our Author have ſaid of this Inſtrument, will, I believe, be ſufficient to ſhew Perſons ſkill'd in the ſeveral practical Parts of Mathematicks, the Manner of uſing this Inſtrument therein.

For the Uſes of the Lines of Numbers, Artificial Sines, and Tangents, as alſo the Lines of Latitude, Hours, and Inclination of Meridians, *See* U S E S *of* Gunter's *Scale.*

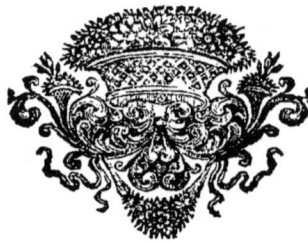

BOOK

Plate VIII   fronting page 76

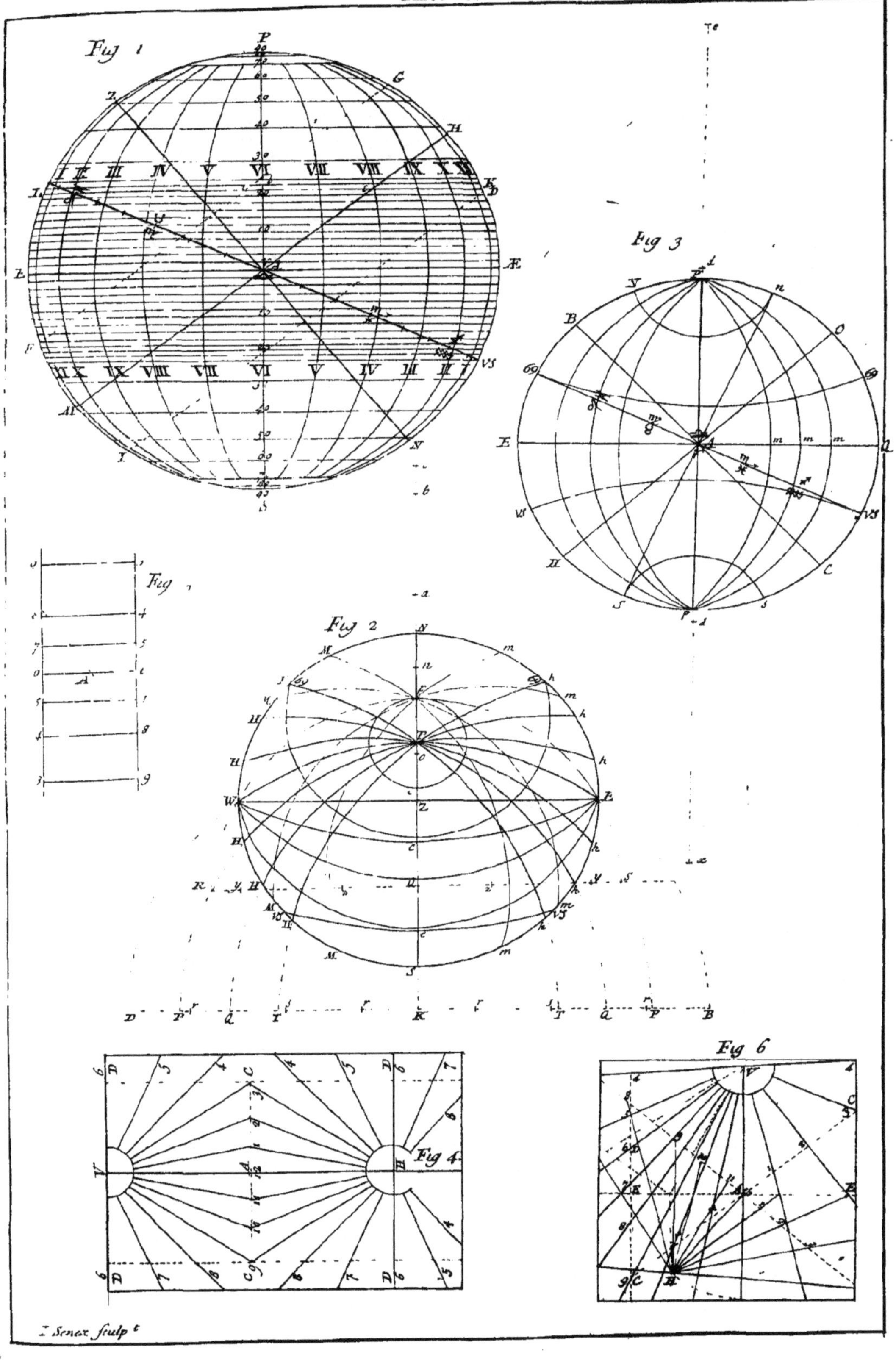

Fig 1

Fig 3

Fig 2

Fig 4

Fig 6

I. Senex sculp.

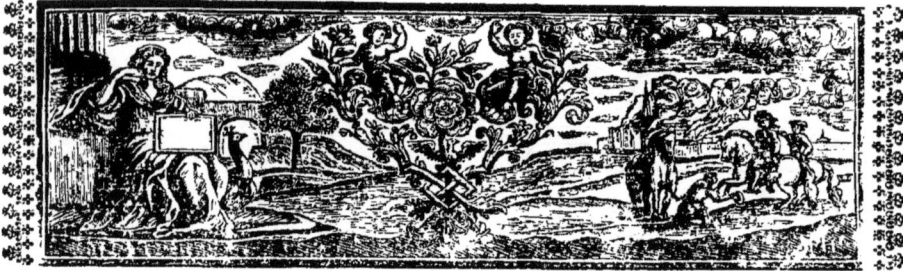

BOOK III.

Of the Construction and Use of several different Sorts of Compasses, and other Curious Instruments.

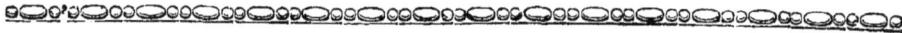

CHAP. I.

Of the Construction and Uses of several Sorts of Compasses.

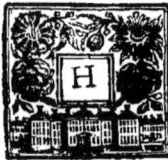

AVING already treated of Common Compasses, usually put into Cases of Instruments, we proceed now to mention some others, sometimes likewise placed in Cases of different Bignesses.

The Construction of Hair-Compasses

These Compasses are so called, because of a Contrivance in the Body of *Plate 9.* them, by means of which an Extent may be taken to a hair's Breadth. **Fig A.**

We have before hinted, that the Goodness of Compasses consists chiefly in having the Motion of their Head sufficiently easy, and that they open and shut very equally, and that they may do so, the Joints ought to be well-slit, and very equal in Thickness.

The Manner of constructing the Joints, is thus. We first, with a Steel-Saw, slit the Head in two Places, so that there remains a Middle-Piece, the Thickness of a Card, then we slit the other Leg of the Compasses, in the middle of the Joint, to receive the Middle-Piece which was reserved for that purpose, afterwards the Joints must be filed and straightned, so that they may be well joined every where. This being done, we drill a round Hole thorow the middle of the Head, in Bigness proportional to that of the Compasses, for the Rivet to go through, the Rivet ought to be very round, and exactly fill the aforesaid Hole When we have rivetted it, the Head of the Compasses must be warmed, and a little yellow Wax poured between the Joints, for lessening the Friction of the Legs in opening and shutting Lastly, we generally put upon the Head two turned Cheeks, serving for Counter-Rivets, and to preserve the Head.

The little Screw at the Bottom of the Body of these Hair-Compasses, is to move the Steel Point backwards or forwards, at pleasure this Point is fastened to the Top of the Compasses by two Rivets, so that in turning the Screw it springs The other Steel Point must be solder'd to the other Leg, as all other Points of Compasses are that are fixed Now to fit these Points for soldering, they must be filed so, as to go into two Slits made in the Bottom of the Body of the Compasses, that there they may be well joined, and the Solder strongly hold them

Note, Solder is commonly made with Silver and Thirds of Copper, that is, twice more Silver than Copper For Example, with one Dram of Silver, we mix half a Dram of Copper, which must be first melted in a Crucible, and afterwards, when cold, hammer'd to about the Thickness of a Card, and cut into small Pieces that it may the sooner run, when there is use for it. Solder is likewise often made with Copper and Zink mixed together, *viz.*

X

In

In melting ½ of Copper, with ⅓ of Zink. In foldering, we ufe Borax finely bruifed, which makes the Solder better run and penetrate the Joints, or any thing elfe to be foldered.

Of the German Compaffes.

Fig. B.

The Legs of thefe Compaffes are fomething bent, fo that, when fhut, the Points only touch each other. One Point of thefe Compaffes may be taken off, and others put on, by means of a fmall fquare Hole made in the Bottom of the Body, for the Points to go in, and a Screw to keep them faft when in: but thefe Points ought very well to fit the aforefaid fquare Hole, that they may not fhake.

The Points generally put on, are,

Firft, A Drawing-Pen Point, by means of which, Lines fine or coarfe may be drawn with Ink, by help of a little Screw near the Point of the Drawing-Pen. This Drawing-Pen Point, as well as the other Points to be put on, has a fmall Joint, almoft like the Head of a Pair of Compaffes, by means of which it may be kept perpendicular to the Paper, according as the Compaffes are more or lefs opened. This Point is reprefented by *Fig. 3*.

Secondly, A Porte-Craion Point, reprefented by *Fig. 2*, for drawing Lines with a Pencil.

And *Laftly*, a Dotting-Wheel Point, (*Fig. 1*) whofe Ufe is to make dotted Lines. What we call a Dotting-Wheel, is a little Wheel of Brafs, or other Metal, about 3 Lines in Diameter, round which is made little pointed Teeth. This Wheel is faftened between two little Pieces of Brafs by a fmall Pin, fo that it may freely turn round, almoft like a Spur; but the faid Teeth muft not be too far diftant from each other, becaufe then the Dots the Wheel makes, will alfo be too far diftant from each other.

The Conftruction of thefe Compaffes as to their Joints, &c. being the fame as thofe before fpoken of, I fhall only add, that fince the Beauty of Compaffes confifts very much in their being well polifhed; for this effect, we firft rub the Compaffes with Slate-Stone dipped in Water, then we rub every part of the Compaffes with a flat Stick of foft Wood, and a Mixture of Emery temper'd with Oil, or fine Tripoly. And laftly, we wipe the Compaffes clean with a Cloth or Piece of Shamoy.

Of the Spring-Compaffes.

Fig. C.

Thefe Compaffes are all made of tempered Steel, which are fo hard every where, that a File cannot touch them; and the Head of thefe Compaffes is rounded, that by its Spring it opens and fhuts itfelf: the Circular Screw fix'd to one of the Legs, ferves to open or fhut it, by means of a Nut. Thefe Compaffes are very fit to take fmall Lengths, and make fmall Divifions; yet they ought to be but fhort, and fo tempered, that they may have a good Spring, and not break.

Of the Clock-makers Compaffes.

Fig. D.

Thefe Compaffes, which are ftrong and folid, ferve to cut Paft-board, Brafs, and other the like things; the Quadrant croffing it, ferves ftrongly to fix it to a propofed Opening, by help of a Screw preffing againft it. The Nut at the End of the faid Quadrant, is to open or fhut the Compaffes at pleafure, in turning the faid Nut, which ought to be fo riveted to the Leg of the Compaffes, that it may make the other Leg move forwards or backwards. The Four Points ought to be made of well tempered Steel. That of *Fig. 1.* is filed flopewife, like a Graving-Tool, to cut Brafs; that of *Fig. 2* is like a pointed Button: and the two other Points are in figure of the fixed Points of common Compaffes, but they muft be very ftrong in proportion to the Compaffes.

There are different ways of tempering the Points of Compaffes, or other Pieces of Steel: For Example; the Points of fmall Compaffes are tempered by means of a Lamp, and a fmall Brafs Pipe: for blowing in the Pipe, caufes a ftrong lively Flame, in which putting the Points, or other Things, to be hardened, and they will become almoft inftantly red hot, and when they are cold, they will be very hard. But the Points of great Compaffes, and other Steel Tools, are tempered with a Charcoal Fire, by blowing thro the aforefaid Pipe, and heating them to a Cherry Colour, and afterwards putting them into Water, and then they will be render'd very hard.

Of the three-legg'd Compaffes.

Fig. E.

The Ufe of thefe Compaffes is to take three Points at once, and fo to form a Triangle, or to lay down three Pofitions of a Map to be copied at once, &c.

The Conftruction of thefe Compaffes doth not much differ from the Conftruction of the others, excepting only that the third Leg has a Motion every way, by means of a turned Rivet, riveted by one End to the two other Legs, and at the other End there muft be a turned Cheek, and a round Plate ferving for a Joint to the third Leg: the little Figure 1 fhows how the Rivet is made.

Of the Sea-Chart Compaffes.

Fig. F.

The Legs of thefe Compaffes are crooked, and widened towards the Head, fo that by preffing the two Legs with your Hand, you may open them. Their Conftruction fufficiently

appears

appears from the Figure, and their Use will be mentioned in the Instruments for Navigation.

Of the simple Proportional Compasses

These Compasses are used in dividing of Lines into 2, 3, 4, or 5 equal Parts, as also to re- Fig G. duce small Figures to greater ones, and contrariwise, &c You must take care in making these Compasses, that the Head be drill'd in a right Line with the Legs, and that the Points are not one forwarder than another Now if you have a mind to make one of these Pair of Compasses to take the ½ of a Line, the Distance from the Center of the Joint to the Ends of either of the longest Legs, must be twice the Length of either of the shortest Legs, and so in proportion for others *Note,* The Compasses of Figure G, are for dividing of Lines into 3 equal Parts, whence the Distance from the Center marked 5, to the Points 2, 2, is three times the Distance from the said Center, to the Points 3 or 4 so that if the third Part of the Line 2, 2, be required, its whole Length must first be taken between the longest Legs of the Compasses, which remaining thus opened, the Distance between the Points of the shortest Legs, will be ⅓ of the given Line

Of the moveable-headed Proportional Compasses

The Use of these proportional Compasses, is to divide a given Line into any Number of Fig H. equal Parts, as also to divide the Circumference of a Circle, so that a regular Polygon may be inscribed therein

These Compasses consist of two equal Legs, each of which is furnish'd with two Steel Points, and are hollow'd in, for a Cursor to slip up and down, in the middle of which Cursor, there is a Screw serving to join the Legs, and to fasten them in divers Places by means of a Nut but the Legs must be hollow'd in exactly in the middle of their Breadth, that so the Center of the Cursor may be in a right Line with the Points of the Legs, and the Cursor slide very exactly along the Legs as also the Head-Screw must exactly fill the Hole in the Cursor, so that nothing may shake when the Legs are fastened with the Nut

Figure 1, represents the Screw, Figure 2, the Nut, Figure 3, half the Cursor, which must be joined by a like half You may see by that little Figure, that there is a Piece in the middle left exactly to fit the Hollow of the Leg of the Compasses the shadow'd Spaces of the said Figure, are to contain the two Sides of the Leg; understand the same of the other half of the Cursor

Figure 1, is one of the Legs separate, upon which are the Divisions for equal Parts for upon one Side of one of the Legs, are the Divisions for dividing of Lines into equal Parts, and upon one Side of the other Leg, are denoted the Numbers shewing how to inscribe any regular Polygon in a proposed Circle.

Now to make the Divisions for dividing Lines into equal Parts, take a well divided Scale, or a Sector, which is better, because it is almost a universal Scale · then take the exact Length of one of the Legs of your proportional Compasses between your Compasses, and having opened the Sector, so that the Distance between 120 and 120 of the Line of Lines be equal to that Extent, take the Distance from 40 to 40, which lay off upon the Leg of your Compasses, and at the End thereof, set the Number 2, which will serve to divide any given Line into two equal Parts The Sector still continuing opened to the same Angle, take the Distance from 30 to 30, on the Line of equal Parts, and lay off upon the aforesaid Leg of the Compasses, where set down the Number 3, and that will give the Division for taking ¼ of any given Line Again, take 24 equal Parts, as before, from the Line of Lines, lay them off upon the Leg, and that will give the Division for dividing a Line into 4 equal Parts

Moreover, take 20 equal Parts, and that will give you the Division upon the Leg of the Compasses, serving to divide a Line into 5 equal Parts the same Opening of the Sector will still serve to divide a Line into 7, 9, and 11 equal Parts But to avoid Fractions, the aforesaid Opening must be chang'd, to make the Division of 6, 8, 10, and 12, upon the Leg but before the said Opening of the Sector be altered, take the Distance from 15 to 15, which will give the Divisions for dividing a Line into 7 equal Parts

Again, take 12, and that will give the Division for dividing a Line into 9 equal Parts, and lastly, the Distance from 10 to 10, will give the Division for dividing any Line into 11 equal Parts

But to make the Division for dividing a Line into 6 equal Parts, take between your Compasses the Length of one of the Legs of the proportional Compasses, and open the Sector so, that the Distance between 140 and 140, on each Line of equal Parts, be equal to the aforesaid Length The Sector remaining thus opened, take the Distance from 20 to 20, on each Line of equal Parts, and lay it off upon the Leg of the Compasses, and that will give the Division for dividing a Line into 6 equal Parts

Again, having taken the Length of the Leg of your Compasses, open the Sector, so that the Distance from 180 to 180, of each Line of equal Parts be equal thereto Then take the Extent from 20 to 20, and that laid off upon the Leg of the Compasses, will give the Division for dividing a Line into 8 equal Parts

Moreover, open the Sector so, that the Distance from 110 to 110, be equal to the Length of the Leg of your Compasses. The Sector remaining thus opened, the Distance

from

from 10 to 10, will give the Diviſion for dividing a Line into ten equal Parts

Laſtly, the Sector being opened, ſo that the Length of the Leg of your Compaſſes be equal to the Diſtance from 130 to 130, and then the Diſtance from 10 to 10 will give the Diviſion for dividing a Line into twelve equal Parts

The Uſe of this Line is eaſy; for ſuppoſe a right Line is to be divided into three equal Parts, firſt puſh the Curſor, ſo that the middle of the Screw may be juſt upon the Figure 3, and having firmly fixed it upon that Point, take the Length of the propoſed Line between the two longeſt Parts of the Legs, then the Diſtance between the two ſhorteſt Parts of the Legs will be ⅓ of the given Line. Proceed thus for dividing a given Line into other equal Parts

Now to make the Diviſions for regualr Polygons, divide the Leg of you. Compaſſes into two equal Parts, and having opened the Sector, let the Diſtance from 6 to 6, on the two Lines of Polygons, be equal to one of thoſe Parts. The Sector remaining thus opened, take the Diſtance from 3 to 3 for a Trigon, and lay it off from the End of the Leg of your proportional Compaſſes, where mark 3. Again, take the Diſtance from 4 to 4 for a Square, upon the Line of Polygons, and that will give the Diviſion for a Square. Moreover, take the Diſtance from 5 to 5, on the Lines of Polygons, and lay off upon the Leg of your Compaſſes, which will give the Diviſion for a Pentagon; proceed thus for the Heptagon, and the other Polygons, to the Dodecagon. It is needleſs to make the Diviſion for a Hexagon, becauſe the Semidiameter of any Circle will divide its Circumference into ſix equal Parts

The Uſe of this Line for the Inſcription of Polygons is very eaſy, for if, for Example, a Pentagon is to be inſcribed in a given Circle, puſh the Curſor ſo, that the middle of the Screw may be againſt the Number 5 for a Pentagon, then with the ſhorteſt Parts of the Legs, take the Semidiameter of the Circle, and the Legs remaining thus opened, the Diſtance between the Points of the longeſt Parts of the Legs, will be the Side of a Pentagon inſcribed in the given Circle

Again, ſuppoſe a Heptagon is to be inſcribed in a Circle, fix the Screw againſt the Number 7, then take the Semidiameter of the Circle between the longeſt Parts of the Legs of your Compaſſes, and the Diſtance between the ſhorteſt Parts of the Legs will be the Side of a Heptagon inſcribed in the ſaid Circle

Of the Beam-Compaſs.

Fig K.

This Compaſs conſiſts of a very even ſquare Branch of Braſs or Steel, from 1 to 3 or 4 Feet in Length. There are two ſquare Braſs Boxes or Curſors exactly fitted to the ſaid Branch, upon each of which may be ſcrewed on Steel, Pencil, or Drawing-Pen Points, according as you have uſe for them. One of the Curſors is made to ſlide along the Branch, and may be made faſt to it by means of a Screw at the Top thereof, which preſſes againſt a little Spring, the other Curſor is fixed very near one End of the Branch, where there is a Nut ſo faſtened to it, that by turning it about the Screw, at the End of the Branch, the ſaid Curſor may be moved backwards or forwards at pleaſure

Theſe Compaſſes ſerve to take great Lengths, as alſo exactly to draw the Circumferences of great Circles, and exactly divide them

Of the Elliptick Compaſſes

Fig L.

This Inſtrument, whoſe Uſe is to draw Ellipſes of any kinds, is made of a croſs Branch of Braſs, very ſtrait and equal, about a Foot long, on which are fitted three Boxes, or Curſors, to ſlide upon it. To one of the Curſors there may be ſcrewed on a Steel-Point, or elſe one to draw with Ink, and ſometimes a Porte-Craion. At the bottom of the two other Boxes are joined two ſliding Dove-Tails (as the little Figure 1 ſhews,) theſe ſliding Dove-Tails are adjuſted in two Dove-Tail Grooves, made in the Branches of the Croſs. The aforeſaid two ſliding Dove-Tails, which are affixed to the Bottoms of the Boxes by two round Rivets, and ſo have a Motion every way, by turning about the long Branch, move backwards and forwards along the Croſs, that is, when the long Branch has gone half way about, one of the ſliding Dove-Tails will have moved the whole Length of one of the Branches of the Croſs, and then, when the long Branch is got quite round, the ſame Dove-Tail will go back the whole Length of the Branch. underſtand the ſame of the other ſliding Dove-Tail.

Note, The Diſtance between the two ſliding Dove-Tails, is the Diſtance between the two Foci of the Ellipſis, for by changing that Diſtance, the Ellipſis will more or leſs ſwell

Underneath the Ends of the Branches of the Croſs, there is placed four Steel-Points, to keep it faſt upon the Paper. The Uſe of this Compaſs is eaſy, for by turning round the long Branch, the Ink, or Pencil-Point, will draw an Oval, or Ellipſis, required. Its Figure is enough to ſhew the Conſtruction and Uſe thereof.

Of Cylindrick and Spherick Compaſſes

Fig M.

Figure M is a Pair of Compaſſes uſed in taking the Thickneſſes of certain Bodies, as Cannon, Pipes, and the like things, which cannot be well done with Compaſſes of but two Points. Theſe Compaſſes are made of two Pieces of Braſs, or other Metal, having two circular Points, and two flat ones, a little bent at the Ends. When you uſe them, one of the

flat

flat Points must be put into the Cannon, and the other without, then the two opposite Points will shew the Thickness of the Cannon

Note, The Head of these Compasses ought to be well drilled in the Center ; that is, if a Line be drawn from one Point to the opposite one, the said Line must exactly pass thro the Center , and when the Compasses are shut, all the Points ought to touch one another

The Figure N is a Pair of Spherick Compasses, which differs in nothing from the Construction of Common Compasses, except only that the Legs are rounded, to take the Diameters of round Bodies, as Bullets, Globes, &c Fig N.

Lastly, the Figure O is another Cylindrical Pair of Compasses, whose Legs are equal The Figure is enough to shew their Construction and Use.

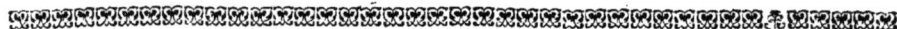

ADDITIONS *to* CHAP. I.

Of the Turn-up Compasses, and the Proportional Compasses, with the Sector Lines upon them.

Of the Turn-up Compasses.

THE Body of these Compasses, is much like the Body of common Compasses, nigh the Fig 1, Bottom of which, and on the outward Faces, are adjusted two Steel Points, one of them having a Drawing-Pen Point at the End, and the other a Porte-Craion at its End, so that they may turn round Nigh the middle of the outward Faces, are two little Steel Spring Catches, to hinder the Points giving way when using The Benefit of this Contrivance, is, that when you want to use a Drawing-Pen Point, or a Pencil, you have no more to do, but turn the Drawing-Pen Point, or the Porte-Craion, until the Steel Points come to the Catch : whereas, in a common Pair of Compasses, you have the trouble of taking off a Steel Point, in order to put either of the aforesaid Points in its place The Figure of this Compass is sufficient to shew its Construction and Use.

Of the Proportional Compasses, with the Sector Lines upon them

These Compasses are made of two equal Pieces of Brass or Silver, of any Length, the Breadth Fig 2, and Thickness of which must be proportionable. Along the greatest Part of their Length are two equal Dove-tail Slits made, in each of which go two Sliding Dove-tails of the same Length, each having a Hole drilled in the Middle, thro which passes a Rivet, with a turned Cheek fixed at one End, (which turned Cheek is fastned to one of the Sliding-Dove-Tails) and a Nut at the other There is another equal turned Cheek, fastened to the other Dove-tail , so that the two Sliding Dove-tails, together with the two turned Cheeks and Rivet, make a Cursor to slip up and down the Slits, and likewise serve as a moveable Joint for the Branches of the Compasses to turn about

At the Ends of the aforesaid Pieces of Brass, or Silver, are fixed four equal Steel-Points, the Lengths of each of which must be such, that when the Cursor is slid as far as it can go, to either of the Ends of the Slits, the Center of the Rivet may be exactly $\frac{1}{4}$ Parts of the Distance from one Point to the other.

At a small Distance from the four Ends of the two Sliding Dove-tails, are drawn across four Lines, or Marks, and when the Center of the Rivet is in the Middle between the Points, the Divisions of the Lines on the Broad-Faces, begin from those Lines, and end at them. But the Divisions on the Side-Faces, begin and end against the Center of the Rivet, when it is in the Middle between the Points

The Lines on the first broad Face of these Compasses, are, 1*st*, the Line of Lines, divided into 100 unequal Parts, every 10th of which are number'd, at the Top of which is writ *Lines.* 2*dly,* A Line of Chords to 60 Degrees, at the Top of which is writ *Chords* On the other broad Face, are, 1*st,* A Line of Sines to 90 Degrees, at the Top of which is writ *Sines.* 2*dly,* A Line of Tangents to 45 Degrees, at the Top of which is writ *Tangents*

On the first Side-Face, are the Tangents from 45 Deg to 71 Deg 34 Min. to which is writ *Tang* and on the second, are the Secants from 0 Deg to 70 Deg 30 Min to which is writ *Sec*

Construction of the Line of Lines on these Compasses.

Draw the Lines A D, C B, of the same Length that you design to have the Branches of Fig. 3, the Compasses, crossing each other in the Middle G , with one Foot of your Compasses in A, and the Distance A D, describe the Arc E D , and with the same Distance in the Point B, describe the Arc C E · thro the Points E, G, draw the right Line E M, which will bisect the Line drawn from C to D, in the Point F, also bisect F D in H, and raise the Perpendicular H R Now if from the Point R, a right Line is drawn to A, it will cut the Line E M in

Y the

the Point *k*, and if with one Foot of your Compaſſes in A, and the Diſtance A *k*, you deſcribe an Arc cutting the Side A D in the Point 50, the ſaid Point 50, on the Side A D, will be the Diviſion for 50 and 50 of the Line of Lines, if the Center of the Curſor was to be ſlid to the Diviſions, when the Compaſs is uſing. But becauſe the Lines drawn acroſs near the Ends of the Sliding Dove-tail, are to be ſlipped to the Diviſions, when the Compaſſes are to be uſed, the Diviſion for 50 muſt be as far beyond the Point 50, as the aforeſaid Line on the Sliding Dove-tail, is diſtant from the Center of the Curſor, which Diſtance ſuppoſe G Q, or G L its Equal. Underſtand the ſame for all other Diviſions, which are found in the manner that I am now going to ſhew.

Divide D H into 50 equal Parts, and from every of which raiſe Perpendiculars to cut the Arc E D (I have only drawn every 10.) Now if from the Point A, to all the Points wherein the Perpendiculars cut the Arc E D, right Lines are drawn, cutting the Line E M, and if the Diſtances of theſe Sections from the Point A, are laid off from the ſame Point on the Line A D, the Diviſions from 0 to 50, for the Line of Lines, will be had, and likewiſe from 50 to 100, which are at the ſame Diſtance from the Center G, in obſerving to place each of them, found out as directed, ſo much further from the Center G, as the Line G Q is diſtant from it.

The Diviſions for the Line of Lines being found, as before directed, they muſt each of them be transfer'd to the Face of your Compaſſes, and be numbered as per Figure.

Conſtruction of the Line of Chords, Sines, Tangents, and Secants

Fig 4

Having taken half of the Line of Lines, and divided the Spaces from 0 to 10, 10 to 20, 20 to 30, 30 to 40, and 40 to 50, into 100 Parts, by means of Diagonals, that half ſo divided, will ſerve as a Scale whereby the Tables of Natural Sines, Tangents, and Secants, and the Diviſions of all the other Lines on this Compaſs, may be eaſily made.

Now having ſlid the Center of the Curſor to the Middle of the Compaſſes, the Beginning and Ending of the Line of Chords muſt be (as in all the other Lines drawn upon theſe Compaſs's, two broad Faces) where the Line drawn acroſs the Sliding Dove-tail cuts the Sides of the Slit: then to find where the Diviſion of any Number of Degrees, or half Degrees, ſuppoſe 10, muſt be, look in the Table of Natural Sines for the Sine of 5 Degrees, which is half 10, and you will find it 871557, which doubled, will give the Chord of 10 Degrees, viz. 1743114: but becauſe the Radius to the Table of Natural Sines, Tangents, and Secants, is 10000, and from the aforeſaid Semi-Line of Lines made into a Diagonal Scale, can be taken but 500 Parts, therefore reject the laſt Figure to the right-hand, together with the Decimals, and you will have 174 for the Chord of 10 Degrees, when the Radius is but 1000 or the Length of the Line of Lines. Now take 174 Parts from the Diagonal Scale, and lay them off from 0, on the Parallels drawn to contain the Diviſions of the Line of Chords, and you will have the Diviſion for 10 Degrees. Again, to find the Diviſion for 20 Degrees, look for the Natural Sine of 10 Degrees, and it will be found 1736482, which doubled, will give the Chord of 20 Degrees, viz. 3472964, and rejecting the laſt Figure to the right-hand, and the Decimals, you will have 347, which being taken from your Diagonal Scale, and laid off from 0 0 on the Parallels, you will have the Diviſion for the Chord of 20 Degrees. In this manner proceed for finding the Diviſions for the Chords of any Number of Degrees, or half Degrees. But note, when you come to the Chord of 29 Degrees, you are got to the furtheſt Diviſion from the Center, becauſe, from the Table of Sines, the Chord of 29 Deg. is half Radius, (or at leaſt near enough half for this Uſe) or 500, and conſequently the Length of your whole Scale: therefore you muſt, for the Diviſions of the Chords of any Number of Degrees above 29, lay off the Parts above 500, taken on the Diagonal Scale, from the Diviſion of 29 Degrees, back again towards the Center, on the other Side the Slit, to 60. As for Example; to find the Diviſion for the Chord of 40 Degrees, the Chord is 684, from which 500 being ſubſtracted, you muſt take the Remainder 184 from your Diagonal Scale, and lay it off towards the Center, on the Parallels drawn on the other Side of the Slit, from a Point over-againſt the Diviſion for the Chord of 29 Degrees, and ſo for any other.

The Lines of Sines, or Tangents, on the other broad Face of theſe Compaſſes, are made in the ſame manner as the Line of Chords is. As, for Example, to make the Diviſion for the Sine of any Number of Degrees, ſuppoſe 10, you will find from the Table of Natural Sines, that the Sine of 10 Degrees is 173, whence lay off 173 Parts, taken on the Diagonal Scale, from the beginning of the Lines drawn to contain the Diviſions, and you will have the Point for the Sine of 10 Degrees. Again, to find the Diviſion for the Sine of 25 Degrees, you will find from the Table, that 422 is the Sine of 25 Degrees, therefore take on your Scale 422 Parts, and lay them off from 0, and you will have the Diviſion for the Sine of 25 Degrees. Thus proceed for the Diviſions of any other Number of Degrees, until you come to 30, whoſe Sine is equal to Half-Radius, and from 30 back again to 90, in obſerving the Directions aforegiven about the Chords, when they return towards the Center.

The Diviſions for the Tangent of any Number of Degrees, ſuppoſe 10, are likewiſe thus found; for the Tangent of 10 Degrees, by the Table, is 176, wherefore taking 176 Parts from your Scale, and laying them off from 0 0 on the Parallels drawn to contain the Diviſions, the Diviſion for the Tangent of 10 Degrees will be had. Again, to find the Diviſion for the Tangent

Tangent

Tangent of 25 Degrees, by the Table of Tangents, the Tangent of 25 Degrees will be found 466, whence taking 466 Parts from your Scale, and laying them off from o o, you will have the Division for the Tangent of 25 Degrees. Thus proceed for the Divisions of the Tangents of any other Number of Degrees, until you come to the Division of the Tangent of 26 Deg. 30 Min. which is half the Radius, and from 26 Deg. 30 Min. back again to 45 Deg. whose Tangent is equal to Radius, in observing the Directions afore-given about the Line of Chords, when they return.

The Construction of the Tangents to a second and third Radius, on the side Face of these Compasses, is thus. Let the Beginning of the second Radius, which is at the Tangent of 45 Degrees, be in the Middle between the Points of the Compasses, because when the Compass is using, a little Notch in the Side of the turned Cheek, which is directly against the Center of the Cursor, is slid to the Divisions. then to make the Divisions for the Tangents of the Degrees, and every 15 Minutes, from the Tangent of 45, to the Tangent of 56 Degrees, and about 20 Minutes, which is half a second Radius, you must look for the respective Tangents in the Table of Natural Tangents, and having cast away the last Figure to the right-hand, and the Decimals, (which always do) substract 1000 from each of them, because that is equal to one of our Radius's, and the Remainders take from your Scale, and lay off from 45, so shall you have the Divisions to the Tangent of 56 Deg. and about 20 Min. Then again, to have the Divisions from 56 Deg. 20 Min. to 63 Deg. and 27 Min. the Tangent of which is equal to 2000, or two of our Radius's, you must substract 1500, which is 2 and a half of our Radius's, from every of the respective Tangents, found and ordered as before directed, and then take each of the Remainders from the Scale, and lay them off from 56 Deg. 20 Min on the Top, and you will have the Divisions of the Tangents of the Degrees, and every 15 Min. from 56 Deg. 20 Min. to 63 Deg. 27 Min. which will fall against 45 Deg. on the Side of the other Branch. Again, to find the Divisions of the Tangents of the Degrees, and every 15 Minutes, from 63 Deg. 27 Min. to 68 Deg. 12 Min. which makes two Radius's and a half, or 2500, you must substract 2000 from each of the Tangents, found and ordered as aforesaid, and the Remainders must be taken off your Scale, and laid off from 63 Deg. 27 Min. and you will have the Divisions for the Tangents of the Degrees, and every 15 Min. from 63 Deg. 27 Min. to 68 Deg. 12 Min. Lastly, to have the Divisions from 68 Deg. 12 Min. to 71 Deg. 34 Min. which ends at 45 Deg. and makes up the third Radius, or 3000: you must substract 2500 from each of the Tangents found in the Table, and ordered as before directed, and take off the Remainders from your Scale, which laid off upwards from 68 Deg. 12 Min. will give the Divisions for the Tangents of the Degrees, and every 15 Minutes, between 68 Deg. 12 Min. and 71 Deg. 34 Min.

The Divisions for the Secants, on the other narrow Face of the Compasses, which run from o Degrees, in the middle between the two Points of the Compasses, to 70 Degrees, 32 Minutes, that is, which are the Secants to a second and third Radius (like as the Tangents last mentioned) are made exactly in the same manner, from the Table of natural Secants, as those Tangents to a second and third Radius are made.

USE *of these Proportional Compasses.*

USE I. *To divide a given right Line into any Number of equal Parts, less than 100.*

Divide 100 by the Number of equal Parts the Line is to be divided into, and slip the Cursor so, that the Line drawn, upon the sliding Dove-Tail, may be against the Quotient on the Line of Lines. then taking the whole Extent of the Line between the two Points of the Compasses, that are furthest distant from the Center of the Cursor, and afterwards applying one of the two opposite Points to the Beginning or End of the given Line, and the other opposite Point will cut off from it one of the equal Parts that the Line is to be divided into.

As, for Example, to divide the Line A B into two equal Parts. 100, divided by 2, gives 50 for the Quotient, therefore slip the Line on the Dove-Tail to the Division 50 on the Line of Lines, and taking the whole Extent of the Line A B between the Points furthest from the Center, then one of the opposite Points set in A or B, and the other will fall on the Point D, which will divide the Line A B in two equal Parts. Fig 5.

Again, to divide a right Line into three equal Parts, divide 100 by 3, and the Quotient will be 33.3, therefore slip the Line of the Dove-Tail to the Division 33, and for the three Tenths conceive the Division between 33 and 34 to be divided into 10 equal Parts, and reasonably estimate 3 of them. Proceed as before, and you will have a third Part of the said Line, and therefore it may easily be divided into 3 equal Parts. Moreover, to divide a given Line into 50 equal Parts, divide 100 by 50, and the Quotient will be 2, therefore slip the Line, on the sliding Dove-Tail, to the Division 2 on the Line of Lines. Proceed as at first, and you will have a 50th Part of the Line proposed, whence it will be easy to divide it into 50 equal Parts.

Note, If each of the Subdivisions, on the Line of Lines, is supposed to be divided into 100 equal Parts, then a Line may, by means of the Line of Lines on these Compasses, be divided into any Number of equal Parts less than 1000. As, for Example, to divide a Line into

into 500 equal Parts   Divide 1000 by 500, and the Quotient will be 2 , therefore flip the Line, on the Dove-Tail, to 2 Tenths of one of the Subdivifions of 100, and proceed, as at firft directed, and you will have the 500th Part of the Line given, which afterwards may eafily be divided into 500 equal Parts   Again , to divide a Line into 200 equal Parts   divide 1000 by 200, and the Quotient will be 50, therefore flip the Line, on the Dove-Tail, to 5 of the Subdivifions of 100, on the Line of Lines, which will now reprefent 50 , proceed as at firft, and you will have the 200th Part of the Line given · therefore it will be eafy to divide it into 200 equal Parts   Moreover, to divide a given Line into 150 equal Parts, divide 1000 by 150, and the Quotient will be 66, wherefore reafonably eftimate 6 of the 10 equal Parts that the firft of the Subdivifions of 100 is fuppofed to be divided into, and flip the Line, on the fliding Dove-Tail, to the 6th , then proceeding as at firft, and the Line may be divided into 150 equal Parts   If a Line be fo long, that it cannot be taken between the Points of your Compaffes, you muft take the half, third, or fourth Part, &c and proceed with that as before directed , then one of the Parts found being doubled, trebled, &c will be the correfpondent Part of the whole Line

USE II   *A right Line being given, and fuppofed to be divided into 100 equal Parts   to take any Number of thofe Parts*

Slip the Line, on the fliding Dove-Tail, to the Number of Parts to be taken, as 10, then the Extent of the whole Line being taken between the Points of the Compaffes, furtheft diftant from the Curfor, if one of the oppofite Points be fet in either Extreme of the given Line, the other will cut off the Part required.

USE III   *The Radius being given , to find the Chord of any Arc under 60 Degrees*

Slip the Line, on the fliding Dove-Tail, to the Degrees fought on the Line of Chords; then take the Radius between the Points of the Compaffes, furtheft diftant from the Center of the Curfor, and the Extent, between the two oppofite Points, will be the Chord fought, if the given Number of Degrees be greater than 29, whofe Chord is Half-Radius , but if the Number of Degrees be lefs than 29, then the Diftance of the two oppofite Points, taken from Radius, will be the Chord of the Degrees required

If the Chord of a Number of Degrees under 60 is given, and the Radius to it be required; you muft flip the Line, on the fliding Dove-Tail, to the Degrees given on the Line of Chords , and taking the Length of the given Chord between the two Points of your Compaffes, that are nigheft the Curfor, the Extent of the two other oppofite Points will be the Radius required

Fig. 6 Example, for the firft Part of this Ufe   Suppofe the Length of the Radius be the Line A B, and the Chord of 35 Degrees be required , Slip the Line, on the fliding Dove-Tail, to 35 Degrees on the Line of Chords , take the whole Extent of the Line A B between the Points of the Compaffes, furtheft diftant from the Curfor , and placing one of the oppofite Points in the Point A, the other Point will give the Extent A D for the Chord of 35 Degrees. Again , to find the Chord of 9 Degrees   Slip the Line, on the fliding Dove-Tail, to 9 Degrees on the Line of Chords   then take the Extent of the Radius, which fuppofe A B, between the two Points of the Compaffes, furtheft diftant from the Center , and placing one of the oppofite Points in the Point A, the other will fall on the Point C, and the Difference between A B and A C, viz CB, will be the Chord of 9 Degrees

USE IV   *The Radius being given, fuppofe the Line* A B, *to find the Sine of any Number of Degrees, as* 50

Fig 7. Slip the Line, on the fliding Dove-Tail, to 50 Degrees on the Line of Sines, then if the Extent A B is taken between the two Points of the Compaffes, furtheft from the Curfor, and one of the oppofite Points be fet in the Point A, the other will give A C for the Sine of 50 Degrees , but if the Sine fought be leffer than the Sine of 30 Degrees, which is equal to Half-Radius, the Difference, between the Extents of the oppofite Points, will be the Sine of the Angle required

USE V   *The Radius being given , to find the Tangent of any Number of Degrees, not above* 71

If the Tangent of the Degrees, under 26 and 30 Minutes, whofe Tangent is equal to Half-Radius, be fought   You muft flip the Line, on the fliding Dove-Tail, to the Degrees propofed on the Line of Tangents , and then take the Radius between the Points of the Compafs, furtheft diftant from the Curfor, and the Difference between the oppofite Points will be the Tangent of the Number of Degrees propofed.

If the Tangent of any Number of Degrees above 26 and 30 Minutes, and under 45, be fought , then you muft flip the Line, on the fliding Dove-Tail, to the Number of Degrees given on the Tangent-Line, and take the Radius between the Points of the Compafs furtheft from the Curfor, then the Diftance, between the two oppofite Points, will be the Tangent of the Degrees required.

If the Tangent required be greater than 45 Degrees, but lefs than 56 Degrees, and about 20 Minutes ; you muft flip the Notch, on the Side of the turned Cheek, to the Degrees of

the

the Tangents upon the Side of the Compass, and take the Radius, between the Points of the Compass, furthest distant from the Cursor, the Difference between the opposite Points, added to Radius, will be the Tangent of the Degrees sought.

If the Tangent required be greater than that of 56 Degrees, 20 Minutes, but less than 63 Degrees, 27 Minutes, you must slip the Notch to the Degrees proposed, and take the Radius, as before, between the Points of the Compass; then the Extent, between the two opposite Points, added to Radius, will be the Tangent required

If the Tangent required be greater than 63 Degrees, 27 Minutes, but less than 68 Degrees; you must slip the Notch, on the Side of the turned Cheek, to the Degrees proposed, and take the Radius between the Points of the Compass, as before; then the Difference between the opposite Points, added to twice Radius, will be the Tangent of the Degrees proposed.

Lastly, If the Tangent be greater than 68 Degrees, but less than 71, you must add the Distance between the opposite Points of the Compass, to two Radius's, and the Sum will be the Tangent of the Degrees sought

The Secant of any Number of Degrees, under 70, by having Radius given, in observing the aforesaid Directions about the Tangents, may be easily found

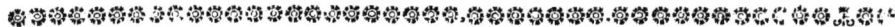

❀ ❀❀❀❀❀❀ ❀❀ ❀❀❀❀❀❀❀❀❀❀❀❀❀.❀❀❀❀❀❀❀.❀❀❀❀❀❀❀❀❀❀❀ ❀

CHAP. II.

Of the Construction of divers Mathematical Instruments.

Of the Sliding Porte-Craion

THIS Instrument is commonly about four or five Inches long, the Outside of which is *Plate* 10. filed into eight Faces, and the Inside perfectly round, in which a Porte-Craion is put, *Fig.* A. which may be slid up and down by means of a Spring and Button, of which we shall speak hereafter   The Compasses of the Figure B is made to screw into one End of this Instrument.

There are commonly drawn, upon the Faces of this Porte-Craion, the Sector-Lines, whose manner of drawing is the same as those on the Sector, and their Use is the same as the Use of those on the Sector, excepting only that they are not so general   For Example, If you have a mind to make an Angle of 40 Degrees upon a given Line, take the Extent of 60 Degrees of the Line of Chords, and therewith describe an Arc upon the given Line: then take the Extent of 40 Degrees, and lay off upon that Arc, and from its Center draw a Line, which will make an Angle of 40 Degrees with the given Line

Note, There are also round Instruments of this kind, whose Outsides are divided into Inches, and each Inch into Lines

This is another Porte-Craion made of Brass, round within, and commonly so without, hav-*Fig.* C. ing the Porte-Craion of Figure D made to slip up and down in it.   In the Ends of the said Porte-Craion are put Pencils, which are made fast by two Rings; and in the middle is placed a well-hammered Brass or Steel Spring, having a Female Screw made in it at 1, in order to receive the Male Screw at the End of the Button E, which goes into a Slit made in the Body of the Instrument   The Figure, and what I have said, is enough to shew the Nature of this Porte-Craion.

Of the Fountain-Pen.

This Instrument is composed of different Pieces of Brass, Silver, &c. and when the Pieces *Fig.* F. F G H are put together, they are about five Inches long, and its Diameter is about three Lines   The middle Piece F carries the Pen, which ought to be well slit, and cut, and screwed into the Inside of a little Pipe, which is soldered to another Pipe of the same Bigness, as the Lid G, in which Lid is soldered a Male Screw, for screwing on the Cover; as likewise for stopping a little Hole at the Place 1, and so hindering the Ink from running through it   At the other End of the Piece F, there is a little Pipe, on the Outside of which the Top-Cover H may be screwed on.   In this Top-Cover there goes a Porte-Craion, that is to screw into the last mentioned little Pipe, and so stop the End of the Pipe at which the Ink is poured in, by means of a Funnel

When the aforementioned Pen is to be used, the Cover G must be taken off, and the Pen a little shaken, in order to make the Ink run freely   *Note,* If the Porte-Craion does not stop the Mouth of the Piece F, the Air, by its Pressure, will cause the Ink all to run out at once. *Note* also, that some of these Pens have Seals soldered at their Ends

Of Pincers for holding Papers together

This little Instrument is made of two well-hammered thin Pieces of Brass, fastened toge-*Fig.* I. ther at top, and having a Brass Spring between them, and a Ferril, that slides up and down, in order to draw them together.   The whole Piece is about two Inches long, and its Figure is enough to shew the Construction and Use thereof.

Z

Of the Pentagraph, or Parallelogram

Fig K

    This Inſtrument, called a *Pentograph*, as ſerving to copy any manner of Deſigns, is compoſed of four Braſs, or very hard Wooden Rulers, very equal in Breadth and Thickneſs , two of them being from 15 to 18 Inches in Length, and the other two but half of their Length, and their Thickneſs is uſually 2 or 3 Lines, and Breadth 5 or 6

    The Exactneſs of this Inſtrument very much depends upon having the Holes made at the Ends, and in the middle of the longeſt Rulers, at an equal Diſtance from the Holes at the Ends of the ſhorteſt Rulers , for this reaſon, that being put together, they may always make a Parallelogram . and when the Inſtrument is to be uſed, there are ſix ſmall Pieces of Braſs put on it

    The Piece 1 is a little turned Braſs Pillar, at one End of which is a Screw and Nut, ſerving to join and faſten the two long Rulers together , and at the other is a little Knob for the Inſtrument to ſlide upon   The Piece 2 is a turned-headed River, with a Screw and Nut at the End , two of which there muſt be for joining the two Ends of the two ſhort Rulers to the middle of the long ones, at the Places 2, 2.   The Piece 3 is a Braſs Pillar, one End of it being hollowed into a Screw, having a Nut to fit it , and at the other End is a Worm to ſcrew into the Table, when the Inſtrument is to be uſed. This Piece holds the two Ends of the ſhort Rulers together, at *Fig* 3.   *Fig* 4 is a Porte-Craion, or Pen, which may be ſcrewed into the Pillar 4, which is fixed on at the Place 4, to the End of the great Ruler. Laſtly, *Fig* 5 is a Braſs Point, ſomething blunt, ſcrewed into a Pillar like one of the former ones, which is ſcrewed on to the End of the other long Ruler   This Inſtrument being put together, and diſpoſed, as *per* Figure, the next thing will be to ſhew its Uſe

    Now when a Deſign, of the ſame Bigneſs as the Original, is to be copied, the Inſtrument muſt be diſpoſed, as in Figure K, that is, you muſt ſcrew the Worm into the Table at the Place 3, and lay the Paper under the Pencil 4, and the Deſign under the Point 5 , then there is no more to do but move the Point 5 over every part of the Deſign 5, and at the ſame time the Pencil, at Figure 4, will mark the ſaid Deſign upon your Paper   But if the Deſign is to be reduced, or made leſs by half, the Worm muſt be placed at one End of the long Ruler, the Paper and the Pencil in the middle, and then you muſt make the Braſs Point paſs over all the Tracts of the Deſign, and the Pencil at the ſame time will alſo have deſcribed all thoſe Tracts , but they will be of but half the Length of the Tracts of the Deſign   for this reaſon , becauſe the Pencil, placed in the manner aforeſaid, moves but half the Length, in the ſame time, as the Braſs Point does   And, for the contrary Reaſon, if a Deſign is to be augmented, for Example, twice the Original, the Braſs Point and the Deſign muſt be placed in the middle, at Figure 3, the Pencil and Paper at the End of one of the long Rulers, and the Worm at the End of the other long Ruler, by this means a Deſign twice the Original may be drawn.

    But to augment or diminiſh Deſigns in other Proportions, there are drilled Holes at equal Diſtances upon each Ruler, *viz.* all along the ſhort ones, and half-way the great ones, in order to place the Pieces carrying the Braſs-Point, the Pencil, and the Worm in a right Line in them , that is, if the Piece carrying the Braſs Point be put into the third Hole, the two other Pieces muſt be likewiſe each put into the third Hole

    Note, If the Point and the Deſign be placed at any one of the Holes of one of theſe great Rulers, and the Pencil with the Paper under one of the Holes of the ſhort Ruler, which forms the Angle, and joins to the middle of the ſaid long Ruler, that then the Copy will be leſs than half the Original . But if the Pencil and Paper be placed under one of the Holes of that ſhort Ruler, which is parallel to the long Ruler, then the Copy will be greater than half the Original. In a word, all theſe different Proportions will be eaſily found by Experience.

Conſtruction of Sizes   To know the Weight of Pearls

Fig. M.

    This little Inſtrument, whoſe Uſe is to find the Weight of very fine and round Pearls, is made of five thin Pieces, or Leaves, of Braſs, or other Metal, about two Inches long, and ſix or ſeven Lines broad   The ſaid Leaves have ſeveral round Holes drilled in them of different Diameters , the Holes in the firſt Leaf ſerve for weighing Pearls from half a Grain to 7 Grains , thoſe in the ſecond Leaf are for Pearls from 8 Grains, which is 2 Carats, to 5 Carats , thoſe in the third for Pearls weighing from $2\frac{1}{2}$ Carats to $5\frac{1}{2}$ Carats , the fourth for Pearls weighing from 6 Carats to 8 , and the fifth for Pearls weighing from $6\frac{1}{4}$ Carats to $8\frac{1}{4}$.

    Now the Diameters of the greateſt and leaſt Holes of each Leaf being found, by weighing of Pearls in nice fine Scales, the Diameters of all the other Holes from thence, by proportion, may be found

    The Hole, ſhewing the Weight of a Pearl of one Grain, is $2\frac{1}{2}$ Lines in Diameter , that ſhowing the Weight of a Pearl of 2 Carats, is $2\frac{1}{2}$ Lines , that ſhowing the Weight of a Pearl of 5 Carats, is 4 Lines , that ſhewing $2\frac{1}{2}$ Carats, is $2\frac{1}{4}$, that of $5\frac{1}{2}$ Carats, is $4\frac{1}{2}$ Lines; that of 6 Carats, is $4\frac{1}{2}$ Lines ; that of 8 Carats, is $4\frac{4}{5}$ Lines , and, Laſtly, the Diameter of that Hole for Pearls weighing $8\frac{1}{4}$ Carats, is $4\frac{1}{4}$ Lines.

The

above the circular Braſs Plate, and another underneath it, both of them being of a convenient Bigneſs, and are ſo faſtened together at the Ends by ſtrong Screws, that there is room enough left between them for the circular Braſs Plate, and alſo for the Touret, or Frame, and a kind of Spring, which carries the Point (of which we ſhall ſpeak preſently) to ſlide freely along the ſquare Iron Ruler 3

Figure 3, repreſents the Side-Draught of the whole Machine put together, whereof the Piece 1, is the Touret, or Frame, placed near the Wheel to be cut, which is repreſented by Number 6 this Wheel is placed in the Center of the Braſs Plate, and is faſtened by the Arbre Screw The Piece 3, is the Iron Ruler along which the Touret of Figure 2 ſlides, as alſo the Spring carrying the Point 4 and Number 5 is a Piece of Iron, by means of which the Machine may be faſtened in a Vice, when it is to be uſed

Figure 4, is a very fine and well-tempered Steel Point, ſcrew'd into the End of a kind of Spring, having a circular Motion, that thereby the ſaid Steel Point may be put into any of the Holes of the Circumferences of either of the concentrick Circles upon the Plate There is likewiſe another Piece joined to the Spring, in order to keep, by means of a Screw, the Point upon any propoſed Diviſion of the Circumference of any of the concentrick Circles, while one Tooth of a Wheel is ſawing

Laſtly, Figure 5, is the Arbre placed in the Center of the Machine, and upon which is put the Wheels to be cut, which are firmly fixed thereon, by means of Screws at the Top and Bottom There are commonly ſeveral Arbres of different Bigneſſes, in proportion to the Holes in the Centers of Wheels to be cut

The Uſe of this Machine is eaſy, for you have no more to do but fix a Wheel to be cut into Teeth, in the Center, (at Number 6) and then fit the Spring (repreſented by *Fig* 4) ſo that its Point may exactly fall upon the Diviſions of that concentrick Circle, which is divided into the ſame Number of equal Parts you deſign your Wheel to have Teeth, and then you muſt move the Touret, with its Saw-Wheel, to cut the Wheel, by means of a Male-Screw (one End of which goes into a round Hole 8, in the Bottom of the Touret, and is there faſtened with a Pin) and a Female-Screw to fit it, at the End of the Iron Ruler, denoted by Number 5, ſo that by turning the ſaid Male-Screw, the Touret may be moved backwards and forwards at pleaſure The Saw-Wheel being thus placed, you muſt turn it 4 or 5 times about, by means of a Bow, whoſe String is put about the Pully, and then one Side of a Tooth will be cut, and having moved the Steel Point 4, to the next Diviſion in the Circumference of that concentrick Circle upon the Plate, whoſe Diviſions are the ſame in Number you deſign your Wheel to have Teeth, give 4 or 5 Strokes with the Bow, and the other Side of the Tooth will be cut and in this manner may all the Teeth be cut, Pinions are alſo thus cut

Note, There are Saw-Wheels of divers Thickneſſes, conformable to the Space there ought to be left between the Teeth of different Wheels.

The Conſtruction of Armour for Load-Stones, as alſo how to cut the ſaid Stones, in order to arm them

The Figures 6, 7, repreſent two armed Load-Stones, the firſt in the Form of a Parallelopipedon, and the ſecond in the Form of a Sphere · But before we ſhew the beſt way of arming them, we will enumerate ſome of the Properties and Virtues of Load-Stones

The Load-Stone is a very hard and heavy Stone, found in Iron Mines, and is almoſt the Colour of Iron, for which reaſon it is reckoned among the Metallick Kind it hath two wonderful Properties, one whereof is to attract Iron, and the other to direct itſelf towards the Poles of the World.

The Load-Stone attracts Iron, and reciprocally Iron attracts the Load-Stone, notwithſtanding any other Body's Interpoſition between them This Stone likewiſe communicates to Iron a Faculty of attracting Iron For Example, an Iron Ring that hath been touch'd with a good Load-Stone, will lift up another Iron Ring by only touching it, and this ſecond a third, &c but the firſt Ring muſt have a greater Degree of Attraction, than the ſecond, and the ſecond than the third, &c

The Blade of a Knife that hath been touch'd with a Load-Stone, will likewiſe lift up Needles, and ſmall Pieces of Iron · alſo ſeveral Sewing-Needles being laid upon a Table in a Row, and a Load-Stone being brought near the firſt, by which receiving the Magnetick Virtue, the ſaid firſt Needle will attract the ſecond, the ſecond the third, &c till they all come together

That Iron reciprocally attracts the Load-Stone, when it can move freely, may be thus ſhewn · For if you put a Load-Stone into a hollow Piece of Cork, and ſet it floating upon the Surface of a Baſon of Water, and bring a Piece of Iron at a convenient Diſtance to it, the Piece of Cork, together with the Stone, will accede to the Iron

That Property of the Load-Stone which is always to reſpect the Poles of the World, may be ſhewn by the following Experiment For having put a Load-Stone into a hollow Piece of Cork, and ſet them both a floating upon the Surface of ſtill Water, (there being no Iron, or other Obſtacle near) the Load-Stone will always ſo diſpoſe itſelf, that one certain Point thereof will regard the North, and the oppoſite Point the South

But

But you muſt note, that the Load-Stone doth not exactly reſpect the North, it having at different Times, and in different Places of the Earth's Superficies, different Declinations, or Variations theretrom, and at this time at *Paris*, varies 12 Deg 15 Min Weſtwards ſo that the South Pole of the Load-Stone varies above 12 Degrees from that of the World, and its Oppoſite ſo likewiſe The Poles of a Load-Stone, are thoſe two Places thereof, that reſpect the two Magnetick Poles of the World, and the principal Axis, is a right Line drawn from one Pole to the other, about which, the greateſt Force of the Load-Stone manifeſts itſelf, and at the two Poles is greateſt Spherical Load-Stones have alſo fictcd Equators, and Meridians, &c from whence they are called Magnetick Spheres.

Now, in order to find the Poles of a Load-Stone, you muſt cut a Hole in a Card of the Figure of the Stone, in which the Stone muſt be put, ſo that its principal Axis may be found in the Plane of the Card This being done, Iron or Steel Filings muſt be ſtrew'd upon it · after which ſtrike the Card ſoftly with a little Stick, ſo that by putting the Filings in Motion, the Magnetick Matter may let them take a Circuit conformable to the way which that Matter takes in moving from a North Pore to another South one, and you will perceive the Filings ranged in the Figure of ſeveral Semi-Circumferences, whoſe oppoſite Ends are the Poles of the Load-Stone

The Poles of a Load-Stone may otherwiſe be found, in plunging it into Iron or Steel Filings, or into very little Bits of Steel Wire, for then they will make different Configurations round the Stone, ſome of them lying flat on it, others half bent, and finally, others quite upright on it and thoſe Places of the Stone where the little Bits of Steel are perpendicular to it, are the Poles, and where they lie along, is the Equator

Having thus found the Poles of a Load-Stone, which is the North or South Pole, may be known in laying the Stone in a hollow Piece of Cork, ſwimming on Water, or by ſuſpending it with a Thread, ſo that its Axis be parallel to the Horizon, for then that Pole of the Stone turning towards the North Pole of the World, will be the South Pole of the Stone, and the oppoſite Point the North Pole

The Poles of a Load-Stone may likewiſe be found by means of a Compaſs, for bringing a touch'd Needle to the Stone, the End that was touch'd, will immediately turn towards that Pole of the Stone agreeing therewith, and the other End of the Needle will likewiſe turn towards the other Pole of the Stone

The Poles of the Stone being found, the next thing will be to cut, and give it a regular Figure, in taking away the Superfluities either with a Saw, and Powder of Emery, or elſe with a Knife-Grinder's Grind-ſtone, preſerving its Axis as long as poſſible, and giving a like Figure to its Poles

Now to make a great many Experiments, it is neceſſary to give to a Load-Stone the moſt regular Figure poſſible, which is determined by the Likeneſs it hath to that of the irregular Maſs it is compoſed of the Cube, the Parallelopipedon, the Oval, and the Round are to be preferr'd, on account of having the principal Axis of the Stone as long as may be If a Load-Stone is to be made in Form of a Sphere, it will not be difficult to find its Poles and Axis, you need only figure it with Powder of Emery in a round Iron Concave, and afterwards finiſh it with find Sand, in a round Braſs Concave

A Load-Stone in Figure of a Sphere, is very fit for many Experiments, and its Poles may be found in manner aforeſaid but it is neceſſary, before any pains be taking in cutting and figuring of a Load-Stone, to be aſſured of its Goodneſs, in obſerving whether it ſtrongly attracts Filings, or little Bits of Steel, and whether there be not other Matter paſſing thro its Pores, which hinders the Magnetical Matter from circulating and paſſing from one Pole to the other

The Goodneſs of a Load-Stone conſiſts in two eſſential Things, which are, firſt, That it be homogenous, having a great Number of Pores filled with Magnetick Matter, which paſſing thro them form about the Stone, as it were, a very extenſive Whirlwind In the ſecond place, its Figure very much contributes to its Force, (as we have already ſaid) for it is certain, that of all Load-Stones of a like Goodneſs, that which hath the beſt Poles, its Axis longeſt, and whoſe Poles meet exactly in the Extremes, will be moſt vigorous

Two Load-Stones placed in two hollow Pieces of Cork, which are both ſet floating upon the Surface of the Water, having their Poles of contrary Denominations turned to each other, will acceed to each other, but if the Poles of the ſame Denomination be turned towards each other, then the Load-Stones will mutually recede from one another

If a Load-Stone be cut into two Pieces, parallel to its Axis, the Sides of the Pieces that were together before the Diviſion, will mutually recede from each other

But if a Load-Stone be cut into two Pieces, according to its Equator, the Sides of the Pieces that were together before they were cut, will be found to have Poles of a contrary Denomination, and will accede to each other

A ſtrong Load-Stone touching a weak one, will attract it with its Pole of the ſame Denomination, &c.

The

The Deſcription of the Armour, or Caping for Load-ſtones

Fig. 6

The Armour for a Loadſtone, cut into the Form of a right-angled Parallelopipedon, is compoſed of two ſquare Pieces of very ſmooth Iron or Steel, but tempered Steel is better than Iron, becauſe its Pores are cloſer, and there are a greater Number of them   Care muſt be taken, that the Armour well encompaſſes, and exactly touches the Poles of the Loadſtone, and that the Armour is in Thickneſs proportionable to the Goodneſs of the Stone   for if ſtrong Armour be put upon a weak Stone, it will produce no Effect, becauſe the magnetick Matter will not have force enough to paſs thro it; and, on the contrary, if the Armour of a ſtrong Stone be too thin, it will not contain all the magnetick Matter it ought, and conſequently the Stone will not produce ſo great an Effect, as when the Armour is thicker

Now, to fit the Armour exactly, you muſt file it thinner by Degrees, and when you find the Effect of the Stone to be augmented as much as poſſible, the Armour will be in its juſt Proportion, and will have its convenient Thickneſs; after which it muſt be ſmoothed within Side, and poliſhed without

The Heads of the Armour (whereon is writ *North* and *South*) muſt be thicker than the other Parts, and cover about ⅗ of the Length of the Axis

The Breadth and Length of the Armour, beſt fitting a Stone, may alſo be found by filing it by little and little, but, above all, Care muſt be taken that the two Heads are equal in Thickneſs, and that their Baſes very exactly meet in the ſame Plane   Number 5 is a Braſs or Silver Girdle fitted about the Stone, ſerving to faſten and hold the Armour, by means of two Screws 1, 1; and at 6 and 6 are two Screws faſtening a round Braſs Plate, carrying the Pendant 4, and its Ring, to the Top of the Armour

Fig 7

The Armour of a ſpherical Loadſtone is compoſed of two Steel Shells, faſtened to the Piece 8 by two Joints 6, 6; of a Girdle 5, 5, of a Pendant and Ring 4, and of a Piece (or *Porte-Poid*) 2, to hold the Hook 3   Great Care muſt be taken that the Shells very exactly join the Superficies of the Stone, and that they well encompaſs the Poles of the Stone, and cover the greateſt part of the Convexity thereof   The convenient Breadth and Thickneſs of this Armour may be found by Trials, as before-mentioned.

It is very wonderful, that two little Pieces of Steel, compoſing the Armour of a Loadſtone, ſhould give it ſuch a Property, that a good Stone, after it is armed, will attract above 150 times more than before it was armed

There are indifferent good Stones, which, unarmed, weigh about three Ounces, and will lift up but half an Ounce of Iron, but being armed, will lift up more than ſeven Pounds.

To preſerve a Loadſtone, you muſt keep it in a dry Place among little Bits of Steel-Wire; for Filings, which are always full of Duſt, make it ruſty.

We ſometimes ſuſpend Loadſtones, ſo that having the liberty to move, they may conform themſelves to the Poles of the World, and if, in this Situation, the Piece carrying the Hook, or *Porte-Poid*, be put on, and the Weight the Stone commonly carries be hung on, and from time to time there be hung to it ſome ſmall Weight more, you will find that, when the Stone has continued ſuſpended ſome Days, that it will lift up a much greater Weight than it did before it was hung up

Several common Experiments made with the Load-ſtone

The firſt and uſefulleſt Experiment made with the Loadſtone, is that of touching the Needles of Sea-Compaſſes, for rightly doing of which, you muſt draw the Needle ſoftly over one of the Poles of the Loadſtone, from its Middle to its End, and then it will receive its Vertue. But, *Note*, that that End of the Needle, which hath been touched with one of the Poles of a Loadſtone, will turn towards the oppoſite Part of the World, to that which that Pole regards, therefore if the End of a Needle is to turn towards the North, it muſt be touched with that Pole of the Stone reſpecting the South. *Note*, The longer Needles are, the leſs will they viberate

This admirable Direction of the Loadſtone and Touched Needle hath not been known in *Europe* much above two hundred Years, by means of which, Navigation hath been almoſt infinitely advanced   But there is one Inconveniency, which is, that a Touched Needle doth not exactly reſpect the Poles of the World, but declines or varies therefrom towards the Eaſt or Weſt, at different Times, and in different Places, variouſly   In the Year 1610, it varied at *Paris* 8 Degrees North-Eaſterly, in 1658, it had no Variation, and in the Year 1716, it varied about 12 Deg. 15 Min. Weſtward

Moreover, the Needle hath alſo an Inclination as well as a Declination, that is, the Needle of a Sea-Compaſs being *in Equilibrio* upon its Pivot, will, when touched, loſe that Equilibrium, and the End that turns North, on this ſide the Equator, will drip or incline towards the Earth, as if it was heavier on that Side; for which reaſon the North Side of a Needle muſt be made lighter, before the Needle be touched, than the South Side, and going towards the Poles, this Inclination grows greater, but in going towards the Equator, it grows leſſer; ſo that under the Equator, the Inclination will be nothing, and in paſſing the Line, the other End of the Needle, reſpecting the South, will begin to incline; ſo that Pilots are obliged to ſtick as much Wax to the End of the Needle, as will make it *in Equilibrio*   *Note*, the

the greater Force that Loadftones, which touch Needles, have, the more will the Needles incline.

There are Needles purpofely made to obferve this Inclination, which at *Paris* is about 70 Degrees.

If a long thin Piece of Steel be drawn over one of the Poles of an armed Loadftone (in the fame manner as was faid before of the Needles) this Piece of Steel will in an inftant acquire the magnetick Virtue, and will not lofe it but by degrees after feveral Months, unlefs it be put in the Fire *Note,* A Piece of Steel, touched by a good Stone, will lift up 14 Ounces

The two Ends of a Steel Blade thus touched will become North and South Poles, that End whofe Contact ends on the South Pole of the Stone, being the North, and the other the South Pole: for if this Piece of Steel be made light enough to fwim, one End thereof will turn to the North, and the other to the South

Again, that End of the Steel Blade where the Contact ended, will attract much ftronger than the other End, and if the faid Blade be once drawn over the Stone the contrary way, it will quite lofe its Virtue, and attract no more. Underftand the fame of the Needle of a Compafs, the Blade of a Knife, &c. two touched Steel Blades will avoid each other, and approach like two Loadftones

A Piece of Steel, in a hollow Piece of Cork fwimming on the Water, may be any ways moved, by bringing the Pole of a Loadftone towards it, or another touched Piece of Steel

A fine Sewing-Needle, fufpended by a Thread, will fhew what is meant by Sympathy and Antipathy, for this Needle will be repelled by one Pole of a Loadftone, and attracted by the other

A Needle may be kept upright, without its touching a Loadftone, fo that there may be put between it and the Stone a Piece of Silver, or other Matter, provided it be not Iron

If, about a Loadftone, fufpended by a String, be circularly placed feveral little touched Needles of a Compafs, upon their Pivots, and the Loadftone be moved any how, you will likewife fee all the Needles move in a pleafant manner, and when the Stone ceafes moving, the Needles will alfo ceafe

What we have already fpoken about ftrewing of Filings about a Loadftone, may be faid alfo of ftrewing them about a Piece of touched Steel.

If Filings be ftrewed upon a Piece of Pafteboard, and a Loadftone be moved under it, the Filings will erect themfelves, and then lie along on that Side from whence the Stone came.

If, inftead of Filings, you lay upon a Piece of Pafteboard feveral Bits of the Ends of broken Needles, by bringing one Pole of a Loadftone towards them, they will erect themfelves upon one of their Ends, and by bringing the other Pole, they will fall, and rife upon their other Ends

It is eafy to feparate a black Powder mixed with white Sand, and propofing it to a Perfon, not knowing the Secret, he will think it impoffible; for if Iron Filings be mixed with fine Sand, they may be feparated from it by a Loadftone, or Piece of touched Steel · for either of them being put into the Mixture, at divers times, you may get all the Filings from among the Sand

A Loadftone will lift up a Whirlegig in Motion, whofe Axis is Steel; and if it be fomething heavy, it will turn a longer time in the Air than upon a Table, where the Friction foon ftops its Motion, and if the Stone be a good one, this Whirlegig may lift up another, and both of them will turn contrary ways. Another diverting Experiment may yet be made, by putting little Steel Fifhes, or Swans, into a flat Bafon of Water; for by moving a good Loadftone under the Bafon, you will fee them prettily fwimming about, and moving the Stone different ways, they will likewife have different Motions, if the Stone be turned round, the Fifhes will alfo turn round, if the Pole of the Stone is turned towards them, they will plunge themfelves, as it were, to join themfelves to the Stone. You may likewife put little Steel Soldiers into the Bafon, which may be made to approach to or recede from each other in form of a Battel; and by bringing the Equator of the Stone towards them, they will fall down

It is pleafant enough to fee a Sewing-Needle threaded, or a little Arrow, faftened by a Hair to the Arc of a *Cupid's* Bow, remain fufpended in the Air eight or ten Lines diftant from a good Loadftone.

There are feveral other Experiments made with the Loadftone, but mentioning them here would take up too much time

The Conftruction of an Artificial Magnet.

This Inftrument, invented by Mr *Joblot,* is compofed of feveral very ftrait Steel Blades Fig. 8, laid upon one another; and to make it paffably hard, there ought to be at leaft 20 of them, (according to the force of the Magnet to be made) each about 10 Inches long, 1 Inch broad, and half a Line in Thicknefs. It is ufelefs to make them thicker, becaufe the magnetick Virtue will not penetrate further into the Steel Blades.

Now thefe Blades being firft touched with a good Stone, are afterwards laid one upon another, having their Poles, of the fame Denomination, turned the fame way, forming a Parallelopipedon, then they are preffed together with four Brafs Stirrups, and as many little Wedges

ges

ges 3, 3, 3, 3, of the ſame Metal, and encompaſſed with Iron Armour of a proper Length, Breadth, and Thickneſs This Armour is held by a Braſs Girdle, and faſtened with the Screws 2, 2 At the Top is placed a Braſs Plate, to which is faſtened the Pendant 4, and its Ring , and at the Bottom is the *Porte-Poids* 5 But, *Note*, that the Baſe of the *Porte-Poids* muſt make the perfecteſt Contact poſſible with the Heads *a, b*, of the Armour. When artificial Magnets are well made, and touched with good Stones, they will have as much Virtue in them as good natural ones, and may be uſed for the ſame Experiments

The Conſtruction of the Spring Steel-yard

Fig. 9.

This Machine, which is portable, and ſerves to weigh any thing from one Pound to about forty, is compoſed of a Braſs Tube or Pipe, open at the Ends, about 4 or 5 Inches long, and 7 or 8 Lines broad, one End whereof is marked 3 ; the reſt being open for ſhewing the Inſide, which is a Spring (2) of tempered Steel-Wire, made like a Worm. *Number 6.* is a little Feril ſcrewed upon the Top of the ſquare Braſs Rod 1, which the Spring croſſes Upon this Rod are the Diviſions of Pounds, and Parts of a Pound, which are made in ſucceſſively hanging on the Hook (4) 1, 2 3, *&c.* Pounds · for the Spring being faſtened by a Screw to the Bottom of the ſquare Rod, the greater the Weight is, that is hung on the Hook, the more will the Spring be contracted , and conſequently a greater part of the Rod will come out of the Tube, thro the ſquare Hole C · therefore if you have a mind to mark the Diviſion for any Number of Pounds upon the Rod, ſuppoſe 10, hang 10 Pounds upon the Hook, and where the Edge of the ſquare Hole C, at the Top of the Tube, cuts the Rod, make a Mark upon the Rod for 10 Pounds, and ſo for any other.

The Uſe of this Inſtrument is very eaſy ; for having ſcrewed the Feril 6 on the Top of the Rod, if you hold the Inſtrument in your Hand by the Hook 5, and hang any thing to be weighed upon the Hook 4, then where the Edge C of the ſquare Hole cuts the Rod, will be the Weight of the thing required

The chief Goodneſs of this Inſtrument conſiſts in having a well-tempered Spring ; ſo that it may fold according to the Force of the Weight it is to carry, and alſo in having a Bigneſs proportionable

The Conſtruction of the Beam Steel-yard.

Fig. 10.

This Inſtrument, which is a kind of Steel-yard, or Balance of Mr *Caſſini*'s Invention, conſiſts of a Rod ſuſpended by a Beam, in its Point of Equilibrium 5, which divides the ſaid Rod into two Arms (like the two Arms of a common Balance) each of which are lengthwiſe divided into equal Parts, beginning from the Point of Suſpenſion or Equilibrium

The Uſe of this Balance is to find both the Weight and Price of Goods at the ſame time. If you uſe it for weighing any thing, the Counter-Weight 4 of one Pound, or one Ounce, muſt be hung to one of the Arms (according as Goods are to be weighed by Pounds or Ounces) ſo that it may ſlide along the Arm, like as in *Roman* Balances ; and on the other Arm muſt be hung on a ſilken Line, for ſuſtaining things to be weighed. Then to weigh any thing, you muſt place the ſil— Line, to which the thing is hung, upon the firſt Diviſion of the Arm, nigheſt the Point of Equilibrium, and moving the Counter-weight upon the other Arm, till it makes an Equilibrium, the Point whereon it falls will ſhow the Weight ſought

To know the Weight of Goods, according to any Price ; for Example, at ſeven Pence an Ounce or Pound , place the Line, ſuſtaining the Goods, upon the Diviſion 7 of the Arm , then placing the Line, carrying the Counter-weight upon the other Arm, ſo that it be in *Equilibrio*, and the Number of Diviſions, from the Point of Suſpenſion to the Line ſuſtaining the Counter-weight, will give the Value of the Goods weighed.

But for Goods that cannot be weighed, unleſs in a Scale, take a Scale of a known Weight, and having hung it upon a Hook to the Arm, proceed as before, and ſubſtract the Weight of the Scale

A *Paris* Pound is 16 Ounces, and is divided into 2 Marks, each of which is 8 Ounces , an Ounce is ſubdivided into 8 Drams, a Dram into 72 Grains, and a Grain, which is nighly the Weight of a Grain of Wheat, is the leaſt Weight uſed.

A Quintal weighs 100 Pounds.

The Paris *Pound compared with thoſe of other Countries.*

The Pound of *Avignon, Lyons, Montpelier*, and *Thouloufe* is 13 Ounces.

The Pound of *Marſeilles* and *Rochell* is 19 Ounces.

The Pound of *Rouen, Beſançon, Straſburgh*, and *Amſterdam* is 16 Ounces, like that of *Paris.*

The Pound of *Milan, Naples*, and *Venice* is 9 Ounce.

The Pound of *Meſſina* and *Genoa* is 9 ½ Ounces.

The Pound of *Florence, Leghorne, Piſa, Sarragoſſa* and *Valence* is 10 Ounces.

The Pound of *Turin* and *Modena* is 10 ⅔ Ounces

The Pound of *London, Antwerp*, and *Flanders* is 14 Ounces.

The Pound of *Baſil, Berne, Frankfort*, and *Nuremburgh* is 16 Ounces and 14 Grains.

That of *Geneva* is 17 Ounces.

Conſtruction

Construction of an Instrument for raising of Weights.

The Instrument of *Fig* 11 consists of two Sheaves, each of which carries eight Pullies, Fig. 11. hollowed in to receive a Rope, which is fastened at one End to the upper Sheave, and after having put it round all the Pullies, the other End of it must be joined to the Power represented by the Hand   Four of the Pullies are carried upon one Axel-Tree, and four upon another, as well in the upper Sheave as in the lower one   At the Top of the upper Sheave is a Ring to hang the Machine in a fixed Place, and at the Bottom of the other, there is another Ring to hang the Weights to

The Use of this Machine is to lift up or draw great Burdens, by multiplying the Force of the Power, which augments, in the Ratio of Unity, to double the Number of the Pullies in the lower Sheave, so that in this Instrument, where the lower Sheave carries eight Pullies, if the Weight (4) weighs 16 Pounds, the Power need be but a little above one Pound to make an Equilibrium, I say, a little above, because of the Friction of the Ropes and Axes' The Pullies of the upper Sheave do not at all contribute to the Augmentation of the Force, but only to facilitate the Motion in taking away the Friction of the Rope, because being as Leavers of the first kind, whose fixed Point is in the middle, the Power will be equal to the Weight, but the Pullies below are as Leavers of the second kind, whose fixed Point is at one of the Ends   for their Diameter is, as it were, fixed at one End, and lifted up at the other, by which each of the Pullies double their Force, since the way moved thro' by the Power, is double to that moved thro' by the Weight

The Construction of the Wind-Cane

This Instrument is about three Foot long, and twelve or fifteen Lines in Thickness   The Fig 12. Tube 3 is made of Brass, very round, and well soldered, from 4 to 6 Lines in Diameter, stopped at one End *a*   At the Place 1 is likewise another larger Tube, so disposed about the former one, that there remains a Space 4, wherein the Air may be closely included   These two Tubes ought to be joined together at one End by a circular Plate *c c*, exactly soldered to them both, for hindering the Air's getting out of the Space 4   The Piece 8 is a Valve stopping a Hole, permitting the Air to pass from 2 towards 1, but not to return from 1 towards 2   There are, moreover, two Holes near the stopped End of the Tube 3; thro one of these Holes, which is marked 6, the Air would come out of the Space 4 into the Tube 3, if it was not hindered by a Spring-Valve opening outwardly   The other Hole is marked 5, thro which there is a Communication with the outward Air, and the Air in the Cavity of the Tube 3, but yet so, that the Air, inclosed in the Space 4, cannot come out thro the Hole 5, it being hindered by a little short Tube soldered to the Tubes 1 and 3   Lastly, the Tube 2 represents the Body of a Syringe, by which as much Air as possible may be intruded into the Space 4; after which having put a Bullet into the Cavity of the Tube 3, near the little Tube 5, the Cane will be charged.   Now, to discharge it, you must push up the Spring-Valve 6, by means of a little Pin exactly filling the Cavity of the little Tube 5, then the compressed Air, in the Cavity 4, will dilate itself, and pass thro' the Hole 6, into the Cavity of the Tube 3, will push the Bullet out with a great force, even to its penetrating thro' a Board of an ordinary Thickness

Note   At Number 7 this Cane may be taken into two Pieces, by unscrewing of it, and the Handle 12 may be taken out, and instead thereof the Head of a Cane put thereon.

The Construction of the Æolipile.

This Instrument is made of hammered Copper, in form of a Ball, or hollow Pear, having Fig. 13. a Neck soldered to it, and a very little Hole drilled at the End of this Neck

The Air in the Ball is first rarefied, by bringing it to the Fire, and afterwards plunging it into cold Water, will condense the Air in it, and the Water will pass thro' the little Hole into the Cavity of the Instrument.

Now having let about as much Water, as will fill ⅞ of the Æolipile, get into it, if it be set upon a good Fire, in the same Situation as in the Figure, the Water, as it grows hot, will dilate itself by little and little, and throw up Vapours into the Space of Air contained between the Surface of the Water, and the little Hole at the End of the Neck, which, together with the Air, will very swiftly crowd thro' the little Hole, and produce a Wind and violent Hissing, continuing till all the Water be evaporated, or the Heat extinguished   *Note*, This Wind has all the Properties of the natural Wind blowing upon the Surface of the Earth.

The Construction of four different Microscopes

This is a Microscope for viewing very minute Objects and Animals that are in Liquors Fig. 14. It is composed of two Plates of Brass, or other Metal, about 3 Inches long, and 8 Lines broad, fastened together, nigh the Ends, by two Screws, 2, 2, which likewise serve to fix the Plates at such a Distance from each other, that a Wheel may turn which has six round Holes, in every of which are flat Pieces of Glass to put different Objects upon, marked 3, 4, 5, &c. Next to the Eye there is a concave Piece of Brass 1, having a Hole in the middle, in which is put a very small *Lens*, or Ball of Glass. This Ball ought to be very convex, and well polished,

in

in order to diſtinguiſh minute Objects The End of the Machine is filed in manner of a Handle to hold it

The Uſe of this Inſtrument is very eaſy ; if the Objects are tranſparent, as the Feet of a Flea, or of Flies, their Wings, the Mites in Cheeſe, or other minute Animals, as likewiſe Hairs of the Head, their Roots, &c. they are put upon the Glaſs Plates on the Wheel, and are held faſt with a little Gum-water : and to ſee the little Animals in ſtale Urine, Vinegar, in Water where there has been infuſed Pepper, Coriander, Straw, Hay, or almoſt any kind of Herbs ; little Drops thereof muſt be taken up with the End of a little Glaſs Pipe, and laid upon the aforeſaid Glaſſes : then the Wheel muſt be turned and raiſed, or depreſſed by means of the Screws 2, 2, and a Spring between the Plates, which ſerves to keep the Wheel in any Situation required, in ſuch manner that a little Drop may be exactly under the Lens Things being thus ordered, take the Microſcope in your Hand, and having placed your Eye to the Concave 1, over the Lens, look ſteadily at the Drop in broad Daylight, or at Night by the Light of a Wax Candle ; at the ſame time turn the Screw at the End by little and little, to bring the Drop nigher, or make it further from the Lens, until the Point be found where the Object will be tranſparent, or the Animals ſwimming in the Drop of Liquor, appear very large and diſtinct

Conſtruction of another Microſcope

Fig 15.

This Microſcope is compoſed of a Braſs Plate about three Inches high, and ¼ an Inch broad, cut in Form of a Parallelogram, at the Bottom of which there is a Handle to hold it The Place marked 1, is a little Groove drilled thro the Middle, in the Hole of which is placed a Lens faſtened in a little Frame ; there may be put into it Lenſes of diverſe Foci, according to the different Objects to be obſerved   *Note,* That the Focus of a Glaſs, is its Diſtance from the Object, and that Lenſes are uſed in theſe Microſcopes, whoſe Foci are from half a Line to four Lines.

On the Backſide of the aforeſaid Plate, (at the Place 2) is fixed a little ſquare Branch of Braſs or Steel, carrying another Plate that ſlides upon it by means of a little Box, a Spring, and a Screw, turned by help of a Wheel, cut into Teeth, which ſerves to bring the ſaid Plate nigher to, or more diſtant from that which carries the Lens. Towards the Top of the ſecond Plate, which has a Hole drilled in it, is alſo a Groove, in which is placed little Pieces of plain Glaſs, and round Concaves to put Liquors on There may be different Glaſſes put in that Groove for viewing different Objects. Laſtly, Obſerve that all the Objects anſwer to the Center of the Lens, and that there muſt be adjuſted on the other Side of the Plate a little Tube (marked 3) of Braſs, about an Inch Diameter, and one or two long, whoſe Center muſt very exactly anſwer to the Center of the Lenſes. It has been found that with ſuch a Tube, theſe Microſcopes will have much more effect upon tranſparent Objects, than without it. The Circulation of the Blood may pretty diſtinctly be obſerved in the Tails of little Fiſhes by this Microſcope, which is, in my Opinion, the moſt commodious of any

The Uſe of this Inſtrument is very eaſy, for having placed the Object over-againſt the Center of the Lens, move it backwards and forwards by means of the Screw, till it be ſeen very diſtinctly

Conſtruction of a ſingle Glaſs Microſcope.

Fig 16.

The little Inſtrument of *Fig 16* is a Microſcope commodious enough, compoſed of a Branch of Braſs, or other Metal, having a Motion towards the Top, for putting it into the Situation as *per Fig.* The Piece, at the End, carries a very convex Lens, magnifying the Object very much : this Branch is ſcrewed into a little Box 5, bored through the Bottom. The Piece 4, is two Springs faſtened to one another in the Middle with a Rivet, to give it a Motion deſired The Branch which carries the Lens, is put through one of the Springs, and through the other there is put a little Branch, carrying at one End the Piece 2, which is white on one Side, and black on the other, for different Objects. The other End 3, is a little kind of Pincer, which opens by preſſing two little Buttons, it ſerves to hold little Animals, or other Bodies. The Foot 5, is about 1 ½ Inch in Diameter, the Branch ſcrews into it, in order to take to pieces the Inſtrument

The Uſe of it is very eaſy, for the Objects being placed upon the little round Piece, or at the End of the Pincer, you muſt bring the Lens towards them, by ſliding the Spring along the Branch, till the Objects be ſeen very diſtinct.

There may likewiſe be diſcovered with this Microſcope, the Animals which are in Liquors, by putting a flat Glaſs in the Place of the little round Piece 2, which unſcrews.

Conſtruction of a Three-Glaſs Microſcope

Fig. 17.

This Inſtrument is compoſed of three Glaſſes, *viz.* the Eye Glaſs 3, the Middle Glaſs 4, and the Object Lens 5 There is a Cover ſcrewed on at the Top to preſerve the Eye Glaſs from Duſt · theſe three Glaſſes are ſet in wooden Circles, and ſcrewed into their Places, for eaſier taking them out to cleanſe The Eye Glaſs, and the middle one, are placed at the Ends of a Tube of Parchment, exactly entering into the outward Tube, in order to lengthen the Microſcope, and place it at its exact Point, according to a Line drawn round about the

afore-

aforesaid Tube. To have this Instrument of a reasonable Bigness, the focal Distance of the Eye Glass ought to be about 20 Lines, that of the middle Glass about 3 Inches, and placed about 3 Inches 3 Lines distant from one another.

The Object Lens is placed at the End of a wooden Tail-piece, glued to the End of the outward Tube, and is enclosed in a little Box, bored through the Bottom, which unscrews in order to change the Object Lenses, and put in others of different focal Distances, which are commonly 2, 3, 4, and 5 Lines in Diameter, and are more or less convex. The Goodness of these Glasses consists in having the concave Brass Basons they are ground in, turned in a just Proportion to the Glasses to be worked, as also in the Motion of the Hand, and the Goodness of the Matter used to construct them, and above all in well polishing them. Brown Freestone is first used to fashion them in the Bason, then fine Sand to smooth them, and Tripoli to polish them. I shall say no more of the Construction of these Glasses, M. Chershm having sufficiently spoken thereof.

The Foot 1, which ought to be pretty heavy to keep the Microscope from falling, is made of Brass 4 or 5 Inches in Diameter, having a Cavity in the Middle, wherein is put a little Piece, white on one Side, and black on the other · black Objects are placed upon the white Side, and white Objects upon the black Side.

The round Brass Branch is fastened at the Edge of the Foot, upon which the Microscope may slide up or down, and turn round by means of the Support or double Square · there is a Circle, or Ring, strongly fastened to the Support, and which very exactly encompasses the outward Tube. There is also a Steel Spring which bears against the Branch, and keeps the Instrument in a required Situation.

Number 6, is a little Brass Frame, having in it a Piece of flat Glass to lay transparent Objects upon. This Frame may slide up and down the Branch underneath the Microscope, and is supported by a double Square.

Lastly, Number 7 is a convex Glass converging the Rays of Light, coming from a Candle under it, and throwing them strongly under the transparent Object on the Glass, makes it be seen more distinctly. The aforesaid Glass is set in a Brass Circle, and rises, falls, and turns by means of a little Arm carrying it, as the Figure shews.

USE *of the aforesaid Microscope*

To use this Instrument, for Example, to observe the Circulation of the Blood in some Animal; a live Fish must be placed upon the Glass 6, so that one part of the Fins of the Tail be exactly opposite to the Object Glass, and over the Ray of the Convex-Glass in broad Daylight, or the Spot of the Candle, in the Night; then place the Microscope exactly to such a Point, and you will see the Blood rise, descend, or circulate.

Number 9, is a little Piece of Lead hollowed, to keep the Fish from any how stirring to hinder the Experiment.

Liquors may also by this Microscope be very well examined, for if you put a little Drop of Vinegar upon the Glass just over the bright Spot, the little Animals in it will very distinctly be observed. The same may be observed of Water in which Pepper or Barley has been infused, &c. as also the Eels and other little Animals observed in standing Water.

A Drop of Blood may be observed by putting it hot over the Speck of the Candle, upon the Glass; after which its Serosity, and little Globules of a reddish Colour, may be discovered therein.

The best way to get a Drop of Blood is to tie a Thread about one's Thumb, and then prick it with a Needle.

The best way to put Liquors upon the Glass, is by taking a Drop of them up with the small End of a little Glass Tube, and then blowing softly at the other End, will make the Liquor descend and drop upon the Glass.

To get a great Number of little Eels in a small Quantity of Liquor, the Liquor must be put into a very narrow-necked Bottle, and always kept full; for by this means, the Animals coming to the Top to get Air, may be sucked into a little Tube in greater Numbers, than if the Neck of the Bottle was wider.

The Eyes of Flies, Ants, Lice, Fleas, and Mites, are put in the Middle of the Foot of the Microscope, as also Sand, Salt, &c. to examine their Colours and Qualities, always observing to lay black Objects upon the white, and white Objects upon the black Side.

I suppose here that the Microscope Glasses are well worked, and placed in their Foci. Note also, that the shorter the Focus of an Object Glass is, the greater will the Object appear, but not altogether so distinct.

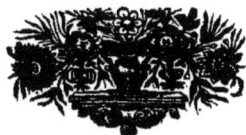

Cc

BOOK

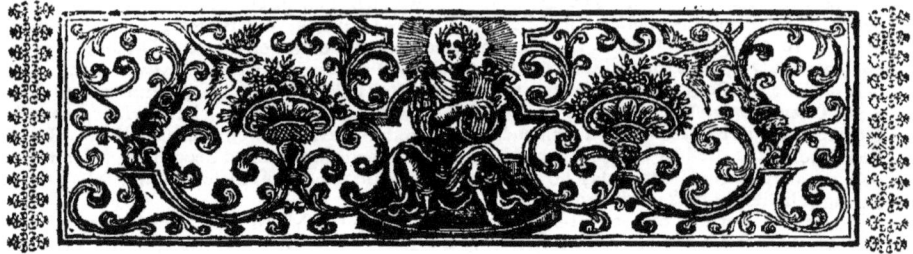

B O O K IV.

Of the Construction and Uses of Mathematical Instru-
ments for measuring and laying out of Land, taking
of Plots, Heights, and Distances; the most usual of
which, are Staffs, Lines, the Toise or Fathom, the
Chain, Surveying-Crosses or Squares, Recipient-
Angles or Measure-Angles, Theodolites, the Qua-
drant, the Semi-circle, and the Compass.

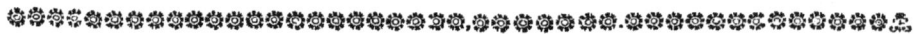

C H A P. I.

Containing the Description and Uses of Staffs, Lines, the Fathom
or Toise, and the Chain.

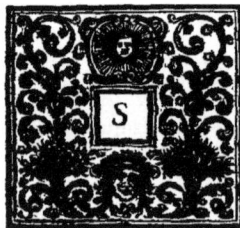

Plate 11.

Fig. A.

Fig B

Fig C

Fig D.

Fig. E.

STAFFS are made of hard Wood, 2 or 3 Foot long, cut pecked at one End, upon which are put pointed Caps of Iron, to make them go easier into the Ground There are sometimes longer ones made, in order to be seen at a great distance

Lines ought to be of good Packthread, or Whipcord, well twisted, and of a convenient Thickness, that they may not easily stretch.

The Toise, or Fathom, is a round Staff 6 Foot long, divided into Feet by little Rings, or Brass Pins, the last Foot being divided into 12 Inches, likewise distinguish'd by little Brass Pins

There are Toises that may be taken into 2, 3, or 4 Pieces, by means of Ferils and Brass Screws at the End of each Piece.

There are also two Brass or Steel Ferils, put upon each End of the Toise, to preserve its Length.

The Chain is composed of several Pieces of thick Iron or Brass Wire, bent at the Ends, each of which is a Foot long, and are joined together with little Rings

Chains are commonly a Perch, or else 4 or 5 Toises in Length, distinguish'd by a great Ring from Toise to Toise These sort of Chains are very commodious, because they will not entangle themselves, as those will that are made with little Iron Rings

In the Year 1668, there was placed a new Toise for a Standard, at the Foot of the Stairs of the *Grand Chatelet* at *Paris*, for having recourse to in case of Need

We have said that a Toise in Length contains 6 Feet, and each Foot 12 Inches

A square Toise contains 36 square Feet, and a square Foot 144 Inches; because 6 times 6 is 36, and 12 times 12 is 144

A

Plate X

I Senex sculp.

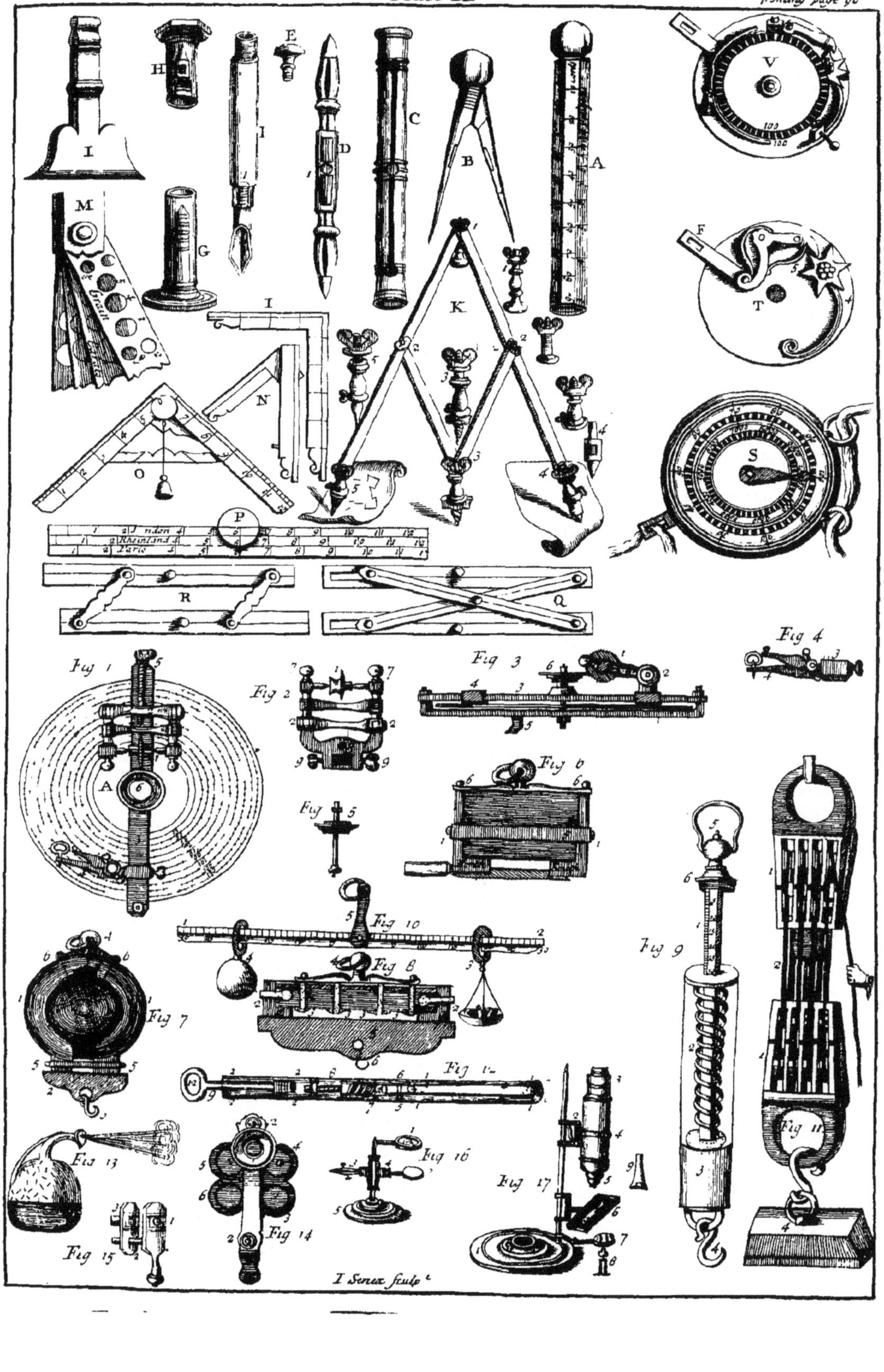

A Cubick Toise contains 216 Cubick Feet, and a Cubick Foot 1728 Cubick Inches, because the Cube of 6 is 216, and the Cube of 12 is 1728

The Length of a Perch is not determined

That of *Paris* is 3 Toises, or 18 Feet, in other Countries it is 20, 22, and 24 Feet

The Perch, used in *France*, to measure Waters and Forests, according to the last Regulation, is 22 Feet long, and consequently a square Perch is 484 square Feet

The Arpent is a superficial Measure, used to measure Ground or Woods

The Arpent of *Paris*, and the adjacent Parts, contains 100 square Perches, or 900 Toises · the Side of which must consequently be 10 Perches, or 30 Toises

A League is a Measure for High-ways, or great Distances; its Length is not determined, being different in different Countries

It is reckoned from the Gate of *Paris*, nigh the *Grand Chatelet*, to the Gate of the Church of *St Dennis*, 2 Leagues, each of which is 2200 Toises

The Gentlemen of the Academy of Sciences have found, that a Degree of a great Circle of the Earth contains 57060 Toises; and giving 25 Leagues to a Degree, each League will contain 2282 Toises.

A Sea-League is greater, for there goes but 20 to make a Degree; therefore it contains about 3000 Toises

The *Italians* reckon by Miles, each of which contains 1000 Geometrical Paces

A Geometrical Pace is five of the antient Feet, one of which the antient *Roman* Palm is three quarters, which may be esteemed about 11 of our Inches, and consequently an *Italian* Mile contains about 769 of our Toises

The *Germans* also reckon by the Mile, but they are much greater than the *Italian* Miles, for one of them contains 3626 Toises

They count by Leagues in *Spain*, one of which contains 2863 Toises, 20 of which exactly make one Terrestrial Degree,

The same may be said of the *English* and *Dutch* Leagues.

USE I. *To draw a right Line thro two Points given upon the Ground, and produce it to any required Length.*

Plant a Staff upon each of the given Points, very upright, and having strained a Line from one Staff to the other, by that Line, as a Guide, draw a Line upon the Ground.

That right Line may be continued by planting a third Staff, so that by placing the Eye to the Edge of the first, the Edges of the two others may be but just seen, and again, the Line may be continued, by taking that Staff, which was the first, and placing it as a third, &c.

USE II. *To measure a right Line upon the Ground*

When a long Line upon the Ground is to be measured, Precaution must be used that we do not mistake, and be obliged to begin again. To do which, two Men must each of them have a Toise, the first having laid down his, must not lift it up, till the second has placed his at the End of the first Man's Toise. The first Man having lifted up his Toise, must loudly count 1, and when he has again laid his down to the End of the second Man's, the second Man must lift up his, and count 2. In thus continuing on to the End, and in order to lay the Toises in a right Line, there must be placed two Staffs, at a Distance before them, to look at; for if there is but one, the Toises cannot be so truly laid in a right Line by help of it

To spare Time and Pains, you ought to have a Chain of 30 Feet, or 5 Toises long, with a Ring at each End, carried by two Men, the first of which carries several Staffs. When the Chain is well extended on the right Line to be measured, the foremost Man must place a Staff at the End of 5 Toises, to the end that the hinder Man may know where the Chain ended; for the whole Matter consists in well counting, and exactly measuring.

USE III. *From a Point given in a right Line, to raise a Perpendicular*

Let the given Line be A B, and the given Point C

Plant a Staff in the Point C, and two others, as E, D, in the same Line, equally distant Fig. 1. from the Point C; then fasten the two Ends of a Line to the two Staves E, D, and fold the Line into two equal Parts in F, afterwards stretch the Line tight, and at the Point F plant a Staff, and the Line F C will be perpendicular to A B

Otherwise, measure 4 Feet, or 4 Toises, from the Point C, on the Line A B, and plant Fig 2. there the Staff G, take a Line containing 8 Feet, or 8 Toises (according as the former are Feet or Toises) fasten one End of the Line to the Staff C, and the other to the Staff G, then stretch the Line, so that 3 of those Parts be next to the Point C, and 5 next to G, plant a Staff in H, and the Line H C will be perpendicular to A B

USE IV. *From a given Point without a Line, to draw a Perpendicular.*

Let the given Line be A B, and the Point F

Fold your Line into two equal Parts, and fix the middle to the Staff F, stretch the two Fig. 3. Halves (which I suppose long enough) to the Line A B, then plant two Staffs, namely, one

to

to each End of your Line, and divide their Distance into two equal Parts, which may be done by folding a Line as long as the Distance A B , plant a Staff in the middle C, and the Line C F will be perpendicular to the Line A B.

USE V *To draw a Line parallel to another, at a given Distance from it*

Fig 4.

Let the given Line be A B, and it is required to draw a Line parallel to it at the Distance of 4 Toises

Raise (by *Use* 3) two Perpendiculars, each of 4 Toises, upon the Points A, B, and upon the Points C, D plant two Staffs, by which draw the Line C D, which will be parallel to A B.

USE VI *To make an Angle on the Ground, at the End of a Line, equal to an Angle given.*

Fig. 5

Let A B C be the given Angle (which suppose is drawn upon Paper)

About the Point B, as a Center, describe upon the Paper the Arc A C, and draw the right Line A C, which will be the Chord of the said Arc. Measure with a Scale, or the Line of equal Parts of the Sector, the Length of one of the equal Legs A B, or B C of the said Angle ; likewise measure, with the same Scale, the Length of the Chord A C, which, for Example, suppose 36 of those equal Parts, whereof the Leg A B contains 30

Now let there be upon the Ground a right Line, as B C, to which it is required to draw another Line F B, making an Angle with B C equal to the proposed one   Plant a Staff in the Point B, and having measured 30 Feet, or 5 Toises, on the Line B C, there plant a Staff, as D, then take two Lines, one of 30 Feet long, which fasten to the Staff B, and the other 36 Feet, which likewise fasten to the Staff D   Draw the Lines tight, and make their Ends meet in the Point F, where again plant a Staff, from which draw the Line F B, which will form, at the Point B, the Angle F B C equal to the proposed one A B C.

USE VII *To draw upon Paper an Angle, equal to a given one upon the Ground.*

Fig 5

This Problem is the Converse of the former.

Let the given Angle upon the Ground be F B C ; measure 30 Feet, or 5 Toises, from B towards C, at the End of which plant the Staff D, measure likewise 30 Feet from B towards F, and there plant another Staff, measure also the Distance of the Staffs F, D, which suppose will be 36 Feet, (as in *Use* VI)

Now let B C be a Line upon the Paper , then about the Point B, as a Center, and with a Length of 30 equal Parts (taken from a Scale) describe the Arc A C , and take 36 of the same Parts, and lay them off from the Point C, upon the Arc C A, and a Line drawn from B to A will make, with the Line B C, the Angle required

If, moreover, the Quantity of the aforesaid Angle be desired, it will be found, by the Protractor, something less than 64 Degrees

The Quantity of Angles (whose Chords are known) in Degrees and Minutes, may more exactly be known by the following Table, which is calculated for Angles, always contained under equal Sides of 30 Feet each

The Use of the said Table is very easy for finding the Quantity of any Plane Angles upon the Ground   for measure 30 Feet upon each of the Lines forming an Angle, and plant a Staff at the End of 30 Feet upon each Line ; then measure the Distance between the two Staffs, which suppose to be 36 Feet (as in the preceding Example) look in the Table in the Column of Bases of 36 Feet, and you will find over against it, in the Column of Angles, 63 Degrees, 44 Minutes, the Quantity of the said Angle

A TABLE of Plane Angles, contained under Sides of 30 Feet.

Bases	Angles D M	Bases	Angles D M	Bases	Angles D M	Bases	Angles D M	Bases	Angles D M	Bases	Angles D M	Bases	Angles D M	Bases	Angles D M	Bases	Angles D M	Bases	Angl. D M
2	0 19	2	6 3	2	11 48	2	17 34	2	23 24	2	29 17	2	35 15	2	41 19	2	47 30	2	53 51
4	0 38	4	6 22	4	12 8	4	17 54	4	23 44	4	29 37	4	35 35	4	41 40	4	47 51	4	54 12
6	0 57	6	6 41	6	12 27	6	18 13	6	24 3	6	29 56	6	35 55	6	41 0	6	48 12	6	54 34
8	1 8	8	7 0	8	12 46	8	18 32	8	24 23	8	30 16	8	36 15	8	42 20	8	48 33	8	54 55
10	1 36	10	7 20	10	13 5	10	18 52	10	24 42	10	30 36	10	36 35	10	44 40	10	48 54	10	55 18
1	1 55	4	7 39	7	13 24	10	19 11	13	25 1	16	30 56	19	36 55	22	43 1	25	49 15	28	55 38
2	2 14	2	7 58	2	13 43	2	19 30	2	25 21	2	31 16	2	37 15	2	43 22	2	49 36	2	56 0
4	2 33	4	8 17	4	14 2	4	19 50	4	25 41	4	31 36	4	37 36	4	43 42	4	49 57	4	56 22
6	2 52	6	8 36	6	14 22	6	20 19	6	26 1	6	31 56	6	37 56	6	44 3	6	50 18	6	56 43
8	3 11	8	8 55	8	14 41	8	20 29	8	26 20	8	32 16	8	38 16	8	44 24	8	50 39	8	57 5
10	3 30	10	9 14	10	15 0	10	20 48	10	26 40	10	32 35	10	38 36	10	44 44	10	51 0	10	57 26
2	3 49	5	9 34	8	15 20	11	21 8	14	26 53	17	32 55	20	38 56	23	45 5	26	51 21	29	57 48
2	4 8	2	9 53	2	15 39	2	21 27	2	27 18	2	33 15	2	39 17	2	45 26	2	51 42	2	58 10
4	4 28	4	10 12	4	15 58	4	21 46	4	27 38	4	33 35	4	39 38	4	45 46	4	52 3	4	58 32
6	4 47	6	10 31	6	16 18	6	22 16	6	27 58	6	33 55	6	39 58	6	46 7	6	52 24	6	58 54
8	5 6	8	10 50	8	16 37	8	22 25	8	28 18	8	34 15	8	40 18	8	46 28	8	52 46	8	59 16
10	5 25	10	11 9	10	16 56	10	22 45	10	28 38	10	34 35	10	40 38	10	46 48	10	53 8	10	59 38
3	5 44	6	11 29	9	17 15	12	23 6	15	28 57	18	34 55	21	40 59	24	47 9	27	53 29	30	60 0

Bases	Angles	Bases	Angles	Bases	Angles	Bases	Angles	Bases	Angles	Bases	Angles	Bases	Angles	Bases	Angles	Bases	Angles	Bases	Angles
2	60 22	2	67 7	2	74 8	2	81 30	2	89 18	2	97 40	2	106 48	2	117 2	2	129 3	2	144 39
4	60 44	4	67 30	4	74 32	4	81 55	4	89 45	4	98 9	4	107 20	4	117 39	4	129 48	4	145 43
6	61 6	6	67 53	6	74 56	6	82 20	6	90 12	6	98 38	6	107 52	6	118 16	6	130 33	6	146 48
8	61 28	8	68 16	8	75 20	8	82 46	8	90 39	8	99 8	8	108 25	8	118 53	8	131 19	8	147 57
10	61 50	10	68 39	0	75 44	10	83 12	10	91 6	10	99 37	10	108 57	10	119 31	10	132 6	10	149 8
31	62 13	34	69 2	37	76 9	40	83 37	43	91 33	46	100 6	49	109 30	52	120 9	55	132 53	58	150 20
2	62 35	2	69 25	2	76 33	2	84 3	2	92 1	2	100 36	2	110 4	2	120 47	2	133 44	2	151 36
4	62 58	4	69 48	4	76 57	4	84 29	4	92 29	4	101 6	4	110 37	4	121 26	4	134 30	4	152 55
6	63 20	6	70 12	6	77 22	6	84 54	6	92 56	6	101 36	6	111 11	6	122 6	6	135 20	6	154 19
8	63 43	8	70 35	8	77 46	8	85 20	8	93 24	8	102 7	8	111 44	8	122 45	8	136 11	8	155 48
10	64 5	10	70 59	10	78 9	10	85 46	10	93 52	10	102 37	10	112 18	10	123 25	10	137 3	10	157 22
32	64 28	35	71 22	38	78 35	41	86 13	44	94 20	47	103 8	50	112 53	53	124 6	56	137 57	59	159 3
2	64 50	2	71 46	2	79 0	2	86 39	2	94 48	2	103 39	2	113 28	2	124 47	2	138 49	2	160 53
4	65 13	4	72 10	4	79 25	4	87 5	4	95 16	4	104 10	4	114 3	4	125 28	4	139 44	4	162 54
6	65 36	6	72 33	6	79 50	6	87 32	6	95 20	6	104 41	6	114 38	6	126 10	6	140 40	6	165 12
8	65 58	8	72 56	8	80 15	8	87 58	8	96 13	8	105 12	8	115 14	8	126 52	8	141 38	8	167 48
10	66 21	10	73 20	10	80 40	10	88 25	10	96 42	10	105 44	10	115 49	10	127 35	10	142 36	10	171 28
33	66 44	36	73 44	39	81 5	42	88 51	45	97 11	48	106 16	51	116 26	54	128 19	57	143 36	60	180 0

Note, That in the Columns of Bases are only set down every 2 Inches, and the Feet from 1 to 60. By means of this Table may be easily and exactly found the Opening and Quantity of any Angle, for suppose your Base be in Length 50 Feet, 3 Inches, and the other 2 Sides each 30 Feet, which they must always be: Seek 50 Feet, 2 Inches, in the Column of Bases; and against it you will find, in the Column of Angles, 113 Deg 28 Min whence by making due Proportion with the Inches and Minutes, the Quantity of the Angle sought will be 113 Deg 44 Min. This Table, together with a well divided Brass Scale, may be used in measuring or laying off Angles upon Paper, with as much Exactness as Lines will do them upon the Ground; because the Sides of equi-angled Triangles are proportional to each other.

This Method of measuring plane Angles, may likewise serve to make Designs of Fortifications, both regular and irregular, to find the Quantities of Angles, as well of Bastions as of the Polygon, formed by the Concourse of the Lines of the Bases, or exterior Sides, either upon Paper or the Ground.

To draw Angles by this Table, seek for the Degrees and Minutes you design an Angle to consist of, which for Example, suppose 54 Deg 34 Min. and against them, in the Column of Bases, is the Number of Feet and Inches corresponding thereto, viz. 27 Feet, 6 Inches; which

D d

which is the Length of the Baſe of the Angle, each of the other Sides of which is 30 Feet, and ſo of others

U S E VIII. *To take the Plan or Plot of a Place within it*

Let the Place whoſe Plan is required, be A B C D E

First, make a Figure upon your Paper, ſomething like the Plan to be taken, and after having meaſured with a Toiſe the Sides A B, B C, C D, D E, and E A, write the Lengths found upon each of their correſponding Lines on the Paper, then inſtead of meaſuring the Angles made by the Sides, meaſure the Diagonals A D, B D, which write down in your Book, and the Figure will be reduced into three Triangles, whoſe Sides are all known, becauſe they have been actually meaſured. Then the Figure muſt be drawn neat in your Book by means of a Scale of equal Parts.

Note, Of all the Ways to take the Plans of Places, that of taking it within is the beſt

U S E IX *To take the Plot of any Place (as a Wood, or marſhy Ground) by meaſuring round about it.*

First draw a rough Sketch of the Figure in your Field-Book if it takes not too much time in going round the Place, then meaſure with a Toiſe, or Chain, all the Sides encompaſſing the Figure propoſed, and ſet the Numbers found upon each correſpondent Line, in your Book, but for the Angles, you muſt meaſure them as follows

To meaſure, for Example, the Angle E F G, produce the Side E F, 5 Toiſes, and plant a Staff at the End K, produce alſo the Side G F, the Length of 5 Toiſes, and plant a Staff at the End L Meaſure the Diſtance L K, and ſuppoſing it 6 Toiſes, 4 Feet, that is 40 Feet, ſet it down upon the Line L K in your Book, by which means the three Sides of the Iſoſceles Triangle L F K will be had, and conſequently the Angle L F K, may be known by the aforementioned Table, or otherwiſe Now the aforeſaid Angle is equal to its oppoſite one E F G, and if you ſeek 40 Feet in the Column of Baſes, the Angle will be found 83 Deg 37 Min

In the ſame manner may the Angle F G H, or any other of the propoſed Figure, be meaſured or elſe thus, Produce the Side H G, the Length of 5 Toiſes, to N, where plant a Staff, make likewiſe G M, 5 Toiſes Meaſure the Diſtance M N, which ſuppoſe, for Example, 6 Toiſes, 2 Feet, or 38 Feet, which write upon the Line M N in your Book

This Number ſought in the Column of Baſes, correſponds to 78 Deg 35 Min for the exterior Angle M G N, whoſe Complement 101 Deg. 25 Min. is the Quantity of the Angle F G H

Then the Figure in your Field-Book muſt be drawn neat by means of a Scale of equal Parts, as well to denote the Lengths of the Sides, as the Baſes of all the Angles, which may exactly be had without the Trouble of taking their Quantities in Degrees and Minutes.

U S E X. *To draw any regular Polygon upon a given Line on the Ground.*

Let, for Example, the given Line be A B, upon which it is required to make an equilateral Triangle

Meaſure 30 Feet upon the Line A B, from A to D, where plant a Staff: then take 2 Lines, each 30 Feet long, one of which faſten to the Staff D, and the other to the Staff A, and ſtretch them till their Ends join in the Point C, where plant another Staff.

Make the ſame Operation at the other End of the given Line, and produce the Lines A C, and B F, till they meet in the Point E, and form the equilateral Triangle A E B required

If a Square be to be made upon the given Line A B, raiſe upon each End A and B, a Perpendicular, (by *U S E* III.)

Then make each of thoſe Perpendiculars equal to the Line given, plant Staffs at their Ends C and D, and draw the Line C D, which will compleat the Square propoſed.

If a Pentagon is required to be drawn upon the given Line A B

You will find that the Angles formed by the Sides of a Pentagon, are each 108 Degrees, (as before has been ſaid, in U S E 3. of the Protractor, and in the third Section, concerning the Line of Polygons of the Sector) therefore ſeek for, in the Table of Plane Angles, the Number that anſwers to 108 Degrees, or nighly approaches it, and you will find 48 Feet, and ſomething above 6 Inches · for that Number anſwers to 107 Deg 52 Min which is leſſer by 8 Min than 108 Degrees, whence 48 Feet, 6 ½ Inches, may be taken for the aforeſaid Baſe

Now meaſure upon the given Line, from the Point A towards B, 30 Feet, and plant a Staff in the Point C, where the ſaid Length terminates then take 2 Lines, one 30 Feet, the End of which faſten to the Staff A, and the other 48 Feet, 6 ½ Inches, which likewiſe faſten to the Staff C, ſtrain the Lines equally, till they join in the Point E, where plant a Staff, and by that means will be had an Angle of 108 Degrees · then produce the Line A E, till it be equal to A B, make the ſame Operation at the End B of the given Line, by which means three Sides A B, A G, B D, of the required Pentagon will be had, which afterwards may be compleated by the ſame Method.

If the Pentagon be not too big, it may be compleated by means of 2 Lines, each equal to the given Side, one faſtened to the Staff D, and the other to the Staff G, for if they are

equally

equally ftrained, they will form the two other Sides of the Polygon, by meeting in the Point H

Any other regular or irregular Polygon, by the fame Method, may be made upon the Ground, by feeking in the before-mentioned Table, the Number of Feet and Inches anfwering to the Angle of the Polygon to be drawn

USE XI *To find the Diftance of two Objects, inacceffible in refpect of each other*

The Diftance, for Example, from the Tower A, to the Windmill B, is required Fig. 11

Plant the Staff C in fome Place from whence it may be eafy to meafure the Diftance in a right Line from it to the Places A and B.

Meafure thofe Diftances exactly, as for Example, from C to A, which fuppofe 54 Toifes, then produce the Line A C to D, likewife 54 Toifes meafure alfo the Line B C, which fuppofe 37 Toifes, and produce it to E, fo that C E may be 37 Toifes likewife, by which means the Triangle C D E, will be formed equal and fimilar to the Triangle A B C, and confequently the Diftance D E will be equal to the propofed inacceffible Diftance from B to A

USE XII *To find the Diftance of two Objects, one of which is inacceffible.*

Let it be propofed, for Example, to find the Breadth A B of a River being at one of its Fig 12. Sides A, plant there a Staff A C, 4 or 5 Feet high, and very upright, make a Slit towards the Top of the Staff, in which put a very ftraight Piece of Steel or Brafs (that may flide up and down) about 3 Inches long, which muft be flipp'd up or down, till the Point B, on the other Side of the River be feen along it, afterwards turn the Staff, and look along (keeping the aforefaid Piece of Brafs in the fame Pofition) the Side of the River upon level Ground, till you fee the Point D, where the vifual Rays terminate The Diftance A D meafured with a Chain, will give the Breadth of the River, to which it is equal.

This Propofition, as fimple as it is, may ferve to know what Length Timber muft be of, to make Bridges over Ditches or Rivers

USE XIII *To draw upon the Ground a right Line from the Point A, to the Point B, between which there is a Building, or other Obftacle, that hinders the continuing of it*

Find, upon very level Ground, a third Point, as C, from which you may fee Staffs planted Fig 13. in the Points A and B, then meafure exactly the Diftance from C to A, and from C to B this being done, take the Half, Third, or any other Part of each of thofe Lines, whereat plant Staffs, as in D bifecting C B, and in E bifecting C A, then draw a right Line from D to E, which produce as is neceffary, and draw a Parallel to it paffing by the Points A and B, by means of Staffs planted between the Point A and the Houfe, as alfo between the Houfe and the Point B, which will fhew the Direction from A to B

USE XIV. *It is required to cut a Paffage thro a Hill from the Point A to B*

Draw on one Side of the Hill a right Line, as D C, and on the other Side another right Fig 14. Line, as E F, parallel to C D, then let fall from the Point A, to the Line C D, the Perpendicular A G, and in fome other Point beyond the Hill, draw another Perpendicular, as C H, equal to A G

Again, from the Point B, let fall upon the Line E F the Perpendicular B I, and from fome other Point beyond the Hill, draw another Perpendicular to the fame Line, as L M, equal to B I, fo that the Diftance I L, may be equal to C G, then draw a right Line from the Staff H, to the Staff M, (and produce it as far as is neceffary) which will be parallel to the Paffage to be made from A to B, therefore any Number of Staffs may be planted at an equal Diftance to that Parallel H M on both Sides the Hill, as O, P, Q, which will ferve as a Guide to pierce the Hill thro from A to B

I fhall again mention the Ufe of the aforefaid Inftruments, in the little Treatife of Fortification, hereafter laid down

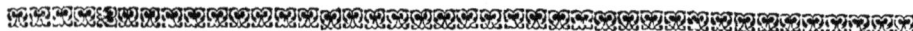

CHAP. II.

Of the Defcription and Ufe of the Surveying-Crofs.

THE Surveying-Crofs is a Brafs Circle of a good Thicknefs, and 4, 5, or 6 Inches Fig 15. Diameter It is divided into 4 equal Parts, by two Lines cutting one another at right Angles in the Center At the four Ends of thefe Lines, and in the Middle of the Limb, there are fixed four ftrong Sights well riveted in fquare Holes, and very perpendicularly flit over the aforefaid Lines, having Holes below each Slit, for better difcovering of diftant Objects the Circle is hollowed to render it more light

Under-

Fig 16.
Underneath, and at the Center of the Inſtrument, there ought to be ſcrewed on a Feril, ſerving to ſuſtain the Croſs upon its Staff of 4 or 5 Feet long, according to the Height of the Obſerver's Eye This Staff muſt be furniſhed with an Iron Point, to go into the Ground the better

All the Exactneſs of this Inſtrument conſiſts in having its Sights well ſlit at right Angles, which may be known by looking at an Object thro' two Sights, and another Object thro' two other Sights then the Croſs muſt be exactly turned upon its Staff, and you muſt look at the ſame Objects through the oppoſite Sights, if they are very exactly in the Direction of the Slits, it is a ſign the Inſtrument is very juſt.

To avoid breaking or damaging the Croſs, the Staff muſt firſt be put in the Ground, and when it is well fixed, the Croſs muſt be ſcrewed upon it

Theſe kinds of Croſſes ſometimes are made with eight Sights, in the ſame manner as the aforeſaid one, and ſerve to take Angles of 45 Degrees, as alſo for Gardeners to plant Rows of Trees by

USE I. *To take the Plot and Area of a Field within it*

Fig 17.
Let the Field propoſed be A B C D E, and having placed at all the Angles Staffs, or Poles very upright, exactly meaſure the Line A C (in the manner we have already laid down, or any other at pleaſure) then make a Memorial, or rough Draught, ſomewhat repreſenting the Field propoſed, on which write all the Dimenſions of the Parts of the Line A C, and of Perpendiculars drawn from the Angles to the Line A C If, for Example, you begin from the Staff A, find the Point F in the Line A C, upon which the Perpendicular E F falls then meaſure the Lines A F and E F, and ſet down their Lengths upon their correſpondent Lines in your Memorial

Now to find the Point F, plant ſeveral Staffs at pleaſure in the Line A C, as alſo the Foot of your Croſs in the ſame Line, in ſuch a manner that you may diſcover thro' two oppoſite Sights, two of thoſe Staffs, and thro' the other two Sights, (which make right Angles with the two firſt ones) you may ſee the Staff E But if in this Station the Staff E cannot be ſeen, remove the Inſtrument backwards or forwards, till the Lines A F, E F, make a right Angle in the Point F, by which means the Plot of the Triangle A F E will be had.

In the ſame manner may the Point H be found, where the Perpendicular D H falls, whoſe Length, together with that of G F, muſt be ſet down in your Memorial, in order to have the Plot of the Trapezium E F H D Again, meaſure H C making a right Angle with H D, and the Plot of the Triangle D H C will be had

Having likewiſe meaſured the whole Line A C, there is no more to do but find the Point G, where the Perpendicular B G falls, and proceeding as before, the Plot of the Triangle A B C may be had, and conſequently the Plot of the whole Field A B C D E The Area of the Field will likewiſe be had, by adding the Triangles and Trapeziums together, which may eaſily be done by the Rules of Planometry, in the following manner:

Suppoſe, for Example, A F is 7 Toiſes, and the Perpendicular E F 10, multiply 7 by 10, and the Product is 70, half of which is 35, the Area of the Triangle A F E

If moreover the Line F H is 14 Toiſes, and the Perpendicular H D 12, add 12 to 10, (which is the Perpendicular F E) the Sum will be 22, half of which being 11, multiplied by 14, will give 154 ſquare Toiſes, for the Area of the Trapezium E F H D, and if the Line H C is 8 Toiſes, multiplying 8 by 12, the Product is 96, whoſe half 48, will be the Area of the Triangle C H D

The whole Line A C is 29 Toiſes, and the Perpendicular B G 10, whence the Product is 290, whoſe half 145, is the Area of the Triangle A B C Finally, adding together 35, 154, 48, and 145, the Sum 382, will be the Number of ſquare Toiſes contained in the Field A B C D E

USE II *To take the Plan of a Wood, Moraſs, &c in which it is not eaſy to enter.*

Fig 18
Let the Moraſs E F G H I be propoſed : Set up Staves at all the Angles, ſo made as to include the Moraſs within a Rectangle, which meaſure, then ſubſtract the Triangles and Trapezia included between the Sides of the Moraſs, and the Sides of the Rectangle, from the ſaid Rectangle, and the Area of the propoſed Moraſs will be had

If, for Example, you begin at the Staff E, produce by help of the Croſs the Line E F, as far as is neceſſary, to which, from the Point G, let fall the Perpendicular G K, ſet up a Staff at K, and produce K G to L, to which, from the Point H, draw the Perpendicular L H, which likewiſe produce as far as is neceſſary: afterwards draw from the Staff E, to the Line H L, produced, the Perpendicular E M: whence the Rectangle E M L K will be had, whoſe Sides muſt be meaſured with a Chain or Toiſe

Suppoſe, for Example, the Line E K, or its Parallel M L (which ought to be equal to it) is 35 Toiſes, and the Line E M, or its Parallel, 10 Toiſes, multiplying theſe two Numbers by one another, there will ariſe 350 ſquare Toiſes for the Area of the Rectangle E M L K. but if F K is 5 Toiſes, and G K 4, by multiplying 4 by 5, the Product is 20, whoſe half 10 Toiſes, is the Area of the Triangle F K G The Line G L, being 6 Toiſes, and H L 4, the Product of 4 by 6 is 24, whoſe half 12 is the Area of the Triangle G L H

After-

Afterwards a Point must be found in the Line H M, where a Perpendicular drawn from the Staff 1 falls, which forms a Triangle and a Trapezium, so that if the Distance H N be 24 Toises, and the Perpendicular N I 4 Toises, 24 by 4 gives 96, whose half 48, is the Area of the Triangle H N I   Lastly, N M being 7 Toises, M E 10, and its Parallel N I 4 Toises, adding 10 to 4, the Sum will be 14, whose half 7, multiplied by 7, produces 49 for the Area of the Trapezium E M N I

Therefore adding together the Areas of the three Triangles, and that of the Trapezium, there will be had 119 Toises, which taken from 350, the Area of the Rectangle, and there remains 231, the Area of the proposed Morass   The same may be done with any other Figure   These two Uses are enough to shew how Surveyors use their Instruments for measuring and taking the Plot of any Piece of Ground.

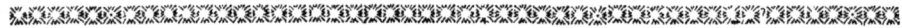

CHAP. III.

Of the Construction and Uses of divers Recipient-Angles.

THERE are several Sorts of Recipient-Angles, but the best and most in use, are those whose Description we are now going to give

The Recipient-Angle A, is composed of two Rules very equal in breadth, for the Insides *Fig A.* of them must be parallel to their Outsides, their Breadth is about an Inch, and their Length a Foot or more   Those two Rulers are equally rounded at the Top, and fastened to one another by means of a Rivet artificially turned, so that the Instrument may easily open and shut   When an Angle is taken with it, the Center of a Protractor must be put to the Place where the two Rulers join each other, and the Degrees cut by the Edge, will shew the Quantity of the Angle, or else the Angle which the two Rulers make, is drawn upon Paper, and then it is measured with a Protractor

The Recipient-Angle B, is made like the precedent one, only there are two Steel Points at *Fig B.* the Ends, in order for it to serve as a Pair of Compasses

The Recipient-Angle C, is different from the others, because it shews the Quantities of *Fig C.* Angles without a Protractor.

It is composed of 2 Brass Rulers of equal Breadth and parallel, about 2 Feet long, and 2 or 3 Inches thick, joined together by a very round Rivet · it has besides a Circle divided into 360 Degrees at the End of one of the Rulers, and a little Index fixed to the Rivet, which shews the Number of Degrees the 2 Rulers contain between them.   I shall not here shew how to divide the Circle, having sufficiently spoken of it in the Construction of the Protractor; only note, that the Degrees are always reckoned from the Middle of the Rule, where the Center is

There are these Sorts of Recipient-Angles made by dividing a Circle upon the under Ruler, and filing the upper one like the Head of a Sector, that thereby the Degrees of the opening of the Legs may be known, by means of the two Shoulders of the upper Leg.

To measure a saliant Angle with any one of the three Recipient-Angles, apply the Insides of the two Rulers, to the Lines forming the Angle, and to measure a rentrant Angle, apply the Outsides of the same Rulers to the Lines forming the Angle.

The Recipient-Angle D, is made of 4 Brass Rules, equal in Breadth, joined together by *Fig. D.* 4 round Rivets, forming an equilateral Parallelogram

At the End of one of the Rules there is a Semi-circle, divided into 180 Degrees.   The other Branch passing upon the Semi-circle, is continued to the Divisions of the Semi-circle, in order to shew the Quantities of Angles

The said Rules are made one or two Feet long, 8 or 10 Lines broad, and of a convenient Thickness, they ought to be drilled very equal in Length, namely, that where the Center of the Semi-circle is (marked 2) and at the other End in the Point 1.   That which serves for an Index, ought to be drilled in the Points 2 and 3   And lastly, the two other Rules in the Point 4   The Rule serving for an Index, must be fastened to the Center of the Semi-circle, and the two other Rules, which are of equal Length, must be fastened underneath the two others, all of them so as their Motion may be very uniform.

When a saliant Angle is to be measured with this Recipient-Angle, the 2 equal Rules must be put underneath the 2 others, so that the End 4 be underneath 2, and thereby the 4 Rules make but 2 to encompass the Angle · but when a rentrant Angle is to be measured, the two Rules must be drawn out, (as *per* Figure) and applied to the Corner of the Angle; and since in every Parallelogram the opposite Angles are equal, the Degrees of the Angle may be known by the Semi-circle

USE I *Of the Recipient-Angle.*

To take the Plan of a Bastion; as, for Example; A B C D E, make a Memorial, and then *Fig. 19* measure, with the Recipient-Angle, the rentrant Angle E, made by the Courtine of the Place,

and

and the flanquant Angle of the propoſed Baſtion, by applying it horizontally, in ſuch manner that one of the Rules may be in the Direction of the ſaid Courtine, and the other in the Direction of the Flank, and having found the Quantity of it in Degrees, ſet it down upon a little Arc in your Memorial, then meaſure the Flank E D, which ſet down upon the Line *e d* in your Memorial. Again, apply the Rules of your Inſtrument to the ſaliant Angle D, and ſet down its Quantity upon a little Arc, meaſure the Length of the left Face C D, take the Quantity of the flanquant Angle C, and of all the other Angles of the Baſtion, as likewiſe the Length of the Faces and Flanks, after which, by help of a Scale, the Plan of the Baſtion may be drawn neat.

But ſince it often happens that theſe Angles, which are commonly made of Free-Stone, are not well cut, by the Negligence of Workmen, who make them either too acute or obtuſe, to remedy this, there muſt be a long Rule horizontally applied to each Wall, whoſe Direction is good, tho' the Angles are not, and putting the Legs of the Inſtrument level upon thoſe two Rules, the Angle to be meaſured may be more exactly had

U S E II *To take the Plot of a Piece of Ground encompaſſed by right Lines*

Fig 20.

Let the Piece of Ground propoſed be A B C D E F G ; meaſure exactly the Length of all the Sides, and ſet them down upon the relative Lines of your Memorial, then take, with any recipient Angle, the Quantity of each Angle, as, for Example, the Angle A G F, and ſet down the Quantity of it upon the relative Angle *a g f*, in the Memorial, meaſure alſo the Angle F E D, by applying the Inſtrument to it (as *per* Figure) and ſet down the Quantity thereof upon the relative Angle of the Memorial, and ſo of all the other Angles, whoſe Quantities being noted in Degrees, as likewiſe the Lengths of all the Lines, the Plot *a b c d e f g* may be neat drawn, and ſimilar to A B C D E F G

In this Plate may be ſeen the Plan of a Pentagon fortified, with the Names of the Parts of its Fortification.

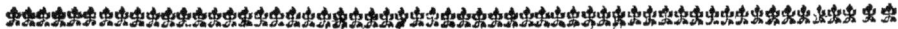

C H A P. IV.

Of the Conſtruction and Uſe of the Theodolite.

Plate 12
Fig. A.

THIS Inſtrument is made of Wood, Braſs, or any other ſolid Matter, commonly circular, and about one Foot in Diameter. In the Center of this Inſtrument is ſet upright a little Braſs Cylinder, or Pivot, about which an Index turns, furniſhed with two Sights, or a Teleſcope, having a right Line, called *The Fiducial Line*, exactly anſwering to the Center of the aforeſaid little Cylinder whoſe Top ought to be cut into a Screw, for receiving a Nut to faſten the Index, upon which is fixed a ſmall Compaſs for finding the Meridian Line

The Limb of the Theodolite is a Circle of ſuch a Thickneſs, as to contain about ſix round Pieces of Paſteboard within it (of which we are going to ſpeak) and of ſuch a Breadth as to receive the Diviſions of 360 Degrees, and ſometimes of every fifth Minute

There are ſeveral round Pieces of Paſteboard, of the Bigneſs of the Theodolite, pierced thro the middle with a round Hole, exactly to fit the Pivot, ſo that the Pivot may be put thro each of the aforeſaid Holes in the Pieces of Paſteboard, and the upper Paſteboard may have the Index moving upon it This upper Paſteboard may be fixed at pleaſure, by means of a little Point faſtened to the Limb of the Inſtrument, and entering a little way into the Paſteboard There is commonly drawn with Ink, upon each of theſe Paſteboards, a Radius or Semidiameter, ſerving for a Station-Line

Underneath the Theodolite is faſtened a Ball and Socket, repreſented by the Figure D, which is a Braſs Ball encloſed between two Shells of the ſame Metal, that may be more or leſs opened by means of a Screw, and a Socket G, in which goes the Head of a three-legged Staff, of which more by and by

Fig A, repreſents the Inſtrument put together We now proceed to ſhew the Conſtruction of the Pieces compoſing it, in beginning with the Diviſion of its Limb.

Firſt, Draw upon the Limb two or three concentrick Circles, to contain the Degrees, and the Numbers ſet at every tenth Degree, then divide one of theſe Circumferences into four very equal Parts, each of which will be 90 Degrees, and dividing each of theſe four Parts into 9 more, the Circumference will be divided into every tenth Degree Again, each of theſe laſt Parts being divided by 2, and each of thoſe ariſing into 5 equal Parts, the whole Circumference will be divided into 360 Degrees. This being done, you muſt draw the Lines of theſe Diviſions upon their convenient Arcs, by means of a Ruler moving about the Center Afterwards Numbers muſt be ſet to every tenth Degree, beginning from the Fiducial Line, which is that whereon the two fixed Sights or Teleſcope is faſtened

A Theodolite thus divided is of much greater Uſe than thoſe whoſe Limbs are not divided ; for it may ſerve exactly to take the Plots of Places, and meaſure inacceſſible Diſtances by Trigonometry.

The

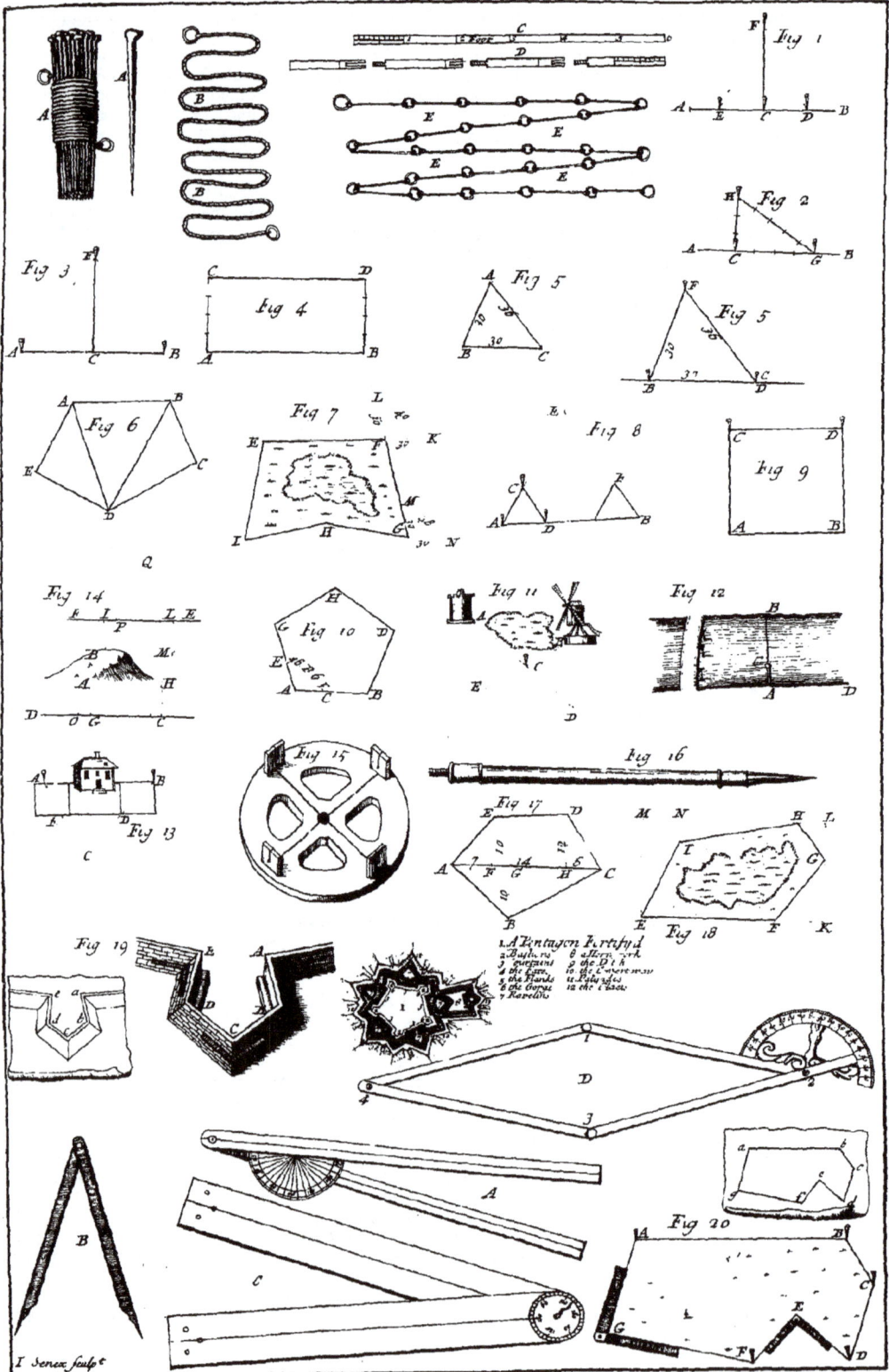

Plate XI

fronting page 116

Fig 1

Fig 2

Fig 3

Fig 4

Fig 5

Fig 5

Fig 6

Fig 7

Fig 8

Fig 9

Fig 14

Fig 10

Fig 11

Fig 12

Fig 13

Fig 15

Fig 16

Fig 17

Fig 18

Fig 19

1. A Pentagon Fortify'd
2. Bastion
3. Curtain
4. the Face
5. the Flanks
6. the Gorge
7. Ravelin
8. a Horn work
9. the Ditch
10. the Counterscarp
11. Palisades
12. the Foss

Fig 20

I Senex sculpt

The Figures B reprefent the Sights which are placed upon different Iiftruments , that to which is placed the Eye, hath a long ftrait Slit, which ought to be very perpendicular, made with a fine Saw , and that which is turned towards the Object, hath a fquare Hole, fo large, that the adjacent Parts of a diftant Object may be perceived thro it · And along the middle of this Hole is ftrained a very fine Gut, in order to vertically cut Objects, when they are perceived thro the Slit of the other Sight But that the Eye may be indifferently placed at any one of the two Sights at pleafure, fo that Objects may be as well perceived thro the Sights on one Side the Inftrument, on which they are placed, as on the other , there is made in each Sight a fquare Hole and a Slit, the Hole in one Sight being below the Slit, and in the other Sight above it, as the little Figures fhew Thefe Sights ought to be exactly placed on the Extremes, and in the fiducial Line, as well of Inftruments as Indexes, and are faftened in little fquare Holes with Nuts underneath, or elfe by means of Screws, according as the Place they are faftened on requires

The little Figure C reprefents the aforefaid Cylinder, or Pivot, with its Nut, for joining the Index to the Theodolite , thofe of Semicircles, and other Inftruments, are made in the fame manner, only they are rivetted underneath

The Figure D reprefents the Ball and Socket for fupporting the Inftrument, and is compofed of a Brafs Ball inclofed between two Shells of the fame Metal, which are made very round, with Balls of tempered Steel cut in manner of a File Thefe Shells are locked more or lefs by means of a Screw, that fo they may prefs the Ball inclofed between them according to neceffity One of thefe Shells is foldered to the Socket G, which is a turned Brafs Feril, in which the Foot of the Inftrument is put Balls and Sockets are made of different Bigneffes, according to the Bigneffes of Inftruments, and are faftened to the Inftruments with Screws, in a Plate rivetted to the Top of the Ball

Conftruction of the Feet for fupporting of Inftruments

We have already mentioned the fimple Feet for fupporting Surveying-Croffes, which are to be forced into the Ground , but thofe whofe Defcription we are now going to give, are not to be forced into the Ground, but are opened or fhut according as the Inequality of the Ground, the Inftrument is to be ufed upon, requires

The Foot E is a triangular Plate, in whofe Middle is a Piece *b*, which is to go into the Socket G

Underneath the aforefaid Plate are faftened three Ferils, or Sockets, moveable by means of Joints, for receiving three round Staves of fuch a Length, that the Obferver's Eye, when the Inftrument is ufing, may commodioufly view Objects thro the Telefcope, or Sights The Extremities of thefe Staves are furnifhed with Ferils and Iron Points, in order to keep the Inftrument firm when it is ufing

The Foot F confifts of four Staves, about two Foot long, whereof that in the middle, called the Shank, hath its Top rounded, that fo it may go into the Socket , the reft of this Staff is cut in Figure of a Triangle, that fo the three Faces thereof may receive upon them three other Staves, faftened by means of three Screws (all of a piece) and fo many Nuts. Thefe three Staves are furnifhed with Ferils and Iron Points, being flat within fide, and have three Faces without

When we have a mind to carry this Foot, we reunite all the Staves together, fo that they make, as it were, but one, and by this means are fhorter by about the half, than when the Foot is ufing

We generally hang to the middle of each of thefe Feet a Thread and Plummet, in order to know the Station-Point.

USE *of the Theodolite*

To take the Map of a Country by this Inftrument, chufe two high Places, for Example, the *Obfervatory*, and the *Salt-Petre Houfe*, from whence the Country nigh *Paris*, a Map of which is to be made, may be feen , then mark round the Center of the upper Pafteboard the Name of the Place chofen for the firft Station, and having fixed it by means of the Point on the Limb of the Theodolite, put the Index upon it, which fufficiently fcrew down by means of the Nut and Screw

Now having placed the Theodolite upon its Foot, planted at the *Obfervatory*, and given it a Situation nearly horizontal, fo that it may remain fteddy while the Index is moving, obferve thro the Sights the Steeple of the Salt-Petre Houfe, and along the fiducial Line of the Index from the Center draw the Station-Line.

Then turn the Index, and obferve fome remarkable Object thro' the Sights, as the Steeple of *Vaugirard*, towards which a Line muft be drawn upon the Pafteboard, from the Center, along the fiducial Line of the Index, and along this Line write the Name of the Place viewed thro the Sights

Again, direct the Index towards fome other Object (as *Mont-rouge*) and draw a Line towards it from the Center, along the fiducial Line, and upon this Line write the Name of the

Fig 1.

Place

Place obferved   Proceed in the fame manner with all the confiderable Places that can be feen from the Obfervatory

Now having removed the Theodolite from its firft Station, having well obferved its Place, and tranfported it to fome other defigned Place, as to the Salt-Petre Houfe, meafure the exact Diftance between the two Stations upon level Ground, the Number of Toifes of which muft be fet down upon your Pafteboard, which muft now be turned, or taken from under the Index, that fo at every different Station, the upper Face of the Pafteboard, upon which the Index is, may be clean   then fet down about the Center of this new Pafteboard, the Name of the Place of your fecond Station, and upon the Bafe Line the Number of Toifes meafured, that fo you may remember this Line is the fame as that on the precedent Pafteboard   The Theodolite being placed here, difpofe it fo, that placing the fiducial Line of the Index upon the Station Line, you may difcover thro' the Sights, the *Obfervatory*, which was your firft Station

The Inftrument remaining firm in this Situation, turn the Index, and fucceffively view thro' the Sights the former Objects obferved from the *Obfervatory*, and draw Lines, as before, upon the Pafteboard, along the Index, from the Center towards the Places view'd, and upon each Line write the correfpondent Name of the Place

If all the Places you have a mind to fet down in your Map, cannot be feen from the two precedent Stations, you muft chufe a third Place from whence they may be obferved, and make as many new Stations, as are neceffary for perceiving each remarkable Object, from two Places fufficiently diftant from each other

Now to reprefent this Map upon a Sheet of Paper, firft draw a right Line at pleafure upon it, for a common Bafe, which divide into the fame Number of equal Parts, as you have meafured Toifes upon the Ground   About one End of this Line, as a Center, defcribe circular Arcs equal to thofe drawn upon the firft Pafteboard, and upon the other Extreme, Arcs equal to thofe drawn upon the fecond Pafteboard, and produce the Lines forming the Arcs till they meet each other, then the Points of Concourfe, will be the Points of Pofition of the Places obferved

The aforefaid Places may be laid down upon the Paper eafier, by placing the Centers of the Pafteboards upon the Extremities of the common Bafe, and noting upon the Paper the Ends of the Lines drawn upon the Pafteboard, and then drawing Lines from the Stations thro' thofe Points till they interfect

By means of this Theodolite may be had in Degrees, or Parts, all the Angles that the Places view'd thro the Sights or Telefcopes, make, with the Places whereat the Inftrument is placed

What we have faid, is fufficient to fhew the Manner of ufing the Theodolite in taking the Pofition of Places, and making of Maps, becaufe the Operations are the fame for all different Places, but for its Ufes, with regard to Trigonometry, they are the fame as thofe of the Semi-circle and Quadrant, of which we are going to treat.

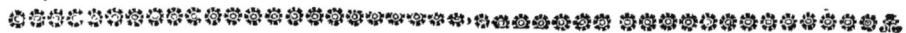

CHAP. V.

Of the Conftruction and Ufes of the Quadrant, and Geometrick Quadrat.

Fig. G.

THE Figure G, reprefents a Quadrant and Geometrick Square, with its Index and Sights

It is commonly made of Brafs, or other folid Matter, 12 or 15 Inches Radius, and an anfwerable Thicknefs   Its Circumference is firft divided into 90 Degrees, and every Degree into as many equal Parts as poffible, without Confufion, and in fuch manner, that the Divifions and Subdivifions may be juft, and very diftinctly marked upon the Limb of the Inftrument

To do which, there muft firft be 2 Arcs drawn nigh the Edge of the Quadrant, about 8 or 9 Lines diftant from each other; and after having divided them into Degrees, draw Diagonal Lines between them, from the firft Degree to the fecond, from the fecond to the third, and fo on to the laft

After which, if you have a mind to fubdivide every Degree into 10 Minutes, there muft 5 other concentrick Arcs be defcribed from the Center of the Inftrument, cutting all the aforefaid Diagonals, but if every Degree is to be fubdivided into Minutes, there muft be 9 concentrick Arcs defcribed between thofe two firft drawn

The Diftances between all thefe Arcs, muft not be all equal, becaufe the Extent of a Degree taken in the Breadth of the Limb, forms a kind of Trapezium, broader towards the outward Arc, and narrower towards the inward one, whence a mean Arc dividing every Degree
gree

gree into 2 equal Parts, muſt be nigher the inward Arc than the outward one, and the o-
thers in proportion.

To make theſe Subdiviſions exactly, the Diagonals muſt be Curve Lines, as B D C, de- Fig H
ſcribed in making the Portion of a circular Arc paſs thro the Center B, the beginning of the
1ſt Degree marked D, upon the inward Arc, and the End C of the ſame Degree, on the outward Arc which is eaſy to do by *Uſe* 18 *Lib* 1 which ſhows how to make a Circle paſs
thro 3 Points given, by which means the Point F, the Center of the Diagonal Curve, paſſing
thro' the firſt Degree, will be found

Afterwards one of theſe Diagonal Curves muſt be divided into equal Parts, and from the
Center of the Inſtrument, there muſt be drawn as many concentrick Arcs, as each Degree is
to have equal Parts

The Reaſon of this Operation is, that the Diagonal Curve being divided into equal Parts,
if from the Center of the Inſtrument there are drawn right Lines thro all the Points of Diviſion of that Arc, there will be had (*per Prop* 27 *Lib* 3 *Eucl*) as many equal Angles in the
Center, becauſe they will be all in the Circumference of the ſame Circle, and ſtand upon
equal Arcs

But ſince it is troubleſome to find the Centers of 90 Arcs, each paſſing thro 3 Points,
ſince it is manifeſt, that all the Centers of theſe Arcs ought to be placed in the Circumference of a Circle whoſe Center is the Point B, there is no more to do but draw a Circle
from the Center B, with the Diſtance B F, and divide its Circumference into 360 equal
Parts, upon every of which, ſetting one Foot of your Compaſſes, you may deſcribe with the
ſame Extent F B, all the Arcs between the Circles A C, D E, and then the circular Arcs,
which are Diagonals, will likewiſe divide the Circumferences, upon the Limb of the Inſtrument, into Degrees. *Note*, Becauſe the Figure is too little, it is divided but into every 5th
Degree

Diagonal Curves may alſo be drawn without transferring the Foot of your Compaſſes from
one Degree to another, upon the aforeſaid Arc, in fixing the Foot of your Compaſſes in only one Point, as F, and letting the Inſtrument be gradually turned about the Center of a large
Circle, whoſe Limb is already divided into Degrees, by means of a Rule ſtrongly faſtened
upon the Inſtrument, and reaching to the Diviſions of the large Circle

Ingenious Workmen may ſhorten their Work by adjuſting a fine Steel Ruler, according to
the Curvature of the firſt Diagonal, which being drawn, by this means they may draw all
the others If Diagonal right Lines are to be drawn from one Degree to the other, the
Lengths of the Radii of each of the Circumferences cutting the Diagonals, may be found by
Trigonometry, an Example of which is as follows

Suppoſe a Quadrant be 6 Inches Radius, which is the ſmalleſt accuſtomed to be divided by
Diagonals Suppoſe alſo you have a Scale of 1000 equal Parts, and that the Diſtance from
the inward Arc to the outward one, is 9 Lines, anſwering to 125 of ſuch Parts, whereof
the Radius is 1000, whence, by Calculation, I find that the right-lined Diagonal, drawn
from one Degree to that which follows it, is 126 of the ſame Parts, and that the Radius of
the inward Arc, which is 5 Inches, 3 Lines, contains 875 of them.

The obtuſe Angle made by the Radius and the Diagonal, is 172 Deg 2 Min and afterwards calculating the Lengths of the Radii of the Circumferences cutting the Diagonals, and
dividing them into every 10 Minutes, I find that the Radius of 10 Min is 894 of the ſame
equal Parts, inſtead of 896 which it would have contained, if the Diſtance between the inward and outward Arc had been divided into 6 equal Parts The Radius of 20 Minutes
ought to contain 913 of them, inſtead of 917, the Radius of 30 Minutes ought to contain
933 of them, inſtead of 938, the Radius of 40 Minutes ought to contain 954 of them, inſtead of 959 Laſtly, the Radius of 50 Minutes ought to contain 977, inſtead of 980, which
it muſt, if the aforeſaid Diſtance be divided into 6 equal Parts

The greateſt Error, which is about 5 Parts, anſwers to about ⅕ of a Line, which may
cauſe an Error of 2 Minutes, but this Error diminiſhes in proportion as the Radius of the
Quadrant augments in reſpect of the Diagonals, ſo that the Error will be leſs by half, if the
Radius of the Quadrant be one Foot, and the Diſtance of the inward and outward Arcs is
but 9 Lines.

What we have ſaid as to the Diviſions of the Quadrant, may likewiſe be applied to Theodolites, Circles, Semi-circles, or any other Portions of Circles to be divided into Minutes.

As to the Geometrick Square, each Side of it is divided into 100 equal Parts, beginning
at the Ends, that ſo the Number 100 may end at the Angle of 45 Degrees Theſe Diviſions
are diſtinguiſh'd by little Lines from 5 to 5, and by Numbers from 10 to 10, all thoſe Diviſions being produced from a kind of Lattice, both ways containing 10000 ſmall and equal
Squares

This Quadrant is furniſhed with two immoveable Sights, faſtened to one of its Semi-diameters, and with a Thread and Plummet fixed to the Center, as likewiſe a moveable Index,
with two other Sights, faſtened to the Center, with a Headed-Rivet. The Sights are nearly
like thoſe belonging to the Theodolite

Inſtead of immoveable Sights, there is ſometimes faſtened to one of the Radius's of the
Quadrant a Teleſcope, and then the 1ſt Point of Diviſion of the Circumference may be

found

it done in the manner as is explained hereafter in the Astronomical Quadrant for this Quadrant is defigned only to take the Heights and Distance of Places on Earth

Upon the under Surface of this Quadrant, is a Ball and Socket faftened with 3 Screws, by means of which it may be put into any Pofition fit for Ufe.

This Inftrument may be put in Ufe in different Situations, for firft, it may be fo difpofed that its Plane may be at right Angles with the Horizon, for obferving Heights and Depths, which may yet be done two different ways, viz. in ufing the fixed Sights, and the Thread and Plummet, and then neither of its Sides will be found parallel to the Horizon, or elfe by keeping the Sights faftened to the Index moveable, and then one of the Semi-diameters of the Quadrant will always be parallel to the Horizon, and the other perpendicular, which may be done by means of a Plummet fufpended in the Center, and then the fixed Sights are ufelefs

Finally, the Quadrant may be placed fo as its Plane may be parallel to the Horizon, for obferving horizontal Diftances with the Index and immoveable Sights, and then the Thread, with its Plummet, is not in ufe.

Ufes of the Quadrant, with two fixed Sights and a Plummet.

USE I   *To take the Height or Depth of any Object in Degrees.*

As fuppofe the Height of a Star or Tower is to be taken in Degrees, place the Quadrant vertically, then place your Eye under that fixed Sight next the Circumference of the Quadrant, and direct it fo, that the vifual Rays paffing through the Holes of the Sights, may tend to the Point of the Object propofed (as to the Sun, it is fufficient that its Rays pafs thro the aforefaid Holes) then the Arc of the Circumference contained between the Thread and its Plummet, and the Semi-diameter on which the Sights are faftened, will fhow the Complement of the Star's Height above the Horizon, or its Diftance from the Zenith : Whence the Arc contained between the Thread, and the other Semi-diameter towards the Object, fhows its Height above the Horizon The fame Arc likewife determines the Quantity of the Angle made by the vifual Ray, and a horizontal Line, parallel to the Bafe of the Tower

But to obferve Depths, as thofe of Wells or Ditches, the Eye muft be placed over that Sight, which is next the Center of the Quadrant.

The whole Operation confifts in calculating Triangles by the Rule of Three, formed in the Porportion of the Sines of Angles, to the Sines of their oppofite Sides, according to the Rules of right-lined Trigonometry, of which we are now going to give fome Examples.

USE II.   *Let it be required to find the Height of the Tower A B, whofe Bafe is acceffible.*

Fig. 2

Having planted the Foot of your Inftrument in the Point C, look at the Top of the Tower thro the fixed Sights, then the Thread of the Plummet freely playing, will fix itfelf upon the Number of Degrees, determining the Quantity of the Angle made at the Center of the Quadrant, by the vifual Ray, and the horizontal Line, parallel to the Bafe of the Tower, accounting the Degrees contained between the Thread and the Semi-diameter next to the Tower

Now fuppofe the Thread fixes upon 35 Deg. 35 Min and having exactly meafured the level Diftance from the Foot of the Tower, with a Chain, to the Place of Obfervation, you will find it 47 Feet; then there will be 3 things given, to wit, the Side BC, and the Angles of the Triangle A B C · for fince Walls are always fuppofed to be built upright, the Angle B is a right Angle, or 90 Deg and confequently the 2 acute Angles A and C, are together equal to 90 Degrees, becaufe the three Angles of any right-lined Triangle, are equal to 180 Degrees, or 2 right Angles

Now the Angle obferved, is 35 Deg 35 Min whence the Angle A is 54 Deg 25 Min therefore you may form this Analogy, As the Sine of 54 Deg 25 Min is to 47 Feet, fo is the Sine of 35 Deg 35 Min to a fourth Term, which will be found $33\frac{1}{2}$ Feet, to which adding 5 Feet, the Height of the Obferver's Eye, and the Height of the propofed Tower will be found $38\frac{1}{2}$ Feet

USE III   *Let it be required to find the Height of the inacceffible Tower D E*

Fig 3

In this Cafe two Obfervations muft be made, as follows :

Place the Foot of your Quadrant in the Point F, and look thro the two immoveable Sights to the Top of the Tower D, then fee on what Degree the Thread of the Plummet fixes, which fuppofe on the 34th This being done, remove the Inftrument, planting a Staff in its Place, and fet it up in fome other Place level to the Place it was in before, as in the Point G, in the fame right Line, and look thro the afore-mentioned Sights, at the Point D of the Tower Note the Point in the Limb of the Quadrant that the Thread cuts, which fuppofe 20 Degrees Meafure likewife very exactly, the Diftance between the two Stations, which fuppofe 9 Toifes, or 54 Feet

This being done, all the Angles of the Triangle D F G will be known, as alfo the Side F G meafured, by which means it will be eafy to find the Side D F, and afterwards the Side E D, by making the following Analogies.

The

The Angle E F D being found 34 Deg. its Complement D F G to 180 Deg will be 146 Deg and the Angle G having been found 20 Deg it follows that the Angle F D G is 14 Deg. therefore say, As the Sine of 14 Deg is to 54 Feet, so is the Sine of 20 Deg to a fourth Term, which will be 76 Feet, and about ¼, for the Side D F. then say, As Radius is to the Hypothenuse F D, so is the Sine of the Angle D F E, to the Side E D, which will be found 42 ¾ Feet, to which adding 5 Feet, the Height of the Center of the Instrument above the Ground, and there will be had 47 ¾ Feet, for the Height of the Tower proposed

These Calculations are much better made with Logarithms, than by common Numbers, because they may be done by only the help of Addition and Substraction, as is more fully explained in Books of Trigonometry

These Propositions, and others the like, may be also geometrically solved, by making Triangles similar to those formed upon the Ground

As to solve the present Question, make a Scale of 10 Toises, that is, draw the right Line A B so long, that the Division of it may be exact, and then divide it into 10 equal Parts, and subdivide one of these Parts into 6 more, to have a Toise divided into Feet

Then draw the indeterminate Line E G, and make with a Line of Chords, or Protractor, an Angle at the Point G of 20 Degrees, and draw the indeterminate Line G D Lay off 9 Toises, or 54 Feet, from G to F, then make at the Point F an Angle of 34 Degrees, and draw the Line F D, cutting the Line G D in some Point as D, from which let fall the Perpendicular D F, which will represent the Height of the proposed Tower, and measuring it with the Scale, you will find it to contain 47 Feet, 8 Inches All the other Sides of these Triangles may likewise be measured with the same Scale.

USE IV *To find the Breadth of a Ditch, or Well, whose Depth may be measured*

Let it be proposed to measure the Breadth of the Ditch C D, which may be approached Fig 4.
Place the Quadrant upon the Brink in the Point A, so that you may see thro' the Sights the Bottom of the Ditch, at the Point D, then find the Angle made by the Thread upon the Limb, which suppose is 63 Degrees, and measure the Depth A C, from the Center of the Quadrant, which suppose 25 Feet, then make a similar right-angled Triangle, one of whose acute Angles is 63 Degrees, (and consequently the other will be 27 Degrees) and the least Side is 25 Parts of some Scale Lastly, measure with the same Scale the Side C D, which will be about 49, therefore the Breadth of the Ditch is 49 Feet.

USE *of the Geometrick Quadrat.*

The Quadrant being vertically placed, and the Sights directed towards the Top of the Fig. G. Tower proposed to be measured, if the Thread of the Plummet cuts the Side of the Quadrat, whereon is writ *right Shadows*, the Distance from the Base of the Tower, to the Point of Station, is less than the Tower's Height if the Thread falls upon the Diagonal of the Square, the Distance is equal to the Height, but if the Thread falls upon the Side of the Square, whereon is writ *versed Shadows*, the Distance of the Tower from you, is greater than its Height

Now having measured the Distance from the Foot of the Tower, its Height may be found by the Rule of Three, in having 3 Terms known, but their Disposition is not always the same, for when the Thread cuts the Side, denoted *right Shadow*, the first Term of the Rule of Three, ought to be that part of the Side cut by the Thread, the second Term will be the whole Side of the Square, and the third, the Distance measured

But when the Thread cuts the other Side of the Square, the first Term of the Rule of Three, must be the whole Side of the Square, the second Term, the Parts of that Side cut by the Thread, and the third, the Distance measured

Suppose, for Example, that looking to the Top of a Tower, the Thread of the Plummet cuts the Side of *right Shadows* in the Point 40, and that the Distance measured is 20 Toises: I order the Rule of Three in the following manner; [40 100 20

Multiplying 20 by 100, and dividing the Product 2000 by 40, there will be found the fourth Term 50, which shews the Height of the Tower to be 50 Toises

But if the Thread of the Plummet falls on the other Side of the Square, as, for Example, upon the Point 60, and the Distance measured is 35 Toises, dispose the three first Terms of the Rule of Three thus, [100 60 35

Multiply 35 by 60, and the Product 2100 being divided by 100, will give 21 for the Height of the Tower

USE *of the Quadrat without Calculation.*

All the aforesaid Operations, with many others, may be made without Calculation, as we shall make manifest by some Examples

USE I Let us suppose (as we have already done) that the Thread falls upon 40 on the Fig G. Side of right Shadows, and that the Distance measured is 20 Toises; seek amongst the little Squares for that Perpendicular to the Side, which is 20 Parts from the Thread, and that Perpendicular will cut the Side of the Square next to the Center in the Point 50, which will be the Height of the proposed Tower in Toises.

USE

USE II But if the Thread cuts the Side of verfed Shadows in the Point 60, and the Diftance is 35 Toifes, count upon the Side of the Quadrant, from the Center, 35 Parts; count alfo the Divifions of the Perpendicular from that Point 35 to the Thread, which will be 21, the Height of the propofed Tower in Toifes

Note, In all Cafes the Height of the Center of the Inftrument above the Ground, muft be added

USE III   *To take an inacceffible Height with the Quadrat*

To do which, there muft be made two Stations, whofe Diftance muft be meafured, and then there will be three Cafes

CASE I   *When the right Shadow is cut in both Stations by the Thread*

Let us fuppofe, for Example, that at the firft Obfervation the Side of right Shadows is cut in the Point 30, and the Inftrument being removed 20 Toifes to a fecond Station, the Side of right Shadows is cut in the Point 70; then note the Pofition of the Thread in thefe two Stations, by drawing a Line upon the Lattice with a Pencil, from the Center to the aforefaid Point 30, and another to the Point 70 Seek between thefe two Lines a Portion of a Parallel, which may have as many Parts as the Diftance meafured has Toifes, which in this Example muft be 20 then the faid Parallel being continued, will meet the Number 50, counting from the Center, whence the Height of the Tower obferved, will be 50 Toifes You will likewife by the fame means find that the Diftance from the Bafe of the Tower, to the firft Station, is 15 Toifes, becaufe there is 15 Parts contained upon the Parallel between the Number 50, and the Line drawn with the Pencil to the Number 30

Inftead of drawing Lines with a Pencil, two Threads faftened to the Center will do, one of which may be the Thread of the Plummet.

CASE II   *When the Side of verfed Shadows is cut at both Stations by the Thread.*

Suppofe, in the firft Station, that the Thread cuts the Side of verfed Shadows in the Point 80, and that being removed 15 Toifes to another Station, the Thread falls upon the Number 50 on the fame Side Mark with a Pencil upon the Lattice, the two different Pofitions of the Thread in both Stations, and find between thefe two Lines, a Portion of a Parallel containing as many Parts as the Diftance meafured contains Toifes, which, in this Example, is 15 Toifes to thefe 15 Parts add 25, which is the Continuation of the fame Parallel to the Side of the Square next to the Center, and the Sum makes 40, whence the Diftance of the Tower, from the fecond Station, is 40 Toifes: and to find its Height, feek the Number 40 upon the Side of the Square next the Center, and count from that Number to the firft Line drawn on the Lattice with the Pencil, the Parts of the Parallel, which in this Example will be found 20, therefore the Height of the Tower is 20 Toifes, by always adding the Height of the Quadrant

CASE III If in one Station the Thread falls upon the Diagonal of the Square, and in the other it cuts the Side of right Shadows, you muft proceed in the fame manner as when the Thread at both Stations falls upon the Side of right Shadows

But when the Thread falls along the Diagonal in one Station, and upon the Side of verfed Shadows in the other, you muft proceed in the fame manner, as when the Thread cuts, at both Stations, the Side of verfed Shadows

The Reafon of all this is, becaufe there is always made upon the Lattice a little Triangle fimilar to a great one, made upon the Ground, altho diverfly pofited The Line made by the Thread and Plummet always reprefents the Vifual Ray, the two other Sides of the little Triangle, which make a right Angle, reprefent the Height of the Tower and its Diftance, and when the Thread cuts the Side of right Shadows, the Height is reprefented by the Divifions of the Sides of the Lattice, which is perpendicular to the Side of the Quadrat, but when the Thread cuts the Side of verfed Shadows, the Diftance is reprefented by the Divifions of the Side diftant from the Center, and the Height by the Perpendicular anfwering to the Number of Divifions of the fame Side.

USE IV   *To find the Depth of a Ditch or Well*

The Breadth of the Ditch (or Well) muft firft be meafured, and afterwards you muft place the Quadrant upon the Brink, and look thro the two Sights, till you fee the oppofite Point, where the Surface of the Water touches the Side of the Ditch, then the Thread will cut the Parallel, anfwering to the Feet or Toifes of the Ditch's Breadth, and that Perpendicular, at which the Parallel ends, will determine the Depth, from which muft be fubftracted the Height of the Inftrument above the Brink of the Ditch

USE *of the Quadrant in taking of Heights and Diftances, by means of an Index and its Sights.*

Place the Quadrant fo that its Plane may be at right Angles with the Plane of the Horizon, and one of its Sides parallel thereto, which will be done when the Plummet, freely hanging, falls along the other Side of the Quadrant   In

In this Situation the two fixed Sights are of no Use, unlefs they are ufed to obferve the Diftance between two Stars, and then the Quadrant muft be inclined, by directing the immoveable Sights towards one Star, and the moveable ones towards the other; and the Number of Degrees, comprehended between them, will be the Diftance of the Stars in Degrees

If it is ufed to obferve an Height, the Center of the Inftrument muft be above the Eye, but if a Depth is to be obferved, the Eye muft be above the Center of the Inftrument.

USE I *To take an Height, as that of a Tower, whofe Bafe is acceffible*

Having placed the Quadrant, as already fhewn, turn the Index, fo that you may fee the Top of the Tower thro' the two Sights, and the Arc of the Limb of the Quadrant, between that Side of it parallel to the Horizon, and the Index, will be the Height of the Tower in Degrees. If afterwards the Diftance from the Foot of the Tower, to the Place where the Inftrument ftands, be exactly meafured, there will be three things given in the Triangle to be meafured, namely, the Bafe, and the two Angles made at its Ends, one of which will be always a right Angle, becaufe the Tower is fuppofed to be built upright, and the other the Angle before obferved, whence the other Sides of the Triangle may be found by the Rules of right-lined Trigonometry, or elfe without Calculation, by drawing a little Triangle fimilar to the great one, whofe Bafe is the Ground, and Perpendicular the Height of the Tower, or otherwife by the Geometrick Square, in obferving, that in *that* Pofition of the Quadrant, the Side of right Shadows ought always to be parallel to the Horizon, and the Side of verfed Shadows perpendicular thereto.

USE II *To find the Height of a Tower, whether acceffible or inacceffible, by means of the Quadrat.*

In the aforementioned Pofition of the Quadrant, there are always formed, in the Quadrat, little fimilar Triangles, whofe homologous Sides are parallel and fimilarly pofited to thofe of the great ones formed upon the Ground, by which means the Operations are rendered more fimple and eafy than in the other Situation of the Quadrant, as we come now to explain, by making three different Suppofitions, according to the different Cafes that may happen

CASE I Let us fuppofe, for Example, that having obferved the Height of a Tower, whofe Bafe is acceffible, thro' the Sights of the Index, the Index cuts the Side of right Shadows in the Point 40, and the Diftance to the Bafe of the Tower is 20 Toifes, feek among the Parallels to the Horizon, from that which paffes thro' the Center to the Index, the Parallel of 20, (becaufe 20 Toifes is the Diftance fuppofed) and you will find that it terminates at the Number 50, on the perpendicular Side of the Square, reckoning from the Center; whence the Height of the Tower is 50 Toifes above the Center of the Inftrument

CASE II Suppofe, in another Obfervation, that the Index cuts the Side of verfed Shadows in the Point 60, and the Diftance meafured is 35 Toifes, count from the Center of the Quadrant upon the Side parallel to the Horizon 35, and from this Point, reckoning the Parts of the Perpendicular, to the Interfection of the Index, and you will find 21, whence the Height of the Tower is 21 Toifes

CASE III *Laftly,* Suppofe the Bafe of the Tower to be inacceffible, and that there muft be made two Stations (as we have faid before), the Height of it may be found without any Diftinction of right or verfed Shadows: for having meafured the Diftance between the two Stations, and drawn two Lines in the Quadrat, fhewing the Situation of the Index in thofe two Stations, find between thofe two Lines a Portion of a Parallel to the Horizon, which fhall have as many Parts, as the Diftance meafured contains Toifes. then if you continue that to the perpendicular Side of the Square diftant from the Center, you will there find a Number expreffing the Height of the Tower, and the Continuation of that Parallel to this Number, will fhow the Diftance to the Bafe of the Tower

Note, In this Situation of the Quadrant, horizontal Diftances are always reprefented in the Quadrat by Lines parallel to the Horizon, and Heights are always reprefented by Lines perpendicular to the Horizon, which renders (as we have already faid) Operations more eafy

It does not happen fo in that other vertical Pofition of the Quadrant, when the fixed Sights are ufed; for if in obferving the Height of an inacceffible Tower, the Thread of the Plummet in one Station falls upon the Side of right Shadows, and in the other Station, on the Side of verfed Shadows, the Diftance between the two Lines drawn with a Pencil on the Lattice, croffes the Squares of the Lattice by their Diagonals, which will not have common Meafures with the Sides, whence it cannot be ufed to find the Height of the propofed Tower

USE *of the Quadrant in meafuring of Horizontal Diftances.*

Altho a Quadrant is not fo proper to meafure horizontal Diftances, as a Semi-circle or whole Circle, becaufe by it obtufe Angles cannot well be taken, yet we fhall here give fome Ufes of it by means of the Quadrat Place the Quadrant upon its Foot nighly parallel to the Horizon, for there is no Neceffity of its Plane being perfectly level, becaufe fometimes it muft be inclined to perceive Objects thro' the Sights.

Then put the Foot of the Inftrument in the Line to be meafured, and make two Obfervations in the following manner, not ufing the Plummet, but the four Sights

G g

Suppofe

Suppose, for Example, the perpendicular Distance A B is to be measured, plant several Staffs in the Line A C D, and the Quadrant in the Point A, in such manner that the two fixed Sights may be in the Line A C, and the Point B may be seen thro' the two moveable Sights, placed at right Angles with the Line A C. then remove the Quadrant, planting a Staff in its place, and measure from A towards B, any Length, as, for Example, 18 Toises at the End of which, having placed the Instrument, so that the two fixed Sights may be in the Line A C, move the Index till you see the Point B thro' its Sights, and you will have upon the Lattice a little Triangle, similar to the great one made upon the Ground, therefore seek amongst the Parallels cut by the Index, that which contains as many Parts as the Distance measured does Toises, that is, in this Example, 18, which will terminate on the Side of the Quadrant, at a Number containing as many Parts as there are Toises in the Line A B proposed to be measured.

The Distance A B may yet otherwise be found, whether perpendicular or not, without making a Station at right Angles with the Point A

Suppose, for Example, that the first Station is made in the Point C, and the second in the Point D, draw upon the Lattice two right Lines with a Pencil, or otherwise, shewing the two different Positions of the Index in both the Stations, and having measured the Distance of the Points C and D, which suppose 20 Toises, seek between the two Lines drawn with a Pencil, a Portion of a Parallel which is 20 Parts, and that will correspond, upon the Semidiameter of the Geometrick Quadrat, to a Number, which, reckoned from the Center, will contain as many Parts as the right Line A B does Toises.

You will likewise find the Lengths of the Distances C B and D B, by the Divisions of the Index, for there is upon the Lattice a little oblique-angled Triangle similar to the great one C D B upon the Ground.

CHAP. VI.

Of the Construction and Uses of the Semi-circle.

Fig I. & K.   **T**HESE Instruments which are also called Graphometers, are made of beaten or cast Brass, from 7 Inches Diameter to 15 ; the Divisions of them are made in the same manner as those of the Theodolite and Quadrant before explained. The simplest of these Instruments, is that of *Fig* K, at the Ends of its Diameter, and in little square Holes made upon the fiducial Line, there is adjusted two fixed Sights, fastened with Nuts underneath, and upon its Center there is a moveable Index furnished with two other Sights, made in the same manner as those before mentioned for the Theodolite, and which is fastened with a Screw. There is a Compass placed in the Middle of its Surface, for finding the North Sides of Planes There is also fixed underneath to its Center, a Ball and Socket, like that mentioned in the Construction of the Theodolite, and for the same Use

Note, These Instruments ought to be well straightned with hammering, then they must be fashion'd with a rough File, and afterwards smoothed with a Bastard-File, and a fine one When they are filed enough, you must see whether they are not bent in filing, if they are, they ought to be well straightned upon a Stone, or very plain Piece of Marble, then they must be rubbed over with Pumice-Stone and Water, to take away the Tracts of the File. To polish Semi-circles well, as also any other Instruments, you must use *German*-Slate Stone, and very fine Charcoal, so that it does not scratch the Work afterwards, to brighten them, you must lay a little Tripoli, tempered in Oil, upon a Piece of Shamoy, and rub it over them

The Semi-circle I, carries Telescopes for seeing Objects at a good Distance, and has the Degrees of its Limb divided into Minutes, by right-lined or curved Diagonals, as in the Quadrant before-mentioned.

There is one Telescope placed underneath along the Diameter of the Semi-circle, whose Ends are B B, and another Telescope adjusted to the Index of the Semi-circle. When the fiducial Line cuts the Middle of the Index, the Telescope fastened to it must be a little shorter than the Index, to the end that the Degrees cut by the fiducial Line may be seen, but the best way is for the Telescopes to be of equal Length, and then the fiducial Line must be drawn from the End C, passing thro' the Center of the Semi-circle, and terminating in the opposite End D The two Ends of the Index are cut so as to agree with the Degrees upon the Limb, as may be seen at the Places C F, G D, in such manner that the Line C F E G D, may be the fiducial Line of the Semi-circle

Note, The Degrees on this Semi-circle do not begin and end at the Diameter, as in others, but at the Lines C F, G D, when the Telescopes are so placed over each other, that the visual Rays agree To make which, the little Frame carrying the cross Hairs, must be moved backwards or forwards by means of Screws The Breadth from the Middle of the Telescope, fcope, to the Points F, G, is commonly about 5 Degrees, and this is the Reason why the Divisions begin further from the Diameter than they end, as may be feen *per* Figure

Thefe Telefcopes have two or four Glaffes, and have a very fine Hair ftrained in the Focus of the Object-Glafs, ferving for a Sight

Telefcopes with four Glaffes fhew Objects in their true Situation, but thofe with two Glaffes invert them, fo that *that* which is on the right Hand appears on the left, and that which is above appears below · but this does not at all hinder the Truth of Operations, becaufe they always give the Point of Direction

Thefe Telefcopes are made with Brafs Tubes foldered, and turned in a Cylindrick Form, as may be feen by the Figure L, which reprefents a Telefcope taken to pieces, the Eye-Glafs, being that to which the Eye is applied to look at Objects, is at the End 1   It is put in another little Tube apart (likewife marked 1) which is drawn out, or flid into the Telefcope, according to different Sights   This little Tube alfo fometimes carries the Hair in the Focus of the Glafs, ferving as a Sight, but it is better for the Hair to be faften'd to a little Piece of Brafs (feen apart) on which there is very exactly drawn a fquare Tract 2, upon which the Hairs are placed   The faid Piece is placed in a Groove made in a little Brafs Frame, foldered to the Tube of the Telefcope at the Place 2, the fmall Screw 5 is to move forwards or backwards, the little Piece carrying the Hairs, the Object-Glafs is placed at the other End of the Telefcope, next to the Object to be feen   It is alfo placed in the little Tube 3, which being put into the Tube of the Telefcope, muft be binded pretty much by it, that it may not eafily change its Place when the Telefcope is adjufted   The Glaffes are convex, which renders their Middle thicker than their Edges, but the Eye-Glafs muft have more Convexity than the Object-Glafs, to the end that Objects may appear greater than by the naked Eye

The Focus of a Convex Glafs is that Place where the Rays, coming from a luminous or coloured Object, unite, after having paffed thro' the Glafs, whence the Picture of Objects, oppofite to the Glafs, are there very diftinctly reprefented   For example, the Point R, at the End of the Cone of the Figure H, is the Focus of the Glafs S, becaufe it is the Point where the Rays, entering at the other End N of the Tube, unite, after having paffed thro' the Glafs S

The Telefcopes moft in Ufe (for Semi-circles) are thofe with two Glaffes, which are fo placed, that their Foci are common, and unite in the fame Point in the Tube of the Telefcope, in which Point the Hairs are placed, if the focal Length of the Object-Glafs is feven or eight times greater than that of the Eye-Glafs, the Object will appear feven or eight times greater than when the Foci of the two Glaffes are equal

The Focus of the Eye-Glafs being common with that of the Object-Glafs, the coloured Rays, which falling upon the Surface of the Object-Glafs, and uniting in the Focus of the Glafs, afterwards continue their way diverging to the Eye-Glafs, and pafs thro it, fo that placing the Eye behind it, Objects may be perceiv'd, whofe Pictures are reprefented in the Focus   for it is the Object that fends forth its Species to the Eye, as may be yet very manifeftly proved by the following Experiment

Darken a Room, by fhutting the Window-Shutters, and make a round Hole in fome Shutter, whofe Window is expofed to a Place on which the Sun fhines in which Hole place a Convex Glafs, and alfo a white Piece of Paper or Sheet in the Room, oppofite to the Hole, and at the Glafs's focal Diftance from it, then a very diftinct Reprefentation of all outward Objects, oppofite to the Hole in the Shutter, will be painted upon the Paper in the Room in an inverted Situation, and this Picture is made by Rays of Light coming from the Objects without   The focal Diftance of the Glafs may be found, by moving the Paper backwards and forwards, till the Reprefentation of the Objects are diftinctly perceived

There is a Ball and Socket belonging to this Semi-circle, which, being well made, in the aforefaid manner, is the moft perfect that can be made

The Inftrument M is a Protractor about 8 or 10 Inches Diameter, with its moveable Index, we make them fometimes as large as Graphometers, and ufe them both in taking Angles in the Field to a Minute, and alfo plotting them upon Paper

The Index of this Protractor turns about a circular Cavity, in the middle of which is a little Point, fhewing the Center of the Protractor   The Divifions of the Limb of this Protractor are made in the fame manner as thofe on the Limb of the Semicircle, and by the Method before explained

USE I   To take the Plot of a propofed Field, as A B C D E, plant a Staff very up- Fig. 6. right, at each Angle of the Field, and meafure exactly, with a Toife, one of its Sides, as A B, which fuppofe 50 Toifes, 2 Feet, then make a Memorial, on which draw a Figure fomething like the Field propofed · This being done, place the Semi-circle; with its Foot, in the Place of the Staff A; fo that looking thro' the fixed Sights of the Diameter, you may fee the Staff B   Afterwards, the Semi-circle remaining fixed in this Pofition, turn the Index, fo that you may fee thro' the Sights the Staff C   Note the Angle made by the fiducial Line with the Side A B, and write down, in your Memorial, the Quantity of the Angle B A C, afterwards turn the Index fo, that you may fee the Staff D thro' the Sights, and write down in your Memorial the Quantity of the Angle B A D . Again, turn the Index ſo that you may ſee thro' the Sights the Staff E, and ſet down the Quantity of the Angle B A E , but every time you look thro' the Sights, Care muſt be taken that the Staff B is in a right Line with the Sights of the Diameter

This being done, remove the Semi-circle with its Foot, and having replanted the Staff A, place the Semi-circle, with its Foot, in the Place of the Staff B, in ſuch manner, that by looking thro' the fixed Sights of the Diameter, you may ſee the Staff A , and the Semi-circle remaining fixed in this Situation, turn, as you have already done, the Index ſo that you may ſucceſſively ſee the Staffs C, D, E, and write down in the Memorial the Quantities of the Angles A B C, A B D, A B E

Finally, Plot the Field exactly with a Semi-circle or Protractor, by laying down all the Angles, whoſe Quantities are marked at the Ends of the Line A B, from whence may be drawn as many right Lines, and from their Interſections other Lines, which will form the Plot of the Field propoſed. The Lengths of all thoſe Sides which have not been meaſured, may be found by a Scale of equal Parts, of which the Line A B is 50½, and the Area of the Field may be found by finding the Area of all the Triangles it may be reduced into

Note, It is proper to meaſure one of the longeſt Sides of the Field, for uſing it as a common Baſe, and making at both its Ends all the Obſervations neceſſary for there forming the Angles of the Triangles required to be made ; for if one of the ſhorteſt Lines be taken for a common Baſe to all the Triangles, the Angles formed by the Interſections of the viſual Rays in looking at the Staffs, will be too acute, and ſo their Interſections very uncertain.

The Meridian Line of Plans may be known by help of the Compaſs, whoſe Meridian is generally parallel to the Diameter of the Semi-circle for ſince the common Baſe of all the Triangles obſerved, is parallel to the ſaid Diameter, you need but note the Angle which it makes with the Needle of the Compaſs, and this may be eaſily done by directing the fiducial Line parallel to the Needle, after which you may draw upon the Plot a little Card in its true Poſition.

       U S E II   *To find the Diſtance from the Steeple* A, *to the Tower* C, *they being ſuppoſed inacceſſible*

Fig 7.

Having choſen 2 Stations, from which the Steeple and Tower may be ſeen, and meaſured their Diſtance ſerving as a Baſe, place the Semi-circle at one of them, as D, and the Staff in the other, as in the Point E, and turn it ſo, that thro the fixed Sights of its Diameter, or thro' the Teleſcope, you may eſpy the Staff E : then move the Index ſo, that thro' its Sights you may ſee the Steeple A , and the Degrees of the Semi-circle between the Diameter and the Index, will give the Quantity of the Angle B D E, being in this Example 32 Deg which note in your Memorial Again, turn the Index till you ſee the Tower C thro' the Sights or Teleſcope, always keeping the Diameter in the Line D E, then the Degrees between the Diameter and Index, will ſhow the Quantity of the Angle C D E, 123 Deg. which likewiſe note in the Memorial Now having removed the Semi-circle from the Station D, and placed a Staff in its Place, meaſure the Diſtance from the Staff D to the Staff E, which ſuppoſe 32 Toiſes, writing it in the Memorial then put the Semi-circle in the Place of the Staff E, ſo that the fixed Sights of the Diameter, or Teleſcope, may be in the Line E D, and turn the Index, that the Tower C may be ſeen thro' its Sights, then the Degrees contained between the Diameter, and the Index, will give the Angle C E D, which in this Example is 26 Degrees Finally, Turn the Index till you ſee the Steeple A thro the Sights, and the Angle A E D will be 125 Degrees, which ſet down in the Memorial, and by help of a Scale and Protractor, the Diſtance A C may be known.

To ſolve the ſame Problem trigonometrically , firſt, We have found by Obſervation in the Triangle D A E, that the Angle A D E is 32 Degrees, and the Angle D E A 125 Degrees, whence the Angle D A E is 23 Degrees (becauſe the three Angles of any right-lined Triangle, are equal to 2 right Angles) and to find the Side A E, make this Analogy As the Sine of 23 Degrees is to 32 Toiſes, ſo is the Sine of 32 Degrees to the Line A E, about 43 Toiſes Likewiſe you will find by Obſervation in the Triangle C D E, that the Angle C D E is 26 Degrees, and the Angle E D C 123 Degrees, whence the Angle D C E is 31 Degrees , and to find the Side C E, make this ſecond Analogy As the Sine of 31 Degrees is to 32 Toiſes, ſo is the Sine of 123 Degrees, or its Complement 57, which is the ſame, to C E 52 Toiſes. Now to find the Diſtance C A, examine the Triangle C A E, whoſe two Sides C E, A E, with the included Angle A E C of 99 Degrees, are known, and conſequently the Sum of the two unknown Angles are equal to 81 Degrees , and to find either of them, make again this Analogy : As the Sum of the two known Sides 95 Toiſes, is to their Difference 9, ſo is the Tangent of 40 Deg. 30 Min half the Sum of the oppoſite Angles, to the Tangent of half their Diſtance, which anſwers to 4 Deg. 37 Min and being added to 40 Deg 30 Min will give the greateſt of the unknown Angles C A E, 45 Deg 7 Min and conſequently the other Angle A C E, will be 35 Deg. 53 Min Laſtly, to find the Length C A, ſay, As the Sine of 35 Deg 53 Min is to 43 Toiſes, ſo is the Sine of 99 Deg to the Diſtance A C, 72 Toiſes, 2 Feet.

USE III　To find the Height of the Tower A B, whose Base cannot be approached because of a Rivulet passing by its Foot, chuse two Stations some where upon level Ground, as in C and D, and place the Semi-circle vertically in the Point D, so that its Diameter may be parallel to the Horizon, which you may do by means of a Thread and Plummet, hung on the Top of a Perpendicular drawn on the backside of the Semi-circle then turn the Index, in order to see the Top of the Tower B thro' the Sights, and take the Quantity of the Angle B D A, which suppose 42 Degrees, noteing it down in your Memorial　Now having removed the Semi-circle, and placed it at the other Station C, measure the Distance D C, which suppose 12 Toises, and after having adjusted the Semi-circle, so that its Diameter may be parallel to the Horizon, turn the Index till you see the Top of the Tower B, and set down the Quantity of the Angle B C D, which suppose 22 Degrees, in the Memorial, then make a similar Figure by means of a Scale and Protractor, and the Height of the Tower A B will be found, which may likewise be found by Calculation in the following manner　The Angle B D A of 42 Degrees, gives the Angle B D C of 138 Degrees, and since the Angle C of 22 Degrees has been measured, the third Angle of the Triangle C B D will be 20 Degrees　Now say, As the Sine of 20 Degrees is to 12 Toises, so is the Sine of 22 Degrees, to the Line B D, about 13 Toises, but B D is the Hypothenuse of the right-angled Triangle B D A, all the Angles of which are known　therefore say by a second Rule of Three, As Radius is to about 13 Toises, so is the Sine of 42 Degrees to the Height A B, 8 Toises, and one Foot

USE IV　*To take the Map of a Country*

First, chuse 2 high Places, from whence a great Part of the Country may be seen, which let be so remote from each other, as that their Distance may serve as a common Base to several Triangles that must be observed for making of the Map, then measure with a Chain the Distance of these two Places　These two Places being supposed A and B, distant from each other 200 Toises, place the Plane of the Semi-circle horizontally, with its Foot in the Point A, in such manner, that you may discover the Point B thro' the fix'd Sights or Telescope　the Instrument remaining fix'd in this Situation, turn the Index, and successively discover Towers, Steeples, Mills, Trees, and other remarkable Things desired to be placed in the Map · examine the Angles which every of them make with the common Base, and set them down together with their proper Names in the Memorial　As, for Example, the Angle B A I 14 Degrees, B A G 47, B A H 53, B A F 68, B A E 83, B A D 107, and lastly, the Angle B A C 130 Degrees　which being done, and the Distance of the two Stations A B set down, place the Semi-circle in the Point B, for a second Station.

The Instrument being so placed that its Diameter may be in the Line B A, turn the Index, and observe the Angles made by the Objects before seen from the Point A, as for Example, the Angle A B C 20 Degrees, A B F 37, A B D 44, A B E 56, A B G 83, A B H 96, and the Angle A B I 133 Degrees, which note down in the Memorial.

If any Object view'd from the Point A, cannot be seen from the Point B, the Base must be changed, and another Point sought, from whence it may be discovered, for it is absolutely necessary for the same Object to be seen at both Stations, because its Position cannot be had but by the Intersection of two Lines drawn from the Ends of the Base, with which they form a Triangle

Note, The Base must be pretty long, in proportion to the Triangles for which it serves, and moreover very streight and level

To make the Map, reduce all those Triangles observed, to their just Proportion, by means of a Scale and Protractor, in the manner as we have already given Directions, in the Use of the Theodolite

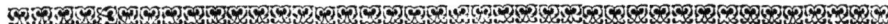

C H A P. VII.

Of the Construction and Use of the Compass.

THIS Instrument is made of Brass, Ivory, Wood, or any other solid Matter, from 2 to 6 Inches in Diameter, being in figure of a Parallelopipedon, in the Middle of which is a round Box, at the Bottom of which is described a Card (of which more in the Construction of the Sea-Compass) whose Circumference is divided into 360 Degrees. In the Center of this Card is fixed a well-pointed Brass or Steel Pivot, whose Use is to carry the touched Needle placed upon it, *in Equilibrio*, so that it may freely turn　This Box is covered with a round Glass, for hindring left the Air should any wise agitate the Needle.

One of the Ends of the Needle always turns towards the North Part of the World, but not exactly, it declining therefrom, and the other towards the South

According to Observations made in *October*, in the Year 1715, in the Royal Observatory, the Needle declined 2 Deg 5 Min. Westwardly

Needles

Needles are made of Pieces of Steel, the Length of the Diameter of the Box, having little Braſs Caps ſoldered to their Middle, hollowed into a conical Figure ſo, that the Needle being put upon the Pivot, may move very freely upon it, and not fall off, they are nicely filed into different Figures, thoſe which are large being like a Dart, and ſmall ones have Rings towards one End, for knowing that End which reſpects the North, as may be ſeen in the little Figures nigh the Compaſs

To touch a Needle well, having firſt got a good Stone, begin your Touch near the Middle of the Needle, and preſſing it pretty hard upon the Pole of the Stone, draw it ſlowly along to the End of the Needle, and lifting your Hand a good Diſtance from the Stone, while you put the Needle forward again, begin a ſecond Touch in the ſame manner, and after that a third, which is enough, only take Care not to rub the Needle to and fro on the Stone, whereby the backward Rubs take away what Virtue the forward ones gave, but lift it out of the Sphere of the Stone's Virtue, when you carry it forward again to begin a new Touch.

This admirable Property, by help of which great Sea-Voyages were firſt undertaken, and vaſt Nations both in the Eaſt and Weſt diſcovered, was not known in *Europe* till about the Year 1260

A Man by means of this Inſtrument, and a Map, may likewiſe go to any propoſed Place, at Land, without enquiring of any body the way, for he need but ſet the Center of the Compaſs, upon the Place of Departure, on the Map, and afterwards cauſe the Needle to agree with the Meridian of this Place upon the Map then if he notes the Angle that the Line leading to the Place makes with the Meridian, he need but in travelling keep that Angle with the Meridian, and that will direct him to the Place deſired

This Inſtrument is alſo very uſeful to People working in Quarries, and Mines under Ground, for having noted upon the Ground the Point directly over that you have a mind to go to, you muſt place the Compaſs at the Entrance into the Quarry or Mine, and obſerve the Angle made by the Needle with the Line of Direction then when you are under Ground, you muſt make a Trench, making an Angle with the Needle equal to the aforeſaid Angle, by means of which you may come to the propoſed Place under ground There are ſeveral other Uſes of this Inſtrument, the principal of which we are now going to ſpeak

USE I. *To take the Declination of a Wall with the Compaſs.*

You muſt remember that there are 4 Points, called Cardinal ones, viz North, South, Eaſt, and Weſt, dividing the Horizon into 4 equal Parts, and when one of theſe Points are found, all the others may likewiſe · for if you have North before you, South will be behind, Eaſt on the right hand, and Weſt on the left

A Wall built upon a Line tending from North to South, will be in the Plane of the Meridian, ſo that one Side thereof will face the Eaſt, and the other the Weſt.

Another Wall, at right Angles with the former, that is one built upon the Line of Eaſt and Weſt, will be parallel to the Prime Vertical, and will not decline at all, and one of its Sides will be directly South, and the other North

Fig 10.

But if a Wall is ſuppoſed to be built upon the Line D E, it is ſaid to decline as many Degrees as is contained in the Arc F, therefore if, for Example, that Arc be 40 Degrees, the Side of the Wall faceing towards the South, declines from the South towards the Eaſt 40 Degrees, and the oppoſite Side of the Wall will decline from the North towards the Weſt 40 Degrees ſo that the Declination of a Wall, is no more than the Angle made by the Wall and the Prime Vertical Another Wall parallel to the Line G H, will decline as many Degrees as is contained in the Arc C, therefore if that Arc be 30 Degrees, the Side of the Wall reſpecting the South, will decline 30 Degrees from the South towards the Weſt, and the other Side will decline 30 Degrees from the North to the Eaſt

In all Operations made with a Compaſs, you muſt take care of bringing it nigh Iron or Steel, and that there be none concealed, for Iron or Steel entirely changes the Direction of the Needle

I ſuppoſe here that the Pivot, upon which the Cap of the Needle is put, is in the Center of a Circle divided into 360 Degrees, or four Nineties, whoſe firſt Degree begins from the Meridian Line, and alſo that the Compaſs be ſquare, as that which is repreſented in the Figure

Apply the Side of the Compaſs where the North is marked, to the Side of the Wall, then the Number of Degrees over which the Needle fixes, will be the Wall's Declination, and on that Side If, for Example, the North Point of the Needle tends towards the Wall, it is a ſign that *that* Side of the Wall may be ſhone on by the Sun at Noon; and if the Needle fixes over 30 Degrees, counting from the North towards the Eaſt, the Declination is ſo many Degrees from South towards the Eaſt. If it fixes over 30 Degrees from the North towards the Weſt, the Declination of the Needle will be ſo many Degrees from the South towards the Weſt

But ſince the Declination of the Needle is at *Paris* 12 Deg 15 Min. N W for correcting that Defect, 12 Deg 15 Min muſt always be added to the Degrees ſhown by the Needle, when the Declination of the Wall is towards the Eaſt, and on the contrary, when the Declination is towards the Weſt, the Declination of the Needle muſt be ſubſtracted

As

As fuppofing, as we have already done, that the Needle fixes over the 30th Degree towards the Eaft, the Declination of the Wall will be 42 Deg 15 Min from the South towards the Eaft; but if the Needle fixes on the Weft-fide of the Wall, over the 30th Degree, the Declination will be 17 Deg 45 Min from the South towards the Weft.

It the South Point of the Needle tends towards the Wall, it is a Sign that the South is on the other Side of the Wall, and confequently that Side of the Wall, whofe Declination is to be found, will not be fhone upon by the Sun at Noon, whence its Declination will be from the North towards the Eaft or Weft, according as it faces towards thofe Parts of the World   This will be more fully explain'd in the Treatife of Dialling

USE II   *To take an Angle with the Compafs*

Let the Angle D A E be propofed to be meafured, apply that Side of the Compafs, where Fig. 11, the North is marked, to one of the Lines forming the Angle, as A D. fo that the Needle may freely turn upon its Pivot, and when it refts, obferve what Number the North Point of the Needle ftands over, and finding it, for Example, 80 Degrees, the Declination of the faid Line will be fo many Degrees.   Afterwards take, in the fame manner, the Declination of the Line A E, which fuppofe 215 Degrees: fubftract 80 Degrees from 215 Degrees, there will remain 135, which fubftract from 180, and there will remain 45 Degrees, the Quantity of the Angle propofed to be meafured

But if the Declination of the Line A D had been, for example, but 30 Degrees, and the Line A E 265 Degrees, the Difference of thofe two Declinations, which would be 235 Degrees, would be too great to fubftract from 180 Degrees, whence in this Cafe 180 Degrees muft be taken from 235 Degrees, and the Remainder 55 Degrees, will be the Angle propofed.

When Angles are meafured with the Compafs, there need not any regard be had to the Variation of the Needle, becaufe the Variation will always be the fame in all the different Pofitions of the Needle, provided at all times there be no Iron near it   and when the Compafs cannot be put nigh the Plane, by means of fome Impediment, it is fufficient to place it parallel, as the Figure fhows, and the Effect will be the fame.

USE III.   *To take the Plot of a Foreft, or Morafs*

Let it be required to take the Plot of the Morafs A B C D E, in which one may enter Fig. 12; To make thefe kind of Operations, there muft be faftened two Sights to the Meridian Line of the Compafs, now plant long Staffs upright, fo that they may be in Lines parallel to the Sides encompaffing the Morafs, and place the Compafs upon its Foot in a horizontal Pofition : then look at two of the Staffs thro the Sights, putting always the Eye to that which is on the South Side of the Compafs, and having drawn a Figure upon Paper fomething reprefenting the Plot of the Morafs, write upon the correfpondent Line the Number of Degrees which the Needle, when fixed, fhows   At the fame time meafure the Length of each Side of the Morafs, and fet down their Lengths upon the correfpondent Lines of your Memorial. When you have gone round the Morafs, the Degrees obferved by the Needle, will ferve to form the Angles of the Figure, and the Length of each Line will determine the Plot of the Morafs propofed.

Let us fuppofe, for Example, that having placed the Compafs along the Side A B, or which is all one, along a Line parallel to that Side, and placing the Eye next to the South Sight of the two Sights, two Staffs fet up in that Line are efpied   If the Needle fixes on the 30th Degree towards the Eaft, fet down the Number 30 upon the Line A B in the Memorial, and alfo 50 Toifes, the Length of the Side A B. afterwards fet the Compafs, with its Foot, along the Side B C, or in the Direction of the Staffs, putting always the Eye next the South Sight   If the Needle fixes on the 100th Degree, I write that Number on the Line B C, and at the fame time 70 Toifes, the Length of the Side B C. doing thus quite round the Morafs, you may fet down upon each correfpondent Line of the Memorial, the Numbers of Degrees and Toifes; by means of which, the Plot may be drawn in the following manner, by help of a Scale and Protractor.

Angles obferved 30 Degrees.		Remaining Angles.	
100		70	Set down, one after the other,
130		30	all the Angles obferved with the
240		110	Compafs, and fubftract the leaft
300		60	from its next greater, as in this Table

Draw the Indefinite Line A B, of 50 equal Parts, reprefenting the 50 Toifes meafured; make the exterior Angle at the Point B 70 Degrees, and draw the indefinite Line B C, on which lay off 70 Toifes from B to C   Make at the Point C an exterior Angle of 30 Degrees, and draw the indefinite Line C D, whofe Length let be 65 Toifes, conformable to the Length meafured.   Make likewife at the Point D an exterior Angle of 110 Degrees, and

draw

draw the Line D E of 70 Toifes Laftly, Make an exterior Angle of 60 Degrees at the Point E, draw the Line A E of 94 Toifes, and the Plot will be compleated.

Note, All the Angles of the Figure taken together, ought to make twice as many right Angles, wanting 2, as the Figure has Sides As, for Example, the Figure of this Ufe, having 5 Sides, all the Angles added together make 540 Degrees, or 6 times 90, which may ferve to prove Operations

This Manner of taking Plots is expeditious enough, but it is very difficult to make Operations exact with a Compafs, becaufe there may be Iron concealed nigh the Places whereat a body is obliged to place the Inftrument

---

CHAP. VIII.

The Ufes of the aforefaid Inftruments, applied to the Fortifications of Places.

Plate 13.

FOrtification is the Art of putting a Place into fuch a State, that a fmall Body of Troops therein may advantageoufly refift a confiderable Army

The Maxims ferving as a Foundation to the Art of Fortification, are certain general Rules eftablifhed by Ingineers, founded upon Reafon and Experience.

The chief Ingineer having examined the Extent and Situation of the Place to be fortified, communicates his Defign in a Plan and Profil, as may be feen in Plate 13 to which he commonly adds a Difcourfe, orderly explaining the Materials imploy'd by the Undertakers · and having fearched the Ground in feveral Parts of the Place propofed, makes a Computation of each Toife of Work, by means of which the Ingineer may nighly eftimate the Charge of the whole Work, the Number of Workmen neceffary to perfect it, and alfo the Time it will be done in

The Plan of a Fortification reprefents, by feveral Lines drawn horizontally, the Inclofures of a Place

This Defign contains feveral Lines drawn parallel to one another; but the firft and principal Tract, which ought to be marked by a Line more apparent than the others, reprefents the chief Inclofure of the Body of the Place between the Rampart and the Ditch; fo that by the Plan and its Scale, the Lengths and Breadths of all the Works compofing the Fortification may be known (*Fig* 1)

The Profil reprefents the principal Tracts appearing upon a plane Surface vertically cutting and feparating all the Works thro' the Middle There is commonly a larger Scale to draw it, than to draw a Plan, for better diftinguifhing their Breadths, Heights, or Depths, (as appears in *Fig.* 3)

The Names of the chief Lines, and principal Angles, forming the Plan.

Fig 1.

The Line A B, is call'd the exterior Side of the Polygon, and L M the interior Side thereof.

L G the Demi-gorge of the Baftion, of which E G is the Flank, A E the Face, and A L the Capital.

G H is the Courtain, and A H the Line of Defence *Razante.*

The Figure A L G E reprefents a Demi-baftion.

The Angle A N B is the Angle of the Center

The Angle K A B is the Angle of the Polygon.

The Angle I A E, made by the two Faces, is the flanquant Angle, or Angle of the Baftion

The Angle A E G made by the Face and the Flank, is called the Angle *de l'Epaule*

The Angle E G H, made by the Flank and the Courtain, is called the Angle of the Flank.

The Angle E G B, made by the Flank and the Line of Defence, is called the interior flanquant Angle

The Angle E D F, made by the two *Razantes* interfecting one another towards the Middle of the Courtain, is called the exterior flanquant Angle, or Angle of the *Tenaille*

The Angle E H G, made by the Courtain and Line of Defence *Razante,* is called the diminifh'd Angle, which is always equal to that made by the Face of the Baftion and the Bafe, or exterior Side

Fundamental Maxims of Fortification.

The principal Maxims may be reduced to fix.

I Every Side round about a Place, muft be flanked or defended with Flanks, for if there be any Side about a Place not feen or defended by the Befieged, the Enemy may there lodge themfelves, and become Mafters of the Place in a fhort time.

It

Plate XII.

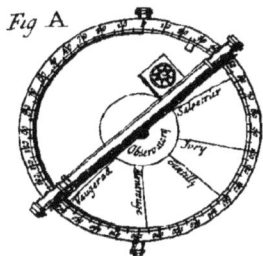

Fig A.

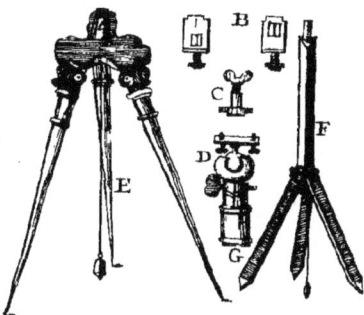

B

C

D

E

F

G

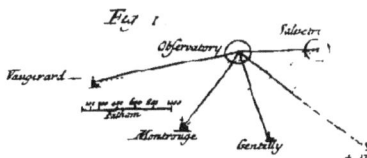

Fig 1

Observatory   Saluerin
Vaugirard
Fathom
Montrouge   Gentilly

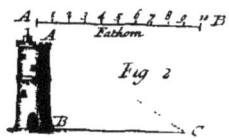

A   B
Fathom
Fig 2
B   C

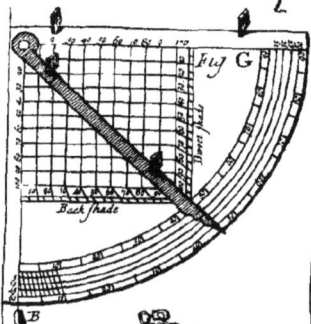

Fig G.
Back shade
B

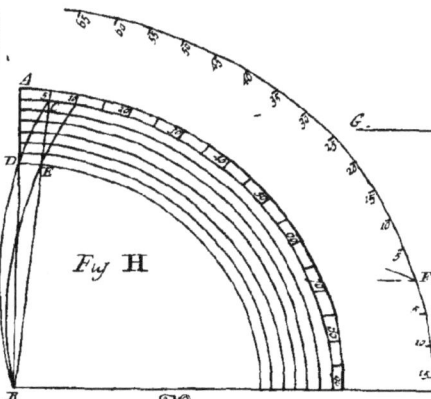

Fig H.
A
D
E
F
B

Fig 3

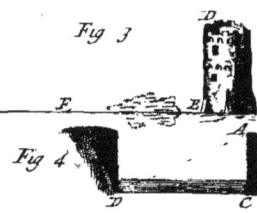

D
G   F   E
A
Fig 4
D   C

B
Fathom
Fig 5

A   C   D

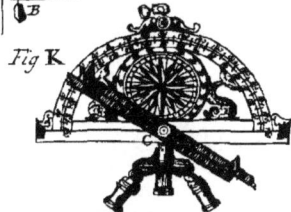

Fig K.

Fig M.

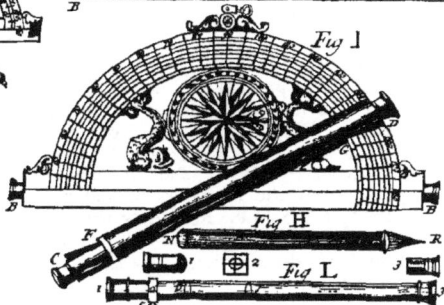

Fig I.

Fig H.

Fig L.

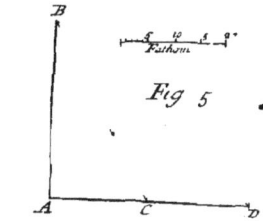

Scale
Fig 7
D   Fathom   E

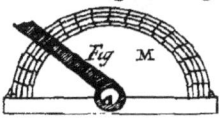

Fathom
Scale
C   D
A   50 Fathom   B

Fig 6

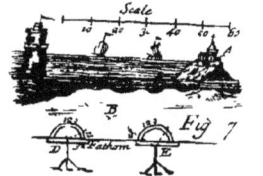

Scale
Fig 8
F   Fathom   D

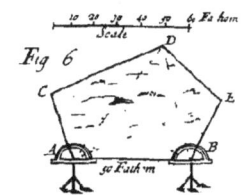

Fig 9
D   H
E
G
C   F
A   200 Fathom   B

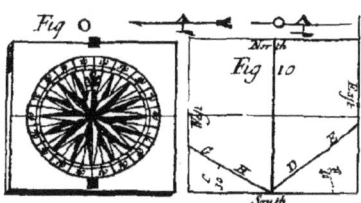

Fig O
North
Fig 10
West   East
South

Fig 11

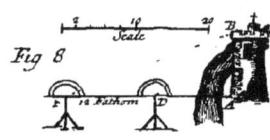

Fig 12

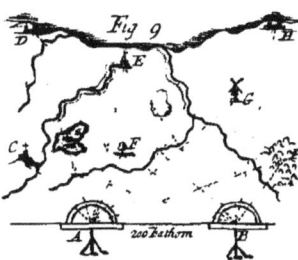

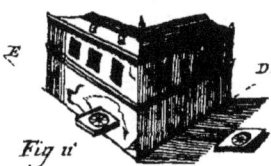

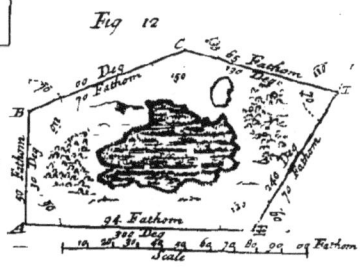

Deg
Fathom
Fathom
Deg
Scale

It follows from this Maxim, that the flanquant Angle, or the Angle made by the Face of the Bastion, being too acute, is defective, because its Point may easily be blunted or broken by the Cannon of the Besiegers, and afterwards Miners may there work safe in working of the Breach

It is also a like Fault to round the Points of Bastions, for the same Reason

II The Force, as much as possible, must be equally distributed every where, for it there be any Side weaker than the rest, that will be it which the Enemy will attack, therefore if from the Nature of the Ground, one Side be weaker than the others, some Work must be there added to augment its Force, in multiplying its Defence

III The flanquant Parts must be no further remote from those which flank them, than a Musquet-shot will do Execution therefore the Line of Defence, or the Distance from the Point of a Bastion to its neighbouring Bastions, ought not much to exceed 125 Toises, which is the Distance that a Musquet, well charged, will do Execution

IV The Flanks of Bastions must be large enough to contain at least 30 Soldiers in Front, and 4 or 5 Pieces of Cannon mounted on their Carriages, in order to defend well the Face of the Bastion attacked by the Enemy , and since the principal Defence arises from Flanks, it is more proper for them to be perpendicular to the Line of Defence, than to have any other Situation This Method was assigned by Count *Pagan*, and has been follow'd by the ablest Ingineers since his Time, and particularly by Monsieur *Vauban*, who, by his singular Services, merited the Esteem of all warlike Nations, and able Ingineers of his Time

V The Fortress must not be commanded by any Side out of the reach of Fire-Arms, which are Musquets and Cannon , but on the contrary, it ought to command all Places round about

VI The Works nighest the Center, must be highest, and command those Places more distant, so that when the Enemy endeavour to make themselves Masters of some Outwork, they may be repulsed by those in the Body of the Place

To draw upon Paper a fortified Plan, according to the Method of Count Pagan

Let it be, for Example, an Hexagon first draw the Line A B 180 Toises, for the exterior Side of the Hexagon, and raise the Perpendicular C D from the Point C of 30 Toises, then draw the Lines A D H, B D G, intersecting each other in the Point D, and take 55 Toises from your Scale, to determine the Length of the Faces A E, B F from the Point E draw the Flank E G, making a right Angle in the Point G, at the end of the Line of Defence B G, and likewise the other Flank F H at right Angles to A H finally, draw the Courtain G H, and you will have one Side of the Hexagon fortified The other Sides are fortified in the same manner About this Side of the Polygon thus fortified, you must draw a Ditch, represented by the Lines A C, C B, parallel to the Faces of the Bastions, meeting each other towards the Middle of the Courtain in the Point C This Ditch ought to be 20 Toises in Breadth, and 3 Toises deep. The Ground taken out in making of the Ditch, serves to form the Rampart with its Parapet, and the Glacis of the Cover'd Way, preferring the finest for the Parapet of the Body of the Place, and the Cover'd Way , for if the Ground be stony, Cannon-Balls, coming from the Besiegers against Parapets made with it, will make the Stones fly about, and annoy the Soldiers defending the Body of the Place On the contrary, when the Ground is fine, the Bullets will but make Holes, and enter therein, provided Parapets have Breadth enough to deaden them by Experience it is found, that Parapets must consist of well-rammed Earth at least 20 Foot thick, to be Proof against Cannon

The Parapet is made upon the Rampart 24 Feet broad, containing the Barquette, or little Bank, made parallel to the Faces, Flanks, and Courtains, forming the Inclosure of the Place

The Base of the Rampart is 15 Toises broad, and is made parallel to the Courtains only, to the end that the Bastions may be full, and that there may be there found Earth in case of need, to make an Intrenchment

When any Bastion is left open, a Mine must be made therein well arched, Bomb proof, and covered with Ground well rammed, and it must be endeavour'd to be made so that the Rain-Water cannot get into it, to the end that Provisions put therein, may be preserved from time to time

The Cover'd Way is made parallel without the Ditch, about 5 Toises broad, and upon it there is a Parapet made 6 Foot high, and a Banquette, at the Foot of the said Parapet, 3 Foot broad, and a Foot and a half high, so that Soldiers may commodiously use their Arms on the Top of the Parapet, whose Top must be *en Glacis*, that is, having a Descent or Slope going down 20 or 30 Toises into the Country

There must be no hollow Places about this *Glacis*, for the Enemy to cover themselves in, therefore when an Ingineer visits the Fortification of a Place, it is requisite for him to examine the adjacent Parts, and have the hollow Places filled up, at least within the reach of a Musquet-shot from the Cover'd Way, and also to have all Places too high levelled, that so those which defend the Place, may discover all the adjacent Parts

Fig. 1

Fig 2.

To draw the Profil of a Fortified Place upon Paper

Draw the indefinite Line O N, representing the Level of the Country, and take 15 Toises, which lay off from O to Q, for denoting the Base of the Rampart, then lay off 20 Toises from Q to R, for the Breadth of the Ditch, over-against one of the Faces of the Bastion, for it is wider over-against the Courtain. lay off 5 Toises from R to P, for the Breadth of the Cover'd Way, and lastly, 20 or 30 Toises from P to N, for the Base of the *Glacis* Note, the longer the Base of the *Glacis* is made, the better will it be

After having determined the Breadths or Thicknesses, the Heights above the Level of the Country, and Depths below, must be as follows

Take 3 Toises from your Scale, and raise from the Points O, Q, Perpendiculars of that Height, for raising above the Level of the Country the Platform or the Rampart, whereof O S is the interior Talud, or Slope, going up from the City to the Platform of the Rampart S T, which Platform ought to be 6 or 7 Toises broad, that so Cannon may be commodiously used thereon, as also the other necessary Munitions for the Defence of the Place

Note, The Rising of the Rampart ought to be very easy over-against the Gorge of the Bastions, for Coaches to go easily there up and down it

The Base of the Talud O Z, is made with new-dug Earth, equal to the Height all along the Courtains, as if the Height be 3 Toises, the Base of the Slope must be also 3 Toises

But at the Entry of the Bastions, the Base must be at least twice the Height, that is, if the Height of the Slope be 3 Toises, the Base of it must be at least 6 or 8 Toises, for Coaches to go up it.

When the Rampart is formed, and the Earth sufficiently raised upon it, which cannot be done but with Time and Precaution, in well ramming it every 2 Feet in Height, and laying Fascines to keep it together, a Parapet is made upon the Earth of the Rampart, 6 Feet of interior Height, and 4 Feet of exterior Height, (for the Top of the Earth to have a Declivity) to discover any thing beyond the Ditch, and being mounted upon the Banquette, the Cover'd Way may be seen, and defended in case of Need

The Base of the Parapet X Y, ought to be about 4 Toises broad, to the end that the Top thereof may be at least 20 Feet broad   At the Bottom of the interior Slope of the Parapet, there is made a little Bank 3 Foot wide, and a Foot and a half high, so that the Parapet will be 4½ Feet above the Bank, which is sufficient for Soldiers to use their Fire-Arms on the Top thereof

Care must be taken to lay Beds of Fascines every Foot in height, between the Earth of the Parapet, and in order to keep the Earth of the said Parapet from crumbling, it is covered with Grass-Turfs, cut with a Turfing-Iron, from some neighbouring Common, about 15 Inches long, and 10 broad.

Now to lay these Turfs, you must place the first Bed, or Row of them, very level all along the Distance of several Toises, and then lay the Turfs of the second Bed so, that the Joints of the first may be covered with them, and the Joints of the second likewise covered with the Joints of the third, &c that so they may all make a good joining

It is sufficient to give 2 Inches of Declivity to one Foot in height, for the interior Slope, and about 4 Inches to one Foot in height, for the exterior Slope of the Parapet. Note, There ought to be Gardiners to cut and lay the Turfs.

At the Foot of the exterior Slope of the Parapet and the Rampart, there is left a little Berm (marked Q,) about 4 Feet wide, for retaining the loose Ground falling down from the Slope

Q B represents the inward Slope of the Ditch, which is 3 Toises deep, and B K is the exterior Slope If the Ground be brittle, they must have more Slope given them, for hindring its falling to the Bottom of the Ditch   The Line K P represents the Platform of the Cover'd Way, which must be 5 Toises broad   P A represents the Parapet of the Cover'd Way, with its Banquette at the Foot thereof.   The whole must be 6 Feet high, for covering those which are on the Cover'd Way

The superior Slope of the *Glacis* A N, ought to be made of fine Earth, the Stones in which, if there be any, must be taken away with an Iron Rake, and buried at the Foot of the *Glacis*, so that Cannon-Balls shot from the Enemy upon the Cover'd Way, may enter therein, without making the broken Pieces of the Stones fly about upon the Cover'd Way

To lay off the Plan of a Fortification upon the Ground

Let, for Example, the Plan of the first Figure be proposed to be drawn upon the Ground.

Instead of a Scale and Compasses, there must be used Staffs, the Toise, and Lines, therefore, after having well examined the Ground, and considered where the Gates and Bastions must be made, which are commonly in the Middle of the Courtains, long Staffs must first be placed, where the flanquant Angles of the Bastions are intended to be

Now having planted a long Staff upright, in the Place fixed on for the Point of the Bastion, (marked A) measure very exactly, with a Toise or Chain, 90 Toises, at the End of which plant a Staff, (marked C)· from the Point C continue that Line 90 Toises more, at the End of which plant another Staff, which will be the Point of the Bastion B. In the

mean

mean time you are measuring with Chains or Lines, some Workmen must follow, and make a little Trench from Staff to Staff, before the Lines are taken away.

After which, a Perpendicular must be drawn from the Staff C, to the Tract A C B

To draw the said Perpendicular, measure two or three Toises from C to A, where plant a Staff, measure likewise from C towards B an equal Number of Toises, at the end of which plant a second Staff. Take two Lines very equal, and having made Loops in the two ends of each of them, put those Loops about each of the Staffs, and holding the two other ends of the Lines in your Hands, stretch them till they join upon the Ground, and in their point of Junction plant a third Staff. Lastly, Fasten a Line tight to the Point C, and that third Staff, by which make a Tract, which will be perpendicular to the Line A C B.

Measure 30 Toises from the Point C along the Tract, at the end of which plant another Staff very upright, which will shew the Point D of the Plan. Return to the Staff A, from which to the Staff D make a Tract, along which from the Point A measure 55 Toises towards D, for the Face of the Bastion A E, plant a Staff in the Point E, for denoting the Angle *de l'Epaule*

Go to the Point B, and there make the same Operations for drawing the Face B F, and plant a Staff at the Angle *de l'Epaule* F

Produce B F from D, towards G, and also A E from D towards H, then measure with the Scale of the Plan the Lines D G, D H, and lay off their Lengths on the Ground from D to G, and from G to H, where plant Staffs. After which it will be easy to draw the Flanks E G, F H, and the Courtain G H

By this means you will have one Front of a fortified Place, drawn on the Ground, the others may be drawn in the same manner by Staffs and Lines

Note, It will not be improper to examine with a Semi-circle or Recipient-Angle, whether the Angles drawn upon the Ground are equal to those taken off of the Plan, and to rectify them before the Works are begun.

Care must likewise from time to time be taken, that the Tracts are followed; for without these Precautions, there will sometimes happen great Deformities.

Of the Construction of the Outworks

The Outworks of a Fortification, are those Works made without the Ditch of a fortified Place, to cover it and augment its Defence

The most ordinary kinds of these Works, are the Ravelins or Half-moons, which are formed between the two Bastions upon the Flanquant Angle of the Counterscarp, and before the Courtain, for covering the Gates and Bridges commonly made in the middle of the Courtains, as the Figures P P show.

The Ravelins are composed of two Faces furnished with one or two little Banks, and a good Parapet raised on the side next the Country, and two Demigorges, without a Parapet, on the side next to the Place, with an Entrance and Slope for mounting the great Ditch on the Platform of the Ravelin

In each Ravelin there is built a *Corps-de-Garde*, to shelter the Soldiers necessary for its Defence, from the Injuries of Weather, but it is proper for the *Corps-de-Garde* to be built in form of a Redoubt, with Battlements all round, for the Soldiers, in case of being attacked, to retire in, and obtain some Capitulation, before they lay down their Arms

To draw a Ravelin before a Courtain, open your Compasses the length of the interior side of the Polygon, and having fixed one of the Points in one of the ends of the Line, with the other Point describe an Arc without the Counterscarp; likewise set one Foot of the Compasses in the other end of the interior side, and with the other Point describe a second Arc, cutting the first in a Point, which will be the Point or Flanquant Angle of the Ravelin. then lay a Ruler on the aforesaid Interfection, and upon each of the ends of the interior side of the Polygon, for drawing the Faces of the Ravelin, which will terminate to the Right and Left upon the edge of the Counterscarp. The two Demigorges are drawn from the end of each Face, to the Rentiant Angle of the Counterscarp

But that the Flanquant Angle may not be too acute, its Capital R S must be but about 40 Toises, and proceed with the rest, as before

Sometimes a similar Work is made before the Point of a Bastion; and since its Gorge is built upon the edge of the Counterscarp, which is commonly rounded over-against the Point of the Bastions, this Work is called a Half-moon, (because its Gorge is in the form of an Arc). They are very often confounded, and the greatest part of the Soldiers give, without distinction, the Name of Half-moons to Ravelins made before the Courtains.

The Defect of this Work is, that it is too distant from the Flanks of the Bastions, for being sufficiently defended by them; therefore a Half-moon must not be made before the Point of a Bastion, unless at the same time there are made other Out-works to the Right and Left before the adjacent Courtains, to defend it

It is proper for these Works to be lined with Walls, as well as the Body of the Place; for when they are not, the Ground must have so great a slope, that it will be easy to mount the Works

In the mean time the new-dug Earth the Works are made with, must settle at least a Year or two before the Walls are built, to the end that the Walls may not be thrown down by it after they are built

Construction of the Hornworks.

Fig 3.

These kind of Works are commonly made before the Courtains, and because the Expence in making them is greater than the Expence in making the Ravelins, they are not made without absolute necessity, they serve to cover some side of the Place, weaker than the others, they likewise serve to occupy an Height, which cannot be done by Persons inclosed in the Body of the Place

Now to draw a Hornwork, first raise the Indefinite Perpendicular 1, 2, on the middle of the Courtain, and to this Line draw two Parallels 3, 4, and 5, 6, from the Angles *de l'Epaules*. These two Parallels, which are called the Whings of the Hornwork, ought to draw their defence from the Faces of the Bastions, whence their length ought not much to exceed 120 Toises, counting from the *Epaules* Thro' the ends of the Whings draw the Line 4, 6, which will be the exterior side of the Hornwork, and is divided into two equal parts in the Point 7, by the Perpendicular 1, 2, then take half that exterior side in your Compasses, and lay it off upon the sides, from 4 to 8, and from 6 to 9, draw the Lines 4, 9, and 6, 8, which interfecting one another in the Point 10, will form the Angle of the *Tenaille*, that represents a Work called the Simple *Tenaille*, which is common enough made before the Courtains, with a little Ravelin without the Ditch, between the two Saliant Angles, and over-against the middle of the Rentrant Angle

But to strengthen this Work, there is added thereto two Demi-bastions, and a Courtain between them, which is better than two simple Rentrant Angles

To draw the Demibastions, bisect the Line 4, 10, in the Point 11, and likewise the Line 10, 6, in the Point 12, then from the Points 11 and 12, draw to the middle of the Courtain of the Place, as at the Point 1, the occult Lines 121, 111, by which means will be had the little Courtain 1314 of the Hornwork, the two Flanks 1113, 1214, and the two Faces 114, 126

The Sides of these Works, which are next to the Country, (as the Demi-bastions, the Courtain, and the Whings of the Hornwork are) ought to be furnish'd with a good Parapet of fine Earth well rammed, 18 or 20 Feet thick, and 6 Feet high before, containing a *Banquette*, like that in the Body of a Place, observing at all times, that the Parapets of the Works nigher the Center of the Place, must be higher above the Level of the Country, than those Works more distant, to the end that when the Besiegers have made themselves Masters of some Outwork, the Besieged, defending the Body of the Place, seeing them altogether uncover'd, may dislodge them therefrom

These Parapets ought to be sustained by a Rampart, whose Platform having a *Banquette*, is three or four Toises wide, but when Earth is wanting, we must be content to make several little Banks upon one another eighteen Inches high, and three or four Feet broad, and the Parapet ought to be about 4 Feet above the highest Bank, for covering the Soldiers the top of the Parapet must be *en Glacis*, gradually descending towards the Country, so that the Besieged may see the Enemy.

The parts of those Works, which are next the Place, must be without a Parapet, and only inclosed with a single Wall, or a Row of Palisadoes, to avoid the Surprizes of the Enemy It is on this side that a Gate must be (for a Communication from the Works to the Body of the Place,) as also the *Corps-de-Garde*, for covering the Soldiers designed for its defence

All these Works ought to be environed with a Ditch 10 or 12 Toises broad, communicating with the Ditch of the Body of the Place, and also as deep

On the outside of that Ditch is made a Cover'd Way five or six Toises broad, with a Parapet, and its Bank, commonly furnished with an enclosure of strong Palisadoes, drove 4 or 5 Feet into the Ground The top of that Parapet must be sloped next to the Country, and if it can be produced 20 or 30 Toises it will be better for a Slope (or Glacis) cannot be too long, because, by means thereof, the Enemy cannot approach the Body of the Place, without being discovered

The Outworks of which we have spoken, are the most common ones There are many other sorts of them, which we shall not mention, it requiring a great Volume

How to measure the Works of Fortifications

The Ground of which the Ramparts and Parapets are formed, is generally taken out of the Ditches made about the Place, to know the quantity of which, measure the Cavity of the Ditches, and reduce it to Cubic Toises As, for example, If the Ditch over-against the Face of a Bastion, be 50 Toises long, 20 broad, and 4 deep, multiply the Length by the Breadth, and the Product will be 1000 square Toises, which multiply'd by 4 the Depth, and there will arise 4000 Cubic Toises

Note, That since there is a necessity to give the Ground a great slope, to keep it from crumbling to the bottom, the Ditch will be wider at the top than at the bottom, whence, if a Ditch be 20 Feet broad in the middle of its Depth, at the top it must at least be 22 Toises broad, and 18 Toises at the bottom: Those 22 Toises added to 18, make 40, whose half 20, is the mean Breadth to be used

The Stone, or Brick-work, keeping together the Earth, ought to have thickness proportionable to its height, and also about a Foot in Talud, the height of every Toise

If, for example, a Wall be built to sustain the Earth of the Rampart of a Place, and it is 6 Toises high, the least thickness that can be given to that height, at the top, must be 3 Feet, and at the bottom, just above the Foundation, 9 Feet, because of its Talud of 1 Foot every Toise in height Now these two thicknesses 9 and 3 make 12, whose half 6 Feet is the mean thickness of the Wall, and consequently, to line the Face of a Bastion, 50 Toises long, 6 Toises high, and one Toise of mean thickness, there must be 300 Cubic Toises of Walling, excluding the Foundation, which cannot be determined without knowing the Ground Besides this, there are commonly made Counter-forts for sustaining the Earth, and hindering its pressing too much against the Walls These Counter-forts ought to be sunk in firm Ground, and enter in the dug Earth, at least a Toise, they are 7 or 8 Feet broad at the Root, that is, on the side where they are fastened to the Wall, and 4 or 5 Feet at the end, going into the Earth of the Rampart, which amounts to one Toise of Surface, in supposing (as we have already) that the Root is 7 Feet, and the end going into the Earth of the Rampart 5 Feet, which makes 12 Feet, half of which being 6, is the mean thickness, and supposing them 4 Toises in height, one with another, each will be 4 Cubic Toises and since there ought to be 10 in the extent of 50 Toises, the Stone or Brick-work of 10 Counter-forts will be 40 Cubic Toises So that there will be about 1000 Cubic Toises to wall the two Faces, and the Flanks of a Bastion, and to wall a Courtain, 80 Toises in length, there must be about 600 Cubic Toises of Stone or Brick-work, whence the Walling for the whole Place may be easily computed

Note, It is better to make an Estimation too great, than too little.

It remains that we say something of the Carpenters Toise, required to construct Bridges and Gates, and other Works of the like Nature

In measuring of Timber, we reduce it to Solives.

A Solive is a Piece of Timber 12 Feet long, and 36 Inches in surface, that is, 6 Inches broad, and 6 thick, which makes 3 Cubic Feet of Timber, being the seventy second part of a Cubic Toise

We shall give here two Ways of Calculation, to the end that the one may prove the other

The first is, to reduce the bigness of the Piece of Timber into Inches, that is, the Inches of its breadth and thickness, and after having multiplied these two Quantities by one another, the Product must be multiplied by the Toises, Feet and Inches of its length, which last Product being divided by 72, the Quotient will give the Number of Solives contained in the Piece of Timber.

The Reason of this is, because 72 Pieces, 1 Inch Base, and a Toise long, make a Solive

Suppose, for example, a great Piece of Timber is to be reduced to Solives, whose length is 2 Toises, 4 Feet, 6 Inches, and 12 by 15 Inches Base, multiply 15 by 12, the Product is 180 square Inches, which again multiplied by 2 Toises, 4 Feet, 6 Inches, and the Product 495, divided by 12, will give 6⅞ Solives.

The second Method is founded upon this, that a Solive contains 3 Cubic Feet

As, for example, If a Piece of Timber (the same as before) be 2 Toises, 4 Feet, 6 Inches long, and Base be 12 by 15 Inches, multiplying 12 by 15, the Product will be 180 square Inches, the 12*th* part of that Number, which is 15, being considered as Feet, makes 2 Toises 3 Feet, which, multiplied by the length 2 Toises, 4 Feet, 6 Inches, make 6 Solives, 5 Feet, and 3 Inches So that there wants but 9 Inches, or the eighth part of a Toise, to make 7 Solives, as in the Calculation of the first Method.

ADDITIONS of ENGLISH INSTRUMENTs.

Of the Theodolite, Plain-Table, Circumferentor, and Surveying-Wheel.

CHAP. I.

Of the Theodolite.

THIS Theodolite confifts of a Brafs Circle, cut in form of the Figure B, ufually about 12 or 14 Inches in Diameter, whofe Limb is divided into 360 Degrees, and each Degree into as many Minutes either Diagonally, or otherwife, as the large-nefs of the Inftrument will admit

Underneath, at the Places *c c* of this Circle, are fixed two little Pillars *d d*, for fupporting an Axis, upon which is fixed a Telefcope with a fquare Brafs Tube, having two Glaffes therein, for better perceiving Objects at a great diftance; whence this Telefcope may be raifed or lowered, according as Objects be Horizontal or not The ends of the aforefaid Pillars are joined by the Piece *g g*, upon the middle of which is folder'd a Socket with its Screw, for receiving the top of the Ball and Socket E. Upon and about the Center of the

Fig. C.

Circle B, muft the Index C move, which is a Circular Brafs Plate, having upon the middle thereof a Box and Needle, or Compafs, whofe Meridian Line anfwers to the Fiducial Line *a a* At the Places *b b* of the Index are fixed two little Pillars for fupporting an Axis, car-rying a Telefcope in the middle thereof, whofe Line of Collimation muft be anfwerable to the Fiducial Line *a a* of the Index This Telefcope hath a fquare Brafs Tube, and two Glaffes therein, and may be raifed or lowered, like that beforemention'd At each end of one of the Perpendicular fides of each Tube of the Telefcopes, are fixed four fmall Sights for viewing nigh Objects thorough them

The ends of the Index *a a* are cut Circular, fo as to fit the Divifions upon the Limb of the Circle B, and when the faid Limb B is Diagonally divided, the Fiducial Line at one end of the Index fhews the Degrees and Minutes upon the Limb But when the Limb is only divided into Degrees, and every 30th Minute, we have a much better Contrivance for find-ing the Degrees, and every 2 Minutes upon the Limb, which is thus Let the half Arc *p a* of one end of the Index contain exactly 8 Degrees of the Limb, then divide the faid half Arc into 15 equal Parts, at every five of which fet the Numbers 10, 20, 30, beginning from the Fiducial Line or middle of the Index Now each of thefe equal Parts will be 32 Minutes· Therefore if you have a mind to fet the Fiducial Line of the Index to any Num-ber of Degrees, and every 2 Minutes upon the Limb, for example, to 40 Degrees 10 Mi-nutes, move the Index fo, the Fiducial Line being between the 40th Degree, and the 40th Degree and 30 Minutes, that the Line of Divifion, numbered 10 upon the Index, may ex-actly fall upon fome Line of Divifion of the Limb, and then the Fiducial Line will fhew 40 Degrees, 10 Minutes.

Again. Suppofe the Fiducial Line being between the 50th Degree and 30 Minutes, and the 51ft, then that Line of Divifion, of equal Parts on the Index, exactly falling upon fome Line of the Divifions of the Limb, will give the even Minutes above 50 Degrees 30 Minutes the Fiducial Line ftands at As fuppofe the 4th Line of Divifion of the Index ftands ex-actly againft fome Line of Divifion of the Limb, then the Minutes above 40 Degrees 30 Mi-nutes will be 8, that the Fiducial Line ftands at · Underftand the fame of others.

Fig. D. is the Brafs Ball and Socket in which goes the Head of the three-legg'd Staff E, for fupporting the Inftrument when ufing: Thefe three Legs are moveable by means of Joints, and may be taken fhorter by half at the Places *a a a*, by means of Screws, for better conveniency of Carriage.

Thus have you the beft Theodolite, as now made in *England*, briefly defcribed

The Ufe thereof will be fufficiently underftood by what our Author fays of the Ufe of the Semi-circle, (which is but half a Theodolite) and I in the Ufe of the Plain-Table, and Circumferentor

Note, There are fome Theodolites that have no Telefcopes, but only 4 Perpendicular Sights two being faftened upon the Limb, and two upon the ends of the Index. Note likewife, That the Index, and Box and Needle, or Compafs of the Theodolite, will ferve for a Circumferentor.

CHAP. II.

Of the Conftruction and Ufe of the Plain-Table, and Circumferentor.

THE Table itfelf is a Parallelogram of Oak, or other Wood, about 15 Inches long, Fig F. and 12 broad, confifting of two feveral Boards, round which are Ledges of the fame Wood, the two oppofite of which being taken off, and the Spangle unfkrewed from the bottom, the aforefaid two Boards may be taken afunder for eafe and conveniency of Carriage For the binding of the two Boards and Ledges faft, when the Table is fet together, there is a Box Jointed-frame, about ⅛ of an Inch broad, and of the fame thicknefs as the Boards, which may be folded together in 6 Pieces. This Frame is fo contrived, that it may be taken off and put on the Table at pleafure, and may go eafily on the Table, either fide being upwards This Frame alfo is to faften a Sheet of Paper upon the Table, by forcing down the Frame, and fqueezing in all the edges of the Paper, fo that it lies firm and even upon the Table, that thereby the Plot of a Field, or other Inclofure, may conveniently be drawn upon it

On both fides this Frame, near the inward edge, are Scales of Inches fubdivided into 10 equal Parts, having their proper Figures fet to them The Ufes of thefe Scales of Inches, are for ready drawing of Parallel Lines upon the Paper, and alfo for fhifting your Paper, when one Sheet will not hold the whole Work

Upon one fide of the faid Box Frame, are projected the 360 Degrees of a Circle from a Brafs Center-hole in the middle of the Table Each of thefe Degrees are fubdivided into 30 Minutes, to every 10th Degree is fet two Numbers, one expreffing the proper Number of Degrees, and the other the Complement of that Number of Degrees to 360 This is done to avoid the trouble of Subftraction in taking of Angles

On the other fide of this Frame, are projected the 180 Degrees of a Semi-circle from a Brafs Center-hole, in the middle of the Table's length, and about a fourth part of its breadth Each of thefe Degrees are fubdivided into 30 Minutes, to every 10th Degree is fet likewife, as on the other fide, two Numbers, one expreffing the proper Number of Degrees, and the other the Complement of that Number of Degrees to 180, for the fame Reafon, as before.

The manner of projecting the Degrees on the aforefaid Frame, is, by having a large Circle divided into Degrees, and every 30 Minutes For then placing either of the Brafs Center-holes on the Table, in the Center of that Circle fo divided, and laying a Ruler from that Center to the Degrees on the Limb of the Circle, where the edge of the Ruler cuts the Frame, make Marks for the Correfpondent Degrees on the Frame

The Degrees thus inferted on the Frame, are of excellent ufe in wet or ftormy Weather, when you cannot keep a Sheet of Paper upon the Table Alfo thefe Degrees will make the Plain-Table a Theodolite, or a Semi-circle, according as what fide of the Frame is uppermoft.

There is a Box, with a Needle and Card, cover'd with a Glafs, fixed to one of the long fides of the Table, by means of a Screw, that thereby it may be taken off This Box and Needle is very ufeful for placing the Inftrument in the fame Pofition upon every remove

There belongs to this Inftrument a Brafs Socket and Spangle, fcrewed with three Screws to the bottom of the Table, into which muft be put the Head of the three-legged Staff, which may be fcrewed faft, by means of a Screw in the fide of the Socket

There is alfo an Index belonging to the Table, which is a large Brafs Ruler, at leaft 16 Inches long, and 2 Inches broad, and fo thick as to make it ftrong and firm, having a floped Edge, called the Fiducial Edge, and two Sights fcrewed perpendicularly on it, of the fame height They muft be fet on the Ruler perfectly at the fame diftance from the Fiducial Edge. Upon this Index it is ufual to have many Scales of equal Parts, as alfo Diagonals, and Lines of Chords.

SECTION

SECTION I.

Of the Construction of the Circumferentor.

Fig G

THIS Instrument consists of a Brass Index and Circle, all of a piece, the Index is commonly made about 14 Inches long, an Inch and half broad, and of a convenient thickness. The Diameter of the aforenamed Circle is about 7 Inches On this Circle is made a Card, whose Meridian Line answers to the middle of the Breadth of the Index That Card is divided into 360 Degrees There is a Brass Ring solder'd on the Circumference of the Circle, on which screws another Ring with a flat Glass in it, so that they make a kind of Box to contain the Needle suspended upon the Pivot placed in the Center of the Circle

There are also two Sights to screw on, or slide up and down the Index, like those beforenamed, belonging to the Index of the Plain-Table, as likewise a Spangle and Socket screw'd on to the back-side of the Circle, for putting the Head of the Staff in

SECTION II.

Of the Use of the Plain-Table and Circumferentor.

BUT first, it is necessary to know how to set the Parts of the Plain-Table together, to make it fit for use.

When you would make your Table fit for use, lay the two Boards together, and also the Ledges at the ends in their due Places, according as they are marked Then lay a Sheet of white Paper all over the Table, which must be stretch'd over the Boards, by putting on the Box Frame, which binds both the Paper to the Boards, and the Boards to one another. Then screw the Socket on the back-side the Table, and also the Box and Needle in its due Place, the Meridian Line of the Card lying parallel to the Meridian or Diameter of the Table; which Diameter is a Right Line drawn upon the Table, from the beginning of the Degrees thro' the Center, and so to the end of the Degrees. Then put the Socket upon the Head of the Staff, and there screw it · Also put the Sights upon the Index, and lay the Index on the Table So is your Instrument prepared for use, as a Plain-Table, Theodolite, or Semicircle

But *Note*, It is either a Theodolite, or Semi-circle, according as the Theodolite or Semi-circular side of the Frame is upwards, for when you use your Instrument as a Plain-Table, you may place your Center in any part of the Table, which you judge most proper for bringing on the Work you intend But if you use your Instrument as a Theodolite, the Index must be turned about upon the Brass Center-hole in the middle of the Table, and if for a Semi-circle, upon the other Brass Center-hole, by means of a Pin or Needle placed therein

If you have a mind to use this Instrument, as a Circumferentor, you need only screw the Box and Needle to the Index, and both of them to the Head of the Staff, with a Brass Screw-Pin fitted for that purpose So that the Staff being fixed in any Place, the Index and Sights may turn about at pleasure, without moving the Staff

USE I. *How to measure the Quantity of any Angle in the Field, by the Plain-Table, considered as a Theodolite, Semi-circle, and Circumferentor*

I *How to observe an Angle in the Field by the Plain-Table*

Plate 14.
Fig 1

Suppose E, K, K G, to be two Hedges, or two Sides of a Field, including the Angle E K G, and it is required to draw upon the Table an Angle equal thereto First place your Instrument as near the Angular Point K as conveniency will permit, turning it about, till the North End of the Needle hang directly over the Meridian Line in the Card, and then screw the Table fast Then upon your Table, with your Protracting-Pin (which is a fine Needle put into a Piece of Box or Ivory, neatly turned) or Compass Point, assign any Point at pleasure upon the Table, and to that Point apply the edge of the Index, turning the Index about upon that Point, till thro' the Sights thereof you see a Mark set up at E, or parallel to the Line E K : And then with your Protracting-Pin, Compass-Point, or Pencil, draw a Line by the side of the Index to the assigned Point upon the Table. Then (the Table remaining immoveable) turn the Index about upon the forementioned Point, and direct the Sights to the Mark set up at G, or parallel thereto, that is, so far distant from G, as your Instrument is placed from K ; and then by the side of the Index draw another Line to the assigned Point. Thus will there be drawn upon the Table two Lines representing the Hedges E K, and K G, and which include an Angle equal to the Angle E K G And tho you know not the Quantity of this Angle, yet you may find it, if required · For in working by this Instrument, it is sufficient only to give the Proportions of Angles, and not their Quantities in Degrees, as in working by the Theodolite, Semi-circle, or Circumferentor. Also in working by the Plain-Table, there needs no Protraction at all, for you will have upon your Table the true

Figure

Plate XIII

Fig. 1

A

Fig. 2

D

C

B

E

F

G

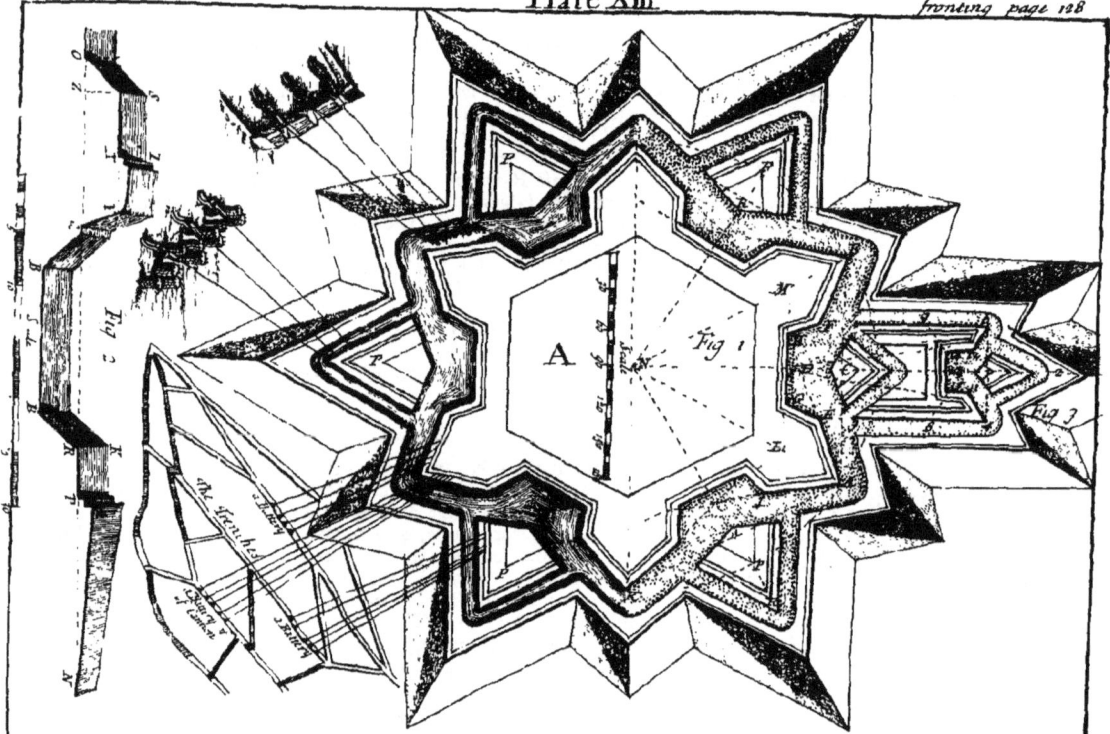

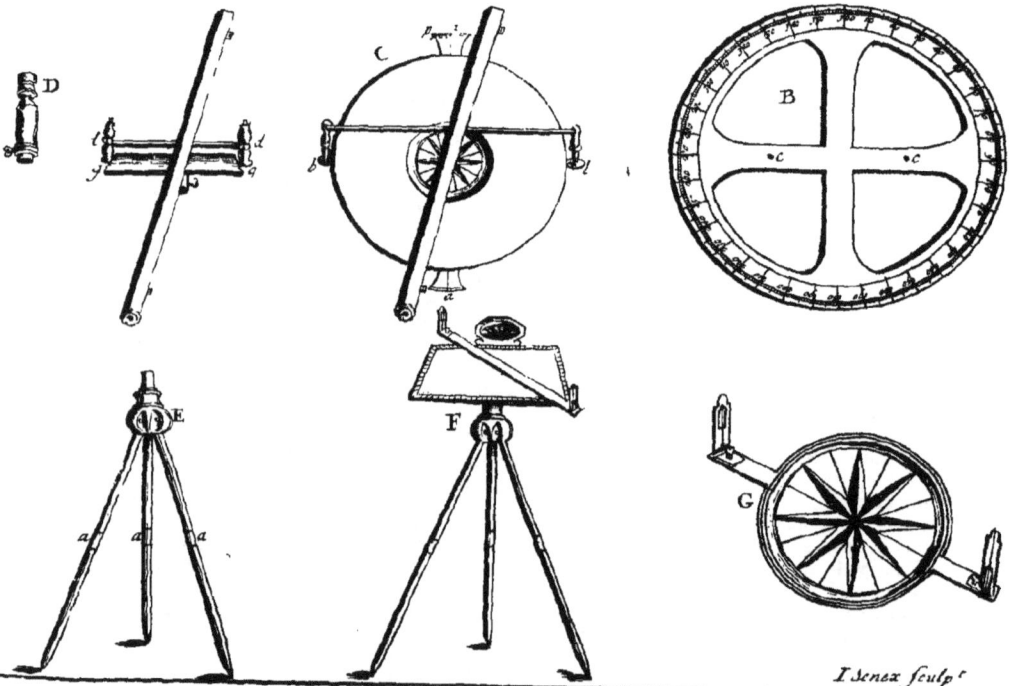

I Senex sculp.

Figure of any Angle or Angles that you obferve in the Field, in their true Pofitions, without any further trouble

II *How to find the Quantity of an Angle in the Field, by the Plain-Table, confider'd as a Theodolite or Semi-circle*

Let it firft be required to find the Quantity of the Angle E K G by the Plain-Table, as a Theodolite Place your Inftrument at K, with the Theodolite fide of the Frame upwards, laying the Index upon the Diameter thereof, then turn the whole Inftrument about (the Index ftill refting upon the Diameter) till thro the S ghts you efpy the Mark at E : Then fcrewing the Inftrument faft there, turn the Index about upon the Theodolite Center-hole in the middle of the Table, till thro the Sights you efpy the Mark at G Then note what Degrees on the Frame of the Table are cut by the Index, and thofe will be the Quantity of the Angle E K G fought **Fig 1.**

You muft proceed in the fame manner for finding the Quantity of an Angle by the Plain-Table as a Semi-circle, only put the Semi-circle fide of the Frame upwards, and move the Index upon the other Center-hole

III *How to obferve the Quantity of an Angle by the Circumferentor.*

If it be required to find the Quantity of the former Angle E K G by the Circumferentor, First, place your Inftrument (as before) at K, with the *Flower-de-luce* in the Card towards you Then direct your Sights to E, and obferve what Degrees are cut by the South-End of the Needle, which let be 296, then turning the Inftrument about (the *Flower-de-luce* always towards you) direct the Sights to G, noting then alfo, what Degrees are cut by the South-End of the Needle, which fuppofe 182 This done (always) fubftract the leffer from the greater, as in this Example 182 from 296, and the remainder is 114 Degrees, which is the true Quantity of the Angle E K G **Fig 2.**

Again, The Inftrument ftanding at K, and the Sights being directed to E, as before, fuppofe the South-End of the Needle had cut 79 Degrees, and then directing the Sights to G, the fame end of the Needle had cut 325 Degrees Now, if from 325 you fubftract 79, the remainder is 246 But becaufe this remainder 246 is greater than 180, you muft therefore fubftract 246 from 360, and there will remain 114, the true Quantity of the Angle fought

This adding and fubftracting for finding of Angles may feem tedious to fome. But here note, that for quick difpatch the Circumferentor is as good an Inftrument as any, for in going round a Field, or in furveying a whole Mannor, you are not to take notice of the Quantity of any Angle, but only to obferve what Degrees the Needle cuts: as hereafter will be manifeft

USE II *How by the Plain-Table, to take the Plot of a Field at one Station within the fame, from whence all the Angles of the fame Field may be feen*

Having enter'd upon the Field to furvey, your firft work muft be to fet up fome vifible Mark at each Angle thereof, which being done, make choice of fome convenient Place about the middle of the Field, from whence all the Marks may be feen, and there place your Table covered with a Sheet of Paper, with the Needle hanging directly over the Meridian Line of the Card, (which you muft always have regard to, efpecially when you are to furvey many Fields together) Then make a Mark about the middle of the Paper, to reprefent that part of the Field where the Table ftands, and laying the Index upon this Point, direct your Sights to the feveral Angles where you before placed Marks, and draw Lines by the fide of the Index upon the Paper Then meafure the diftance of every of thefe Marks from your Table, and by your Scale fet the fame diftances upon the Lines drawn upon the Table, making fmall Marks with your Protracting-Pin, or Compafs-Point, at the end of every of them. Then Lines being drawn from the one to the other of thefe Points, will give you the exact Plot of the Field, all the Lines and Angles upon the Table being proportional to thofe of the Field **Fig 2**

Example, Suppofe the Plot of the Field A B C D E F was to be taken. Having placed Marks in the feveral Angles thereof, make choice of fome proper Place about the middle of the Field, as at L, from whence you may behold all the Marks before placed in the feveral Angles, and there place your Table. Then turn your Inftrument about, till the Needle hang over the Meridian Line of the Card, denoted by the Line N S

Your Table being thus placed with a Sheet of Paper thereon, make a Mark about the middle of your Table, which fhall reprefent the Place where your Table ftands Then, applying your Index to this Point, direct the Sights to the firft Mark at A, and the Index refting there, draw a Line by the fide thereof to the Point L. Then with your Chain meafure the diftance from L, the Place where your Table ftands, to A, the firft Mark, which fuppofe 8 Chains, 10 Links Then take 8 Chains 10 Links from any Scale, and fet that diftance upon the Line from L to A

Then directing the Sights to B, draw a Line by the fide of the Index, as before, and meafure the diftance from your Table at L, to the Mark at B, which fuppofe 8 Chains 75

L l   Links.

Links This diftance taken from your Scale, and apply'd to your Table from L to C, will give the Point C, reprefenting the third Mark

Then direct the Sights to the third Mark C, and draw a Line by the fide of the Index, meafuring the diftance from L to C, which fuppofe 10 Chains 65 Links This diftance being taken from your Scale, and apply'd to your Table from L to C, will give you the Point C, reprefenting the third Mark

In this manner you muft deal with the reft of the Marks at D, E, and F, and more, if the Field had confifted of more Sides and Angles

Laftly, When you have made Obfervations of all the Marks round the Field, and found the Points A B C D E and F upon your Table, you muft draw Lines from one Point to another, till you conclude where you firft begun As, draw a Line from A to B, from B to C, from C to D, from D to E, from E to F, and from F to A, where you begun, then will A B C D E F, be the exact Figure of your Field, and the Line N S the Meridian

Note, Our Chains are commonly 4 Poles in Length, and are divided into one hundred equal Parts, called Links, at every tenth of which are Brafs Diftinctions numbering them

U S E III *To take the Plot of a Wood, Park, or other large Champain Plain, by the Plain-Table, in meafuring round about the fame*

Suppofe A B C D E F G to be a large Wood, whofe Plot you defire to take upon the Plain-Table

Fig. 3

I Having put a Sheet of Paper upon the Table, place your Inftrument at the Angle A, and direct your Sights to the next Angle at B, and by the fide thereof draw a Line upon your Table, as the Line A B Then meafure by the Hedge-fide from the Angle A to the Angle B, which fuppofe 12 Chains 5 Links Then from your Scale take 12 Chains 5 Links, and lay off upon your Table from A to B Then turn the Index about, and direct the Sights to G, and draw the Line A G upon the Table But at prefent you need not meafure the diftance

II Remove your Inftrument fiom A, and fet up a Mark where it laft ftood, and place your Inftrument at the fecond Angle B Then laying the Index upon the Line A B, turn the whole Inftrument about, till thro the Sights you fee the Mark fet up at A, and there fcrew the Inftrument Then laying the Index upon the Point B, direct your Sights to the Angle C, and draw the Line B C upon your Table Then meafuring the diftance B C 4 Chains 45 Links, take that diftance from your Scale, and fet it upon your Table from B to C

III Remove your Inftrument from B, and fet up a Mark in the room of it, and place your Inftrument at C, laying the Index upon the Line C B, and turn the whole Inftrument about, till thro the Sights you efpy the Mark fet up at B, and there faften the Inftrument Then laying the Index on the Point C, direct the Sights to D, and draw upon the Table the Line C D Then meafure from C to D 8 Chains 85 Links, and fet that diftance upon your Table from C to D

IV. Remove the Inftrument to D, (placing a Mark at C, where it laft ftood) and lay the Index upon the Line D C, turning the whole Inftrument about, till thro the Sights you fee the Mark at C, and there faften the Inftrument Then lay the Index on the Point D, and direct the Sights to E, and draw the Line D E Then with your Chain meafure the diftance D E 13 Chains 4 Links, which lay off on the Table from D to E

V Remove your Inftrument to E, (placing a Mark at D, where it laft ftood) and laying the Index upon the Line D E, turn the whole Inftrument about, till thro the Sights you fee the Mark at D, and there faften the Inftrument Then lay the Index on the Point E, and direct the Sights to F, and draw the Line E F Then meafure the diftance E F 7 Chains 70 Links, which take from your Scale, and lay off from E to F

VI Remove your Inftrument to F, placing a Mark at E, (where it laft ftood) and lay the Index upon the Line E F, turning the Inftrument about, till you fee the Mark fet up at E, and there faften the Inftrument. Then laying the Index on the Point F, direct the Sights to G, and draw the Line F G upon the Table, which Line F G will cut the Line A G in the Point G Then meafure the diftance F G 5 Chains 67 Links, and lay it off from F to G.

VII Remove your Inftrument to G, (fetting a Mark where it laft ftood) and lay the Index upon the Line F G, turning the whole Inftrument about, till thro the Sights you fee the Mark at F, and there faften the Inftrument Then laying the Index upon the Point G, direct the Sights to A, (your firft Mark) and draw the Line G A, which, if you have truly wrought, will pafs directly thro the Point A, where you firft began

In this manner may you take the Plot of any Champain Plain, be it never fo large And here note, that very often Hedges are of fuch a thicknefs, that you cannot come near the Sides or Angles of the Field, either to place your Inftrument, or meafure the Lines Therefore in fuch Cafes you muft place your Inftrument, and meafure your Lines parallel to the Side thereof, and then your Work will be the fame as if you meafured the Hedge itfelf

NOTE

N O T E alſo, That in thus going about a Field, you may much help your ſelf by the Needle   For looking what Degree of the Card the Needle cuts at one Station, if you remove your Inſtrument to the next Station, and with your Sights look to the Mark where the Inſtrument laſt ſtood, you will find the Needle to cut the ſame Degree again, which will give you no ſmall Satisfaction in the proſecution of your Work   And tho there be a hundred or more Sides, the Needle will ſtill cut the ſame Degree at all of them, except you have committed ſome former Error   therefore at every Station have an Eye to the Needle.

Of Shifting of Paper

In taking the Plot of a Field by the Plain-Table, and going about the ſame, as before di- Fig 4. rected, it may ſo fall out, if the Field be very large, and when you are to take many Incloſures together, that the Sheet of Paper upon the Table will not hold all the Work   But you muſt be forced to take off that Sheet, and put another clean Sheet in the room thereof and, in Plotting of a Manner or Lordſhip, many Sheets may be thus changed, which we call Shifting of Paper   The Manner of performing thereof is as follows

Suppoſe in going about to take the Plot A B C D E F G, as before directed, that you having made choice of the Angle at A for the Place of the beginning, and proceeded from thence to B, and from B to C, and from C to D, when you come to the Angle at D, and are to draw D E, you want room to draw the ſame upon the Table   Do thus.

Firſt, thro the Point D draw the Line D O, which is almoſt ſo much of the Line D E, as the Table will contain   Then near the edge of the Table H M, draw a Line parallel to H M, by means of the Inches and Subdiviſions on the oppoſite ſides of the Frame, as P Q, and another Line at Right Angles to that thro the Point O, as O N   This being done, mark this Sheet of Paper with the Figure (1) about the middle thereof, for the firſt Sheet Then taking this Sheet off your Table, put another clean Sheet thereon, and draw upon it Fig 5. a Line parallel to the contrary edge of the Table, as the Line R S   Then taking your firſt Sheet of Paper, lay it upon the Table ſo, that the Line P Q may exactly lie upon the Line R S, to the beſt advantage, as at the Point O (*Fig 5*)   Then with the Point of your Compaſſes draw ſo much of the Line O D upon the clean Sheet of Paper as the Table will hold   Having thus done, proceed with your Work upon the new Sheet, beginning at the Point O ; and ſo going forward with your Work, as in all Reſpects has before been directed , as from O to E, from E to F, from F to G, and from G to A, (by this direction) ſhifting your Paper as often as you have occaſion.

U S E IV   *How to take the Plot of any Wood, Park, &c. by going about the ſame, and making Obſervations at every Angle thereof, by the Circumferentor*

Suppoſe A B C D E F G H K is a large Field, or other Incloſure, to be Plotted by Fig.6. the Circumferentor

1   Placing your Inſtrument at A, (the *Flower-de-luce* being towards you) direct the Sights to B, the South-end of the Needle cutting 191 Degrees, and the Ditch, Wall, or Hedge, containing 10 Chains 75 Links   The Degrees cut, and the Line meaſured, muſt be noted down in your Field-Book.

2   Place your Inſtrument at B, and direct the Sights to C, the South-end of the Needle cutting 279 Degrees, and the Line B C containing 6 Chains 83 Links , which note down in your Field-Book

3   Place the Inſtrument at C, and direct the Sights to D, the Needle cutting 216 Deg 30 Min   and the Line C D containing 7 Chains 82 Links

4   Place the Inſtrument at D, and direct the Sights to E, the Needle cutting 327 Degrees, and the Line D F containing 9 Chains 96 Links

5   Place the Inſtrument at E, and direct the Sights to F, the Needle cutting 12 Deg 30 Min   and the Line F E 9 Chains 71 Links

6   Place the Inſtrument at F, and direct the Sights to G, the Needle cutting 342 Deg 30 Min   and the Line F G being 7 Chains 54 Links

7   Place the Inſtrument at G, and direct the Sights to H, the Needle cutting 98 Deg 30 Min   and the Line G H containing 7 Chains 52 Links

8   Place the Inſtrument at H, and direct the Sights to K, the Needle cutting 71 Deg and the Line H K containing 7 Chains 78 Links.

9   Place the Inſtrument at K, and direct the Sights to A, (where you began) the Needle cutting 161 Deg 30 Min   and the Line K A containing 8 Chains 22 Links.

Having gone round the Field in this manner, and collected the Degrees cut, and the Lines meaſured, in the Field-Book, you will find them to ſtand as follows, by which you may protract and draw your Field, as preſently I ſhall ſhew.

Degrees

	Degrees.	Minutes	Chains	Links
A	191	00	10	75
B	297	00	6	83
C	216	30	7	82
D	325	00	6	96
E	12	30	9	71
F	324	30	7	54
G	98	30	7	54
H	71	00	7	78
K	161	30	8	22

In going about a Field in this manner, you may perceive a wonderful quick Diſpatch; for you are only to take notice of the Degrees cut once at every Angle, and not to uſe any Back-Sights, that is, to look thro the Sights to the Station you laſt went from   But to uſe Back-Sights with the Circumferentor, is beſt to confirm your Work · For when you ſtand at any Angle of a Field, and direct your Sights to the next, and obſerve what Degrees the South-end of the Needle cuts; if you remove your Inſtrument from this Angle to the next, and look to the Mark or Angle where it laſt ſtood, the Needle will there alſo cut the ſame Degrees as before

So the Inſtrument being placed at A, if you direct the Sights to B, you will find the Needle to cut 191 Degrees, then removing your Inſtrument to B, if you direct the Sights to A, the Needle will then alſo cut 191 Degrees

Notwithſtanding the quick Diſpatch this Inſtrument makes, one half of the Work will almoſt be ſaved, if, inſtead of placing the Inſtrument at every Angle, you place it but at every other Angle   An Inſtance of which take in the aforegoing Example

1 Placing the Inſtrument at A, and directing the Sights to B, you find the Needle to cut 191 Degrees   Then,

2 Placing the Inſtrument at B, directing the Sights to C, you find the Needle to cut 279 Degrees   And,

3 Placing the Inſtrument at C, and directing the Sights to D, you find the Needle to cut 216 Degrees

Now, having placed your Inſtrument at A, and noted down the Degrees cut by the Needle, which was 191, you need not go to the Angle B at all, but go next to the Angle C, and there place your Inſtrument, and directing your Sights backwards to B, you will find the Needle to cut 279 Degrees, which are the ſame as were before cut when the Inſtrument was placed at B ſo that the Labour of placing the Inſtrument at B is wholly ſaved. Then (the Inſtrument ſtill ſtanding at C) direct the Sights to D, and the Needle will cut 216 Degrees, as before, which note in your Feld-Book. This done, remove your Inſtrument to E, and obſerve according to the laſt directions, and you will find the Work to be the ſame as before   Then remove the Inſtrument from E to G, from G to K, and ſo to every ſecond Angle

I now proceed, to ſhew the Manner of Protracting the former Obſervations.

Fig 7.
According to the largeneſs of your Plot provide a Sheet of Paper, as L M N O, upon which draw the Line L M, and parallel thereto draw divers other Lines quite thro the whole Paper, as the pricked Lines, in the Figure, drawn between L M and N O   Theſe Parallels thus drawn, repreſent Meridians   Upon one or other of theſe Lines, or parallel to one of them, muſt the Diameter of your Protractor be always laid

1 Your Paper being thus prepar'd, aſſign any Point upon any of the Meridians, as A, upon which place the Center of the Protractor, laying the Diameter thereof upon the Meridian Line drawn upon the Paper.   Then look in your Field-Book what Degrees the Needle cuts at A, which was 191 Degrees   Now, becauſe the Degrees were above 180, you muſt therefore lay the Semi-circle of the Protractor downwards, and keeping it there, make a Mark with the Protracting-Pin againſt 191 Degrees, thro which Point, from A, draw the Line A B, containing 10 Chains 75 Links

2 Lay the Center of the Protractor on the Point B, with the Diameter in the ſame Poſition as before directed, (which always obſerve) And becauſe the Degrees cut at B were more than 180, viz. 279, therefore the Semi-circle of the Protractor muſt lie downwards, and ſo holding it, make a Mark againſt the 279 Degrees, and thro it draw the Line B C, containing 6 Chains 83 Links

3. Place the Center of the Protractor on the Point C. Then the Degrees cut by the Needle at the Obſervation in C, being above 180, namely, 216 Degrees 30 Minutes, the Semi-circle of the Protractor muſt lie downwards   Then making a Mark againſt 216 Deg 30 Min thro it draw the Line C D, containing 7 Chains 82 Links

4 Lay the Center of the Protractor upon the Point D, the Degrees cut by the Needle at that Angle being 325 which being above 180, lay the Semi-circle downward, and againſt 325 Degrees make a Mark, thro which Point, and the Angle D, draw the Line D E, containing 6 Chains 96 Links.

5 Remove

5 Remove your Protractor to E   And becaufe the Degrees cut by the Needle at this Angle were lefs than 180, namely, 12 Degrees 30 Min therefore lay the Semi-circle of the Protractor upwards, and make a Mark againft 12 Degrees 30 Minutes, thro' which draw the Line E F, containing 9 Chains 71 Links

6 Lay the Center of the Protractor upon the Point F; and becaufe the Degrees to be protracted are above 180, viz 342 Degrees 30 Minutes, lay the Semi-circle of the Protractor downwards, and make a Mark againft 342 Degrees 30 Minutes, drawing the Line F G, containing 7 Chains 54 Links

And in this Manner muft you protract all the other Angles, G, H, and K, and more, if the Field had confifted of more Angles.

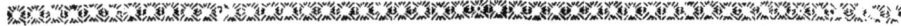

CHAP. III.

Of the Conftruction and Ufe of the Surveying-Wheel.

THIS Inftrument confifts of a wooden Wheel, fhoe'd with Iron, to prevent its wear- Fig 8. ing, exactly two Feet feven Inches and a half in Diameter, that fo its Circumference may be eight Feet three Inches, or half a Pole

At the end of the Axle-tree of this Wheel, on the Left fide thereof, is, at Right Angles to the Axle-tree, a little Star, about three fourths of an Inch Diameter, having eight Teeth   Now the Ufe of this Star is fuch, that when the Wheel moves round, the faid Star's Teeth, by falling at Right Angles into the Teeth of another Star of eight Teeth, fixed at one end of an Iron Rod (Q) caufes the Iron Rod to move once round in the fame time the Wheel hath moved once round   Therefore every time you have drove the Wheel half a Pole, the Iron Rod goes once round

This Iron Rod, lying along a Groove in the fide of the Body of the Inftrument, hath on the other end a fquare hole, in which goes the fquare end *b* of the little Cylinder P   This Cylinder is faftened underneath the upper Plate H, of a Movement, covered with a Glafs, placed in the Body of the Inftrument at B, yet fo, that Fig. 9. it may be moveable about its Axis, having the end *a* cut into a fingle threaded perpetual Screw, which falling into the Teeth of the Wheel A, being thirty two in Number, when you drive the Inftrument forwards, caufes the Wheel A to go once round at the end of each 16th Pole   The Pinion B hath fix Teeth, which falling into the Teeth of the Wheel C, whofe Number is fixty, caufes that to move once round at the end of each 160th Pole, or half Mile   This Wheel carries round a Hand, once in 160 Poles, over the Divifions of an Annular Plate, fixed upon the Plate H, whofe outmoft Limb is divided into 160 equal Parts, each tenth of which is numbered, and fhews how many Poles the Inftrument is drove

Again, the Pinion D, which is fixed to the fame Arbre as the Wheel C is, hath twenty Teeth, which by their falling into the Teeth of the Wheel E, which hath forty Teeth, caufes the faid Wheel E to go round once in 320 Poles, or one Mile, and the Pinion F, of twelve Teeth, falling into the Teeth of the Wheel G, whofe Number is 72, caufes the Wheel G to go once round in 12 Miles   This Wheel G carries another lefser Hand once round in 12 Miles, over the Divifions of the innermoft Limb of the aforefaid Annular Plate, which is divided into twelve equal Parts for Miles, and each Mile fubdivided into halves and quarters, (that is, into eight equal Parts, for Furlongs) with Roman Characters numbering the Miles

The Ufe of this Inftrument is fuch, that by driving the Wheel before you, the Number of Miles, Poles, or both, you have gone, is eafily fhewn by the two Hands   And fo this Inftrument, together with a Theodolite or Circumferentor, for taking of Bearings, is of excellent Ufe in Plotting of Roads, Rivers, &c   For having placed your Wheel and Circumferentor at the beginning of the Road you defign to plot, which call your firft Station, caufe fome Perfon to go as far along the Road as you find it ftraight, and then take a Bearing to him, which fet down.   This being done, drive the Wheel before you to the Place where the Man ftands, which call the fecond Station, and note, by the Hands of the Dial-Plate, the diftance from the firft Station to the fecond, which fet down   Again, having placed your Circumferentor at the fecond Station, caufe the Man to go along the Road till he comes to another Bend therein   And from the fecond Station take a Bearing to the Man at the third, which fet down.   Then drive the Wheel from the fecond Station to the third, and note the diftance, which fet down   And in this Manner proceed till you come to your Journey's end   Then in Plotting the Road, you muft obferve the fame Directions, as are given in Plotting the Example of Ufe IV of the laft Chapter.

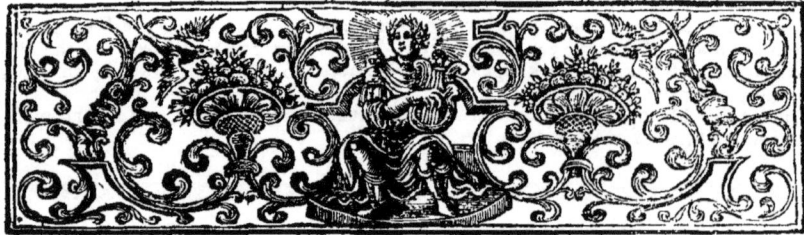

BOOK V.

Of the Conſtruction and Uſes of Levels, for conducting of Water; as alſo of Inſtruments for Gunnery.

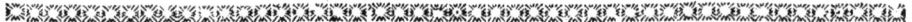

C H A P. I.

Of the Conſtruction and Uſes of different Levels.

Conſtruction of a Watu Level

Plate 15
Fig A

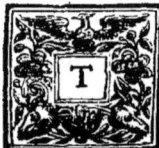

THE firſt of theſe Inſtruments is a Water Level, compoſed of a round Tube of Braſs, or other ſolid Mattei, about 3 Feet long, and 12 or 15 Lines Diameter, whoſe ends are turned up at Right Angles, for receiving two Glaſs Tubes, 3 or 4 Inches long, faſtened on them with Wax or Maſtick At the middle and underneath this Tube, is fixed a Ferril, for placing it upon its Foot.

There is as much common or coloured Water poured into one end of it, as that it may appear in the Glaſs Tubes

This Level, altho very ſimple, is very commodious for Levelling ſmall Diſtances.

It is founded upon this, that Water always naturally places itſelf level, and therefore the height of the Water in the two Glaſs Tubes will be always the ſame, in reſpect to the Center of the Earth

Fig. B.

The Air Level B, is a very ſtraight Glaſs Tube, every where of the ſame thickneſs, of an indetermined Length, and Thickneſs in proportion, being filled to a drop with Spirit of Wine, or other Liquor, not ſubject to freeze. The ends of the Tube are hermetically ſealed, that is, the end through which the Spirit of Wine is poured muſt afterwards be cloſed, by heating it with the Flame of a Lamp, blown thro a little Braſs Tube, to make the heat the greater, and then when the Glaſs is become ſoft, the end muſt be cloſed up

When this Inſtrument is perfectly Level, the Bubble of Air will fix itſelf juſt in the middle, and when it is not Level, the Bubble of Air will riſe to the top

Conſtruction of an Air Level

Fig. C.

This Inſtrument is compoſed of an Air Level 1, about 8 Inches long, and 7 or 8 Lines in Diameter, ſet in a Braſs Tube 2; which is left open in the middle for ſeeing the Bubble of Air at the top

It is carried upon a very ſtrong ſtraight Rule, about a Foot long, at the ends of which are placed two Sights exactly of the ſame height, and like that of Number 3, which has a ſquare hole therein, having two Filets of Braſs very finely filed, croſſing one another at Right Angles, in the middle of which Filets is drilled a little hole There is faſten'd a little thin Piece of Braſs to this Sight, with a ſmall Headed-Rivet, to ſtop the ſaid Square opening,
when

Plate XIV

fronting page 174

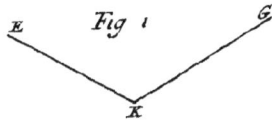

Fig 1

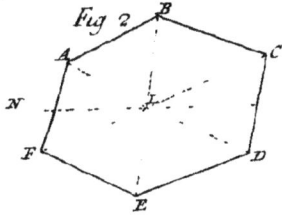

Fig 2

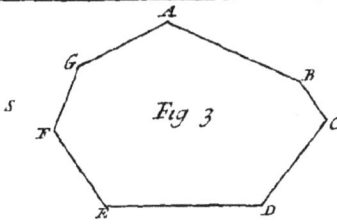

Fig 3

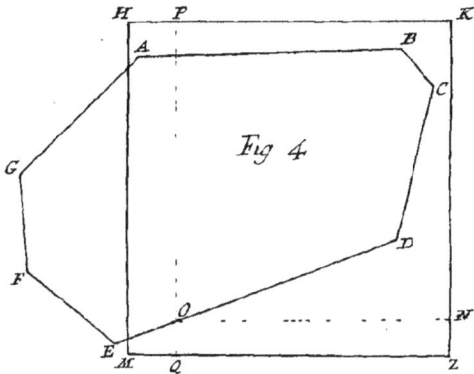

Fig 4

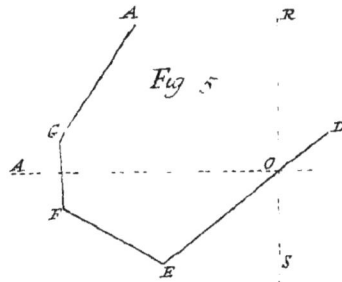

Fig 5

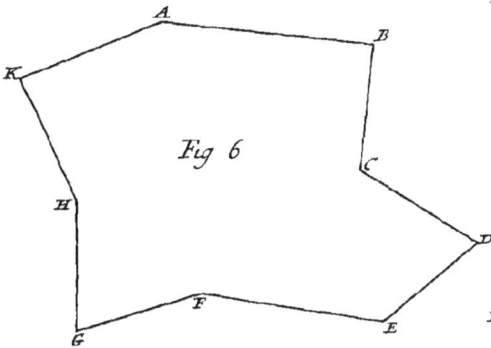

Fig 6

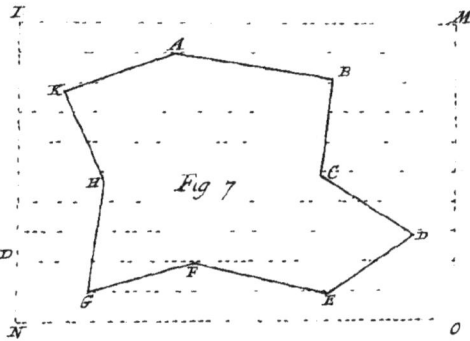

Fig 7

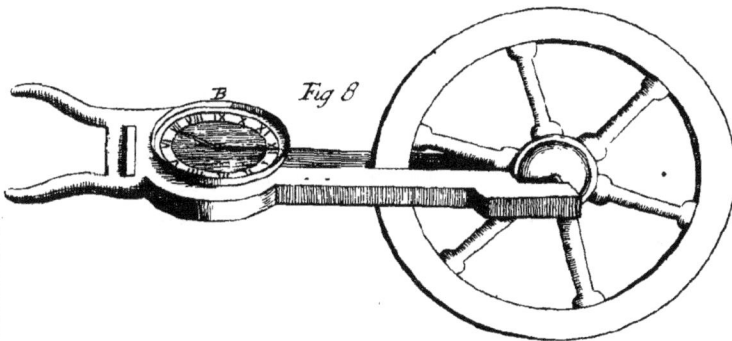

Fig 8

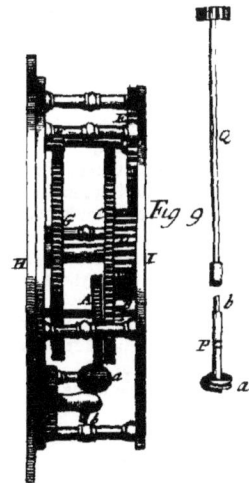

Fig 9

I Senex Sculp.

when there is occasion, and having a little hole drilled thro it, answering to that which is in the middle of the Filets The Brass Tube is fastened upon the Rule, by means of two Screws, one of which marked 4, serves to raise or depress the Tube at pleasure, for placing it level, and making it agree with the Sights

The top of the Ball and Socket is riveted to a little Rule, that springs, one of whose ends is fastened with two Screws to the great Rule, and at the other end there is a Screw 5, serving to raise or depress the whole Instrument when it is nearly level

The Manner of adjusting this Level is easy, for you need but place it upon its Foot, so that the Bubble of Air may be exactly in the middle of the Tube, then shutting the Sight next to the Eye, and opening the other, the Point of the Object which is cut by the horizontal Filet is level with the Eye, and to know whether the Air Level agrees well with the Sights, you must turn the Instrument quite about, and shut the Sight which before was opened, and open the other Then looking through the little hole, if the same Point of the Object before observed be cut by the horizontal Filet, it is a sign the Level is just, but if there be found any difference, the Tube must be raised or depressed by means of the Screw 4, till the Sights agree with the Level, that is, that looking at an Object, the Bubble of Air being in the middle, and afterwards turning the Instrument about, the same Object may be seen

The Level D is a little Glass Tube inclosed within a Brass Tube, fastened upon a Rule Fig D perfectly equal in thickness, and serves to know whether a Plane be level, or not

Construction of a Telescope Air Level

This Level is like the Level C, but instead of Sights, it carries a Telescope to discover Fig E Objects at a good distance This Telescope is in a little Brass Tube, about 15 Inches long, fastened upon the same Rule as the Level, which ought to be of a good thickness, and very straight

At the end of the Tube of the Telescope, marked 1, enters the little Tube 1, carrying the Eye Glass, and a human Hair horizontally placed in the Focus of the Object Glass 2 This little Tube may be drawn out or pushed into the great one, for adjusting the Telescope to different Sights

At the other end of the Telescope is placed the Object Glass, whose Construction is the same as that before mentioned, belonging to the Semi-circle

The whole Body of the Telescope is fastened to the Rule, as well as the Level, with Screws, upon two little square Plates, soldered towards the ends of each Tube, which ought to be perfectly equal in thickness

The Screw 3, is for raising or lowering, the little Fork carrying the human Hair, and making it agree with the Bubble of Air, when the Instrument is level, and the Screw 4, is for making the Bubble of Air agree with the Telescope

Underneath the Rule there is a Brass Plate with Springs, having a Ball and Socket fastned thereto

The Level F, is in form of a Square, having its two Branches of equal length, at the Fig F. junction of which there is made a little hole, from which hangs a Thread and Plummet, playing upon a Perpendicular Line, in the middle of the Quadrant, often divided into 90 Degrees Its Use is very easy, for the ends of the Branches being placed upon a Plane, we may know that the Plane is level when the Thread plays upon the Perpendicular in the middle of the Quadrant

Construction of a Telescope Plumb-Level

This Instrument is composed of two Branches, joined together at Right Angles, whereof Fig G. *that* carrying the Thread and Plummet, is about a Foot and a half, or two Foot long

This Thread is hung towards the top of the Branch, at the Point 2 The middle of the Branch, where the Thread passes, is hollow, that so it may not touch in any Place but towards the bottom, at the Place 3, where there is a little Blade of Silver, on which is drawn a Line perpendicular to the Telescope

The said Cavity is covered by two Pieces of Brass, making as it were a kind of Case, lest the Wind should agitate the Thread, for which reason there is also a Glass covering the Silver Blade, to the end that we may see when the Thread and Plummet play upon the Perpendicular The Telescope 1, is fastened to the other Branch, which is about two Feet long, and is made like the other Telescopes of which we have already spoken All the Exactness of this Instrument consists in having the Telescope at Right Angles with the Perpendicular

This Instrument has a Ball and Socket fastened behind the aforesaid Branch, for placing it upon its Foot

There are some of these sort of Levels made of Brass or Iron, whose Telescope and the Cavity, in which is included the Thread carrying the Plummet, is about 4 or 5 Feet long, in order to level great Distances at once

The Telescope is about 1 Inch and a half Diameter, and the Case in which the Thread, carrying the Plummet, is inclosed, is about 2 Inches wide, and half an Inch thick This Case is fastened with

with Screws in the middle, to the Teleſcope, ſo that they may be at Right Angles with one another And at the two ends of the Teleſcopes are adjuſted two broad Circles, in which the Teleſcope exactly turns, which Circles, being flat underneath, are faſtened to a ſtrong Iron Rule

This Level is ſupported by two Feet almoſt like that of Figure E, *Plate* 12, faſtened with Screws to the Extremities of the Iron Rule Alſo there are two Openings, covered with Glaſſes, incloſed in little Braſs Frames, which open, that ſo the Thread and Plummet may be hung to the top of the Caſe, and play upon two little Silver Blades, in a Line drawn on them perpendicular to the Teleſcope Theſe Blades are placed againſt the Openings of the Caſe, and the Teleſcope is like that before ſpoken of, in ſpeaking of the Semi-circle

All the Exactneſs of this Inſtrument conſiſts in having the Teleſcope at Right Angles to the Perpendiculars drawn upon the Silver Blades.

To prove this Level, you muſt place it upon its Foot, in ſuch manner that the Thread may exactly play upon the Perpendicular, and note ſome Object cut by the Hair in the Focus of the Teleſcope Then taking off the Thread and Plummet, turn the inſtrument upſide down, and hanging the Thread and Plummet to the Hook at the bottom of the Caſe, which will now be uppermoſt, look thro the Teleſcope at the aforeſaid Object, and if the Thread exactly plays upon the Perpendicular, it is a ſign the Inſtrument is exact, but if it does not, you muſt remove the little Hook to the Right-hand or Left, till you make the Thread fall upon the Perpendicular, both before you have turned the Inſtrument upſide down, and afterwards You may likewiſe raiſe or lower the Teleſcope, by means of a Screw *Note,* Ingenious Workmen may eaſily ſupply what I have omitted in this brief Deſcription.

Fig H The Inſtrument H is a little ſimple Level, founded on the ſame Principle as the three precedent ones, the Figure thereof is ſufficient to ſhew its Conſtruction and Uſe

Fig I The Level I places itſelf, and is compoſed of a pretty thick Braſs Rule, about one Foot long, and an Inch broad, having two Sights of the ſame height placed at the ends of the Rule, and in the middle there is a kind of Beam (almoſt like thoſe of common Scales) for freely ſuſpending the Level.

At the bottom of the ſaid Rule is ſcrew'd on a Piece of Braſs, likewiſe carrying a pretty heavy Ball of Braſs All the Exactneſs of this Inſtrument conſiſts in a perfect *Equilibrium*, to know which, it is eaſy for holding the Inſtrument ſuſpended by its Ring, and having eſpied ſome Object thro the Sights, you need but turn the Inſtrument about, and obſerve whether the aforeſaid Object appears of the ſame height thro the Sights, and if it does, the Inſtrument is perfectly *in equilibrio* but if the Object appears a little higher or lower, you may remedy it by removing the Piece of Braſs carrying the Ball till it be exactly n the middle of the Point of Suſpenſion, and then it muſt be fixed with a Screw, becauſe, by experience, the Inſtrument was found to be level

Conſtruction of a Level of Mr Hugens's

Fig K. The principal part of this Inſtrument, is a Teleſcope *a*, 15 or 18 Inches long, being in form of a Cylinder, and going thro a Ferril, in which it is faſtened by the middle. This Ferril has two flat Branches *b b*, one above and the other below, each about a fourth part of the Teleſcope in length At the ends of each of theſe two Branches are faſtened little moving Pieces, which carry two Rings, by one of which the Teleſcope is ſuſpended to a Hook, at the end of the Screw 3, and by the other a pretty heavy Weight is ſuſpended, in order to keep the Teleſcope *in equilibrio* This Weight hangs in the Box 5, which is almoſt filled with Linſeed Oil, Oil of Wallnuts, or any thing elſe that will not coagulate, for more aptly ſettling the Ballances of the Weight and Teleſcope

This Inſtrument carries ſometimes two Teleſcopes cloſe and very parallel to each other, the Eye Glaſs of one being on one ſide, and the Eye Glaſs of the other on the oppoſite ſide, that ſo one may ſee on both ſides, without turning the Level If the Tube of the Teleſcope being ſuſpended, be not found level, as it will often happen, put a Ferril or Ring 4 upon it, which may be ſlid along the Tube, for placing it level, and keeping it ſo And this muſt be, if there be two Teleſcopes

There is a human Hair horizontally ſtrained and faſtened to a little Fork in the Focus of the Object Glaſs of each Teleſcope, which may be raiſed or lower'd, by means of a little Screw, as has been already mentioned

For proving this Level, having ſuſpended it by one of the Branches, obſerve ſome diſtant Object through the Teleſcope, with the Weight not hung on, and very exactly mark the Point of the Object cut by the Hair of the Teleſcope Now hanging the Weight on, if the horizontal Hair anſwers to the ſame Point of the ſaid Object, it is a ſign the Center of Gravity of the Teleſcope and Weight, is preciſely in a Right Line joining the two Points of Suſpenſion, which continued would paſs thro' the Center of the Earth.

But if it otherwiſe happens, you muſt remedy it, by ſliding the little Ring backwards or forwards Having thus adjuſted the Teleſcope, that the ſame Point of an Object be ſeen, as well before the Weight is hung on, as afterwards, you muſt turn it upſide down, by ſuſpending it to the Branch that was lowermoſt, and hanging the Weight upon the other Then if the Hair in the Teleſcope cuts the aforeſaid Point of the Object, it is manifeſt, that that

Point

Point of the Object is in the horizontal Plane, with the Center of the Tube of the Telefcope. but if the Hair does not cut that Point of the Object, it must be raifed or lowered
by means of the Screw till it does   *Note*, You muft every now and then prove this Inftrument, for fear leaft fome Alteration has happen'd thereto

The Hook on which this Inftrument is hung, is fixed to a flat wooden Crofs, at the Ends
of each Arm of which, there is a Hook ferving to keep the Telefcope from too much Agitation, when the Inftrument is ufing, and for keeping it fteady when it is carrying, in lowering the Telefcope by means of the Screw 3, which carries it

There is applied to the faid flat Crofs, another hollowed Crofs faftened with Hooks, which
ferves as a Cafe for the Inftrument.   But note, the two Ends of the Crofs are left open, that
fo the Telefcope being covered from Wind and Rain, may be always in a Condition to ufe.

The Foot fupporting the Inftrument, is a round Brafs Plate fomething concave, to which
is faftened three Brafs Ferrils, moveable by means of Joints, wherein are Staves of a convenient Length put   The Box at the Bottom of the Level is placed upon this Plate, and may
be any ways turned, fo that the Weight, which ought to be Brafs, may have a free Motion
in the Box, which muft be fhut by means of a Screw, that fo the Oil may be preferved in
Journeys.

Conftruction of another Level.

This Inftrument is a Level almoft like that whofe Defcription we have laft given, but it is Fig. L.
eafier to carry from place to place

Number 1 Is the Cafe in which the Telefcope is enclofed

2 Is a kind of Stirrup, where the Screw, ferving for the Point of Sufpenfion, paffes, at
the End of which is a Hook, upon which the Ring, at the End of the Plate carrying the
Telefcope, is hung

3 Are the Screws above and below for fixing the Telefcope, when the Inftrument is carrying

4 Are the Hooks for keeping the Cafe fhut.

5 Is one End of the Telefcope

6 Is the End of the Plate whereon a great Brafs Ball is hung, ferving to keep the Telefcope level

There are three Ferrils 8, well fixed to the Bottom of the Stirrup, ferving as a Foot to
fupport the whole Inftrument   *Note*, There are fometimes put two Telefcopes on this Level, as well as in that other of which we have laft fpoken.

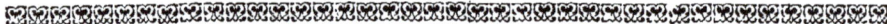

C H A P. II.

Of the Ufes of the aforefaid Inftruments in Levelling.

LEvelling is an Operation fhowing the Height of one Place in refpect to another   One
Place is faid to be higher than another, when it is more diftant from the Center of the
Earth   A Line equally diftant from the Center of the Earth, in all its Points, is called the
Line of true Level, whence, becaufe the Earth is round, that Line muft be a Curve, and
make a part of the Earth's Circumference, as the Line B C F G, all the Points of which are Fig. 1.
equally diftant from the Center A of the Earth: but the Line of Sight, which the Operations
of Levels give, is a right Line perpendicular to the Semi-diameter of the Earth A B, raifed
above the true Level, denoted by the Curvature of the Earth, in proportion as it is more extended, for which Reafon, the Operations which we fhall give, are but of the apparent Level, which muft be corrected to have the true Level, when the Line of Sight exceeds 50
Toifes

The following Table, in which are denoted the Corrections of the Points of apparent
Level, for reducing them to the true Level, was calculated by help of the Semi-diameter of
the Earth, whofe Length may be known by meafuring one Degree of its Circumference   The
Gentlemen of the Academy of Sciences, have found by very exact Obfervations, that one De-
gree of the Circumference of a great Circle of the Earth, as the Meridian, contains 57060
Toifes, and giving 25 Leagues to a Degree, a League will be $2282\frac{2}{5}$ Toifes

Now the whole Circumference of the Earth will be 9000 of the fame Leagues, and its
Diameter 2865 of them, from whence all Places on the Superficies of the Earth, will be diftant from its Center $1432\frac{1}{2}$ Leagues

The Line A B reprefents the Semi-diameter of the Earth, under the Feet of the Obferver   The right Line B D E, reprefents the vifual Ray, whofe Points D and E are in the
apparent Level of the Point B   This Line of apparent Level, ferves for determining a Line
of true Level, which is done by taking from the Points of the Line of apparent Level, the
Height they are above the true Level in refpect to a certain Point, as B; for it plainly appears
from the Figure, that all the Points D, E, of the apparent Level, are farther diftant from the

N n   Center

Center of the Earth, than the Point B; and to find the Difference, you need but confider the right-angled Triangle A B D, whose two Sides A B, B D, being known, the Hypothenufe A D, may be found from which fubftracting the Radius A C, the Remainder C D will fhow the Height of the Point D of apparent Level, above the Point of true Level

A T A B L E *fhewing the Corrections of the Points of apparent Level, for reducing them to the true Level, every 50 Toifes.*

Diftances of the Points of apparent Level	Corrections.	
	Inches.	Lines
50 Toifes	0.	0
100	0	1 $\frac{1}{3}$
150	0.	3
200	0	5 $\frac{1}{3}$
250	0.	8 $\frac{1}{3}$
300	1	0
350	1.	4 $\frac{1}{3}$
400	1	9 $\frac{1}{3}$
450	2	3
500	2.	9
550	3.	6
600	4	0
650	4	8
700	5.	4
750	6.	3
800	7	1
850	7	11 $\frac{1}{2}$
900	8.	11
1950	10.	0
000	11.	0

The Rule ferving to calculate this Table, is to divide the Square of the Diftance by the Diameter of the Earth, which is 6,538,694 Toifes, for which Reafon the Corrections are to one another, as the Squares of the Diftances. Altho the Foundation of this Calculation be not ftrictly Geometrical, yet it is nigh enough the Truth for Practice

If the Points of apparent Level fhould be taken inftead of the Points of true Level, a body would err in conducting the Water of a Source, which let be, for Example, at the Point B, for this Source will not run along the Line B D E, but will remain in the Point B, for if it fhould run along the Line B E, it would run higher than it is, which is impoffible, becaufe it cannot be endued with any other Figure but a circular one, equally diftant from the Center of the Earth On the contrary, a Source in D will have a great Defcent down to the Point B, but it cannot run further, becaufe it muft be elevated higher than the Source, if it continues its way in the fame right Line, which cannot be done, unlefs it be forced by fome Machine.

How to rectify Levels.

To rectify Levels, as, for Example, the Air Level, you muft plant two Staffs, as A B, about 50 Toifes diftant from each other, becaufe of the Roundnefs of the Earth; (take care of exceeding that Diftance) then efpying from the Station A, the Point B, the Level being placed horizontally, and the Bubble of Air being in the Middle of the Tube, you muft raife or lower a Piece of Pafteboard upon the Staff B, in the Middle of which is drawn a black horizontal Line, till the vifual Ray of the Obferver's Eye meets the faid Line, after which muft be faftened another Piece of Pafteboard to the Staff A, the Middle of which let be the Height of the Eye, when the Piece of Pafteboard B was feen then removing the Level to the Staff B, place it to the Height of the Center of the Pafteboard, and the Level being horizontally pofited for obferving the Piece of Pafteboard A, if then the vifual Ray cuts the Middle of the Piece of Pafteboard, it is a fign the Level is very juft, but if the vifual Ray falls above or below, as in the Point C, you muft, by always keeping the Eye at the fame Height, lower the Telefcope or the Sight, till the Middle of the vifual Ray falls upon the Middle of the Difference, as in D, and the Telefcope thus remaining, the Tube of the Level muft be adjufted till the Bubble of Air fixes in the Middle, which may be done by means of the Screw 4.

Again, return to the Staff A, and place the Level the Height of the Point D, for looking at the Piece of Pafteboard B, and if the vifual Ray falls upon the Middle of the Piece of Pafteboard, it is a fign the Telefcope agrees with the Level if not, the fame Operations muft be repeated, until the vifual Rays fall upon the Centers of the two Pieces of Pafteboard.

Another way to rectify Levels

Knowing two Points diftant from each other, and perfectly level, place the End of the Telefcope carrying the Eye-Glafs to the exact Height of one of thofe two Points, the Bubble of Air being fixed in the Middle of its Tube, then by looking thro it, if it happens that
the

Fig. 2.

the Hair of the Teleſcope cuts the ſecond Point, it is a ſign the Level is juſt, but if the Hair falls above or below the Point of Level, you muſt, in always keeping the Eye at the ſame height, raiſe or lower the end of the Level where the Object Glaſs is, until the Viſual Ray of the Teleſcope falls upon the exact Point of Level, and leaving it thus, raiſe or depreſs the Tube carrying the Level, ſo that the Bubble of Air may remain in the middle

What we have ſaid concerning the Rectification of this Level, may ſerve likewiſe for the Rectification of others, the difference is only to change the Plummets and the Hairs of the Teleſcopes, according to their Conſtructions

The Manner of Levelling

To find, for Example, the height of the Point A on the top of a Mountain, above the Fig 3. Point B at its foot, place the Level about the middle diſtance between the two Points, as in D, and plant Staffs in A and B Alſo let there be Perſons inſtructed with Signals, for raiſing or lowering upon the ſaid Staffs ſlit Sticks, at the ends of which are faſtened pieces of Paſte-Board · The Level being placed upon its foot, look towards the Staff A E, and cauſe one of the Perſons to raiſe or lower the Paſte-Board, until the upper edge or middle appears in the viſual Ray, then meaſure exactly the perpendicular Height of the Point A above the Point E, which, in this Example, ſuppoſe 6 Feet 4 Inches, which ſet down in a Memorial Then turn the Level horizontally, ſo that it may always be at the ſame height, for the Eye Glaſs of the Teleſcope to be next to the Eye, but if it be a Sight Level, there is no neceſſity of turning it about, and cauſe the Perſon at the Staff B to raiſe or lower the piece of Paſte-Board, until the upper edge of it be ſeen, as at C, which ſuppoſe 16 Feet 6 Inches, which ſet down in the Memorial above the other Number of the firſt Station, whence to know the height of the Point A above the Point B, take 6 Feet 4 Inches from 16 Feet 2 Inches, and the remainder will be 10 Feet 2 Inches, for the heighth of A above B

Note, If the Point D, where the Obſerver is placed, be in the middle between the Point A and the Point B, there is no neceſſity of regarding the height of the apparent Level above the true Level, becauſe thoſe two Points being equally diſtant from the Eye of the Obſerver, the viſual Ray will be equally raiſed above the true Level, and conſequently there needs no Correction to give the height of the Point A above the Point D.

Another Example of Levelling

It is required to know, whether there be a ſufficient Deſcent for conducting of Water Fig 4. from the Source A to the Vaſe B of a Fountain Now becauſe the diſtance from the Point A to B is great, there are ſeveral Operations required to be made Having choſen a proper height for placing the Level, as at the Point I, plant a Pole in the Point A near the Source, on which ſlide up and down another, carrying the piece of Paſte-Board L, meaſure the diſtance from A to I, which ſuppoſe 1000 Toiſes Then the Level being adjuſted in the Point K, let ſomebody move the Paſte-Board L up or down, until you can eſpy it thro the Teleſcope or Sights of the Level, and meaſure the height A L, which ſuppoſe 2 Toiſes, 1 Foot, 5 Inches But becauſe the diſtance A I is 1000 Toiſes, according to the aforementioned Table, you muſt ſubſtract 11 Inches, and the height A L will conſequently be but 2 Toiſes 6 Inches, which note down in the Memorial

Now turn the Level about, ſo that the Object Glaſs of the Teleſcope may be next to the Pole planted in the Point H, and the Level being adjuſted, cauſe ſome Perſon to move the piece of Paſte-Board G up and down, until the upper edge of it may be eſpied thro the Teleſcope, meaſure the height H G, which ſuppoſe 3 Toiſes, 4 Feet, 2 Inches, meaſure likewiſe the Diſtance of the Points I, H, which ſuppoſe 650 Toiſes, for which diſtance, according to the Table, you muſt ſubſtract 4 Inches 8 Lines from the height H G, which conſequently will then be but 3 Toiſes, 3 Feet, 9 Inches, 4 Lines, which ſet down in the Memorial

This being done, remove the Level to ſome other Eminence, from whence the Pole H G may be diſcovered, and the Angle of the Houſe D, the Ground about which is level with the Vaſe B of the Fountain

The Level being adjuſted in the Point E, look at the Staff H, and the viſual Ray will give the Point F, meaſure the height H F, which ſuppoſe 11 Feet 6 Inches, likewiſe meaſure the diſtance H E, which ſuppoſe 500 Toiſes, for which diſtance the Table gives 2 Inches 9 Lines of abatement, which being taken from the height H F, and there will remain 11 Feet, 3 Inches, 3 Lines, which ſet down in the Memorial Laſtly, Having turned the Level for looking at the Angle of the Houſe D, meaſure the height of the Point D, where the Viſual Ray terminates above the Ground, which ſuppoſe 8 Feet 3 Inches Meaſure alſo the diſtance from the Point D, to the ſaid Houſe, which is 450 Toiſes, for which diſtance the Table gives 2 Inches 3 Lines of abatement, which being taken from the ſaid height, there will remain 8 Feet 9 Lines, which ſet down in the Memorial.

How to ſet down all the different Heights in the Memorial.

Having found proper Places (as we have already ſuppoſed) for placing the Level between two Points, you muſt write on the Memorial, in two different Columns, the obſerved Heights, namely, under the firſt Column thoſe obſerved by looking thro the Teleſcope, when the Eye was next to the Source A, and under the ſecond Column, thoſe obſerved when the Eye was next to the Vaſe B of the Fountain, in the following manner

First Column.						Second Column.				
	Toiſes.	Feet.	Inches.	Lines.			Toiſes	Feet.	Inches	Lines
First Height						Second Height				
Corrected	2	0	6	0			3	3	9	4
Third Height	1	5	3	3		Fourth Height	1	2	0	9
	3	5	9	3			4	5	10	1

Having added together the Heights of the firſt Column, and afterwards thoſe of the ſecond, ſubſtract the firſt Additions from the ſecond

Toiſes	Feet.	Inches.	Lines.
4	5	10	1
3	5	9	3
1	0	0	10

Whence the Height of the Source A above the Vaſe B is 1 Toiſe and 10 Lines

If the Diſtance be required, you need but add all the Diſtances meaſured together, namely,

The Firſt of	1000	Toiſes
The Second	650	
The Third	500	
The Fourth	450	

The whole Diſtance 2600 Toiſes.

Laſtly, Dividing the Deſcent by the Toiſes of the Diſtance, there will be for every 100 Toiſes, about 2 Inches 9 Lines of Deſcent, nighly.

CHAP. III.

Of the Conſtruction and Uſe of a Gauge for Meaſuring of Water.

Fig M.

THIS Gauge ſerves to know the Quantity of Water which a Source furniſhes, and is commonly a Rectangular Parallelopepidon of Braſs well ſolder'd, about a Foot long, 8 Inches broad, and as many in height, more or leſs, according to the Quantity of Water to be meaſured, having ſeveral round holes very exactly drilled in it, an Inch in Diameter, and others for half an Inch of Water to paſs thro, and alſo others for a quarter of an Inch of Water to paſs thro them All of which ought to be drilled ſo as their Centers may be at the ſame height. The upper Extremes of the Inch-holes muſt be within two Lines of the top of the Gauge; and the holes are ſtopped with little ſquare Braſs Plates, adjuſted in the Grooves 1, 2, and 3. There is a Braſs Partition, croſſing the Veſſel at the place 4, fixed about an Inch from the bottom, and drilled with ſeveral holes, for the Water to paſs more freely This Partition is made to receive the ſhock of the Water falling from the Source into the Gauge, and hindering it from making of Waves, ſo that it may more naturally run out thro the holes.

Note, The holes which give a Cylindric Inch of Water, ought to be exactly 12 Lines in Diameter, that giving half an Inch ought to be 8½ Lines, and that giving a quarter of an Inch muſt be exactly 6 Lines. This may be eaſily found by Calculation

To uſe this Inſtrument, it muſt be placed ſo as its bottom may be parallel to the Horizon, and then let the Water of the Source run thro a Pipe into the Gauge, (as *per* Figure) and when it wants about a Line of the top, open one of the holes (for Example) of an Inch Then if the Water always keeps the ſame height in the Gauge, it is manifeſt that there **runs** as much into it as goes out of it, and ſo the Source will furniſh an Inch of Water

But

But if the Water in the Gauge rises, there must be another hole opened, either of an Inch, half an Inch, or a quarter of an Inch, so that the Water may keep to the same height in the Gauge, that is, to a Line above the holes of an Inch, and then the number of Holes opened will give the Quantity of Water furnished by the Source

The little Vessel receiving the Water running out of the Gauge, is to shew how much Fig. N. Water the Source furnishes in a determinate space of Time · For having a Pendulum which swings Seconds, note how many Seconds there will be in the time that this Vessel, set under the hole giving an Inch of Water, is filling, and exactly measuring the Quantity of Water it contains, you may have the Quantity of Water the Source furnishes in an Hour

There has several very exact Experiments been made upon this Subject from whence it has been found, that a Source giving one Inch of Water, will fill 14 Pints of *Paris*, in a Minute

It follows from hence, that an Inch of Water gives in an Hour 8 *Paris* Muids, and in 24 Hours, 72 Muids

If, for Example, a Cubic Vessel be placed under the Gauge, containing a Cubic Foot; and if the Water runs thro the hole giving an Inch of Water, that Vessel will be filled in two Minutes and a half From whence it follows, that it gives 14 Pints in a Minute, because it furnished 35 Pints in two Minutes and a half

By this means we may know the Inches of Water a Spring or Running-Stream gives · As if, for Example, the Spring gives 7 Pints of Water in a Second, then it is said to furnish an Inch of Water If it should give 21 Pints, then it is said to furnish 3 Inches of Water and so of others.

To measure the Running-Water of an Aqueduct or River, which cannot be received in a Gauge, you must put a Ball of Wax upon the Water, made so heavy with some other Matter, as that there may be but a small part of the Ball above the Surface of the Water, that so the Wind can have no power on it And after having measured a Length of 15 or 20 Feet of the Aqueduct, you may know by a Pendulum in what time the Ball of Wax will be carried that distance, and afterwards multiplying the Breadth of the Aqueduct or River by the height of the Water, and that Product by the space which the Ball of Wax has moved, this last Product will give all the Water passed, in the noted time, thro the Section of the River Example, Suppose in an Aqueduct two Feet wide, and one Foot deep, a Ball of Wax moves, in 20 Seconds, 30 Feet, which will be one Foot and a half in a Second But because the Water moves swifter at the Top than the Bottom, you must take but 20 Feet, which will be one Foot in a Second, the Product of one Foot deep, by 2 Feet broad is 2 Feet, which multiply'd by 20, the Length, gives 40 Cubic Feet, or 40 times 35 Pints of Water, which makes 1400 Pints in 20 Seconds, and if 20 Seconds give 1400 Pints, 60 Seconds will give 4200 Pints, and dividing 4200 by 14, which is the Number of Pints an Inch of Water gives, in a Minute or 60 Seconds, the Quotient 300 will be the Number of Inches which the Water of the Aqueduct furnishes

Mr *Mariotte*, who has learnedly wrote about the Motion of Water, is of opinion that Springs are nothing but Rain Water, which passing thro the Earth, meets with Hassock or Clay, which it cannot penetrate, and therefore is obliged to run along the Sides, and so form a Spring For supporting this Hypothesis, he brings the following Experiment

Having set a Cubic Vessel about a Foot high in a proper place to catch Rain-Water for several Years, he observed that the Water arose in the Vessel each Year, one with another, 18 Inches, but he thought it better to make it but 15 Inches · whence a Toise will receive in a Year 45 Cubic Feet of Water, for multiplying 36 Feet by 15 Inches, the Product will be 45 Cubic Feet

The same Author likewise computes the Extent of Ground which supplies the River *Seine* with Water, and has found that the *Seine* is not the sixth part as big as it might be He has again observed, that it has but 10 Inches of Descent in 1000 Toises over-against the *Invalids* He saith likewise, that, according to this supposition, the greatest Spring of *Montmartre*, when it is most abounding, doth not furnish over and above Water, since the Ground overwhelming it ought to send Water thereto Whence he concludes, that there is a great deal of Water lost in the Earth

To know the Shock Water produces, Experience has shown that Water accelerates its Motion, according to the odd Numbers 1, 3, 5, 7, &c that is, if in a fourth part of a Second it descends one Foot in a Pipe, it will descend 3 Feet in the next fourth of a Second

The Quantities of Water spouting out thro equal holes made at the Bottoms of Reservatories, of different heights, are to each other in the subduplicate *Ratio* of the heights The following Table shews the different Expences of Water at different heights

Heights of Reſervatories.	A Table of the Expence of Water in a Minute, the Diameter of the Ajutage being three Lines in different Heights of a Reſervatory.		Expence of Water 3 Lines in Ajut.	Diameters of different Ajutages.	A Table of the Expence of Water thro different Ajutages at the ſame Height of the Reſervatory		Expence of Water.	Heights of Jets.	A Table of the Height of Jets at different Heights of Reſervatories.			Heights of Reſervatories.
	Feet.	Pints			Lines.	Pints			Feet	Pints	Inches	
	6	9			1	1			6	5	1	
	9	11			2	6			10	10	4	
	12	14			3	14			20	21	4	
	18	16			4	25			30	33	0	
	25	19			5	39			40	45	4	
	30	21			6	56			50	58	4	
	40	24			7	76			60	72	0	
	52	28			8	110			70	86	4	

You may ſee by this Table, that an Ajutage, double another in Diameter, will expend four times the Water as that other will Example, that of three Lines will expend in a Minute 14 Pints, and that of 6 Lines will expend 56 Pints Note, The Ajutages muſt not be made Conical, but Cylindrical.

CHAP. IV.

Of the Conſtruction and Uſes of Inſtruments for Gunnery.

Conſtruction of the Callipers.

Fig. O.

THIS Inſtrument is made of two Branches of Braſs, about ſix or 7 Inches long when ſhut, each Branch being four Lines broad, and three in thickneſs The Motion of the Head thereof is like that of the Head of a two-Foot Rule, and the ends of the Branches are bent inwards, and furniſhed with Steel at the Extremes.

There is a kind of Tongue faſtened to one of the Branches, whoſe Motion is like that of the Head, for raiſing or lowering it, that ſo its end, which ought to be very thin, may be put into Notches made in the other Branch, on the inſide of which are marked the Diameters anſwerable to the Weights of Iron Bullets, in this manner· Having gotten a Rule, on which are denoted the Diviſions of the Weights, and the Bores of Pieces (the Method of dividing of which will be ſhown in ſpeaking of the next Inſtrument) open the Callipers, ſo that the inward ends may anſwer to the diſtance of each Point of the Diviſions ſhewing the weights of Bullets : And then make a Notch at each opening with a triangular File, that ſo the end of the Tongue entering into each of theſe Notches, may fix the opening of the Branches exactly to each Number of the Weights of Bullets. We commonly make Notches for the Diameters of Bullets weighing from one fourth of a Pound to 48 Pounds, and ſometimes to 64 Pounds. And then Lines muſt be drawn upon the ſurface of this Branch againſt the Notches, upon which muſt be ſet the Correſpondent Numbers denoting the Pounds.

The Uſe of this Inſtrument is eaſy, for you need but apply the two ends of the Branches to the Diameter of the Bullet to be meaſured, and then the Tongue being put in a convenient Notch, will ſhow the weight of the Bullet.

There ought always to be a certain Proportion obſerved in the breadth of the Points of this Inſtrument , ſo that making an Angle (as the Figure ſhews) at each opening, the inſide may give the weight of Bullets, and the outſide the Bores of Pieces, that is, that applying the outward ends of thoſe Points to the Diameter of the Mouths of Cannon, the Tongue, being placed in the proper Notch, may ſhow the weights of Bullets proper for them.

Conſtruction of the Gunners Square

Fig. P.

This Square ſerves to elevate or lower Cannons or Mortars, according to the Places they are to be levelled at, and is made of Braſs, one Branch of which is about a Foot long, 8 Lines broad, and one Line in thickneſs ; the other Branch is 4 Inches long, and of the ſame Length and Breadth as the former Between theſe Branches there is a Quadrant divided into 90 Deg. beginning from the ſhorteſt Branch, furniſhed with a Thread and Plummet

The

The Use of this Instrument is easy, for there is no more to do but to place the longest Branch in the Mouth of the Cannon or Mortar, and elevate or lower it, till the Thread cuts the Degrees necessary to hit a proposed Object.

There are likewise very often denoted, upon one of the Surfaces of the longest Branch, the Division of Diameters and Weights of Iron Bullets, as also the Bores of Pieces

The making of this Division is founded upon one or two Experiments, in examining, with all possible Exactness, the Diameter of a Bullet, whose Weight is very exactly known For Example, having found that a Bullet, weighing four Pounds, is three Inches in Diameter, it will be easy to make a Table of the Weights and Diameters of any other Bullets, because, *per Prop* 18 *lib* 12. *Eucl.* Bullets are to one another as the Cubes of their Diameters; from whence it follows, that the Diameters are as the Cube Roots of Numbers, expressing their Weights.

Now having found, by Experience, that a Bullet, weighing four Pounds, is three Inches in Diameter; if the Diameter of a Bullet weighing 32 Pounds be required, say, by the Rule of Three, As 4 is to 32, so is 27, the Cube of 3, to a fourth Number, which will be 216; whose Cube Root, 6 Inches, will be the Diameter of a Bullet weighing 32 Pounds

Or otherwise, seek the Cube Root of these two Numbers 4 and 32, or 1 and 8, which are in the same Proportions, and you will find 1 is to 2, as 3 is to 6, which is the same as before

But since all Numbers have not exact Roots, the Table of homologous Sides of similar Solids (in the Treatise of the Sector) may be used It now, by help of that Table, the Diameter of an Iron Bullet, weighing 64 Pounds, be required, form a Rule of Three, whose first Term is 397, the Side of the fourth Solid; the second 3 Inches, or 36 Lines, the Diameter of the Bullet weighing four Pounds, and the third Term 1000, which is the Side of the 64th Solid: the Rule being finished, you will have 90 $\frac{3}{4}$ Lines for the Diameter of a Bullet weighing 64 Pounds Afterwards to facilitate the Operations of other Rules of Three, always take, for the first Term, the Number 1000, for the second 90 $\frac{3}{4}$ Lines, and for the third the Number found in the Table, over against the Number expressing the Weight of the Bullet. As to find the Diameter of a Bullet weighing 24 Pounds, say, As 1000 is to 90 $\frac{3}{4}$ Lines, so is 721, to 65 Lines, which is 5 Inches and 5 Lines for the Diameter sought By this Method the following Table is calculated.

A TABLE, *containing the Weights and Diameters of Iron Bullets, and the Bores of the most common Pieces used in the Artillery.*

Weights of Bullets. Pounds.	Diameters Inches.	Lines.	Bores of Pieces.	Inches	Lines.
$\frac{1}{4}$	1	2 $\frac{1}{4}$	$\frac{1}{4}$	1	3
$\frac{1}{2}$	1	6	$\frac{1}{2}$	1	6 $\frac{3}{4}$
1	1	10 $\frac{5}{8}$	1	1	11 $\frac{5}{8}$
2	2	4 $\frac{1}{2}$	2	2	5 $\frac{3}{4}$
3	2	8 $\frac{3}{4}$	3	2	10
4	3	0	4	3	1 $\frac{1}{4}$
5	3	2 $\frac{3}{4}$	5	3	4 $\frac{1}{4}$
6	3	5	6	3	6 $\frac{7}{8}$
7	3	7 $\frac{1}{4}$	7	3	9 $\frac{1}{8}$
8	3	9 $\frac{3}{8}$	8	3	11 $\frac{1}{8}$
9	3	11	9	4	1 $\frac{1}{4}$
10	4	$\frac{3}{4}$	10	4	2 $\frac{3}{4}$
12	4	3 $\frac{3}{4}$	12	4	5 $\frac{3}{4}$
16	4	9	16	4	11 $\frac{1}{2}$
18	4	11 $\frac{1}{3}$	18	5	1 $\frac{2}{3}$
20	5	1 $\frac{1}{2}$	20	5	4
24	5	5	24	5	8
27	5	8 $\frac{7}{8}$	27	5	10 $\frac{1}{2}$
30	5	10 $\frac{1}{2}$	30	6	1 $\frac{1}{2}$
33	6	$\frac{1}{4}$	33	6	3 $\frac{1}{2}$
36	6	2 $\frac{1}{4}$	36	6	5 $\frac{3}{4}$
40	6	5 $\frac{1}{2}$	40	6	8 $\frac{1}{2}$
48	6	10	48	7	1 $\frac{3}{4}$
50	6	11 $\frac{1}{2}$	50	7	2 $\frac{3}{4}$
64	7	6 $\frac{3}{4}$	64	7	10 $\frac{1}{4}$

Of the Curved-Pointed Compasses.

These Compasses do not at all differ in Construction from the others, of which we have Fig. Q. already spoken, excepting only that the Points may be taken off, and curved ones put on, which

which ſerve to take the Diameters of Bullets, and then to find their Weights, by applying the Diameters on the Diviſions of the before-mentioned Rule. But when you would know the Bores of Pieces, the curve Points muſt be taken off, and the ſtrait ones put on, with which the Diameters of the Mouths of Cannon muſt be taken, and afterwards they muſt be applied to the Line of the Bores of Pieces, which is alſo ſet down upon the aforeſaid Rule, by which means the Weights of the Bullets, proper for the propoſed Cannon, may be found

Conſtruction of an Inſtrument to level Cannon and Mortars

Fig. R.

This Inſtrument is made of a Triangular Braſs Plate, about four Inches high, at the Bottom of which is a Portion of a Circle, divided into 45 Degrees, which Number is ſufficient for the higheſt Elevation of Cannon or Mortars, and for giving Shot the greateſt Range, as hereafter will be explained. There is a Piece of Braſs ſcrewed on the Center of this Portion of a Circle, by which means it may be fixed or movable, according to Neceſſity

The End of this Piece of Braſs muſt be made ſo, as to ſerve for a Plummet and Index, in order to ſhew the Degrees of different Elevations of Pieces of Artillery. This Inſtrument hath alſo a Braſs Foot to ſet upon Cannon or Mortars, ſo that when the Pieces of Cannon or Mortar are horizontal, the whole Inſtrument will be perpendicular

The Uſe of this Inſtrument is very eaſy, for place the Foot thereof upon the Piece to be elevated, in ſuch manner that the Point of the Plummet may fall upon a convenable Degree, and this is what we call levelling of a Piece

Of the Artillery Foot-Level

Fig S.

The Inſtrument S is called a Foot-Level, and we have already ſpoken of its Conſtruction, but when it is uſed in Gunnery, the Tongue, ſerving to keep it at right Angles, is divided into 90 Degrees, or rather into twice 45 Degrees from the middle. The Thread, carrying the Plummet, is hung in the Center of the aforeſaid Diviſion, and the two Ends of the Branches are hollowed, ſo that the Plummet may fall perpendicular upon the middle of the Tongue, when the Inſtrument is placed level.

To uſe it, place the two Ends upon the Piece of Artillery, which may be raiſed to a propoſed Height, by means of the Plummet, whoſe Thread will give the Degrees

Upon the Surface of the Branches of this Square, which opens quite ſtrait like a Rule, are ſet down the Weights and Diameters of Bullets, and alſo the Bores of Pieces, as we have before explained in ſpeaking of the Gunner's Square

Fig T

The Inſtrument T is likewiſe for levelling Pieces of Artillery, being almoſt like R, except only the Piece, on which are the Diviſions of Degrees, is movable, by means of a round Rivet, that is, the Portion of the Circle (or Limb) may be turned up and adjuſted to the Branch, ſo that the Inſtrument takes up leſs room, and is eaſier put in a Caſe. The Figure thereof is enough to ſhew its Conſtruction, and its Uſes are the ſame as thoſe of the precedent Inſtrument.

Explanation of the Effects of Cannon and Mortars

Fig V

The Figure V repreſents a Mortar upon its Carriage, elevated and diſpoſed for throwing a Bomb into a Citadel, and the Curve-Line repreſents the Path of the Bomb thro the Air, from the Mouth of the Piece to its Fall. This Curve, according to Geometricians, is a Parabolic Line, becauſe the Properties of the Parabola agree with it, for the Motion of the Bomb is compoſed of two Motions, one of which is equal and uniform, which the Fire of the Powder gives it, and the other is an uniform accelerate Motion, communicated to it by its proper Gravity. There ariſes, from the Compoſition of theſe two Forces, the ſame Proportion, as there is between the Portions of the Axis and the Ordinates of a Parabola, as is very well demonſtrated by M. *Blondel*, in his Book, entitled, *The Art of throwing Bombs*

Maltus, an *Engliſh* Engineer, was the firſt that put Bombs in practice in *France*, in the Year 1634 all his Knowledge was purely experimental, he did not, in the leaſt, know the Nature of the Curve they deſcribe in their Paſſage thro the Air, nor their Ranges, according to different Elevations of Mortars, which he could not level but tentively, by the Eſtimation he made of the Diſtance of the Place he would throw the Bomb to, according to which he gave his Piece a greater or leſs Elevation, ſeeing whether the firſt Ranges were juſt or not, in order to lower his Mortar, if the Range was too little, or raiſe it, if it was too great, uſing, for that effect, a Square and Plummet, almoſt like that of which we have already ſpoken

The greateſt Part of Officers, which have ſerved the Batteries of Mortars ſince *Maltus*'s time, have uſed his Elevations, they know, by Experience, nearly the Elevation of a Mortar to throw a Bomb to a given Diſtance, and augment or diminiſh this Elevation in proportion, as the Bomb is found to fall beyond or ſhort of the Diſtance of the Place it is required to be thrown in

Yet there are certain Rules, founded upon Geometry, for finding the different Ranges, not only of Bombs, but likewiſe of Cannon, in all the ſorts of Elevations, for the Line, deſcribed in the Air by a Bullet ſhot from a Cannon, is alſo a Parabola in all Projections, not only oblique ones, but right ones, as the Figure W ſhews.

A

A Bullet going out of a Piece, will never proceed in a ſtraight Line towards the Place it is levelled at, but will riſe up from its Line of Direction the moment after it is out of the Mouth of the Piece For the Grains of Powder nigheſt the Breech, taking fire firſt, preſs forward, by their precipitated Motion, not only the Bullet, but likewiſe thoſe Grains of Powder which follow the Bullet along the Bottom of the Piece ; where ſucceſſively taking fire, they ſtrike as it were the Bullet underneath, which, becauſe of a neceſſary Vent, has not the ſame Diameter as the Diameter of the Bore and ſo inſenſibly raiſe the Bullet towards the upper Edge of the Mouth of the Piece, againſt which it ſo rubs in going out, that Pieces very much uſed, and whoſe Metal is ſoft, are obſerved to have a conſiderable Canal there, gradually dug by the Friction of Bullets Thus the Bullet going from the Cannon, as from the Point E, raiſes itſelf to the Vertex of the Parabola G, after which it deſcends by a mixed Motion towards B

Ranges, made from an Elevation of 45 Deg are the greateſt, and thoſe made from Elevations equally diſtant from 45 Deg are equal . that is, a Piece of Cannon, or a Mortar, levell'd to the 40th Deg will throw a Bullet, or Bomb, the ſame diſtance, as when they are elevated to the 50th Degree , and as many at 30 as 60, and ſo of others, as appears in Fig X

Fig X

The firſt who reaſoned well upon this Matter, was *Galilæus*, chief Ingineer to the Great Duke of *Tuſcany*, and after him *Torricellius* his Succeſſor

They have ſhewn, that to find the different Ranges of a Piece of Artillery in all Elevations, we muſt, before all things, make a very exact Experiment in firing off a Piece of Cannon or Mortar, at an Angle well known, and meaſuring the Range made, with all the exactneſs poſſible : for by one Experiment well made, we may come to the Knowledge of all the others, in the following manner

To find the Range of a Piece at any other Elevation required, ſay, As the Sine of double the Angle under which the Experiment was made, is to the Sine of double the Angle of an Elevation propoſed, ſo is the Range known by Experiment, to another

As ſuppoſe, it is found by Experiment that the Range of a Piece elevated to 30 Deg is 1000 Toiſes to find the Range of the ſame Piece with the ſame Charge, when it is elevated to 45 Deg you muſt take the Sine of 60 Degrees, the double of 30, and make it the firſt Term of the Rule of Three , the ſecond Term muſt be the Sine of 90, double 45 , and the third the given Range 1000 : Then the fourth Term of the Rule will be found 1155, the Range of the Piece at 45 Degrees of Elevation

If the Angle of Elevation propoſed be greater than 45 Deg there is no need of doubling it for having the Sine as the Rule directs, but inſtead of that, you muſt take the Sine of double its Complement to 90 Degrees · As, ſuppoſe the Elevation of a Piece be 50 Degrees, the Sine of 80 Degrees, the double of 40 Deg muſt be taken

But if a determinate Diſtance to which a Shot is to be caſt, is given, (provided that Diſtance be not greater than the greateſt Range at 45 Deg. of Elevation) and the Angle of Elevation to produce the propoſed Effect be required ; as ſuppoſe the Elevation of a Cannon or Mortar is required to caſt a Shot 800 Toiſes , the Range found by Experiment muſt be the firſt Term in the Rule of Three, as for Example 1000 Toiſes, the propoſed Diſtance : 800 Toiſes, muſt be the ſecond Term , and the Sine of 60 Degrees, the third Term The fourth Term being found, is the Sine of 43 Deg 52 Min. whoſe half 21 Deg 56 Min is the Angle of Elevation the Piece muſt have, to produce the propoſed Effect ; and if 21 Deg 56 Min be taken from 90 Deg you will have 68 Deg 4 Min for the other Elevation of the Piece, with which alſo the ſame Effect will be produced

For greater Facility, and avoiding the trouble of finding the Sines of double the Angles of propoſed Elevations, *Galilæus* and *Torricellius* have made the following Table, in which the Sines of the Angles ſought are immediately ſeen

A TABLE *of Sines for the Ranges of Bombs.*

Degrees.	Degrees	Ranges	Degrees.	Degrees	Ranges.
90	0	0	66	24	7431
89	1	349	65	25	7660
88	2	698	64	26	7880
87	3	1045	63	27	8090
86	4	1392	62	28	8290
85	5	1736	61	29	8480
84	6	2709	60	30	8660
83	7	2419	59	31	8829
82	8	2556	58	32	8988
81	9	3090	57	33	9135
80	10	3420	56	34	9272
79	11	3746	55	35	9397
78	12	4067	54	36	9511
77	13	4384	53	37	9613
76	14	4695	52	38	9703
75	15	5000	51	39	9781
74	16	5299	50	40	9848
73	17	5592	49	41	9903
72	18	5870	48	42	9945
71	19	6157	47	43	9976
70	20	6428	46	44	9994
69	21	6691	45	45	10000
68	22	6947			
67	23	7193			

The Use of this Table is thus : Suppose it be known by experience, that a Mortar elevated 15 Degrees, charged with three Pounds of Powder, throws a Bomb at the distance of 350 Toises, and it is required with the same Charge to cast a Bomb 100 Toises further; seek in the Table the Number answering to 15 Degrees, and you will find 5000 Then form a Rule of Three, by saying, As 350 is to 450, so is 5000 to a fourth Number, which will be 6428 Find this Number, or the nighest approaching to it, in the Table, and you will find it next to 20 Deg. or 70 Deg which will produce the required Effect, and so of others.

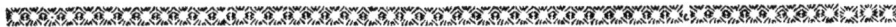

Of the Construction and Use of the Englifh Callipers.

Fig Y

THESE Callipers or Gunners Compasses, consist of two long thin Pieces of Brass, join'd together by a Rivet in such a manner, that one may move quite round the other The Head or End of one of these Pieces is cut Circular, and the Head of the other Semicircular, the Center of which being the Center of the Rivet The length of each of those Pieces from the Center of the Rivet is six Inches; so that when the Callipers are quite opened, they are a Foot long

One half of the Circumference of the Circular Head, is divided into every 2 Degrees, every tenth of which are numbered And on part of the other half, beginning from the Diameter of the Semi-circle, when the Points of the Callipers are close together, are Divisions from 1 to 10, each of which are likewise subdivided into four parts The Use of these Divisions and Subdivisions, is, that when you have taken the Diameter of any round thing, as a Cannon-Ball, not exceeding 10 Inches, the Diameter of the Semi-circle will, amongst those Divisions, give the Length of that Diameter taken between the Points of the Callipers in Inches and 4th Parts

From this Use, it is manifest how the aforesaid Divisions for Inches may be easily made : For, first, set the Points of the Callipers together, and then make a Mark for the beginning of the Divisions, then open the Points one fourth of an Inch, and where the Diameter of the Semi-circle cuts the Circumference, make a Mark for one fourth of an Inch Then open the Points half an Inch, and where the Diameter of the Semi-circle cuts the Circumference, make another Mark for half an Inch In this manner proceed for all the other Subdivisions and Divisions to Ten

Upon

Upon one of the Branches, on the fame fide the Callipers, are, Firft, half a Foot or fix Inches each, fubdivided into ten Parts Secondly, a Scale of unequal Divifions beginning at two, and ending at ten, each of which are fubdivided into four Parts The Conftruction of this Scale of Lines will be very evident, when its Ufe is fhown, which is thus If you have a mind to find how many Inches, under 10, the Diameter of any Concave, as the Diameter of the Bore of any Piece of Ordnance is in length, you muft open the Branches of the Callipers, fo that the two Points may be outwards, then taking the Diameter between the faid Points, fee what Divifion or Subdivifion, the outward Edge of the Branch with the Semicircular Head, cuts on the aforefaid Scale of Lines, and that will be the Number of Inches, or Parts, the Diameter of the Bore of the Piece is in length. Therefore the Divifions on this Scale may be made in the fame manner as I have before directed, in fhowing how to make the Divifions for finding the Diameters of round Convex Bodies.

Thirdly, The two other Scales of Lines on the fame Face of the fame Branch, fhew when the Diameter of the Bore of a Piece of Cannon is taken with the Points of the Callipers outward, the Name of the Piece, whether Iron or Brafs, that is, the Weight of the Bullets they carry, or fuch and fuch a Pounder, from 42 Pounds to 1. The Conftruction of thefe Scales are from experimental Tables in Gunnery.

On the other Branch, the fame fide of the Callipers, is, Firft, fix Inches, every of which is fubdivided into 10 Parts Secondly, a Table fhewing the Weight of a Cubic Foot of Gold, Quick-filver, Lead, Silver, Copper, Iron, Tin, *Purbec*-Stone, Chryftal, Brimftone, Water, Wax, Oil and dry Wood

On the other fide of the Callipers, is a Line of Chords to about three Inches Radius, and Fig. Z. a Line of Lines on both Branches, the fame as on the Sector

There is alfo a Table of the Names of the following Species of Ordnance, *viz* a Falconet, a Falcon, a Three-Pounder, a Minion, a Sacker, a Six-Pounder, an Eight-Pounder, a Demi-culverin, a Twelve-Pounder, a Whole-Culverin, a Twenty-four-Pounder, a Demi-Cannon, Baftard-Cannon, and a Whole-Cannon. Under thefe are the Quantities of Powder neceffary for each of their Proofs, and alfo for their Service

Upon the fame Face is a Hand graved, and a Right Line drawn from the Finger towards the Center of the Rivet Which Right Line fhews, by cutting certain Divifions made on the Circle, the Weight of Iron-fhot, when the Diameters is taken with the Points of the Callipers, if they are of the following Weights, *viz* 42, 32, 24, 18, 12, 9, 6, 4, 3, 2, 1, $1\frac{1}{2}$, 1, Pounds. Thefe Figures are not all fet to the Divifions on the Circumference, for avoiding Confufion The aforefaid Divifions on the Circumference may be thus made Firft, When the Points of the Callipers are clofe, continue the Line drawn from the Finger on the Limb, to reprefent the beginning of the Divifions. Now becaufe from experience it is found, that an Iron Ball or Globe weighing one Pound is 1 8 of an Inch, open the Callipers, fo that the diftance between the two Points may be 1.8 of an Inch, and then, where the Line drawn from the Finger cuts the Circumference, make a Mark for the Divifion 1 Again, to find where the Divifion 1 5 muft be, fay, As 1 is to the Cube of 1 8, fo is 1 5 to the Cube of the Diameter of an Iron Ball weighing 1 5 Pounds, whofe Root extracted will give 2 23 Inches. Therefore open the Points of the Callipers, fo that they may be 2 23 Inches diftant from each other, and then, where the Line drawn from the Finger cuts the Circumference, make a Mark for the Divifion 1 5 The Reafon of this is, becaufe the Weights of Homogeneous Bodies, are to each other as their Magnitudes, and the Magnitudes of Globes and Spheres, are to each other as the Cubes of their Diameters

Proceed in the aforefaid manner, in always making 1 the firft Term of the Rule of Three, and the Cube of 1 8 the fecond, *&c* and all the Divifions will be had.

Upon the Circle or Head, on the fame fide of the Callipers, are graved feveral Geometrical Figures, with Numbers fet thereto There is a Cube whofe fide is fuppofed to be 1 Foot or 12 Inches, and a Pyramid of the fame Bafe and Altitude over it On the fide of the Cube is grav'd 470, fignifying that a Cubic Foot of Iron weighs 470 Pounds, and on the Pyramid is graved $156\frac{1}{3}$, fignifying that the Weight of it is fo many Pounds

The next is a Sphere, fuppofed to be infcribed in a Cube of the fame Dimenfions, as the former Cube, in which is writ $246\frac{1}{4}$, which is the Weight of that Sphere of Iron The next is a Cylinder, the Diameter and Altitude of which is equal to the fide of the aforefaid Cube, and a Cone over it, of the fame Bafe and Altitude, there is fet to the Cylinder $369\frac{1}{14}$, fignifying, that a Cylinder of Iron of that Bignefs, weighs $369\frac{1}{14}$, and to the Cone $121\frac{7}{14}$, fignifying, that a Cone of Iron of that Bignefs weighs $121\frac{7}{14}$ Pounds

The next is a Cube infcribed in a Sphere of the fame Dimenfions as the aforefaid Sphere There is fet to it the Number $90\frac{1}{2}$, fignifying, that a Cube of Iron infcribed in the faid Sphere, weighs $90\frac{1}{4}$ Pounds

The next is a Circle infcribed in a Square, and a Square in that Circle, and again a Circle in the latter Square There is fet thereto the Numbers 28, 11, 22 and 14, fignifying, that if the Area of the outward Square is 28, the Area of its infcribed Circle is 22, and the Area of the Square infcribed in the Circle 14, and the Area of the Circle infcribed in the latter Square 11.

The

The next and laft, is a Circle croffed with two Diameters at Right Angles, having in it the Numbers 7, 22, 113 and 355 ; the two former of which reprefent the Proportion of the Diameter of a Circle to its Circumference ; and the two latter alfo the Proportion of the Diameter to the Circumference.   But fomething nearer the Truth.

I have already, as it were, fhewn the Ufes of this Inftrument ; but only of the Degrees on the Head, which is to take the Quantity of an Angle, the manner of doing which is eafy: For if the Angle be an inward Angle, as the Corner of a Room, &c apply the two outward Edges of the Branches to the Walls or Planes forming the Angles, and then the Degrees cut by the Diameter of the Semi-circle, will fhew the Quantity of the Angle fought But if the Angle be an outward Angle, as the Corner of a Houfe, &c you muft open the Branches till the two Points of the Callipers are outwards ; and then apply the ftraight Edges of the Branches to the Planes, or Walls, and the Degrees cut by the Diameter of the Semi-circle, will be the Quantity of the Angle fought, reckoning from 180 towards the Right Hand.

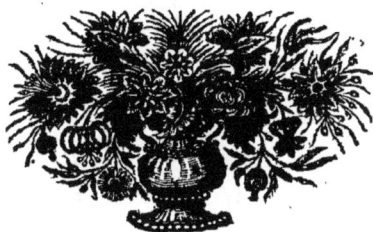

BOOK

Plate XV

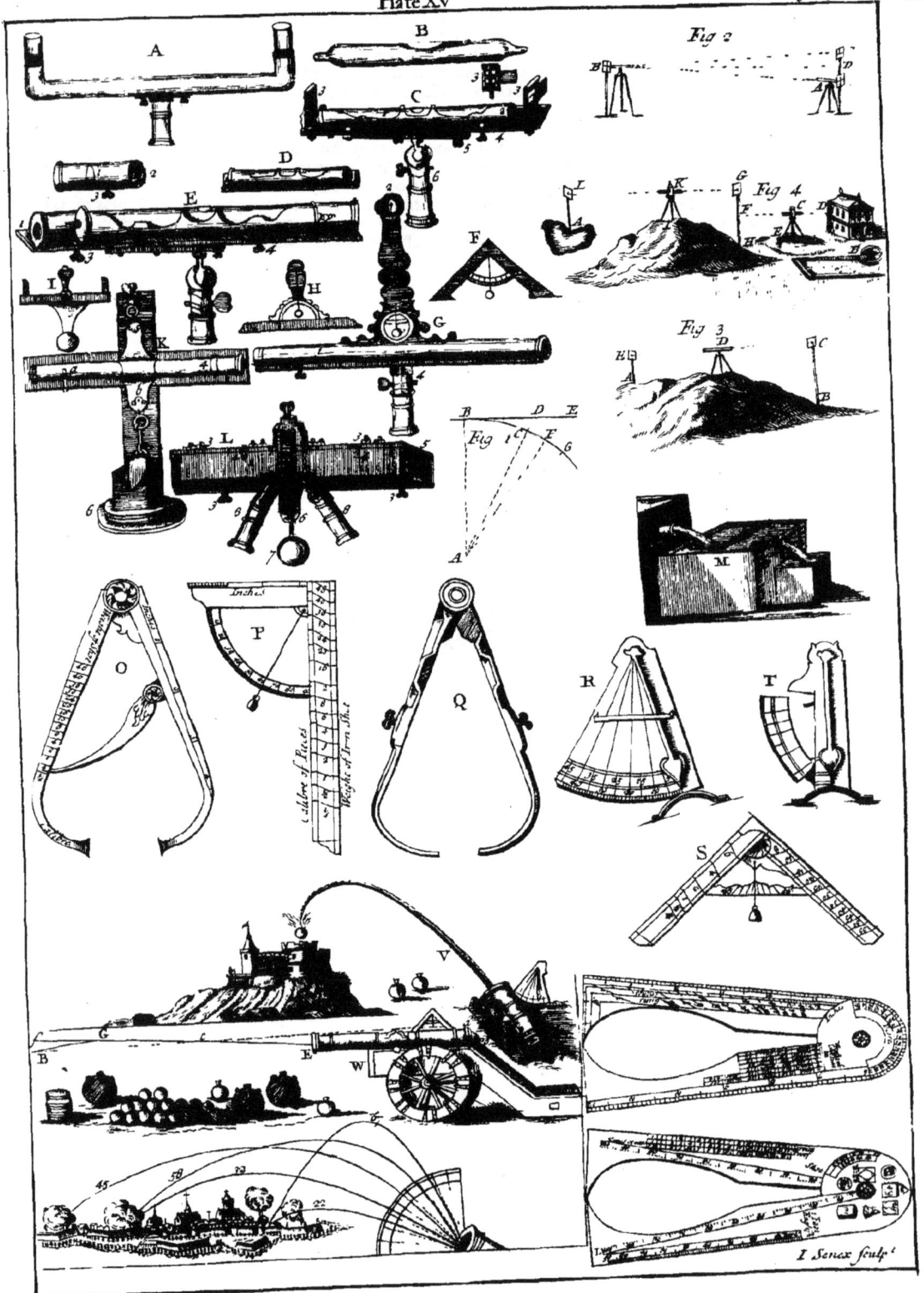

I Senex sculp.t

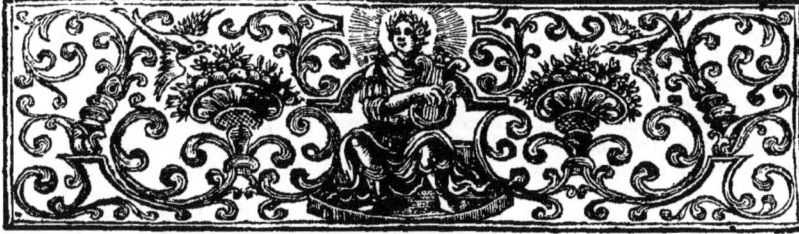

BOOK VI.

Of the Construction and Uses of Astronomical Instruments.

Taken from the Astronomical Tables of M de la Hire, and the Observations of the Academy of Sciences.

C H A P. I.

Of the Construction and Uses of the Astronomical Quadrant.

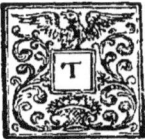

THE Quadrants used by Astronomers for Celestial Observations, are usually three Feet, or three Feet and a half (of *Paris*) Radius, that so they may be easily managed and carried from Place to Place   Their Limbs are divided into Degrees and Minutes, that so Observations made with them may be very exact

This Instrument is composed of several pretty thick Iron or Brass Rules, *Plate* 16 whose Breadths ought to be parallel to its Plane   There are moreover other Fig 1. Iron or Brass Rules, so adjusted and joined behind the former ones, that their Breadths are perpendicular to the Plane of the Quadrant   These Rules are joined together by Screws, by means of which the whole Conjunction of the Instrument is made, which ought to be very strait every way, firm, and pretty weighty   The Limb is likewise strengthen'd with a curved Brass, or Iron Ruler.   There is a thick strong circular Blade placed in the Center, serving for the Uses hereafter mentioned , which circular Blade and the Limb must be raised something higher than the Plane of the Instrument, both of which must be covered with well-polished thin Pieces of Brass   But you must take great care that the Surfaces of these Pieces of Brass be both in the same Plane

The aforesaid circular Iron Blade in the Center must have a round Hole in the middle thereof, about $\frac{1}{5}$ of an Inch in Diameter, in which is placed a well-turned Brass Cylinder, raised something above the central thin Piece of Brass

This Cylinder, which is represented in Figure 2, hath the Point of a very fine Needle ad-Fig 2. justed in the Center of its Base, which is supported in going into a little Hole in the Center of the Base, and by lying along a semicircular Cavity, and is kept therein by means of a little Spring pressing against it , so that when the Needle is taken away, and we have a mind to put it there again, it may exactly be placed in the little Hole in the Center of the said Cylinder   This little Hole ought to be no bigger than a Hair, but it must be something deep, that so the Point of the Needle may go far enough into it, that at the shaking of the Quadrant it may not come out.   At the Point of this Needle is hung a Hair, by means of a Ring made with the same Hair big enough, for fear lest the Knot of the Ring should touch the central Plate, and the Motion of the Hair be disturbed   *Note,* The Base of the central Cylinder A, represented in this Figure, must be such, that the Ring of the Hair, hung

Qq

on

on the Point of the Needle, may not touch the ſaid Baſe otherwiſe than in its Center, when there is a Plummet hung to the End of the Hair, of about half an Ounce in weight

The Conſtruction of this central Cylinder ought to be ſuch, that it may be taken away and preſerved, and another placed inſtead thereof, of the ſame Thickneſs therewith, but ſomething longer, which coming out beyond the central Blade, ſuſtains the Rule of the Inſtrument, in ſuch manner as we are going to explain

There is moreover, at the central Braſs Blade, which covers the Iron one, a plane Ring A, turning about the Center, but not touching the central Cylinder, in ſuch manner, that the outward Surface thereof is even with the Surface of the ſaid Braſs Blade Upon this Ring is faſtened, with two Screws, a flat Tube M, which moves freely along with the Hair and Plummet, which it covers, and ſo preſerves it from the Wind when the Inſtrument is uſing.

This Tube carries a Glaſs, placed againſt the Diviſions of the Limb of the Quadrant, in order to ſee what Point of Diviſion the Hair falls upon Behind and nigh to the Center of Gravity of the Quadrant, is firmly fixed, with three or four Screws, to the Rules of the Inſtrument, the Iron Cylinder I, whoſe Length is 8 Inches, and Diameter of its Baſe two Inches This Cylinder being perpendicular to the Plane of the Quadrant, may be called its Axis

Now becauſe the principal Uſe of this Inſtrument is for taking the Altitudes of the Sun or Stars, it muſt be ſo ordered, that its Plane may be eaſily placed in a vertical Situation; therefore an Iron Ruler M N muſt be prepared, whoſe Thickneſs is three Lines, Length eight Inches, and Breadth one Inch, or thereabouts On one Side of this Ruler are adjuſted two Iron Rings Z Z, open a-top with Ears, each of which has a Screw to draw the Ears cloſer together, which have a Spring The Bigneſs of theſe Rings is nearly equal to the Thickneſs of the Cylinder I, or Axis of the Quadrant, which being put thro them, is made faſt with the Screws, ſo that the Axis and Quadrant, which it is fixed to, may remain firm in any Poſition the Quadrant is put into

On the other Side of the ſaid Ruler M N is ſoldered an Iron Cylinder O, of ſuch a Length and Breadth, as to go into the Tube Q, of which we are going to ſpeak

Now when the Inſtrument is to be placed ſo, that its Plane may be horizontal, for uſing an Index or moveable Arm to take the Diſtances of Stars or Places upon Earth, the Cylinder I muſt be put into the Tube Q, by which means the Quadrant may be eaſily turned to what part you pleaſe

Fig. 5. The Foot, or Support of the whole Inſtrument, is commonly compoſed of an Iron Tube Q, whoſe upper Part is capable of containing the Cylinder O, and its lower Part goes thro the middle of an Iron Croſs, and is faſtened in it by four Iron Arms, at the four Ends of which Croſs are four great Screws, to raiſe or lower the Quadrant, and put it in a convenient Situation. But Monſieur *de la Hire* propoſes a Triangular Support in his Tables, which is compoſed of an Iron or Braſs Tube, big enough to contain the Cylinder O, faſtened with two Screws to three Iron Rulers R S, bent towards their Tops, and of a pretty good Thickneſs, which are adjuſted and well fixed to a Tee or double Square T X Y The Screw V, in the middle of the Tube Q, is for fixing the Cylinder O, according to Neceſſity

Now when the Meridian Altitudes of Stars are to be obſerved, the Ruler T Y ought to be placed in the Meridian Line, and of the three Screws T X Y, which ſuſtain the weight of the whole Inſtrument, that which is in X ſerves to lower the Plane of the Inſtrument, till it anſwers to the Plane of the Meridian, according as the Obſerver would have it, and the other two are for raiſing or lowering the Inſtrument by little and little, until the Plumb-Line falls upon the requiſite Altitude But it often happens in turning the Screws that are in T and Y, that the Quadrant diſplaces itſelf from its true Poſition; whence, if the Defect be ſome Minutes, this may be remedied, by hanging a moveable Weight to the Back-ſide of the Branches of the Inſtrument, which may alter the Center of Gravity, as likewiſe change the Inclination of the Quadrant, for the Rulers compoſing the Foot are not entirely free from Elaſticity Now the nigher to the Foot the Place of Suſpenſion of the Weight is, the leſs Force will it have to ſhake the Inſtrument *Note*, The Height of the Foot is commonly four Feet and a half, or thereabouts, and the ſame Uſe is equally made of the four Branch Support

Fig. 6. The Diviſions on the Limb of this Quadrant ought to be made with great Care, that ſo Obſervations may thereby be exactly taken Each Degree is divided into 60 Minutes, by means of 11 concentrick Circles, and 6 Diagonal right Lines, as in Figure 6 may be ſeen Theſe Diagonal Diſtances are equal between themſelves, but thoſe of the Concentrick Circles are unequal, yet this Inequality is not ſenſible, if the Radius of the Quadrant be three Feet, and the Diſtance between the two outmoſt Concentrick Circles be one Inch, for if the Arc A E, of the outmoſt Circle be 10 Minutes, and there are drawn, from the Center C of the Quadrant, the Radii A D C, E B C, meeting the inner Concentrick Circle in the Points D, B, the Arc D B will be likewiſe 10 Minutes. *Note*, Figure 6 is ſuppoſed to be put upon the Limb of the Inſtrument, Figure 1.

But

But if the Right-lined Diagonals A B, D E, are drawn interfecting each other in the Point F, I say F is the middle Point of Division thro which the middle Circle ought to pass · For the Arcs A E, B D, which may be taken for strait Lines, are to each other, as A F is to F B: for it is evident, that C A is to C B, as the Divisions of the Bafe A B of the Right-lined Triangle A C B, but since C A is to C B as A E is to D B, therefore A E is to D B, as the Divisions of the Bafe A B made by a Radius, bifecting the Angle A C B and confequently the Point F, before found in the Right-lined Diagonal A B, will be the middle Point of the Divisions

Now let us fuppofe, that A C is to C B, as 36 Inches is to 35, then A B is to A F, as 71 is to 36 Therefore if the breadth of one Inch, or 12 Lines, which is the fuppofed meafure of A B, is divided into 71 equal Parts, the part A F will be 36 of them, which will be greater by half, or about $\frac{1}{2}$ of a Line, than half of A B, which is but $35\frac{1}{2}$ This Difference is of no confequence, and may, without any fenfible Error, be neglected in the Divifion of the middle, and much more in the other Divifions, where it is lefs

Inftead of making Right-lined Diagonals, we may make then Portions of Circles paffing thro the Center of the Inftrument, and the firft and laft Point of the fame Diagonal, then we need but divide the firft Circular Portion into ten equal Parts, and the exact Points will be had thro which the eleven Concentrick Circles muft pass.

The Radius of this firft Portion may be eafily found, and then if a thin Ruler be bent into the Curvature thereof, all the other Portions may be drawn by means of it, as we have already mentioned in fpeaking of the Divifions of Quadrants, Semicircles, &c

Note, It will be proper to leave, at the Bottom of the Limb, the Points that were made for drawing every 10th Minute, for thefe will be a means to take the Correfpondent Altitudes of the Sun, Morning and Evening, much exacter than can be done by the Diagonals, becaufe of the Eftimation thereby avoided Moreover, there may be fome fault in the Diagonals which there cannot be in the Points, if care be taken in making them · for it is difficult enough to draw the Diagonals exactly thro thofe Points they fhould pass For which reafon, if a Micrometer be joined to the fixed Telefcope of the Inftrument, the Diagonals need not be ufed, and the aforefaid Points will be fufficient, fince the Micrometer will give, by means of a moveable Hair, the Interval between the neareft of one of the aforefaid Points, at every 10th Minute, and the Plummet And this is done by raifing or lowering the moveable Hair above or below the horizontal Hair, 10 Minutes of a Degree, or a little more The Chevalier *de Louville*, of the Academy of Sciences, hath fatisfactorily ufed a Quadrant for his Obfervations, conftructed in this manner

We now come to fpeak of Telefcopes, and the Manner of finding the firft Point of the Divifions of the Limb of the Quadrant

Thefe Telefcopes have each two Glaffes, one of which is the Object-Glafs, placed towards the vifible Object, and near to the Center of the Quadrant, and the other is the Eye-Glafs, placed at the other end of the Telefcope, next to the Eye of the Obferver

The Object-Glafs is firmly faftened in an Iron Frame, which is fix'd with Screws about the Center of the Inftrument Near the Eye-Glafs are placed two fine Hairs, croffing each other at Right Angles, in an Iron Frame, to which they are faftened with Wax upon a little piece of Brafs, fo that the one is perpendicular to the Plane of the Inftrument, and the other parallel thereto

The Eye-Glafs muft be placed in a Tube, that fo it may be moved backwards or forwards, according to different Sights, and the diftance between the Object-Glafs and Crofs-hairs, muft be the faid Glafs's Focal Length, that is, the Crofs-hairs muft be placed in the Focus of the Object-Glafs Thefe Telefcopes muft be fo difpofed, that the Surfaces of the Lenfes (as Planes) and the Planes in which are the Crofs-hairs, be parallel to each other, and perpendicular to Right Lines drawn thro the Centers of the Lenfes, and the Points wherein the Hairs crofs each other Thefe Telefcopes are adjufted behind the Quadrant, that fo the divided Brafs-Limb may not be incumbered by them

Between the Frames fuftaining the Glaffes, is a Brafs or Iron Tube, compofed of two Parts, one of which is inchafed in the other, that fo they may eafily be taken from between the Frames, by means of Ferrils keeping them together

The Convex Eye-Lens muft be brought nearer, or removed further from the Crofs-hairs, according to the diverfe Conftitutions of Obfervators Eyes, that fo diftant Objects may be diftinctly perceived, as likewife the Crofs-hairs This Eye-Glafs is placed in another little moveable Tube, the greateft part of which lies concealed in another Tube, as may be feen in *Fig 7*

When the Eye-Glafs wants cleanfing, or the Crofs-hairs are broken or diforder'd, and others to be put in their place, the beforementioned Brafs or Iron Tube muft be taken from between the Frames

But the Conftruction of the Eye-Glafs will be much more convenient, if, inftead of a Frame *Fig 7.* only, you ufe a little fquare Box, about four Lines in thicknefs, whofe two oppofite Sides, which are parallel to the Limb of the Quadrant, have Grooves along them, in which may move a little Plate of a mean thicknefs, drilled thro the middle with a round hole of a convenient bignefs

Upon

Upon the Surface of this Plate, reprefented by the Figure *a*, are continued out two Diameters of the aforefaid hole, croffing each other at Right Angles, one of which is parallel to the Limb, and the other perpendicular thereto, upon which are placed the Crofs-hairs. This Plate is very ufeful for moving the faid Crofs-hairs, ftrained at Right Angles a-crofs the middle of the hole, backwards or forwards, according to neceffity. And when the Hairs are placed as they fhould be, the aforefaid Plate is fixed to the Box with Wax, which ought to be furnifhed with a fliding Cover, for keeping the Crofs-hairs from Accidents.

The infide of the Tube ought to be blackened with the Smoke of Rofin, in order to preferve the Eye from too ftrong Rays which come from a luminous Object, that fo the appearance thereof may be more perfect. *Note*, Inftead of having Crofs-hairs in the beforementioned Box, a little piece of plain Glafs may be ufed, having two fine Lines drawn upon it at Right Angles with the Point of a Diamond.

The Telefcope being prepared and placed in a convenient Situation parallel to the Radius, or fide of the Quadrant; the next thing to be done, is to find the firft Point of the Divifions of the Limb of the Quadrant, which is 90 Degrees diftant from the Line of Collimation or Sight of the Telefcope, or a Line parallel to it, paffing thro the Center of the Quadrant. But, Firft, it will be neceffary to fay fomething concerning this Line of Collimation, or Sight, about which M *de la Hire* fays, he had formerly a long Controverfy, with very celebrated and great Aftronomers, who, for want of duly confidering Dioptricks, maintained, that it is impoffible to find a fettled and conftant Line of Collimation in thefe kind of Telefcopes.

It is now manifeft, that all the Rays proceeding from any one Point of an Object, after having paffed thro the Glafs Lens, will all concur in one and the fame Point, which is called the Focus, provided that the Diftance of the Radiating Point from the *Lens* be greater than the Semidiameter of either of the Convexities of the *Lens*, which here we fuppofe equal; that befides, among the Rays coming from a Radiating Point, and falling upon the anterior Surface of the Glafs, that which concurs with a Line paffing thro the Centers of the Convexities, will fuffer no Refraction at its going in or coming out of the Glafs, therefore the Points of Objects that are in that Right Line, are reprefented in the fame Line, which is called the Axis of the Optick Tube, and the Point of the Axis which is in the middle of the Glafs's thicknefs, is called the Center of the *Lens*.

If the Right Line paffing thro the Center of the *Lens*, and the Point where the Hairs crofs one another, agrees with the Axis of the faid Optick Tube, it will be the Line of Collimation of the Telefcope, and an Object very diftant, placed in the Axis produced, will appear in the fame Point where the Hairs crofs one another: juft as in common Indexes, where we take for the Line of Sight, the Right Line, that paffing thro the flits of the Sights, tends to the Object. But altho it almoft never happens in the Pofition of Telefcopes, which we have eftablifhed, that the Right Line tending from the Object to the Point wherein the Hairs crofs, and whereat the Object is reprefented, coincides with the Optick Axis; neverthelefs we fhall not defift finding that Line of Collimation tending from the Object to its Picture, reprefented in the Point wherein the Hairs crofs each other, which may be done in the following manner.

Fig S   Let X V be a Glafs *Lens*, its Axis A C B, and its Center C; let F be the Point wherein the Hairs crofs one another without the Axis A C B. If from the Point F, which by Conftruction is at the Focal Diftance from the *Lens*, Rays pafs thro the Glafs, they will fuffer a Refraction at their entrance into the Glafs, and a fecond Refraction at their going out thereof; after which, they will continue their way parallel to one another. Now there is one of thefe Rays, namely, F E, which coming from the Point F, after the firft Refraction in the Point E, paffes thro the Center C; for after a fecond Refraction at its going out of the Glafs in the Point D, it will continue its way from D to O, parallel to F E, according to Dioptrick Rules. But all the Rays feparated at their going out of the Glafs may be taken as parallel, if they tend to a very diftant Point O, therefore they are alfo parallel to the Ray F E O, which is produced from the Object directly to the Point O, and it is this Right Line F E O, which we call the *Line of Collimation*, in the aforefaid Pofition of Telefcopes, and it will always remain the fame, if the Situation of the Glaffes be not changed, that is, if the *Lens* and the Crofs-hairs are in the fame Pofition and Diftance. The Object O being in one of the extreme Points of the Right Line F E O, will be reprefented in the Point F.

Note, The Diftance between the principal Ray O D, falling from the Point O of the Object upon the *Lens*, and its refracted Ray E F, is always leffer than the thicknefs of the faid *Lens* D E, which is infenfible, and of no importance, in the Diftance of a very diftant Object, and the Diftance of the parallel Rays O D, O E F, will be fo much the lefs, as the *Lens* is more directly turned towards the Pofition of the Crofs-hairs.

We come now to fhew how to find the firft Point of the Divifions of the Limb of the Quadrant, which is thus: Having fixed the Plane of the Quadrant in a vertical Pofition, by means of the Plumb-Line C D, direct the Telefcope towards a very diftant vifible Point, nigh to the Senfible Horizon, in refpect the Place where the Telefcope of the Inftrument is placed, which may be firft known by marking the Point B upon the Limb, in the Radius C B; parallel to the Axis of the Tube, which may be nearly done, and by taking the Point D, diftant from the Point B 90 Degrees: for when the Plumb-Line falls upon the Point D,

the

the Object appearing in the Point wherein the Hairs crofs one another, will be nigh to the Horizon, for the Senfible Horizon muft be at Right Angles with the Plumb-Line C D   But fince we are not yet certain whether the Telefcope be perfectly Horizontal, the Inftrument muft be turned upfide down, fo that the Point D may be above, and the Center below, but it is neceffary in this Tranfpofition, that the Line of Collimation be at the fame height as it was in the firft Pofition   Having again directed the Telefcope towards the Point firft obferved, fo that it may appear in the Point wherein the Hairs crofs, and having adjufted the Cylinder in the Center of the Inftrument, faften the Plumb-Line with Wax upon the Limb in the Point D, and if it exactly falls upon the Center C, it is certain that the *Line of Collimation* is horizontal.   For this *Line of Collimation* will remain the fame in both Situations of the Quadrant, and produced with the Vertical Line C D, the Point D will be the beginning of the Divifions of the Limb

But if, after having turned the Inftrument upfide down, the Plumb-Line, fufpended at the Point D, does not precifely fall upon the Center C, you muft move it till it does pafs thro it, not any wife changing the Pofition of the Quadrant, nor the Glaffes of the Telefcope; and then the Point E, upon which the Plumb-Line falls, muft be marked in the circular Arc D E, defcribed about the Center C, paffing thro the Point D

Now, I fay, if the Arc D E be bifected in the Point O, this Point will be the firft Point of the Divifions of the Limb, and the Radius C O will be at Right Angles with the *Line of Collimation*   This Operation is very manifeft, for the *Line of Collimation*, or the Radius C B, parallel to it, will not be changed in either of the Pofitions of the Quadrant, if the Angle B C D, in the natural Situation of the Inftrument, be greater than a Right Angle, that is, if the Point of an Object the Telefcope is directed to, be under the Horizon, it is manifeft that the Vertical Line C D produced, anfwering to the Plumb-Line, makes with the *Line of Collimation* an Angle lefs than a right one, *viz* the Complement of the Angle B C D, which is equal to the Angle B C E, therefore the Angle B C O, which is a Mean between that which is greater than a right one, and that leffer, made by the Radius C O, and the *Line of Collimation*, will be a right Angle, which was to be proved

We may yet otherwife have the firft Point of the Divifions of the Limb, by knowing a Point perfectly level with the Eye, then placing the Telefcope in that Point, and that place of the Limb upon which the Plumb-Line plays, will give the firft Point of Divifion

The Proof of this Operation is juftified, if (the Plumb-Line paffing thro the Point O) a very diftant Object appears in the Point wherein the Hairs crofs one another   For having inverted the Inftrument, and the Telefcope being always directed towards the fame Object, the Plumb-Line will pafs thro the Points O and C, otherwife there will be fome Error in the Obfervations

Being well affured of the firft Point of the Divifions of the Limb, you muft draw about the Center C two Portions of Circles, an Inch diftance from each other, between which the Divifions of the Limb are to be included, to do which, you muft ufe a Beam-Compafs, whofe Points are very fine, one of which, next to the end, moves backwards or forwards, by help of a Screw and Nut, which is adjufted to the end of the Branch of the Compafs

Then one of the Points of the Compafs being placed in O, the firft Point of the Divifions of the Limb, and the other being diftant therefrom the length of the Radius of one of the faid Concentrick Arcs, make a Mark upon the correfpondent Concentrick Arc, which exactly divide into two equal parts, one of which being laid off beyond the Mark, will give the Point B, and fo the Quadrant O B will be divided into three equal Parts, each being 30 Degrees.

Thefe Parts being each divided into three more, and each of thefe laft into two, and, finally, each of the Parts arifing into five more equal ones, the Quadrant will be divided into 90 Degrees, each of which being again divided into fix equal Parts, every 10th Minute will be had

The outward and inward Concentrick Arcs of the Limb being very exactly divided, as we have directed, very fine Lines muft diagonally be drawn thereon, that is, from the firft Point of Divifion of the inward Arc, to the fecond Point of Divifion of the outward Arc, and fo on from one Divifion in the inward Arc to the next enfuing Divifion of the outward Arc, as appears in *Fig 6*   This being done, the diftance between the outward and inward Arcs muft be divided into 10 equal Parts, thro each Point of Divifion of which, muft nine Concentrick Arcs be drawn about the Center of the Quadrant C, which will divide the Diagonals into ten Parts, and fo the Limb of the Inftrument will be divided into Degrees and Minutes.   Great care ought to be taken, that fo the Divifions may be very exactly drawn equal, and that they may be as exact as poffible, very good and fine Compaffes exquifitely to draw the Lines and Circles muft be ufed, and in making the feveral Divifions, we ufe fine Spring Compaffes, whofe Points are as fine as a Needle, and a good dividing Knife   *Note*, The Divifions of the Limb of the Quadrant for certain Ufes, are continued about 5 Degrees beyond the Point O.

After this Instrument hath been carried in a Coach or on Horseback, &c care ought to be taken to prove it, for fear left the Glasses of the Telescope should have been disorder'd, or the Cross-hairs removed, which often happens. Likewise when the Tube of the Telescope, if the Instrument be not convey'd as aforesaid, is exposed to the Heat of the Sun, the Cross-hairs are too much stretched, and afterwards when the Sun is absent, they relax and become slack, and so are not very fit to be used. yet nevertheless, if you think the Cross-hairs have not been moved, there is no necessity of proving the Telescope, because the Object-Glass remains immoveable, and always the same, and the Cross-hairs, which by the moisture of the Air are slacken'd, will often become tight again in fine Weather

NOTE, If a Telescope be placed to an Instrument already divided, it is very difficult to make it agree with the Divisions of the Limb, therefore having proved it, according to the Directions before given, we shall find how much greater or lesser than a Right Angle the Telescope makes, with a Radius passing thro the first Point of the Divisions of the Limb, and this Difference must be regarded in all Observations made with the Instrument. For if the Angle be greater than a Right one, all Altitudes observed will be greater than the true ones by the quantity of the said Difference, and contrariwise, if the aforenamed Angle be lesser than a Right Angle, the true Altitudes will be greater than the observed ones. Notwithstanding this, the Cross-hairs may be so placed, that the *Line of Collimation* of the Telescope may make a Right Angle with the Radius passing thro the first Point of Division of the Quadrant, in applying the Cross-hairs on a moveable Plate, as we have mentioned in the Construction. But because in conveying this Instrument to distant places, the Proof thereof must be often made, and since the Method already laid down is subject to great Inconveniencies, as well on account of the difficulty of inverting the Instrument, so that the Tube of the Telescope may be at the same height, as because of the different Refractions of the Atmosphere near the Horizon, at different Hours of the Day, as likewise because of the Agitation and Undulation of the Air, and other the like Obstacles : Therefore we shall here shew two other ways of rectifying these Instruments, that so any one may chuse that which appears most convenient for him

Now the first of these Methods is this. You must chuse some Place from whence a distant Object may be perceived distinctly, at least 1000 Toises, and whose Elevation above the Horizon does not exceed the Number of Degrees of the Limb of the Quadrant continued out beyond the beginning of the Divisions. Now after you have observed the Altitude of the said Object, as it appears by the Degrees of the Limb, a Pail brim-full of Water, or some broad-mouth'd Vessel, must be placed before, and as nigh to the Quadrant as possible, which must be raised or lower'd until the said Object be perceived thro the Telescope upon the Surface of the Water, as in a Looking-Glass, which will not be difficult to do, provided the Surface of the Water be not disturbed by the Wind, whence the Depression of the said Object will be had in Degrees by Reflexion, and it will appear in an erect Situation, because the Telescope is composed of two Convex Glasses, which represent Objects inverted. But by Reflexion inverted Objects appear erect, and erect Objects inverted

But you ought to observe, that when the Angle made by the Line of Collimation, and the Radius passing thro the first Point of the Divisions of the Limb, is greater than a right one, the Depression of the aforesaid Object will appear as an Altitude, that is, when you look thro the Telescope at the Image of the Object in the Surface of the Water, the Plumb-Line of the Quadrant will fall on the left Side of the first Point O of the Divisions of the Limb, and not on the Divisions continued out beyond the Point O. And contrariwise, in other Cases, when the Angle the Line of Collimation makes with the Radius passing thro the first Point of the Divisions of the Limb, is lesser than a right one, the Altitude of the Object will appear by the Divisions of the Limb, as tho it was depressed, that is, when you look at the aforesaid Object thro the Telescope, the Plumb-Line of the Quadrant will fall upon the Divisions of the Limb continued out beyond the Point O. But in all Cases, without regarding the Degrees of Altitude or Depression, denoted by the Plumb-Line, when the Object and its Image, in the Surface of the Water, is espied thro the Telescope, the exact middle Point between the two places whereon the Plumb-Line falls at both Observations on the Limb, is vertical, and answers to the Zenith with respect to the Line of Collimation of the Telescope.

Now having found the Error of the Instrument, that is, the difference between the first Point of the Divisions of the Limb, and the said middle Point answering to the Zenith, you must try to place the Cross-hairs in their true Position, if you can conveniently, but if not, regard must be had to the Error in all Observations, whether of Elevation, or Depression

But note, if the Object be near, and elevated some Minutes above the Horizon, the true Error of the Instrument may be found in the following manner

We have three things given in a Triangle, one of which is the known Distance between the Place of Observation and the Object, the other the Distance between the middle of the Telescope, and the Point of the Surface of the Water, upon which a reflected Ray falls, and the last, the Angle included between those two Sides ; that is, the Arc of the Limb contained between the two places of the Limb upon which the Plumb-Line falls in, observing, as aforesaid, the Object and its Image on the Surface of the Water thro the Telescope. I say, we

have

have the said two Sides and included Angle given, to find the Angle opposite to the lesser Side This being done, if the Arc of the Limb included between the two places whereon the Plumb-Line falls, in observing, as aforesaid, be diminished, on the Side of the Limb produced, by the Quantity of the Angle found, the middle of the remaining Arc will be the true vertical Point Note, To find the Distance between the middle of the Tube of the Telescope, and the Point of the Surface of the Water upon which the reflected Rays fall, you may use a Rod or Thread prolonged from the said Tube to the Surface of the Water

The other way (which is very simple, but yet not easy) of proving whether the Line of Collimation of the fixed Telescope be right, is thus · We suppose in this Method, that the Limb of the Quadrant is continued out, and divided into some few Degrees beyond 90 Now in some serene still Night, we take the Meridian Altitude of some Star near the Zenith, having first turned the divided Face of the Limb of the Quadrant towards the East This being done, within a Night or two after, we again observe the Altitude of the same Star, the divided Face of the Limb being Westward. Then the middle of the Arc of the Limb between the Altitudes at each Observation, will be the Point of 90 Deg that is, a Point thro which a Radius of the Quadrant passes, parallel to the Line of Collimation of the Telescope Note, This Method is very useful for proving the Position of Telescopes, which are adjusted not only to Quadrants, but principally to Sextants, Octants, &c for by means thereof may be found which of the Radii of the several Instruments are parallel to the Lines of Collimation of the Telescope

We shall hereafter shew the Manner of taking the Altitudes of Celestial Bodies, as likewise how to observe them thro Telescopes

Of the Index, or moveable Arm of the Quadrant

I shall conclude this Chapter in saying something concerning the Construction and Use of this Index, which is no more than a moveable Alidade, with a Telescope adjusted thereto, which produces the same effect as the Alidades of other Instruments do, that is, to make any Angle at pleasure with the Telescope fixed to the Quadrant. The principal part of this Index is an Iron or Brass Ruler, drill'd at one end, and is so adjusted to the Central Cylinder, of which we have already spoken, that it has a circular Motion only

Upon this Ruler are fastened two Iron or Brass Frames, in one of which, viz that which is next to the Center of the Instrument, the Object-Glass is placed, and in the other, the Eye-Glass and Cross-hairs, which together make up a Telescope, alike in every thing to the other fixed Telescope of the Quadrant

At the end of the Index joining to the Limb, is a little Opening about the bigness of a Degree of the Limb, thro the middle of which is strained a Hair, which is continued to the Center of the Quadrant. But because in using the Index the said Hair is subject to divers Inconstancies of the Air, it is better to use a thin piece of clear Horn, or a flat Glass, adjusted to the aforesaid little Opening in a Frame, having a Right Line drawn upon that Surface thereof next to the Limb, so that it tends to the Center of the Instrument Note, The Frame is fastened in the little Opening by means of Screws

Now the Index being fastened to the Center before it is used, the Telescope must be proved, that so it may be known whether the fixed Telescope agrees therewith To do which, having placed the Plane of the Instrument horizontally, and directed the fixed Telescope to some Point of a visible Object, distant at least 500 Toises, afterwards the moveable Telescope must be pointed to the same Object, that so one of the Cross-hairs, viz that which is perpendicular to the Plane of the Quadrant, may appear upon the aforesaid Point of the Object for it matters not whether the Intersection of the Hairs appear thereon, or the perpendicular Hair only Then, if the Line drawn upon the Horn or Glass on the Index falls upon the 90th Degree of the Limb of the Quadrant, the Telescopes agree if not, either the Horn or Glass must be removed till the Line drawn thereon falls upon the 90th Degree of the Divisions of the Limb, and then it must be fastened to the Index, or else regard must be had, in all Observations, to the difference between the first Point of the Divisions of the Limb, and the Line drawn upon the said piece of Horn or Glass

CHAP. II.

Of the Construction and Use of the Micrometer.

THE *Micrometer* is an Instrument of great Use in Astronomy, and principally in measuring the apparent Diameters of the Planets, and taking small Distances not exceeding a Degree, or Degree and a half This Instrument is composed of two rectangular Brass Frames, one of which, viz. A B C D, is commonly 2½ Inches long, and 1½ broad, having the Sides
A B

A B and C D, divided into equal Parts, about four Lines distant from each other (for this is according to the Turns of the Screw, as shall be hereafter explain'd) but in such manner, that the Lines drawn thro each Division be perpendicular to the Sides A B and C D, and having human Hairs strain'd from Division to Division, fastened with Wax to the places 2, 2, &c

The other Frame E F G H, whose Length E F is one Inch and a half, is so adjusted to the former Frame, that the Sides E F and G H of the one, may move along the Sides A B and C D of the other, without being separated therefrom, which is done by means of Dove-tail Grooves. The Face of this second Frame next to the divided Face of the former, is likewise furnish'd with a Hair, strain'd at the place 4, so that when the Frame is moving, the said Hair may be always parallel to the Hairs on the other Frame. The Screw I, whose Cylinder is about four or five Lines in Diameter, goes thro, and turns in the Side B D of one of the Frames, which for this purpose is made thicker than the other Sides. The end of this Screw is cut so as to go thorow a round hole made in the Side F H of the lesser Frame, which for this purpose is likewise made thicker than the other Sides; there is also a little Pin K put thro a hole made in the end of the Screw, that so the lesser Frame can no ways move, but in turning the Screw to the right or left, according as you would have the Frame move forwards or backwards. M N is a circular Plate about an Inch in Diameter, fastened with two Screws to the Side B D of the Frame. This Plate is commonly divided into 20 or 60 equal Parts, which serve to reckon the Revolutions and Parts of the Screw, by means of the Index M, which is adjusted under the Neck of the said Screw, and turns with it. Now the Divisions of the Sides of the Frame A B C D, are made according to the Breadth of the Threads of the Screw, for if, for example, the Divisions are desired to be 10 Turns of the Screw distant from each other, turn the said Screw ten times about, and note how far the Frame hath moved; if it has moved four Lines, the Divisions must be four Lines distant from each other, and so of others.

Now because Hairs are subject to divers Accidents by Heat, and otherwise, therefore M *de la Hire* proposes a very thin and smooth piece of Glass to be used instead of them, adjusted in Grooves made in the Sides of the Frame, and having very fine parallel Lines drawn thereon, which produce the same effect as the parallel Hairs. All the difficulty consists in chusing a very fine and well polished Piece of Glass, and drawing the Lines extremely nice, for the Defaults will grosly appear, when the said Lines are perceived in a Telescope.

Note, These Lines must be very lightly drawn upon the Glass with a small Diamond, whose Point is very fine.

This Instrument is joined to a Telescope, by means of the prominent Pieces L, L, which slide in a kind of parallelogramick Tin-Box, at the two Sides of which are two Circular Openings, wherein are solder'd two short Tubes, that on one Side being to receive the Tube carrying the Eye-Glass, and that on the other Side, the Tube carrying the Object-Glass, so that the Micrometer may be in the Focus of the said Object-Glass.

Use of the Micrometer.

In order to use this Instrument, a lively Representation of Objects appearing thro the Telescope must be made in the Point whereat the parallel Hairs are placed, therefore if the Object-Glass be placed at its Focal Distance from the Micrometer, more or less, according to the Nature and Constitution of the Eyes of the Observator, the Objects and the parallel Hairs will appear distinctly in the said Focus.

If then the Focal Length of the Object-Glass be measured in Lines or 12th Parts of Inches, or, which is all one, the Distance from the Center of the Object-Glass to the parallel Hairs of the Micrometer, be measured, this Distance is to the Length of four Lines, which is the Interval between two fixed parallel Hairs nighest each other, as Radius is to the Tangent of the Angle, subtended by the two nearest parallel Hairs. This is evident from Dioptricks: for the Distance between the Object and the Observator's Eye, is supposed to be so great, that the Focal Length of the Object-Glass, compared therewith, is of no consequence, so that the Rays proceeding from the Points of the Object directly pass thro the Center of the Object-Glass in the same manner, as tho the Observator's Eye was placed in the said Object-Glass. This may be shewn by Experience thus:

Draw two black Lines parallel upon a very smooth and white Board, whose Interval let be such, that at the Distance of 200 or 300 Toises, they may be met with or embraced by two parallel Hairs of the Micrometer. This being done, remove the Table in a convenient place (there being no Wind stirring) so far from the Telescope, until the Lines drawn thereon, which must be perpendicular to a Right Line drawn from the Table to the Micrometer, be catched by two fixed parallel Threads of the Micrometer, and then the Distance between the Table and the Object-Glass will have the same proportion to the Distance between the Lines on the Table, as Radius is to the Tangent of the Angle subtended by two Hairs of the Micrometer.

Now move the Frame E F G H, by means of the Screw, till its Hair exactly agrees with one of the parallel Hairs of the other Frame, and when this is done, observe the Situation of the Index of the Screw, then turn the Screw until the said Hair of the Frame E F G H

agrees

agrees with the next nearest fixed Hair of the other Frame, or, which is the same thing, move the Frame E F G H the Length of four Lines, or one third of an Inch, which may be easily known by means of the Object-Glass, which magnifies Objects, and count the Revolutions and Parts of the Screw, compleated in moving the said Frame that Length. Finally, make a Table, shewing how many Revolutions, and parts of a Revolution of the said Screw, are answerable to every Minute and Second, by having the Angle subtended by the two black Lines on the Board given, and taking the Revolutions proportional to the Angles; that is, if a certain Number of Revolutions give a certain Angle, half this Number will give half the Angle, &c. And this Proportion is exact enough in these small Angles

Now the manner of taking the apparent Diameters of the Planets, is thus · Having directed the Telescope, and its Micrometer, towards a Planet, dispose the Hairs, by the Motion of the Telescope, in such a manner, that one of the fixed parallel Hairs do just touch one edge of the Planet, and turn the Screw till the moveable Hair just touches the opposite edge of the said Planet. Then, by means of the Table, you will know how many Minutes or Seconds correspond to the Number of Revolutions or Parts, reckoning from the Point of the Plate over which the Index stood when the fixed Hair touched one edge of the Planet, to the Point it stands over when the moveable Hair touches the opposite edge, and consequently, the apparent Diameter of the said Planet will be had. And in this manner may small Angles on Earth be taken, which may be easier done than those of the Celestial Bodies, because of their Immobility

This Method is convenient enough for measuring the apparent Diameters of the Planets, if the Body of any one of them moves between the parallel Hairs. Yet it ought to be observed, that the Sun and Moon's Diameters appear very unequal upon the account of Refraction, for in small Elevations above the Horizon, by the space of 30 Minutes, the vertical Diameters appear something lesser than they really are in the Horizon, and the horizontal Diameters cannot be found, unless with much trouble, and several repeated Observations, as likewise the Distance between two Stars, or the Horns of the Moon, because of their Diurnal Motions, which appear thro the Telescope very swift

If two Stars of different Altitudes pass by the Meridian at different times, the Difference of their Altitudes will be the Difference of their Distances from the Equator towards either of the Poles, which is called their Difference of Declination, and by their Difference of Time in coming to the Meridian, the Difference of their Distance from a determinate Point of the Equator, that is, the first Degree of *Aries* will be had, and this is their Difference of Right Ascension

If the two Stars are distant from each other, we have time enough, in the Interval of their Passage by the Meridian and Micrometer, to finish the Operations regarding the first, before proceeding to those of the second, but if they be very near each other, it is extremely difficult to make both the Observations at the same time, that so the two Stars may be precisely catched in the Meridian. But M *de la Hire* shews how to remedy this Inconveniency, by only using the common Micrometer for the Observation of the Passage of Stars between, or upon the Hairs of the Micrometer, will give, by easy Consequences, their Difference of Right Ascension and Declination, without even supposing a Meridian known or drawn

But if the Difference of Declination and Right Ascension of two Stars that cannot be taken in between the Hairs of the Micrometer be required, this may be found in the following manner.

We adjust a Cross-hair to the Micrometer, cutting the parallel ones at Right Angles, Fig. 10· which we fasten with Wax to the middle of the Sides A C and B D. Then the Telescope, and its Micrometer, being fixed in a convenient Position, so that the Stars may successively pass by the parallel Hairs, as the Stars A and S, in Figure 10, we observe, by a second Pendulum Clock, the time wherein the first Star A touches the Point in which the aforementioned Cross-hair A S crosses some one of the parallel Hairs, as A *d*. The Micrometer being disposed for this Observation, which is not difficult to do, reckon the Seconds of time elapsed between the Observations made in the Point A, and the arrival of the said Star to the Point B, being the concourse of another parallel Hair B D. We likewise observe the Time wherein the other Star S meets the Cross-hair at the Point S, and then at the Point D of the parallel Hair B D. *Note*, It is the same thing if the Star S first meets the parallel Hair in D, and afterwards the Cross-hair in S

Now as the Number of Seconds the Star A is moving thorow the space A B, is to the Number of Seconds the Star S is moving thorow the space S D, so is the Distance A C, known in Minutes and Seconds of a Degree in the Micrometer, to the Distance C S, in Minutes and Seconds of a Degree. But the Horary Seconds of the Motion thorow the space A B, must be converted into Minutes and Seconds of a great Circle, by the Rule of Proportion

Having first converted the Seconds of the time of the said Motion from A to B, which may be here esteemed as a Right Line, or an Arc of a great Circle, into Minutes and Seconds of a Circle, in allowing 15 Minutes of a Circle to every Minute of an Hour, and

S f   the

the same for Seconds: We say, by the Rule of Proportion, As Radius is to the Sine Complement of the Stars known Declination, so is the Number of Seconds in the Arc A B also known, to the Number of Seconds of the same kind contained in the Arc C A, as an Arc of a great Circle

Moreover, in the Right-angled Triangle C A B, the Sides C A, and A B being given, as likewise the Right Angle at C, we find the Angle C A B, and supposing C P R perpendicular to the Line A B, A B will be to C A as C A is to A P

But in the Right-angled Triangle C A P, we have (besides the Right Angle) the Angle A, as likewise the Side C A given, therefore as Radius is to C A, so is the Sine of the Angle C A P, to C P. And as the Number of horary Seconds of the Motion from A to B, is the horary Seconds in the Motion from S to D, so is C P to C R Then taking C R from C P, or else adding them together, according as A B or S D is next to the Point C, and we shall have the Quantity of P R in parts of a great Circle, which will be the Difference of the two Stars Declinations We have no regard here to the Difference of Motion thorow the spaces A B and S D, caused by the difference of Declination, because it is of no consequence in the Difference of Declinations, as they are observed by the Micrometer

Finally, As A B is to A P, so is the Number of horary Seconds of the observed Motion of the Star A thorow the space A B, to the Number of Seconds of the Motion of the said Star thorow the space A P Wherefore the time when the Star A comes to P, will be known But as the Number of Horary Seconds of the Motion thorow the Space A B is to the Number of Horary Seconds of the Motion thorow the Space S D, so is the Number of Horary Seconds of the Motion thorow the Space A P, to the Number of Horary Seconds of the Motion thorow S R.

Moreover, The Time when the Star S is in S is known, to which if the Time of the Motion thorow S R be added, when A and S are on the same side the Point C, or substracted if otherwise, and the time when the Star is in R will be had Now the difference of Time between the arrivals of the Stars in P and R, that is, the difference of the Times wherein they come to the Meridian, will be the difference of their Right Ascensions, which by the Rule of Proportion may be reduced into Degrees and Minutes *Note*, We have no regard here to the proper Motion of the Stars

From hence it is easy to know how, instead of the parallel Hair A B, to use another parallel one, passing thro A, or any other, as also a moveable Parallel, provided that they form Similar Triangles, as will be easily conceiv'd by what hath been already said

The aforesaid Operation may yet be done by another Method For the parallel Hairs of the Micrometer being so disposed, that the first of the Stars may move upon one of them, and if the time wherein the said Star crosses the Cross-hair of the Micrometer be observed, and if moreover the time wherein the other Star crosses the said Cross-hair be observed, and at the same time the moveable parallel Hair be adjusted to the second Star, no ways altering the Micrometer, we shall have, by means of the Distance between that parallel Hair, the first Star moved upon, and the moveable parallel Hair, the Distance between two parallel Circles, to the Equator, passing thro the places of the said Stars, which is their Difference of Declination And if moreover, the Difference of the Times between the passages of each of the Stars by the Cross-hair of the Micrometer be converted into Minutes and Seconds of a Degree, the said Stars ascensional Difference will be had This needs no Example

But if this be required between some Star, and the Sun or Moon, as for Example, *Mercury* moving under the Sun's Disk, place the Micrometer so, that the Limb of the Sun may move along one of the parallel Hairs, and observe the times when the Sun's antecedent and consequent Limbs, and the Center of *Mercury*, touch the Cross-hair, then the Difference of *Mercury*'s Declination, and the Sun's Limb, by means of the moveable Hair, will be had, the Micrometer remaining fixed And if to the time of the Observation of the Sun's antecedent Limb, half the time elapsed between the Passages of the antecedent and consequent Limb be added, we shall have the time of the Passage of the Sun's Center by the Cross-hair of the Micrometer, and by this means the difference of the times between the Passage of the Sun's Center and *Mercury* over the Cross-hair, that is, by the Meridian, will be obtained And this Difference of time being converted into Degrees and Minutes, will give their ascensional Difference

Moreover, since the Sun's Center is in the Ecliptick, if in the same time as the said Center passes over the Cross-hair, (the Sun's true place being otherwise known) you seek in Tables, the Angle of the Ecliptick with the Meridian, you will likewise have the Angle that the Ecliptick makes with the Sun's Parallel, as in *Fig. 11* the Angle O C R, of the Ecliptick O C B, and of the Parallel to the Equator R C Let P C be the Meridian, *Mercury* in M, the Center of the Sun in C, M R parallel to P C, and C R the difference of Right Ascension between the Center of the Sun C, and *Mercury* in M Now the Minutes of the Difference of the Right Ascension C R in the Parallel, being reduced to Minutes of a great Circle, say, As Radius is to the Sine Complement of the Sun's or *Mercury*'s Declination, so is the Number of Seconds of the Difference of Right Ascension, to the Number of

Seconds

Fig. 11.

Seconds C R, as the Arc of a great Circle. Then in the Triangle C R'T, Right-angled at R, we have the Side C R (now found), as also the Angle R C T, *viz* the Difference between the Right Angle, and the Angle made by the Ecliptick and Meridian, whence the Hypothenuse C T, and the Side R T may be found. And if R T be taken from M R, which is the difference of Declination of *Mercury* in M, and the Center of the Sun in C, there will remain T M. Again, as C T is to T R, so is T M to T O, M O will be the Latitude of *Mercury* at the time of Observation. And adding T O to the Side C T, we shall have C O, the difference of Longitude between *Mercury* and the Sun's Center. Therefore the Sun's Longitude being known, that of *Mercury*'s may also be found.

It moreover, two or three Hours after the first Observation of *Mercury* in M, the difference of Declination and Right Ascension thereof be again observed, when he is come to N, we shall find, as before, N Q the Latitude of *Mercury*, and C Q the difference of Longitude of him and the Sun's Center C, whence the place of the apparent Node of *Mercury* will be had. But note, the Point of Concourse A, in the Right Line M N, with the Ecliptick C B, is not the place of the said Node, with regard to the Point C, because between the Observations made in the Points M and N, the Sun by its proper Motion is moved a few Minutes forwards, according to the Succession of Signs, which notwithstanding we have not regarded in the Observations. Therefore say, As the difference of the Latitudes M O and N Q, to O Q, *in aus* the proper Motion of the Sun, between the Observations made in M and N, so is M O to the Distance O A, whence the true Distance from the Sun's Center C to *Mercury*'s Node A will be had. Note, The proper Motion of the Sun between the Observations must be taken from O Q, because during that time *Mercury* is Retrograde, but if its Motion had been direct, the Sun's Motion must have been added to O Q.

In the Observations of *Mercury*'s Passage under the Sun's Disk, we have had no regard to the proper Motion of the Sun, as being of small consequence, but if it is required to be brought into Consideration, C O and C Q must be diminished by so much of the Sun's proper Motion, as is performed in the Interval of time between the Passage of the Sun's Center and *Mercury*, by the Meridian.

By the same Method, the Distances of Planets from each other, or from fixed Stars near the Ecliptick, may be observed, nevertheless, excepting some Minutes, not only upon the account of the proper Motions of the Stars, but also because of their Distance from the Ecliptick or too great Latitude. Note, This second Method for finding the Difference of Declination and Right Ascension is not exacter than the former, altho it is perform'd with less Calculation, for it is so difficult to dispose the Hairs of the Micrometer according to the Parallel of the Diurnal Motion, that it cannot be done, but by several uncertain trials.

M *de la Hire* hath also invented another Micrometer, whose Construction is easy, for it Fig 12. is only a pair of proportional Compasses, whose Legs on one Side, are, for example, ten times longer than those on the other Side. The shortest Legs of these Compasses must be put thro a slit made in the Tube of the Telescope, and placed so in the Focus of the Object-Glass, that the two Points, which ought to be very fine, may be apply'd to all Objects represented in the said Focus. Then if the Angle subtended by the Distance of two Objects in the Focus of the Object-Glass be required to be found by means of these Compasses, you must shut or open the two shortest Legs till their Points just touch the Representations of the Objects, and keeping the Compasses to this opening, if the longest Legs be apply'd to the Divisions of a Scale, the Minutes and Seconds contained in the Angle subtended by the Distance of the aforesaid Objects will be had. The Manner of dividing the said Scale, is the same as that for finding the Distances of the parallel Hairs of the other Micrometer, in saying by the Rule of Proportion, As the Number of Lines contain'd in the Focal Length of the Object-Glass, is to one Line, so is Radius to the Tangent of the Angle subtended by one Line in the Focus, therefore if the longest Legs be ten times longer than the others, ten Lines on the Scale will measure the said Angle subtended by one Line, which being known, it will be easy to divide the Scale for Minutes and Seconds.

This Micrometer may be used for taking the apparent Diameters of the Planets, as also to take the Distances of fixed Stars which are near each other, and measure small Distances on Earth.

C H A P. III.

Of making Celestial Observations.

OBservations of the Sun, Stars, &c. made in the Day-time with long Telescopes, are easy, because the Cross-hairs in the Focus of the Object-Glass may then be distinctly perceived, but in the Night the said Cross-hairs must be enlightened with a Link, or

Candle,

Candle, that so one may see them with the Stars, thro the Telescope : and this is done two ways

First, We enlighten the Object-Glass of the Telescope, in obliquely bringing a Candle near to it, that so its Smoke or Body do not hinder the Progress of the Rays coming from the Star But if the Object-Glass be something deep in the Tube, it cannot sufficiently be enlightened, without the Candle's being very near it, and this hinders the Sight of the Star, and if the Telescope is above six Feet long, it will be difficult sufficiently to enlighten the Object-Glass, that so the cross Hairs be distinctly perceived

Secondly, We make a sufficient opening in the Tube of the Telescope near the Focus of the Object-Glass, thro which we enlighten with a Candle the cross Hairs placed in the Focus

But this Method is subject to several Inconveniencies, for the Light being so near the Observator's Eyes, he is often incommoded thereby And moreover, since the cross Hairs are by that opening uncovered and exposed to the Air, they lose their Situation, become slack, or may be broken

Besides this, the said second Method is liable to an Inconveniency for which it ought to be entirely neglected, and that is, that it is subject to an Error, which is, that according to the Position of the Light illuminating the cross Hairs, the said Hairs will appear in different Situations because, for example, when the Horizontal Hair is enlightened above, we perceive a luminous Line, which may be taken for the said Hair, and which appears at its upper Superficies And contrariwise, when the said Hair is enlightened underneath, the luminous Line will appear at its lower Superficies, the Hair not being moved, and this Error will be the Diameter of the Hair, which often amounts to more than six Seconds But M *de la Hire* hath found a Remedy for this Inconveniency For he often found, in Observations made in Moonshine Nights, in Weather a little foggy, that the cross Hairs were distinctly perceived, whereas, when the Heavens were serene, they could scarcely be seen : whence he bethought himself to cover that End of the Tube next to the Object-Glass with a Piece of Gawze, or very fine white silken Crape, which succeeded so well, that a Link placed at a good distance from the Telescope so enlightened the Crape, that the cross Hairs distinctly appeared, and the Sight of the Stars was no way obscured

Solar Observations cannot be made without placing a smoked Glass between the Telescope and the Eye, which may thus be prepared Take two equal and well polished round Pieces of flat Glass, upon the Surface of one of which, all round its Limb, glew a Pasteboard Ring, then put the other Piece of Glass into the Smoke of a Link, taking it several times out, and putting it in again, for fear lest the Heat of the Link should break it, until the Smoke be so thick thereon, that the Link can scarcely be seen thro it but the Smoke must not be all over it of the same Thickness, that so that Place thereof may be chosen answering to the Sun's Splendor This being done, this Glass thus blackened, must be glewed to the before mentioned Pasteboard Ring, with its blacken'd Side next to the other Glass, that so the Smoke may not be rubbed off

Note, When the Sun's Altitude is observed thro a Telescope, consisting of but two Glasses, its upper Limb will appear as tho it were the lower one

There are two principal kinds of Observations of Stars, the one being when they are in the Meridian, and the other when they are in Vertical Circles

If the Position of the Meridian be known, and then the Plane of the Quadrant be placed in the Meridian Circle, by means of the plumb Line suspended at the Center, the Meridian Altitudes of Stars may be easily taken, which are the principal Operations, serving as a Foundation to the whole Art of Astronomy The Meridian Altitude of a Star may likewise be had by means of a Pendulum Clock, if the exact Time of the Star's Passage by the Meridian be known Now it must be observed, that Stars have the same Altitude during a Minute before and after their Passage by the Meridian, if they be not in or near the Zenith ; but if they be, their Altitudes must be taken every Minute, when they are near the Meridian, which we suppose already known, and then their greatest or least Altitudes will be the Meridian Altitudes sought

As to the Observations made without the Meridian in Vertical Circles, the Position of a given Vertical Circle must be known, or found by the following Method

First, The Quadrant and its Telescope remaining in the same Situation wherein it was when the Altitude of a Star, together with the Time of its Passage by the Intersection of the cross Hairs in the Focus of the Object-Glass, was taken, we observe the Time when the Sun, or some fixed Star, whose Latitude and Longitude is known, arrives to the Vertical Hair in the Telescope, and from thence the Position of the said Vertical Circle will be had, and also the observed Star's true Place.

But if the Sun, or some other Star, does not pass by the Mouth of the Tube of the Telescope, and if a Meridian Line be otherwise well drawn upon a Floor, or very level Ground, in the Place of Observation, you must suspend a Plumb-Line to some fixed Place, about three or four Toises distant from the Quadrant, under which upon the Floor must a Mark be made in a right Line with the Plumb-Line. This being done, you must put a thin Piece of Brass, or Pasteboard, very near the Object-Glass, in the middle of which there is a small Slit vertically placed, and passing thro the Center of the Circular Figure of the Object-Glass Now by means of this Slit, the beforementioned Plumb-Line may be perceived thro the Telescope, which before could not be seen, because of its Nearness thereto. Then the Plumb-Line must be removed and suspended, so that it be perceived in a right Line with the vertical Hair in the Focus of the Object-Glass, and a Point marked on the Floor directly under it. And if a right Line be drawn thro this Point, and that marked under the Plumb-Line before it was removed, the said Line will meet the Meridian drawn upon the Floor, and so we shall have the Position of the vertical Circle the observed Star is in, with respect to the Meridian, the Angle whereof may be measured in assuming known Lengths upon the two Lines from the Point of Concourse, for if thro the Extremities of these known Lengths, a Line or Base be drawn, we shall have a Triangle, whose three Sides being known, the Angle at the Vertex may be found, which will be the Angle made by the Vertical Circle and Meridian

The Manner of taking the Meridian Altitudes of Stars

It is very difficult to place the Plane of the Quadrant in the Meridian exactly enough to take the Meridian Altitude of a Star, for unless there be a convenient Place and a Wall, where the Quadrant may be firmly fastened in the Plane of the Meridian, which is very difficult to do, we shall not have the true Position of the Meridian, proper to observe all the Stars, as we have mentioned already Therefore it will be much easier, and principally in Journeys, to use a portable Quadrant, by means of which the Altitude of a Star must be observed a little before its Passage over the Meridian, every Minute, if possible, until its greatest or least Altitude be had Now, tho by this means we have not the true Position of the Meridian, yet we have the apparent Meridian Altitude of the Star

Altho this Method is very good, and free from any sensible Error, yet if a Star passes by the Meridian near the Zenith, we canot have its Meridian Altitude, by repeated Observations every Minute, unless by chance, because in every Minute of an Hour the Altitude augments about fifteen Minutes of a Degree and in these kind of Observations, the inconvenient Situation or the Observator, the Variation of the Star's Azimuth several Degrees in a little time, the Alteration that the Instrument must have, and the Difficulty in well replacing it vertically again, hinders our making of Observations oftner than in every fourth Minute of an Hour, during which Time the Difference in the Star's Altitude will be one Degree Therefore in these Cases it will be better to have the true Position of the Meridian, or the exact Time a Star passes by the Meridian, in order to place the Instrument in the said Meridian, or move it so that one may observe the Altitude of the Star the moment it passes by the Meridian

Of Refractions

The Meridian Altitudes of two fixed Stars, which are equal, or a small matter different, the one being North, and the other South, being observed, and also their Declination otherwise given, to find the Refraction answering to the Degrees of Altitude of the said Stars, and the true Height of the Pole, or Equator, above the Place of Observation.

Having found the apparent Meridian Altitude of some Star near the Pole (by the aforegoing Directions) if the Complement of the said Star's Declination be added thereto, or taken therefrom, we shall have the apparent Height of the Pole After the same manner may also the apparent Height of the Equator be found, by means of the Meridian Altitude of some Star near the Equator, in adding or substracting its Declination

Then these Heights of the Pole and Equator being added together, their Sum will always be greater than a Quadrant, but 90 Degrees being taken from this Sum, the Remainder will be double the Refraction of either of the Stars observed at the same height : and therefore taking the said Refraction from the said apparent Height of the Pole, or Equator, we shall have their true Altitude

Example

Let the Meridian Altitude of a Star observed below the North Pole, be 30 deg 15 min. and the Complement of its Declination 5 deg whence the apparent Height of the Pole will be 35 deg 15 min Also let the apparent Meridian Altitude of some other Star, observed near the Equator, be 30 deg 40 min and its Declination 40 deg 9 min whence the apparent Height of the Equator will be 54 deg 49 min. Therefore the Sum of the Heights of the Pole and Equator thus found, will be 90 deg 4 min from which substracting 90 deg. and there remains 4 min which is double the Refraction at 30 deg 28 min of Altitude, which is about the middle between the Heights found · therefore at the Altitude of 30 deg 15 min the Refraction will be something above 2 min viz. 2 min 1 sec. and at the Altitude of 30 deg. 40 min the Refraction will be 1 min 59 sec.

Lastly, If 2 min 1 sec. be taken from the apparent Height of the Pole 35 min 15 sec the Remainder 35 deg 12 min 59 sec. will be the true Height of the Pole, and so the true Height of the Equator will be 54 deg 47 min 1 sec as being the Complement of the Height of the Pole to 90 deg

Note,

Note, The Refraction and Height of the Pole found according to this way, will be so much the more exact, as the Altitude of the Stars is greater, for if the Difference of the Altitudes of each Star should be even 2 deg when their Altitudes are above 30 deg we may by this Method have the Refraction, and the true Height of the Pole, because in this Case the Difference of Refraction in Altitudes differing two Degrees, is not sensible

Another Way of observing Refractions

The Quantity of Refraction may also be found by the Observations of one Star only, whose Meridian Altitude is 90 deg or a little less, for the Height of the Pole or Equator above the Place of Observation being otherwise known, we shall have the Star's true Declination, by its Meridian Altitude, because Refractions near the Zenith are insensible

Now if we observe by a Pendulum the exact Times when the said Star comes to every Degree of Altitude, as also the Time of its Passage by the Meridian, which may be known by the equal Altitudes of the Star being East and West, we have three things given in a spherical Triangle, *viz.* the Distance between the Pole and Zenith, the Complement of the Star's Declination, and the Angle comprehended by the aforesaid Arcs, namely, the Difference of mean Time between the Passage of the Star by the Meridian and its Place, converted into Degrees and Minutes; to which must be added the convenable proportional Part of the mean Motion of the Sun in the Proportion of 59 min 8 sec per Day: therefore the true Arc of the Vertical Circle between the Zenith and the true Place of the Star may be found

But the apparent Arc of the Altitude of the Star is had by Observation, and the Difference of these Arcs will be the Quantity of Refraction at the Height of the Star. By a like Calculation the Refraction of every Degree of Altitude may be found

The same may be done by means of the Sun, or any other Star, provided its Declination be known, to the end that at the time of Observation the true Distance of the Sun or Star from the Zenith may be found

The Refractions of Stars being known, it will then be easy to find the Height of the Pole, for having observed the Meridian Altitude of the Polar Star, as well above as below the Pole, the same Day, and having diminished each Altitude by its proper Refraction, half of the Difference of the corrected Altitudes, added to the lesser Altitude corrected, or substracted from the greater Altitude thus corrected, will give the true Height of the Pole

M *de la Hire* has observed with great Care for several Years the Meridian Altitudes of fixed Stars, and principally of *Sirius*, and *Lucida Lyra*, with Astronomical Quadrants very well divided, and very good Telescopes at different Hours of the Day and Night, and at different Seasons of the Year, and he assures us, that he never found any Difference in their Altitudes, but what proceeded from their proper Motion

And because *Sirius* comes to about the 26th Degree of the Meridian, we might doubt whether in the lesser Altitudes the Refractions in the Winter would be greater than those in the Summer, hence he also observed, with the late M *Picard*, the lesser Meridian Altitudes of the Star *Capella*, which is about 4½ Degrees at several different Times of the Year

Having compared these different Observations together, and made the necessary Reductions, because of the proper Motion of that Star, there was scarcely found one Minute of Difference, that could proceed from any other Cause but Refraction. Therefore he made but one Table of the Refraction of the Sun, Moon, and the Stars, for all Times of the Year, conformable to the Observations that he made from them

Notwithstanding this, one would think that Refractions nigh the Horizon are subject to divers Inconstancies, according to the Constitution of the Air, and the Nature of high or low Grounds, as M *de la Hire* has often found, for observing the Meridian Altitudes of Stars at the Foot of a Mountain, which seemed to be even with the top of it, they appeared to him a little higher, than if he had observed them at the top · But if the Observations of others may be depended upon, Refractions are greater, even in Summer, in the frozen Zones, than in the temperate Zones.

How to find the Time of the Equinox and Solstice by Observation

Having found the Height of the Equator, the Refraction and the Sun's Parallax at the same Altitude, it will not afterwards be difficult to find the Time in which the Center of the Sun is in the Equator, for if from the apparent Meridian Altitude of the Center of the Sun, the same Day as it comes to the Equinox, be taken the convenient Refraction, and then the Parallax be added thereto, the true Meridian Altitude of the Sun's Center will be had Now the Difference of this Altitude, and the Height of the Equinoctial, will shew the Time of the true Equinox before or after Noon and if the Sum of the Seconds of that Difference be divided by 59, the Quotient will shew the Hours and Fractions which must be added or substracted from the true Hour of Noon, to have the Time of the true Equinox

The Hours of the Quotient must be added to the time of Noon, if the Meridian Altitude of the Sun be lesser than the height of the Equator about the time of the vernal Equinox , but they muſt be ſubſtracted, if it be found greater   You muſt proceed contrariwiſe, when the Sun is near the autumnal Equinox

Example   The true Height 41 deg. 10 min of the Equator being given, and having obſerved the true Meridian Altitude 41 deg 5 min 15 ſec of the Sun, found by the apparent Altitude of its upper or lower Limb, corrected by its Semidiameter, Refraction, and Parallax, and the Difference will be 4 min 45 ſec or 285 Seconds, which being divided by 59, the Quotient will be 4⁴⁵, that is, 4 Hours 48 Minutes, which muſt be added to Noon, if the Sun be in the vernal Equinox, and conſequently the time of the Equinox will happen 4 Hours 48 Minutes after Noon   But if the Sun was in the autumnal Equinox, the time of the ſaid Equinox would happen 4 Hours 48 Minutes before Noon, that is, at 12 Minutes paſt Seven in the Morning

As to the Solſtices, there is much more Difficulty in determining them than the Equinoxes, for one Obſervation only is not ſufficient , becauſe about this time the Difference between the Meridian Altitudes in one Day, and the next ſucceeding Day, is almoſt inſenſible

Now the exact Meridian Altitude of the Sun muſt be taken, 12 or 15 Days before the Solſtice, and as many after, that ſo one may find the ſame Meridian Altitude by little and little , to the end that by the proportional Parts of the alteration of the Sun's Meridian Altitude, we may more exactly find the time wherein the Sun is found at the ſame Altitude, before and after the Solſtice, being in the ſame Parallel to the Equator

Now having found the time elapſed between both the Situations of the Sun, you muſt take half of it, and ſeek in the Tables the true place of the Sun at theſe three times This being done, the Difference of the extreme Places of the Sun muſt be added to the mean Place, in order to have the mean Place with Compariſon to the Extremes , but if the mean Place found by Calculation, does not agree with the mean Place found by Compariſon, you muſt take the Difference, and add to the mean Time, the Time anſwering to that Difference, if the mean Time found by Calculation be leſſer, but contrariwiſe, it muſt be ſubſtracted if it be greater, in order to have the Time of the Solſtice

Example   The laſt Day of *May*, the apparent Meridian Altitude of the Sun was found at the Royal Obſervatory, 64 deg 47 min 25 ſec and the 22d Day of *June* following, the apparent Meridian Altitude was found 64 deg 28 min 15 ſec from whence we know, by having the Difference of Declination at thoſe times, that the Sun came to the Parallel of the firſt Obſervation, the 22d of *June*, at 4 Hours 12 Minutes in the Morning, and conſequently the mean Time between the Obſervations, was on the 22d of *June*, at 2 Hours 6 Minutes in the Morning

Now by Tables, the true place of the Sun at the time of the firſt Obſervation, was 2 Signs 18 deg 58 min 23 ſec and at the time of the laſt it was 3 Signs, 11 deg 4 min. 52 ſec and in the middle time 3 Signs, 1 min 56 ſec   But the Difference of the two extreme Places is 22 deg 6 min 29 ſec half of which is 11 deg. 3 min 15 ſec which added to the mean Place, makes 3 Signs, 1 min 38 ſec which is the mean Place with compariſon to the Extremes   Again, The Difference between the mean Place, by calculation 3 Signs, 1 min 56 ſec and the mean Place by Compariſon, is 18 Seconds, which anſwers to 7 min 18 ſec. of Time, which muſt be taken from the mean Time, becauſe the mean Place by Calculation is greater than the mean Place by Compariſon   Therefore the Time of the Solſtice was the 11th of *June*, at 1 Hour, 58 min 18 ſec in the Morning

Note, The Error of a few Seconds, in the obſerved Altitude of the Sun, will cauſe an alteration of an Hour in the true time of the Solſtice , as in the propoſed Example, 10 Seconds, or thereabouts, in Altitude, will cauſe an Error of an Hour, whence the true Time of the Solſtice cannot be had but with Inſtruments well divided, and ſeveral very exact Obſervations

Obſervations made in the Royal Obſervatory at Paris, *about the Time of the Solſtice for finding the Height of the Pole, and the Sun's greateſt Declination or Obliquity of the Ecliptick*

	Deg.	Min	Sec
The apparent Meridian Altitude of the upper Limb of the Sun at the time of the Summer Solſtice, gathered from ſeveral Obſervations, is found —	64	55	24
Refraction to be ſubſtracted ————	00	00	33
Parallax to be added ————	00	00	01
True Altitude of the upper Limb of the Sun ————	64	54	52
Semidiameter of the Sun ————	00	15	49
True Meridian Altitude of the Sun's Center ————	64	39	03
At the time of the Winter Solſtice, the apparent Meridian Altitude of the upper Limb of the Sun	18	00	24
Refraction to be ſubſtracted ————	00	03	12
Parallax to be added ————	00	00	05
True Altitude of the Sun's upper Limb ————	17	57	17
Semidiameter of the Sun ————	00	16	21

True

	Deg	Min	Sec
True Meridian Altitude of the Sun's Center ———	17	40	56

Then the true Diſtance of the Tropicks is ———	46	58	7
The half, which is the greateſt Declination of the Sun, is ——	23	29	3½
The Height of the Equator above the Obſervatory ———	41	09	59½
Its Complement, which is the Height of the Pole ———	48	50	00½

Obſervations of the Polar Star

By divers Obſervations of the greateſt and leaſt apparent Meridian Altitudes of the Polar Star, which is in the end of the Tail of the Little Bear, it is concluded that the apparent Altitude of the Pole, as M *Picard* has denoted it in his Book of the Dimenſions of the Earth, between *St James's* and *St Martin's* Gates (about *S Jaques de la Boucherie,* at *Paris*) is 48 deg 52 min 20 ſec

	Deg	Min	Sec
The Reduction being made according to the Diſtance of the Places, the apparent Height of the Pole at the Royal Obſervatory will be ———	48	52	02
The Convenable Refraction to that Height ———	00	01	04
Then the true Height of the Pole at the Obſervatory ———	48	52	58
For which let us take ———	48	50	00
And conſequently the Height of the Equator will be ———	41	10	00

The true or apparent Time in which a Planet or fixed Star paſſes by the Meridian, being given, to find the Difference of Right Aſcenſion between the fixed Star, or Planet, and the Sun

The given Time from Noon to or from the time of the Paſſage of the Star or Planet by the Meridian, muſt be converted into Degrees, and what is required will be anſwered

Example *Jupiter* paſſed by the Meridian at 10 Hours, 23 min 15 ſec in the Morning, whoſe Diſtance in time from Noon, which is 1 Hour, 36 min 45 ſec being converted into Degrees of the Equator, will give 24 deg 11 min 15 ſec for the Difference of Right Aſcenſion between the Sun and *Jupiter*, in that moment the Center of *Jupiter* paſſed by the Meridian

In this, and the following Problem, we have propoſed the true or apparent Time, and not the mean Time, becauſe the true Time is eaſier to know by Obſervations of the Sun, than the mean Time We ſhall explain what is meant by mean Time, as likewiſe true or apparent Time, in the next Chapter

The true Time between the Paſſages of two fixed Stars by the Meridian being given, or elſe of a fixed Star and a Planet, to find their Aſcenſional Difference

The given Time between their Paſſages by the Meridian muſt be converted into Degrees of the Equator, and the Right Aſcenſion of the true Motion of the Sun anſwering to that time, muſt be added thereto, then the Sum will be the Aſcenſional Difference ſought

Example Suppoſe between the Paſſages of the Great Dog, called *Sirius,* by the Meridian, and the Heart of the Lion named *Regulus,* there is elapſed 3 Hours, 20 min. of time, and the Right Aſcenſion of the true Motion of the Sun, let be 7 min 35 ſec

Whence converting 3 Hours, 20 min into Degrees of the Equator, and there will be had 50 deg to which adding 7 min 35 ſec and the Sum 50 deg 7 min 35 ſec will be the Aſcenſional Difference between *Sirius* and *Regulus*

You muſt proceed thus for the Aſcenſional Difference of a fixed Star and a Planet, or of two Planets, yet note, if the proper Motion of the Planet or Planets be conſiderable between both their Paſſages by the Meridian, regard muſt be had thereto

How to obſerve Eclipſes.

Amongſt the Obſervations of Eclipſes, we have the Beginning, the End, and the Total Emerſion, which may exactly enough be eſtimated by the naked Eye, without Teleſcopes, except the Beginning and the End of Eclipſes of the Moon, where an Error of one or two Minutes may be made, becauſe it is difficult certainly to determine the Extremity of the Shadow But the Quantity of the Eclipſe, that is, the eclipſed Portion of the Sun and Moon's Diſk, which is meaſured by Digits, or the 12th parts of the Sun and Moon's Diameter, and Minutes, or the 60th parts of Digits, cannot be well known without a Teleſcope joined to ſome Inſtrument For an Eſtimation made with the naked Eye is very ſubject to Error, as it is eaſy to ſee in Hiſtory of ancient Eclipſes, altho they were obſerved by very able Aſtronomers.

The Aſtronomers who firſt uſed Teleſcopes furniſhed with but two Glaſſes, namely, a Convex Object-Glaſs, and a Concave Eye-Glaſs, in the Obſervations of Eclipſes, obſerved thoſe of the Sun in the following manner They cauſed a hole to be made in the Window-ſhutter of a Room, which Room in the Day-time, when the Shutters were ſhut, was darkened thereby; thro which hole they put the Tube of a Teleſcope, in ſuch manner, that the Rays of the Sun, paſſing thorow the Tube, might be received upon a white

piece

piece of Paper, or a Table-Cloth, upon which was first described a Circle of a convenable bigness, with five other Concentric Circles, equally distant from one another, which, with the Center, divided a Diameter of the outward Circle into 12 equal Parts. Then having adjusted the Table-Cloth perpendicular to the Situation of the Tube of the Telescope, the luminous Image of the Sun was cast upon the Table-Cloth, which would still be greater according as the Table-Cloth was more distant from the Eye-Glass of the Telescope, whence by moving the Tube forwards and backwards, they found a place where the Image of the Sun appeared exactly equal to the outward Circle, and at that Distance they fixed the Table-Cloth, with the Tube of the Telescope, which composed the Instrument for the said Observation. Afterwards they moved the Tube according to the Sun's Motion, to the end that the luminous Limb of its Disk might every where touch the outward Circle described upon the Table-Cloth, by which means the Quantity of the eclipsed Portion was seen, and its greatest Obscurity measured by the Concentric Circles, they denoted the Hour of every Phase, by a Second Pendulum Clock, rectified and prepared for that purpose. The same Method is still observed by many Astronomers, who use also a Circular Reticulum, made with six Concentric Circles upon very fine Paper, which must be oiled, to render the Sun's Image more sensible. The greatest of the Circles ought exactly to contain the Image of the Sun in the Focus of the Object-Glass of a Telescope of 40 or 60 Feet, the six Circles are equally distant, and divide the Diameter of the Sun in twelve equal Digits. When the Paper is placed in the Focus of a great Telescope, the enlightened part of the Sun will very distinctly be seen, then the Eye-Glass is not used.

There are others who use a Telescope furnished with two Convex-Glasses, from whence the same effect follows. But altho the Use of a Telescope in this manner be very proper to observe Eclipses of the Sun, yet it is not fit to observe Eclipses of the Moon, because its Light is not strong enough. Lastly, Others place a Micrometer in the common Focus of the Convex Lenses. Besides the Quantity of the Phases of the Eclipses of the Sun and Moon, (easily known by the said Micrometer) we may have the Diameters of the Luminaries, and the proportion of the Earth's Diameter to the Moon's, as well by the obscure Portion of its Disk, as by the luminous Portion and the Distance between its Horns.

The Method of observing Eclipses by means of the Micrometer will be much better, if the Divisions to which the parallel Hairs are applyed be made so, that six Intervals of the Hairs, may contain the Diameter of the Sun or Moon. For the moveable Hair posited in the middle of the Distance between the immoveable ones, (which is not difficult to do) will shew the Digits of the Eclipse.

The same Telescope and Micrometer may serve for all the other Observations, and to measure Eclipses, as, to observe the Passage of the Earth's Shadow over the Spots of the Moon, in Lunar Eclipses.

There yet remains one considerable Difficulty, and that is, to make a new Division of the Micrometer serving as a common Reticulum for all Observations, for it scarcely happens in an Age in two Eclipses, that the apparent Diameters of the Sun and Moon are the same.

Therefore M. *de la Hire* has invented a new Reticulum, which having all the Uses of the Micrometer, may serve to observe all Eclipses, it being adapted to all apparent Diameters of the Sun and Moon, and its Divisions are firm and solid enough to resist all the Vicissitudes of the Air, altho they are as fine as Hairs.

The Construction and Use of this Reticulum is thus. First, Take two Object Lenses of Telescopes of the same Focus, or nighly the same, which join together. As for example, The Focus of two Lenses together of eight Feet, which is the fit length of a Telescope for observing Eclipses, unless the Beginning and the End of Solar ones, which require a longer Telescope exactly to determine them.

Secondly, We find from Tables, that the greatest Diameter of the Moon at the Altitude of 90 deg is 34 min. 6 sec. To which adding 10 sec and there will arise 34 min 16 sec. Therefore say, As Radius is to the Tangent of 17 min. 8 sec (the half of 34 min 16 sec) so is 8 Feet, or the focal Length of the two Lenses to the parts of a Foot, which doubled will subtend an Angle of 34 min 16 sec in the Focus of the Telescope, and this will be the Diameter of the said Circular Reticulum.

Thirdly, Upon a very flat, clear, and well polished piece of Glass, describe lightly with the point of a Diamond, fastened to one of the Legs of a pair of Compasses, six Concentric Circles, equally distant from each other. The Semidiameter of the greatest and last let be equal to the fourth Term before found. Likewise draw two Diameters to the greatest Circle at Right Angles. The flat piece of Glass being thus prepared and put into the Tube, of which we have before spoken, and in the Focus of the Telescope, will be a very proper Reticulum for observing Solar and Lunar Eclipses, and it will divide all the apparent Diameters into twelve equal Parts or Digits, as we are now going to explain.

It is manifest from Dioptricks, that all Rays coming from Points of a distant Object, after their Refraction by two Convex Lenses, either join'd or something distant from each other, will be painted in the common Focus of the said Lenses, which will appear so much the greater according as the Lenses be distant from one another; so that they will appear the

U u

smallest

fmalleft when the Lenfes are joined together Therefore if the Object-Glaffes ufed in this Conftruction, be each put into a Tube, and one of thefe Tubes ilides within the other, then the faid Lenfes being thus joined, the Image of a diftant Object, whofe Rays fall upon the Lenfes under an Angle of 34 min 16 fec will exceed the Moon's greateft apparent Diameter by 10 fec Therefore in moving the Lenfes by little and little, fuch a Pofition may be found, wherein the Diameter of the greateft Circle on the Reticulum pofted in the Focus, will anfwer to an Angle of 34 min 16 fec For the Image of an Object perceived under a lefs Angle, may be equal to the Image of the fame Object perceived under a greater Angle, according to the different Lengths of the Foci But the Reticulum is in a feparate Tube, and fo it may be removed at a diftance at pleafure from the Object Glaffes We now proceed to lay down two different Ways of finding the Pofitions of the Lenfes and Reticulum, proper to receive the different Diameters of the Sun and Moon

Firft, In a very level and proper Place for making Obfervations with Glaffes, place a Board, with a Sheet of Paper thereon, directly expofed to the Tube's Length, having two black Lines drawn upon it parallel to each other, and at fuch a Diftance from each other, that it fubtends an Angle of 34 min 6 fec. fo that the Diftance of the faid two Lines, reprefented in the Focus of the Object-Glafles, may likewife fubtend an Angle of 34 min 6 fec And this may be found in reafoning thus, (as we have already done for the Micrometer) As Radius is to the Tangent of 17 min 3 fec fo is the Diftance from the Tube of the Object-Glaffes to the Board, to half of the Diftance that the parallel Lines on the Paper muft be at And thus we fhall find by Experience the Place of each Object-Glafs, and the Reticulum in the common Focus, in fuch manner that the Reprefentation of the two black Lines on the Paper, embaraffes entirely the Diameter of the greateft Circle of the faid Reticulum Now we fet down 34 min 6 fec upon the Tubs, in each Pofition of the Lenfes and their Foci, or the Reticulum, that fo the Lenfes and Reticulum may be adjufted to their exact Diftance, every time an Angle of 34 deg 6 min is made ufe of

Again, Let the faid Board and white Paper be placed further from the Tube, in fuch manner, that the Diftance between the parallel Lines on the Paper fubtend, or is the Bafe of an Angle of 33 min for example, whofe Vertex is at the Lenfes of the Telefcope which may be done, in faying, As the Tangent of 16 min 30 fec is to Radius, fo is half the Interval of the parallel Lines on the Paper, to the Diftance of the Board from the Lenfes Now in this Pofition of the Telefcope and Board, the Pofition of the Lenfes and Reticulum between themfelves muft be found, fo that the Reprefentation of the parallel Lines, which appear very diftinctly in the Focus of the Lenfes, occupies the whole Diameter of the greateft Circle on the Reticulum This being done, the Number 33 min muft be made upon the Tubes, in the Places wherein each of the Lenfes and Reticulum ought to be Proceed in this manner for the Angles of 32 min 31 min 30 min and 29 min

If the Diftances, denoted upon the Tubes between the different Pofitions of the Lenfes and the Reticulum, anfwering to a Minute, be divided into 60 equal Parts, we fhall have their Pofitions for every Second, and by this means the fame Circle of the Reticulum may be accommodated to all the different apparent Diameters of the Sun and Moon, and the Diameter of the greateft Circle being divided into 12 equal Parts, it will ferve to meafure the Quantities of all folar and lunar Eclipfes

The fecond Method taken from Opticks, being not founded upon fo great a Number of Experiments as the former, may perhaps appear eafier to fome Perfons, for the Foci of both the Lenfes being known, fay, As the Sum of the focal Lengths of the Lenfes (whether they be equal or not) lefs the Diftance between the Lenfes, is to the focal Length of the outward Lenfes, lefs the Diftance between the Lenfes; fo is this fame Term, to a fourth which being taken from the focal Length of the outward Lens, there remains the Diftance from the outward Lens, to the common Focus of the Lenfes, which is the Place of the Reticulum

The Pofition of the common Focus of the Lenfes may alfo be known by this Method, when they be joined, in ufing the aforefaid Analogy, without having any regard to the Diftance between the Lenfes, which is computed from the Places of the Lenfes Centers; therefore in fuppofing feveral different Diftances between the Object-Lenfes, the Length of their Foci will be had, that is, the Place of the Reticulum, correfpondent to each Diftance

Again, fay, As the known focal Length is to the Semidiameter of the Reticulum, be it what it will, fo is Radius, to the Tangent of the Angle anfwering to the Semidiameter of the Reticulum. By this Method we may likewife have the Magnitude of the faid Reticulum, in faying, As Radius is to the Tangent of an Angle of 17 min 3 fec fo is the focal Length of the Lenfes, to the Semidiameter of the outward concentrick Circle Having thus found the Minutes and Seconds fubtended by the Diameter of the greateft Circle of the Reticulum, according to the different Intervals of the Lenfes, they muft be wrote upon each Tube of the Lenfes and Reticulum, and the Diftances between the Terms found, divided into Seconds, as is mentioned in the former Method And thus may the Pofitions of the Lenfes and Reticulum be foon found, which fhall contain the apparent Diameters of the Sun or Moon, according as they appear If it be found very difficult to draw exactly the

concentrick

concentrick Circles upon the Piece of Glaſs, you need but draw thirteen right Lines there-on with the Point of a Diamond, equally diſtant and parallel to each other, with another right Line perpendicular to them, but the Length of this Perpendicular between the two extreme Parallels, muſt be equal to the Diameter of the Reticulum, found in the manner aforeſaid. This Reticulum may be uſed inſtead of one compoſed of Hairs.

A plain thin Piece of Glaſs, having Lines drawn thereon with a very fine Point of a Dia-mond, may likewiſe be uſed in an Aſtronomical Teleſcope, &c. for if it be adjuſted in its proper Frame, in the manner as is directed in the Micrometer, the Lines drawn thereon may be uſed inſtead of the parallel Hairs. I am of opinion, that the aforeſaid Reticula are very uſeful in practical Aſtronomy, they not being ſubject to the Inconſtancies of the Air, of being gnaw'd by Inſects, or to the Motions of the Inſtrument, which the Hairs are.

There are thoſe who prefer Hairs, to Lines drawn upon a piece of Glaſs, whoſe Surface may cauſe ſome Obſcurity to the Objects, or if it be not very flat, there may ſome Error ariſe, but if they have a mind to avoid theſe Difficulties, which are of no conſequence, as we know by Experience, they may uſe ſtraight Glaſs-Threads, inſtead of Hairs; for ſome of theſe may be procured as fine as Hairs, and of Strength enough to reſiſt the Inconſtancies of the Air.

Altho the Phaſes or Appearances of the Eclipſes of the Moon, apply'd by Aſtronomers to Aſtronomical and Geographical Uſes, may be obſerved much eaſier and exacter by our Reticulum, than by the antient Methods, yet it muſt be acknowledged, that the Immerſions into, and Emerſions of the Moon's Spots out of the Earth's Shadow, may more conve-niently be obſerved, becauſe of their great Number, than the Phaſes, and that there is leſs Preparation in uſing a Teleſcope, which need be only ſix Feet in length; and in order for this, a Map of the Moon's Disk, when it is at the full, muſt be procured, wherein are denoted the proper Names of the Spots, and principal Places appearing on its Disk. This may be found in the reformed Aſtronomy of *R P Riccioli*, &c.

There are great Advantages ariſing from Obſervations of Eclipſes, for if the exact Time of the Beginning of an Eclipſe of the Moon, of its total Immerſion in the Shadow, of its Emerſion and its End, as likewiſe of the Paſſage of the Earth's Shadow by the Spots on its Surface, be obſerved, we ſhall have the Difference of Longitude of the two Places wherein the Obſervations are made, this is known to all Aſtronomers. But ſince Lunar Eclipſes ſeldom happen, ſo as that the Difference of Longitude may thereby be concluded, the E-clipſes of *Jupiter*'s Satellites may be obſerved inſtead of them, but principally of the firſt, whoſe Motion about *Jupiter* being very ſwift, one may make ſeveral Obſervations thereof during the ſpace of one Year, and from thence the Difference of Longitude of the two Pla-ces, wherein the ſaid Obſervations are made, may be had.

Nevertheleſs you muſt take notice, that Lunar Eclipſes may much eaſier be obſerved, than the Eclipſes of *Jupiter*'s Satellites, which cannot be eaſily and exactly done without a Teleſcope of twelve Feet in length, whereas the Phaſes of the Beginning or End, or of the Immerſion and Emerſion of Lunar Eclipſes, may be obſerved without a Teleſcope, and the Immerſions and Emerſions of its Spots with one of an indifferent length.

M *Caſſini*, a very excellent Aſtronomer of the Academy of Sciences, publiſhed in the Year 1693, exact Tables of the Motions of *Jupiter*'s Satellites; therefore in comparing the Times of the Immerſion or Emerſion of *Jupiter*'s firſt Satellite, found by the Tables fitted for the Obſervatory (at *Paris*) with the Obſervations thereof made in any other Place, we ſhall have, by the Difference of Time, the Difference of Longitude of the Obſervatory, and the Place wherein the Obſervations were made; which may be confirmed in obſerving the ſame Phenomena in both Places.

It is proper here to inform Obſervators of one Caſe, which often hinders an exact Ob-ſervation of *Jupiter*'s Satellites, which is, that in a ſerene Night, we often find the Light of *Jupiter* and its Satellites, obſerved thro the Teleſcope, to diminiſh by little and little, ſo that it is impoſſible to determine exactly the true Times of the Immerſion and Emerſion of the Satellites. Now the Cauſe of this Accident proceeds from the Object-Glaſs of the Teleſcope, which is covered over with Dew, and thereby a great Number of Rays of Light, coming from *Jupiter* and its Satellites, is hinder'd from coming thro the Object-Glaſs to the Eye. A very ſure Remedy for this, is, to make a Tube of blotting Paper, that is, a Tube about two Feet long, and big enough to go about the End of the Tube of the Teleſcope next to the Object-Glaſs, muſt be made, in rolling two or three Sheets of ſinking Paper upon each other. This Tube being adjuſted about the Tube of the Te-leſcope, will ſuck in, or drink up the Dew, and hinder its coming to the Object-Glaſs; and by this Means we may make our Obſervations conveniently.

CHAP.

CHAP. IV.

Of the Construction and Use of an Instrument shewing the Eclipses of the Sun and Moon, the Months and Lunar Years, as also the Epacts.

Fig 13.

THIS Instrument was invented by M. *de la Hire*, and is composed of three round Plates of Brass, or Pieces of Pasteboard, and an Index which turns about a common Center upon the Face of the upper Plate, which is the least   There are two circular Bands, the one blue, and the other white, in which are made little round Holes, the outward of which shews the New Moons, and the Image of the Sun , and the inward ones, the Full Moons, and the Image of the Moon   The Limb of this Plate is divided into 12 lunar Months, each containing 29 Days, 12 Hours, 44 Minutes, but in such manner, that the End of the 12th Month, which makes the Beginning of the second lunar Year, may surpass the first New Moon by the quantity of 4 of 179 Divisions, denoted upon the middle Plate

Upon the Limb of this Plate is fastned an Index, one of whose Sides, which is in the *fiducial Line*, makes part of a right Line, tending to the Center of the Instrument , which Line also passes thro the middle of one of the outward Holes, shewing the first New Moon of the lunar Year. *Note*, The Diameter of the Holes is equal to the Extent of about 4 Degrees.

The Limb of the second Plate is divided into 179 equal Parts, serving for so many lunar Years, each of which is 354 Days, and about 9 Hours.   The first Year begins at the Number 179, at which the last ends

The Years accomplished are each denoted by their Numbers 1, 2, 3, 4, &c at every fourth Division, and which make four times a Revolution to compleat the Number 179, as may be seen in the Figure of this Plate   Each of the lunar Years comprehend four of the aforesaid Divisions   So that in this Figure they anticipate one upon the other four of the said 179 Divisions of the Limb.

Upon the Limb of the same Plate, under the Holes of the first, there is a space coloured black, answering to the outward Holes, and which shews the Eclipses of the Sun, and another red Space, answering to the innermost Holes, shewing the Eclipses of the Moon   The Quantity of each Colour appearing through the Holes, shows the Bigness of the Eclipse   The middle of the two Colours, which is the middle of the Moon's Node, answers on one side to the Division marked $4\frac{3}{7}$ of a Degree , and on the other side it answers to the opposite Number

The Figure of the coloured Space is shown upon this second Plate, and its Amplitude or Extent shews the Limits of Eclipses

The third and greatest Plate, which is underneath the others, contains the Days and Months of common Years.   The Divisions begin at the first Day of *March*, to the end that a Day may be added to the Month of *February*, when the Year is *Bissextile*   The Days of the Year are described in form of a Spiral, and the Month of *February* goes out beyond the Month of *March*, because the lunar Year is shorter than the solar one , so that the 15th Hour of the 10th Day of *February* answers to the Beginning of *March*   But after having reckoned the last Day of *February*, you must go back again to have the first of *March*   There are thirty Days marked before the Month of *March*, which serve to find the Epacts

Note, That the Days, as they are here taken, are not accomplished pursuant to the Use of Astronomers, but as they are vulgarly reckoned, beginning one a Minute, and ending at the Minute of the following Day   Therefore every time that the first Day, or any other of a Month is spoken of, we understand the Space of that Day marked in the Divisions , for we here reckon the current Days according to vulgar Use.

In the middle of the upper Plate are wrote the *Epochs*, shewing the Beginning of the lunar Years, with respect to the solar Years, according to the *Gregorian* Calendar, and for the Meridian of *Paris*   The Beginning of the first Year, which must be denoted by o, and answers to the Division 179, happened in the Year 1680 at *Paris*, the 29th of *February* at $14\frac{1}{2}$ Hours   The End of the first lunar Year, being the Beginning of the second, answers to the Division marked 1, which happened at *Paris* in the Year 1681, the 27th of *February*, at $23\frac{1}{2}$ Hours, in counting successively 24 Hours from one Minute to the other   And lest there should be an Error in comparing the Divisions of the Limb of the second Plate with the Divisions of the *Epochs* of lunar Years answering them, we have put the same Numbers to them both.

We

We have set down successively the *Epochs* of all the lunar Years, from the Year 1700 to the Year 1750, to the end that the Use of this Instrument may more easily serve to make each of the aforesaid solar and lunar Years agree together. As to the other Years of our Cycle of 179 Years, it will be easy to render it compleat, in adding 354 Days, 8 Hours, 48 ½ Minutes for each lunar Year.

The Index extending it self from the Center of the Instrument to the Limb of the greatest Plate, serves to compare the Divisions of one Plate with those of the two others. And if this Instrument be apply'd to a Clock, a perfect and accomplished Instrument in all its Parts will be had.

The Table of *Epochs*, which is fitted for the Meridian of *Paris*, may easily be reduced to other Meridians, if for the Places eastward of *Paris*, the Time of the Difference of Meridians be added, and for Places westward, the Time of the Difference of Meridians be substracted.

It is proper to place the Table of *Epochs* in the middle of the upper Plate, to the end that it may be seen with the Instrument.

How to make the Divisions upon the Plates

The Circle of the greatest Plate is so divided, that 368 deg 2 min 42 sec may comprehend 354 Days, and something less than 9 Hours, from whence it is manifest, that the Circle must contain 346 Days, 15 Hours, which may without sensible Error be taken for ¾ of a Day. Now to divide a Circle into 346 ¾ equal Parts, reduce the whole into third Parts, which in this Example make 1040, then seek the greatest Multiple of 3 less than 1040, which may be halved. Such a Number will be found in a double Geometrical Progression, whose first Term is 3, as for example, 3, 6, 12, 24, 48, 96, 192, 384, 768.

Now the 9th Number of this Progression is the Number sought. Then substract 768 from 1040, there will remain 272, and find how many Degrees, Minutes and Seconds this remaining Number makes, by saying, as 1040 is to 360 deg so is 272 to 94 deg 9 min 23 sec.

Therefore take an Angle of 94 deg 9 min 23 sec. from the said Circle, and divide the remaining part of the Circle always into half, after having made 8 Subdivisions, you will come to the Number 3, which will be the Arc of one Day, by which likewise dividing the Arc of 94 deg 9 min 23 sec the whole Circle will be found divided into 346 ¾ Days, for there will be 256 Days in the greatest Arc, and 90 ¾ Days in the other. Each of these Spaces answer to 1 deg 2 min 18 sec as may be seen in dividing 360 by 346 ¾, and ten Days make 10 deg 23 min. And thus a Table may be made, serving to divide the Plate.

Those Days are afterwards distributed to each of the Months of the Year, according to the Number corresponding to them, in beginning at the Month of *March*, and continuing on to the 15th Hour of the 10th of *February*, which answers to the beginning of *March*, and the other Days of the Month of *February* go on farther above *March*.

The Circle of the Second Plate must be divided into 179 equal Parts; to do which, seek the greatest Number which may be continually bisected to Unity, and be contained exactly in 179: you will find 128 to be this Number, which take from 179, and there remains 51. Now find what part of the Circumference of the Circle the said Remainder makes; in saying, As 179 Parts is to 360 deg so is 51 Parts to 102 deg 34 min 11 sec.

Therefore having taken from the Circle an Arc of 102 deg 34 min 11 sec divide the remaining part of the Circle always into half, and after having made seven Subdivisions, you will come to Unity. whence this part of the Circle will be divided into 128 equal Parts, and then the remaining 51 Parts may be divided, by help of the last opening of the Compasses. Wherefore the whole Circumference will be found divided into 179 equal Parts, every of which answers to 2 deg 40 sec as may be seen in dividing 360 by 179.

Lastly, To divide the Circle of the upper Plate, take one fourth of its Circumference, and add to it one of the 179 Parts or Divisions of the Limb of the middle Plate, the Compasses opened to the extent of the Quadrant thus augmented, being turned four times over, will divide the Circle in the manner as it ought to be: for in subdividing every of the Quarters into three equal Parts, one will have twelve Spaces for the twelve Lunar Months, in such manner, that the end of the 12th Month, which makes the beginning of the Lunar Year, exceeds the first New Moon by 4 of the 179 Divisions, marked upon the middle Plate.

Use of this Instrument

A Lunar Year being proposed, to find the Days of the Solar Year corresponding to it, in which the New and Full Moons, together with the Eclipses, ought to happen.

For example, Let the 24th Lunar Year of the Table of *Epochs* be proposed, which answers to the Division 24 of the middle Plate. Fix the Fiducial Line of the Index on the upper Plate, over the Division marked 24, in the middle Plate, wherein the beginning of the 25th Lunar Year is, and seeing by the Table of *Epochs*, that that beginning falls upon the 14th Day of *June*, of the Year 1703, at 9 Hours, 52 Minutes, turn the two upper

X x Plates

Plates together, in the Position they are in, till the Fiducial Line of the Index, fastened to the upper Plate, answers to the 10th Hour, or thereabouts, of the 14th of *June*, denoted upon the undermost Plate, at which time, the first New Moon of the proposed Lunar Year happens for then the Fiducial Line passes thro the middle of the hole of the first New Moon of the said Lunar Year

Afterwards, without changing the Situation of the three Plates, extend a Thread from the Center of the Instrument, or the moveable Index, making it pass thro the middle of the hole of the first Full Moon, and the Fiducial Line will answer to the beginning of the 29th Day of *June*, at 4 hours and a quarter, which is the time that *that* Full Moon was totally Eclipsed, as appears by the red Colour quite filling the hole, showing the Full Moon.

By the same means we may know, that at the time of the Full Moon, which happened about the third Hour in the Morning, of the 14th of *July*, there was a partial Eclipse of the Sun.

If we proceed farther, the Eclipses may be known which happened in the Month of *December*, in the Year 1703, and towards the beginning of the following Year But because the 10th New Moon goes out beyond the 28th day of *February*, having brought the Index to the 28th day of *February*, move the two upper Plates backwards, conjointly with the Index (in the Posture they are found in) until the Fiducial Line happens over the beginning of *March*, whence moving the Index over all the holes of the New and Full Moons, and the last Plate will shew the times in which the Eclipses ought to happen

But because the 13th New Moon is the first of the succeeding Lunar Year, which answers to the Number 25 of the Divisions of the middle Plate, leave the two undermost Plates in the posture they are found, and move forwards the upper Plate till the Fiducial Line meets with the Number 25 of the middle Plate, at which Point it will shew upon the greatest Plate, the first New Moon of the 26th Lunar Year, according to the order of our Epoch, which happened the 2d Day of *June*, 18 hours 40 minutes of the Year 1704, and afterwards moving the Index over the middle of the holes of the New and Full Moons, it will shew upon the last Plate the Days they happened on, as well as the Eclipses to the end of *February* after which, the same Operation must be made for the preceding Year, that is, that after having come to the last Day of *February*, you must proceed backwards to the first Day of *March*

We might likewise find the beginnings of all the Lunar Years without using the Table of Epochs, but since it is not possible to adjust the Plates and the Index so exactly one upon another, as that some Error may not happen, which will augment itself from Year to Year, the said Table of Epochs will serve to rectify the Use of this Instrument

In placing the Fiducial Line of the Index upon the Moon's Age, between the Days of the Lunar Months, denoted upon the Limb of the upper Plate, the correspondent Days of the common Months will be shewn, and the Hours nearly, upon the Limb of the lower Plate.

Note, That the Calculations of the Table of Epochs are made for the mean Time of the Full Moons, which supposes the Motions of the Sun and Moon always equable, from whence there will be found some Difference between the apparent Times of the New Moons, Full Moons and Eclipses, as they appear from the Earth, and the times found by that Table

The proper Motions of the Sun and Moon, as well as those of the other Planets, appear to us sometimes swift, and sometimes slow, which apparent Inequality in part proceeds from their Orbits being not concentric with the Earth, and in part from hence, that the equal Arcs of the Ecliptick, which are oblique to the Equator, do not always pass thro the Meridian with the equal Parts of the Equator Astronomers, for the ease of Calculation, have fitted a Motion which they call mean or equable, in supposing the Planets to describe equal Arcs of their Orbits, in equal Times That Time which they call true or apparent, is the measure of true or apparent Motion, and mean Time is the measure of mean Motion They have likewise invented Rules for reducing mean Time to true or apparent Time, and contrariwise, for reducing true or apparent Time to mean Time

To find by Calculation whether there will happen an Eclipse at the time of the New or Full Moon

For an Eclipse of the Sun, multiply by 7361, the Number of Lunar Months accomplished from that which begun the 8th of *January*, 1701, according to the *Gregorian* Calendar, to that which you examine, and add to the Product the Number 33890, then divide the Sum by 43200; and after the Division, without having regard to the Quotient, examine the Remainder, or the difference between the Divisor and the Remainder. for if either of them be less than 4060, there will happen an Eclipse of the Sun

But to find an Eclipse of the Moon, likewise multiply by 7361, the Number of Lunar Months, accomplished from that which begun the 8th of *January*, 1701, to the New Moon preceding the Full Moon examined; add to the Product 37326, and divide the Sum by 43200. The Division being made, if the Remainder, or the difference between the Remainder and the Divisor be less than 2800, there will be an Eclipse of the Moon

Note,

Note, An Eclipse of the Sun or Moon will be so much the greater, as the Remainder or Difference is leffer, and contrariwife

Example of an Eclipfe of the Sun.

It is required to find, whether at the New Moon of the 22d of *May,* in the Year 1705, there happened an Eclipfe of the Sun

From the 8th of *January,* 1701, to the 22d of *May,* 1705, there was accomplifhed 54 Lunations Multiply, according to the Rule, the Number 54 by 7361, and add to the Product 33890. the Sum being divided by 43200, there will remain 42584, which is greater than 4060, and the Difference between the Remainder 42584, and the Divifor 43200, is 616, which is lefs than 4060 therefore there was then an Eclipfe of the Sun

Example of an Eclipfe of the Moon.

It is required to find whether the Full Moon of the 27th of *April,* in the Year 1706, was eclipfed

From the 8th of *January,* in the Year 1701, to the New Moon preceding the Full Moon in queftion, there were 65 Lunar Months accomplifhed, therefore having multiplied, according to the Rule, the Number 65 by 7361, and added to the Product 37326, the Sum will be 515791, which being divided by 43200, without having any regard to the Quotient, the Remainder will be 40591, greater than 2800 The Difference between the Divifor and the Remainder is 609, which is lefs than 2800, therefore there was an Eclipfe of the Moon the 27th day of *April,* 1706

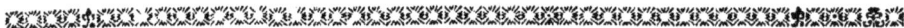

CHAP. V.

The Defcription of a Second Pendulum Clock for Aftronomical Obfervations.

THE Figure here adjoined, fhews the Compofition of a Second Pendulum Clock, *Plate* 17. whofe two Plates A A and B B, are about half a Foot long, and two Inches and a Fig. 1. half broad, having four little Pillars at the four Corners, that fo they may be an Inch and a half diftant from each other Thefe Plates ferve to fuftain the Axes of the principal Wheels, the firft of which being the loweft, and figured C C, hath 80 Teeth The Axis of this Wheel hath a little Pulley, having feveral Iron Points D D round about the fame, in order to hold the Cord to which the Weights are hung, in the manner as we fhall explain by and by The Wheel C C, being turned by the Weight, likewife turns the Pinion E of eight Teeth, and fo moves the Wheel F, which is faftened to the Axis of the Pinion E, this Wheel hath forty-eight Teeth, which falling into the Teeth of the Pinion G, whofe Number is eight, moves the Wheel H, (made in figure of a Crown) confifting of forty-eight Teeth Again, The Teeth of this laft Wheel fall into the Teeth of the Pinion I, whofe Number is twenty-four, and the Axis thereof being upright, carries the Wheel K of 15 Teeth, which are made in Figure of a Saw: Over this Wheel is a crofs Axis, having two Palats L L, fuftained by the Tenons N, Q and P, which are faftened to the Plate B B. It muft be obferved, that as to the Tenons N and Q, the lower part Q appearing, hath a great hole drilled therein, that the Axis L M may pafs thro it, this part Q, which is faftened to the lower part of the Tenon N, likewife holds the Wheel K, and the Pinion I There is a great Opening in the Plate B B, in order for the Axis and the Palats to go out beyond it One end of this Axis (as I have already mentioned) goes into the Tenon P, and fo moves eafier than if it was fuftained by the Plate B B, and then go out beyond the faid Plate, which it muft neceffarily do, that fo the little Stern S, fixed thereto, may freely vibrate with the faid Axis, and the Teeth of the Wheel K alternately meet the Palats L L, as in common Clocks

The lower part of the little Stern S is bent, and a flit made therein, thro which goes an Iron-Rod, ferving as a Pendulum, having the Lead X at the end thereof. This Rod is faftened in V to a very thin piece of Brafs or Steel, which vibrates between two Cycloidal Cheeks T T, (one of which is feen in Fig. 1. and both in Fig. 2) of which more hereafter.

It is eafy to perceive in what manner this Clock goes by the force of the Wheels carried round by the Weight · for the Motion is continued by the Pendulum V X, when the faid Pendulum is fet a going, becaufe the little Stern S, altho very light, being in motion, not only goes with the Pendulum, but likewife by its Vibrations ftill affifts the Motion fome fmall matter, and fo renders it perpetual, which otherwife by Friction and the Air's refiftance, would come to nothing. But becaufe the Property of the Pendulum is to move equably always, provided its length be the fame, the faid Pendulum will caufe the

Wheel

Wheel K to go neither too faſt nor too flow, (as happens to Clocks not having Pendulums) every Tooth is obliged to move equably, therefore the other Wheels, and the Hands of the Dial-plate, are neceſſarily conſtrained to perform their Revolutions equably Whence if there ſhould be ſome Default in the Conſtruction of the Clock, or if the Axes of the Wheels do not move freely on account of the Intemperance of the Air, provided the Clock does not ſtand ſtill, we have nothing to fear from theſe Inequalities, for the Clock will always go true

As to the Hands for ſhewing the Hours, Minutes, and Seconds, we diſpoſe them in the following manner. The third Plate Y Y is parallel to the two precedent ones, and is three Lines diſtant from A A We deſcribe a Circle about the Center *a*, which is the middle of the Axis, carrying the Wheel C, continued out beyond the Plate A A This Circle is divided into 12 equal Parts, for the Hours We likewiſe deſcribe another Circle about the ſaid Center, and divide it into 60 equal Parts, for the Minutes in an Hour We place the Wheel *b* upon the Axis R, continued out beyond the Plate A A, faſtened to a little Tube, going out beyond the Plate Y Y to *e* This Tube is put about the Axis R, and turns about with it, in ſuch manner neverthelefs, that it may be turned only when there is neceſſity We place the Hand ſhewing the Minutes in *e*, which makes one Revolution in an Hour The beforementioned Wheel *b* moves the Wheel *b*, having the ſame Number of Teeth as that, *viz* 30, and the Teeth of the Wheel *f* falls into the Teeth of the Pinion *h*, whoſe Number is 6, and they have a little Axis common to them, which is partly ſuſtained by the Tenon *d* This Pinion moves round the Wheel *f*, having 72 Teeth, faſtened to a little Tube *g*, which is put about the Tube carrying the Wheel *b* Now the Hand ſhewing the Hours muſt be placed upon the Extremity of the Tube *g*, and will be ſhorter than that denoting the Minutes But that one may not be deceived in reckoning of Seconds, we place a round Plate *m m* upon the Extremity of the Axis of the Wheel H, divided into 60 equal Parts, and make an opening Z in the Plate Y, in the upper part of which Opening is a ſmall Point *o*, which, as the ſaid Plate turns about, ſhews the Seconds The Diſpoſition of the Hands and Circles will be eaſier ſeen in Figure 3, which repreſents the Outſide of the Clock

Now having ſpoken of the Diſpoſition of the Wheels, the next thing is to determine the Length of the Pendulum, which muſt be ſuch, that every of its Vibrations be made in a Second of Time. This Length muſt be 3 Feet 8 ½ Lines (of *Paris*) from the Point of Suſpenſion, which is the Center of the Cycloidal Cheeks, to the Center of the Weight X.

We now proceed to ſay ſomething concerning the Times of the Revolutions of the Wheels and the Hands, in order to confirm what we have already ſaid of the Number of Teeth Now one Revolution of the Wheel C C, makes ten Revolutions of the Wheel F, ſixty of the Wheel H, and one hundred and twenty of the upper Wheel K, which having 15 Teeth, and alternately puſhing the Palats L L, makes thirty Vibrations, which are ſo many goings and comings of the Pendulum V X Whence 120 Revolutions of the Wheel K, is equal to 3600 Viberations of the Pendulum, which are the Seconds contained in one Hour, and ſo the Wheel C makes one Revolution in an Hour, and the Hand *e* faſtened thereto, ſhews the Minutes, and becauſe the Wheel *b* makes its Revolution in the ſame time, (*viz* an Hour) the Wheel *b* hath the ſame Number of Teeth as *b*, and the Pinion on the ſame Axis hath ſix Teeth, and ſince the Number of Teeth of the Wheel *f* is twelve times greater, the ſaid Wheel will go round once in 12 Hours, as likewiſe the Hand *g* faſtened thereto Finally, Becauſe the Wheel H is making ſixty Revolutions in the ſame time the Wheel C C is making one, therefore the circular Plate Z, having the Seconds denoted thereon, will move once Round in a Minute, and ſo every 60th part of the ſaid Plate will ſhew one Second

The Weight X, at the end of the Pendulum, muſt weigh about 3 Pounds, and be of Lead covered with Braſs Regard muſt not only be had to its Weight, but likewiſe to its Figure, which is of conſequence, becauſe the leaſt Reſiſtance of the Air is prejudicial thereto, whence we make it in form of a Convex Cylinder, whoſe ends are pointed, as appears in Figure 3 wherein the Pendulum is repreſented, tho the Weights at the end of the Pendulums made for theſe Clocks uſed at Sea are in the Figure X, in form of a Lens, this Figure being found more proper than the other

Fig 3. In the ſame Figure may likewiſe be ſeen the manner of the Diſpoſition of the Weight *b*, in order to ſo move the Clock, that it may not ſtand ſtill while the Weight *b* is drawing up, and this is done by means of a Cord, one end of which muſt firſt be faſtened to a piece of Iron fixed to the Plate A A, (of Figure 1) and then it muſt be put about the Pulley *c*, of the Weight *b*, afterwards over the Pulley *d*, (which hath Iron Points round it in figure of the Teeth of a Saw, for hindering, leſt the Weight *b* ſhould pull the Cord down all at once) then about the Pulley *f* of the Weight *g*, and laſt of all the other end of the ſaid Cord muſt be fixed to ſome proper Place. Things being thus diſpoſed, it is manifeſt that half of the Weight *b* moves the Wheels round, and that the Motion of the Clock doth not ceaſe, when the Cord *e* is pulled with one's Hand in order to draw the Weight *b* up. *Note*, The Weight *g* is for ſuſtaining the Weight *b*, and need not be near ſo big

The

Plate XVI.   *Fenning pag. 175*

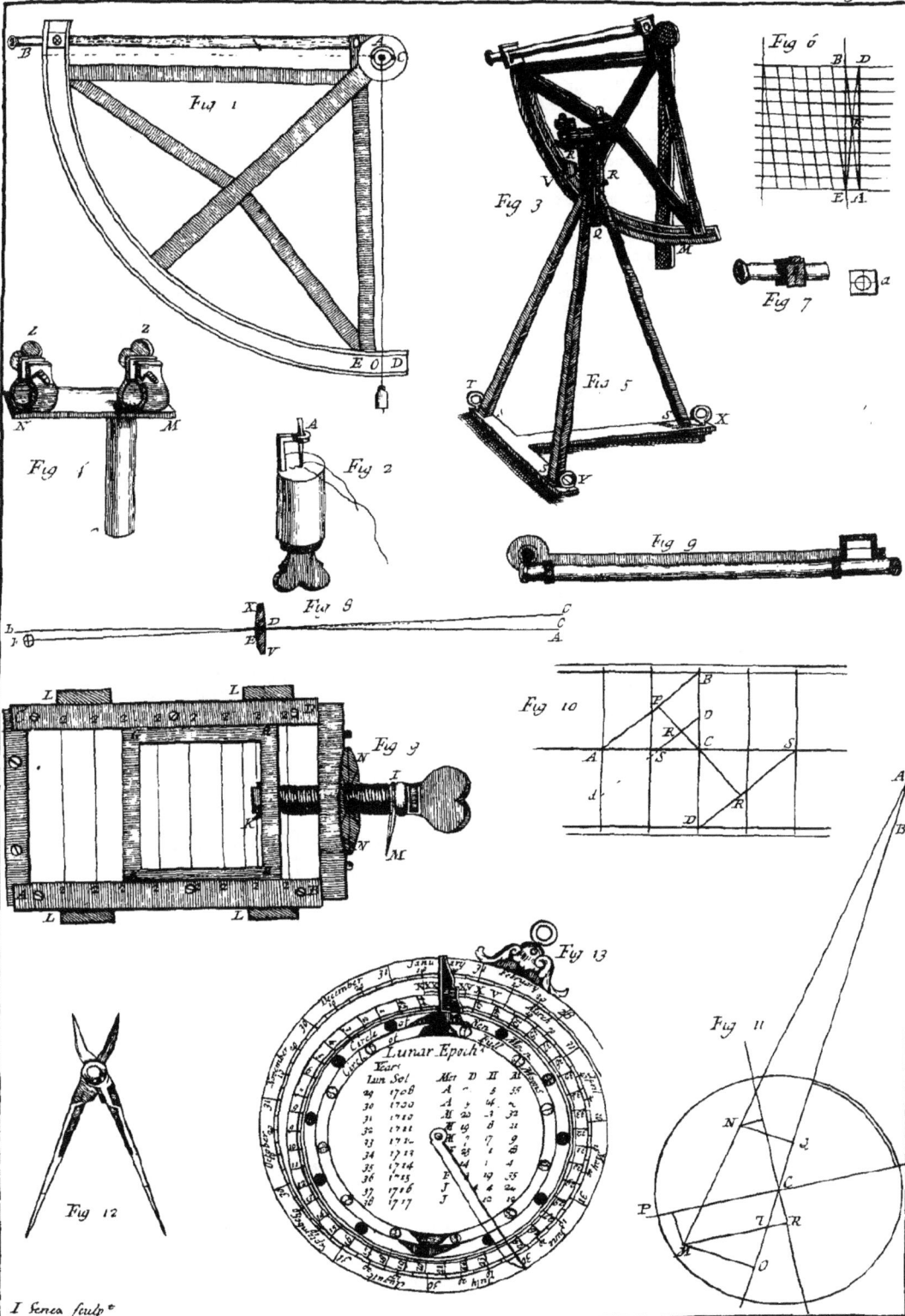

Fig 1

Fig 3

Fig 6

Fig 7

Fig 5

Fig 4

Fig 2

Fig 8

Fig 9

Fig 9

Fig 10

Fig 13

Lunar Epoch

Fig 12

Fig 11

I Senex sculp.

The Weight of *b* cannot be certainly determined by Reasoning, but the less it is the better, provided it be sufficient to make the Clock go They weigh generally about six Pounds in the best kind of these Clocks that have yet been made, whereof the Diameter of the Pulley D is one Inch, the Weight of the Pendulum X three Pounds, and its Length three Feet 8 ½ Lines. *Note,* It this Clock be at the height of a Man above the Ground, it will go 30 Hours

We now proceed to shew the manner of making the Cycloidal Cheeks between which the Fig. 4. Pendulum swings, and in which the whole Exactness of the Clock consists In order to do which, describe the Circle A F B K, whose Diameter A B let be equal to half of the Length of the Pendulum , assume the equal Parts of the Circumference A C, C D, D E, E F and A G, G H, H I, I K, and draw the Lines G C, H D, I E and K F, from one Division to the other, which Lines will be parallel. Now make the Line L M equal to the Arc A F, which divide into the same Number of equal Parts as A F, and assume one of these Parts, which lay off upon the Line C G, from C to N, and G to O Again, Lay off two of the said equal Parts of the Line L M, upon the Line D H, from D to P, and from H to Q Moreover, Assume three of the said equal Parts upon the Line L M, which lay off upon I E from E to R, and I to S And finally, Assume four of the said Parts (which is the whole Length of the Line L M) and lay off upon K F, from F to T, and K to V; and so of other Parts, if there had been more of them assumed upon the Periphery of the Circle A F B K Now if the Points N, P, R, T, as also O, Q, S, V, be joined, we shall have the Figure of the Cycloidal Cheeks, (between which the Pendulum swings) which must be afterwards cut out in Brass To draw the Line L M equal to the Arc A F, assume the two Semi-Chords of the Arc A F, which lay off upon the Line X V, from X to Y; this being done, take the whole Chord of the Arc A F, and lay off from X to Z, and divide Z Y into three equal Parts, one of which being laid off from Z to V, and the Line X V will be nearly the Length of the Arc A F

The Use of this Instrument sufficiently appears from what hath been already said

The principal Instruments that an Astronomer ought to have, besides a good Quadrant, and Pendulum Clock, is a Telescope seven or eight Foot long, having a Micrometer adjusted thereto, for observing the Digits of Solar and Lunar Eclipses, as likewise another of 15 or 16 Foot, for the Observation of *Jupiter's* Satellites , and, if possible, a Parallactick Instrument to take the Parallaxes of the Stars

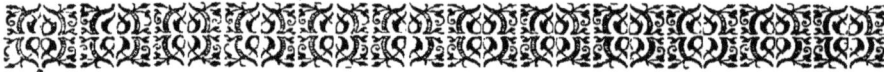

ADDITIONS of *English* Instruments.

Of Globes, Spheres, the Astronomical Quadrant, a Micrometer, and Gunter's Quadrant.

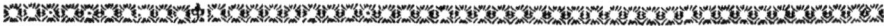

CHAP. I.
Of the GLOBES.

SECTION I.

OF Globes there are two kinds, *viz.* Celestial and Terrestrial The first is a Re-Fig. 5. & 6. presentation of the Heavens, upon the Convex Surface of a material Sphere, containing all the known Stars, after the manner that Astronomers, for the easier knowing them, have divided them into Constellations, or Figures of Men, Beasts, Fowls, Fishes, &c. according to the resemblance they fancied each select Number of Stars formed. The other is the Terrestrial Globe, which is the Image of the Earth, on the Convex Surface of a material Sphere, exhibiting all the Kingdoms, Countries, Islands, and other Places situated upon it, in the same Order, Figure, Dimensions, Situation, and Proportion, respecting one another as on the Earth itself.

There are ten eminent Circles upon the Globe, six of which are called *greater,* and the four other *lesser Circles*

A leſſer Circle is that which is parallel to a *greater*, as the Tropicks and Polar Circles are to the Equator, and as the Circles of Altitude are to the Horizon

The great Circles are,

I The *Horizon*, which is a broad wooden Circle encompaſſing the Globe about, having two Notches, one in the North, the other in the South part thereof, for the *Brazen Meridian* to ſtand, or move round in, when the Globe is to be ſet to a particular Latitude

There are uſually reckoned two *Horizons* Firſt, The *Viſible* or *Senſible Horizon*, which may be conceived to be made by ſome great Plane, or the Surface of the Sea, and which divides the Heavens into two *Hemiſpheres*, the one above, the other (apparently) below the Level of the Earth

This Circle determinates the Riſing and Setting of the Sun, Moon, or Stars, in any particular Latitude for when any one of them comes juſt to the Eaſtern edge of the *Horizon*, then we ſay it Riſes, and when it doth ſo at the Weſtern edge, we ſay it Sets And from hence alſo is the Altitude of the Sun or Stars reckoned, which is their height in Degrees above the Horizon

Secondly, The other *Horizon* is called the *Real* or Rational Horizon, and is a Circle encompaſſing the Earth exactly in the middle, and whoſe Poles are the *Zenith* and *Nadir*, that is, two Points in its Axis, each 90 deg diſtant from its Plane, (as the Poles of all Circles are) the one exactly over our Heads, and the other directly under our Feet This is the Circle that the wooden Horizon on the Globe repreſents

On which *Broad Horizon* ſeveral Circles are drawn, the innermoſt of which is the Number of Degrees of the *Twelve Signs* of the Zodiack, viz 30 to each Sign for the ancient Aſtronomers obſerved the Sun in his (apparent) *Annual Courſe*, always to deſcribe one and the ſame Line in the Heavens, and never to deviate from this *Tract* or *Path* to the North or South, as all the other Planets did, more or leſs and becauſe they found the Sun to ſhift as it were backwards, thro all the Parts of this Circle, ſo that in one whole Year's Courſe he would *Riſe*, Culminate, and *Set*, with every Point of it, they diſtinguiſhed the fixed Stars that appeared, in or near this Circle, into 12 Conſtellations or Diviſions, which they called *Signs*, and denoted them with certain Characters, and becauſe they are moſt of them uſually drawn in the form of Animals, they called this Circle by the Name of *Zodiack*, which ſignifies an *Animal*, and the very middle Line of it the *Ecliptick*, and ſince every Circle is divided into 360 Degrees, a twelfth part of this Number will be 30, the Degrees in each Sign

Next to this you have the Names of thoſe Signs; next to this the Days of the Months, according to the *Julian* Account, or Old Stile, with the Calender, and then another *Calender*, according to the *Foreign Account* or New Stile

And without theſe, is a Circle divided into thirty two equal Parts, which make the 32 Winds or Points of the Mariners Compaſs, with the Names annexed.

The Uſes of this Circle in the Globe are,

1 To determine the Riſing and Setting of the Sun, Moon, or Stars, and to ſhew the time of it, by help of the Hour Circle and Index; as ſhall be ſhewn hereafter

2 To limit the Increaſe and Decreaſe of the Day and Night for when the Sun riſes due Eaſt, and ſets Weſt, the Days are equal.

But when he Riſes and Sets to the North of the Eaſt and Weſt, the Days are longer than the Nights, and contrariwiſe, the Nights are longer than the Days, when the Sun Riſes and Sets to the Southwards of the Eaſt and Weſt Points of the Horizon.

3. To ſhow the Sun's Amplitude, or the Amplitude of a Star, and alſo on what Point of the Compaſs, it Riſes and Sets

II The next Circle, is the *Meridian*, which is repreſented by the brazen Frame or Circle, in which the Globe hangs and turns. This is divided into four Nineties or 360 Degrees, beginning at the Equinoctial

This Circle is called the Meridian, becauſe when the Sun comes to the South part of it, it is Meridies, Mid-day, or High-noon, and then the Sun hath its greateſt Altitude for that Day, which therefore is called the *Meridian Altitude* The Plane of this Circle is perpendicular to the *Horizon*, and paſſeth thro the South and North Parts thereof, thro the *Zenith* and *Nadir*, and thro the Poles of the World In it each way from the *Equinoctial* or the *Celeſtial Globe*, is accounted the North or South Declination of the Sun or Stars, and on the *Terreſtrial*, the Latitude of a Place *North* or *South*, which is equal to the elevation or height of the Pole above the Horizon Becauſe the Diſtance from the *Zenith* to the *Horizon*, being the ſame as that between the *Equinoctial* and the *Poles*, if from each you imagine the Diſtance from the Pole to the Zenith to be taken away, the Latitude will remain equal to the Pole's Altitude.

There are two Points of this Circle, each 90 Degrees diſtant from the Equinoctial, which are called the *Poles* of the World, the upper one the North Pole, and the under one the South Pole. A Diameter continued thro both the Poles in either Globe and the Center, is called the Axis of the Earth or Heavens, on which they are suppofed to turn about

The Meridians are various, and change according to the Longitude of Places, for as foon as ever a Man moves but one Degree, or but a Point to the Eaft or Weft, he is under a New Meridian But there is or fhould be one fixed, which is called the firft *Meridian*

And this on fome Globes, paffes thro one of the *Azores* Iflands but the *French* place the firft Meridian at *Ferro*, one of the *Canary* Iflands

The Poles of the Meridian are the Eaft and Weft Points of the Horizon On the *Terreftrial Globe*, are ufually drawn 24 Meridians, one thro every 15 Degrees of the *Equator*, or every 15 Degrees of Longitude

The Ufes of the Meridian Circle are,

Firft, To fet the Globe to any particular Latitude, by a proper Elevation of the Pole above the Horizon of that Place And, Secondly, To fhew the Sun or Stars Declination, Right Afcenfion, and greateft Altitude, of which more hereafter

III The next great Circle, is the *Equinoctial Circle*, as it is called on the *Celeftial*, and the *Equator*, on the Terreftrial Globe This is a great Circle whofe Poles are the Poles of the World: it divides the Globe into two equal Parts or Hemifpheres as to North and South, it paffes thro the Eaft and Weft Points of the Horizon, and at the Meridian is always as much raifed above the Horizon, as is the Complement of the Latitude of any particular Place Whenever the Sun comes to this Circle, it makes equal Days and Nights all round the Globe, becaufe it then Rifes due Eaft, and Sets due Weft, which it doth at no other time of the Year All Stars alfo which are under this Circle, or which have no Declination, do always Rife due Eaft, and Set full Weft

All People living under this Circle (which by Navigators is called the *Line*) have their Days and Nights conftantly equal And when the Sun is in the Equinoctial, he will be at Noon in their *Zenith*, or directly over their Heads, and fo their erect Bodies can caft no Shadow

From this Circle both ways, the Sun, or Stars Declination on the Celeftial, or Latitude of all Places on the *Terreftrial Globe*, is accounted on the Meridian and fuch leffer Circles as run thro each Degree of Latitude or Declination parallel to the Equinoctial, are called Parallels of Latitude or Declination

Through every 15 Degrees of this Equinoctial, the Hour-Circles are drawn at Right Angles to it on the *Celeftial Globe*, and all pafs thro the Poles of the World, dividing the Equinoctial into 24 equal Parts

And the Equator on the *Terreftrial Globe*, is divided by the Meridians into 36 equal Parts; which Meridians are equivalent to the Hour-Circles on the other Globe

IV. The *Zodiack* is another *great Circle* of the *Globe*, dividing the Globe into two equal Parts (as do all great Circles) : When the Points of *Aries* and *Libra* are brought to the Horizon, it will cut *that* and the Equinoctial obliquely, making with the former an Angle equal to 23 Degrees 30 Minutes, which is the Sun's greateft Declination. This Circle is accounted by Aftronomers as a kind of broad one, and is like a Belt or Girdle Through the middle of it is drawn a Line called the *Ecliptick*, or *Via Solis*, the *Way of the Sun*, becaufe the Sun never deviates from it, in its annual Courfe

This Circle is marked with the Characters of the *Twelve Signs*, and on it is found out the Sun's place, which is under what Star or Degree of any of the *Twelve Zodiacal Conftellations*, he appears to be in at Noon By this are determined the four Quarters of the Year, according as the Ecliptick is divided into four equal Parts, and accordingly as the Sun goes on here, he has more or lefs Declination

Alfo from this Circle the Latitude of the Planets and fixed Stars are accounted from the Ecliptick towards the Poles.

The Poles of this Circle are 23 Degrees, 30 Minutes diftant from the Poles of the World, or of the Equinoctial, and by their Motion round the Poles of the World, are the Polar Circles defcribed

V If you imagine two great Circles both paffing thro the Poles of the World, and alfo one of them thro the Equinoctial Points *Aries* and *Libra*, and the other thro the *Solftitial Points*, *Cancer* and *Capricorn* Thefe are called the two *Colures*, the one the *Equinoctial*, and the other the *Solftitial Colure*. Thefe will divide the Ecliptick into four equal Parts, which are denominated according to the Points they pafs thro, called the four Cardinal Points, and are the firft Points of *Aries*, *Libra*, *Cancer* and *Capricorn*

Thefe are all the great Circles

VI If you fuppofe two Circles drawn parallel to the Equinoctial at 23 Degrees 30 Minutes, reckoned on the Meridian, thefe are called the *Tropicks*, becaufe the Sun appears, when in them, to turn backward from his former Courfe, the

one

one the Tropick of *Cancer*, the other the Tropick of *Capricorn*, becaufe they are under thefe Signs

VII If two other Circles are fuppofed to be drawn thro 23 Degrees 30 Minutes, reckoned in the Meridian from the Polar Points, thefe are called the *Polar Circles* : The Northern is the Arctick, and the Southern the Antartick Circle, becaufe oppofite to the former

Thefe are the four leffer Circles

And thefe on the *Terreftrial Globe*, the Ancients fuppofed to divide the Earth into five *Zones*, *viz* two *Frigid*, two *Temperate*, and the *Torrid Zone*

Befides thefe ten Circles already defcribed, there are fome other neceffary Circles to be known, which are barely imaginary, and only fuppofed to be drawn upon the Globe

1. *Meridians* or *How-Circles*, which are great Circles all meeting in the Poles of the World, and croffing the Equinoctial at right Angles, thefe are fupply'd by the brazen meridian Hour-Circle and Index

2. *Azimuths* or *Vertical Circles*, which likewife are great Circles of *the Sphere*, and meet in the *Zenith* and *Nadir*, as the Meridians and Hour-Circles do in the Poles, thefe cut the Horizon at right Angles, and on thefe is reckon'd the Sun's Altitude, when he is not in the Meridian They are reprefented by the Quadrant of Altitude, by and by fpoken of, which being fixed at the Zenith, is moveable about the Globe thro all the Points of the Compafs

3. There are alfo *Circles of Longitude* of the Stars and Planets, which are great Circles paffing thro the Poles of the Ecliptick, and in that Line determining the Stars or Planets Place or Longitude, reckoned from the firft Point of *Aries*

4. *Almicanters*, or *Parallels of Altitude*, are Circles having their Poles in the Zenith, and are always drawn parallel to the Horizon Thefe are leffer Circles of the Sphere, diminifhing as they go further and further from the Horizon In refpect of the Stars, there are alfo Circles fuppofed to be *Parallels of Latitude*, which are Parallels to the Ecliptick, and have their Poles the fame as that of the Ecliptick

5. *Parallels of Declination* of the Sun or Stars, are leffer Circles, whofe Poles are the Poles of the World, and are all drawn parallel to the Equinoctial, either North or South, and thefe (when drawn on the *Terreftrial Globe*) are called *Parallels of Latitude*

VIII There are belonging to Globes a Quadrant of Altitude, and Semicircle of Pofition. The firft is a thin pliable piece of Brafs, whereon is graduated 90 Degrees anfwerable to thofe of the Equator, a fourth part of which it reprefents, with a Nut and Screw, to faften it to any part of the brazen Meridian as occafion requires There is or fhould be likewife a Compafs belonging to a Globe, that fo it may be fet North and South

The Semicircle of Pofition is a narrow Plate of Brafs, infcribed with 180 Degrees, and anfwerable to juft half the Equator

Laftly, The Brafs Circle, faftened at right Angles on the brazen Meridian, and the Index put on the Axis, is called the Index and Hour-Circle

SECTION II.

Having now defcribed the Circles of the Globes, I proceed to their Conftruction.

The Body of the Globe is compofed of an *Axle-Tree*, two *Paper-Caps* fewed together, a Compofition of Plaifter laid over them, and laft of all globical Papers or Gores (of which more by and by) ftuck or glewed on the Plaifter

The *Axle-Tree* is a piece of Wood which runs thro the middle of the Globe, turned fometimes of an equal Thicknefs, but oftner fmaller in the Middle than at the Ends, where two pieces of thick hardened Wire are ftruck in, which is the Axis, that appears without the Globe, on which it turns within the brazen Meridian.

The Paper-Caps inclofe this *Axle-Tree*, and are made in the following manner You muft have a Ball of Wood turned round, about a quarter of an Inch lefs in Diameter, than the Size you intend to make your Globe of, with two Pieces of Wire ftuck into it, diametrically oppofite to each other, for Conveniency of turning in a Frame, which may be made of two Pieces of Stick fixed upright in a Board, with Notches on the Tops to lay the Wire in Round this wooden Ball you muft pafte wafte Paper, both brown and white, till you judge it to be of the Thicknefs of Pafteboard, and before it be quite dry, cut it in the middle, fo that it may come off in two Hemifpheres to prevent the Paper from fticking, let the Ball at firft making be thick painted, and every time before you pafte Paper on it, greafe or oil it a little

The Holes at the Tops of the Caps, occafioned by the *Axis* on which the Ball turned, are very convenient for the *Axis* of the Globe to go thro in covering of it Then having faftened the Top of the Caps with fmall Nails to each end of the wooden Axle-Tree, few them clofe together in the middle with ftrong Twine.

That

That the Caps may meet exactly, obferve two things· 1ft, That the *Axletree* be juft in the Diameter of the Ball. 2dly, That before you take the Caps off the Ball, you make Scores a-crofs the parting all round, about an Inch afunder, whereby to bore the Holes for fewing them even together, and leave a Mark to direct how to join them again in the fame Points. for inftance, make a Crofs over any one of the Scores in the upper Cap, and another Crofs upon the fame Score in the under Cap; and when you clofe them, bring the two Croffes together, by which means the Caps in fewing will come as clofe together as before they were parted. This Care muft be taken, that there may be no Openings between, in which cafe, Paper muft be cramb'd in to ftop up the Gaps. but whether there be any Gaps or no, there muft be Paper pafted all over its fewing, to prevent any of the Plaifter from falling in.

The Plaifter is made with Glue, diffolved over the Fire in Water and Whitening mixed up thick, with fome Hemp fhred fmall, the Ufe of which is to bind the Plaifter, and keep it from cracking (as Hair is put into Mortar for the fame end:) a Handful will ferve two or three Gallons of Stuff. There is no neceffity for mixing the whole over the Fire, except the Whitening runs into Lumps not eafily to be broken with the Hand.

For laying on this Plaifter over the Caps in a globular Form, you muft have a Steel Semicircle exactly half the Circumference you intend the Globe to have, fixed flat-ways in a level Table made for that purpofe, with a Notch at each end for the *Axis* (which muft nicely fit it) to turn in, and two Buttons to cover it, to prevent the *Axis* from being forced out of the Notches, when the Globe is clogg'd with Plaifter, and fo requires fome Violence to turn it.

Then fixing your Paper-Sphere within this Semicircle, lay Plaifter on it with your Hands, turning the Globe eafily round, till it be covered fo as to fill the Semicircle· But before it comes to touch the Semicircle in all its Parts, and be equally fmooth all round, it will require a great many Layings on of the Plaifter, letting it dry between every fuch Application.

The fecond or third time of laying on Stuff, it will begin to touch the Semicircle in fome parts, and to appear round, the fourth time it will touch in more parts, and look rounder, till at laft it will touch in all parts, and become perfectly round and fmooth, like a Ball of polifhed Marble.

The next thing to be done is to poife the Globe, for it generally happens, by reafon of the Plaifter lying thicker in one place than in another, that fome fide weighs ftill downwards. To remedy this, a Hole muft be cut in that part, and a convenient Quantity of Shot put in, in a Bag, to bring it to a due Ballance with the reft, after which the Place muft be ftopped up with a Cork, and covered again with Plaifter. The Bag that holds the Shot may be glewed or fewed to the Cap within, or faftened to the Cork: fometimes after one part is ballanced, the Weight will incline to another, in which cafe the fame Remedy muft be apply'd again, as often as there will be neceffity.

This done, by help of another Semicircle, divided into 18 equal Parts, draw the Equator and Parallels of Latitude, placing a Black-lead Pencil at the Graduation, and turning the Globe againft the Point of it to make a Line. Then divide the Equator with a pair of Compaffes into fo many parts as there are globical Papers or Gores to lay on, and draw Lines thro each from Pole to Pole by the fide of the Semicircle. Within each of thefe Spaces fo marked out, you have only to lay one of the Gores, which (being cut out fo exact, as neither to lap over, nor leave a Vacancy between them) by the Affiftance of the Lines drawn upon the Plaifter, may be fitted, fo as to fall in with each other with the greateft Exactnefs. In applying the Gores, you may ufe a good binding Pafte, but Mouth Glue is better.

SECTION III.

Conftruction of the Circles of the Globe on the Globical Papers or Gores.

As 7 is to 22, fo is the Diameter of a Globe to the Circumference of any one of its greateft Circles. The Diameter of the Globe is ufually given, from whence it often happens that the Circumference confifts of odd Numbers and Parts. Whereas if the Circumference was given in even Numbers, as Inches, it might more eafily be divided into Parts. For example, if the Circumference was 36 Inches, each 10 Degrees of Longitude on the Equator will be one Inch; if the Circumference be 54, each 10 Degrees will be one Inch and a half, if 72, every 10 Degrees of Longitude will be two Inches.

The Diameter of a Globe being given, fuppofe 24 Inches, to find the Circumference, fay, As 7 is to 22, fo is 24 to 75 43 Inches, the Length of the Circumference fought.

The Length of each Gore, from the North Pole to the South Pole, will be exactly half the Circumference of the Globe, which is 37 71 Inches, and the Length from the Equator to either Pole will be ½, viz. 18 86 Inches.

If each of the Globical Papers contain in their greatest Breadth 30 Degrees of the Equator, 12 of them will cover the Globe, and by Dividing the Circumference 75 43 by 12, the Quotient will give 6 28 Inches for the Breadth of the Gore.

If 18 of the Gores go to cover the Globe, the Breadth of each will be 20 Degrees of the Equator, or 4 19 Inches

If 24, each will contain 15 Degrees of the Equator, or 3 14 Inches of the Circumference.

If 36, each Paper will contain 10 Degrees of the Circumference, or 2 09 Inches.

If the Globe be so large as to take up 360 Papers, that is, one to every Degree of Longitude, then will the Breadth of each Gore be 23 parts of an Inch.

Again, If the Circumference of a Globe be given, suppose 72 Inches, divide it by 2 (for the Length of the Gores from Pole to Pole) and the Quotient will be 36 Inches, and consequently half that Length, or the Distance from the Equator to either Pole, will be 18 Inches · as the Distance from N. to S. taken from a supposed Scale of Inches, is 36 Inches, or one half of the Circumference of the Globe, and the Distance from C to N or S, 18 Inches, or ¼ of the Circumference

If each Gore contains 30 Degrees of the Equator in Breadth, or $\frac{1}{12}$ of the Circumference, it will take up 6 Inches thereof as I K.

If 18 of the Gores go to cover a Globe of the aforesaid Circumference, each will contain 20 Degrees in Longitude of the Equator, or 4 Inches, as L M.

If your Papers be $\frac{1}{24}$ of the Circumference, each will contain 15 Degrees of the Equator, or 3 Inches, as *a b.*

If they be $\frac{1}{36}$ of the Circumference, each will contain 10 Degrees of the Equator, or 2 Inches, as *c d.*

If there be 72 Papers for covering the Globe, each will contain 5 Degrees of the Equator, or 1 Inch, that is $\frac{1}{72}$ of the Circumference

If, lastly, the Globe requires 360 Papers, each will contain 1 Degree, or ¼ of an Inch

This being premised, I now proceed to give the Manner of drawing the Circles of the Globes upon the aforesaid Gores.

Fig 7. Draw the Diameter W E, and cross it with another at right Angles to it, as N S. From the Scale of Inches set off from C to N, and to S, (the North and South Poles) 18 Inches, or ¼ of the Circumference, which divide into 9 equal parts, each of which likewise subdivide into 10 more (for the 90 Degrees of North and South Latitude) upon C, as a Center, describe the Circle N E, S W, and divide each Quadrant into 90 Degrees, numbering each 10th Degree with Figures from the Equator towards the Poles, as 10, 20, 30, &c Thus the three Points are found, thro which the parallel Circles to the Equator must be drawn, *viz.* two of them are in the Quadrants N E, N W, and S E, S W, and the third is in the Diameter N S

To find the Centers of any of the said Parallels, suppose of the Parallel of 60 Degrees, set one Foot of your Compasses in the Point 60, or F, of the Quadrant N E, and extend the other to the Point 60, or D, in the Diameter N S; then describe the little Arcs A, B, and removing the Foot of your Compasses to the Point D, describe two other Arcs, cutting those before described, and thro the Points of Intersection draw a right Line, which will cut the Diameter C N, produced in the Point G, the Center of the 60th Parallel. Having thus found the Centers of all the Parallels, and drawn them in the Northern Hemisphere, transfer the central Points in the Line C N continued, into the Line C S continued also, and draw the Parallels of the Southern Hemisphere Note, That whether the polar Papers extend to the 80th or 70th Parallel, those Circles in the meridional Papers, or those that encompass the Body of the Globe, must be described as is here ordered; but in the polar Papers the Pole must be the Center, as you see in the Figure, where one Point of the Compasses being set in the South Pole S, and the other extended to the 80th or 70th Degree of Latitude in the Diameter, strikes those Parallels in the polar Papers See more concerning the polar Papers hereafter

Then because the polar Circles and Tropicks are but Parallels 23 deg. 30 min distant from the Poles and Equator; at those Distances describe double Lines, representing such Circles, to distinguish them from other Parallels.

To draw the Meridians.

Having chosen one of the Proportions beforementioned for the Breadth of each Paper on the Equator, suppose $\frac{1}{12}$ of the Equator, which is the common Proportion in globical Papers, and the greatest Breadth that can be allowed them, let the Globe be of what Magnitude soever, then because $\frac{1}{12}$ of the Equator contains 30 Degrees, which in the Gores for a Globe of 72 Inches Circumference, are six Inches in Breadth, from a Scale of Inches take three Inches between your Compasses, and lay them off on the Diameter W C E, from C to K, and from C to I, the Length from I to K being six Inches, or 30 Degrees of the Equator, into which it must be divided, and numbered at each 5th or 10th Degree, with the Degrees of Longitude

Now

Now becaufe a fingle Degree cannot be well divided into Parts in fo fmall a Projection, and feeing that any Number of Degrees of Longitude in any Parallel has the fame Proportion to one Degree in that Parallel, as the fame Number of Degrees of Longitude under the Equator has to one Degree of Longitude; therefore take 15 Degrees of the Equator, *viz.* I C or I K, in your Compaffes, and having divided it feparately, as you would a fingle Degree, into 60 equal Parts, look in the following Table what Proportion a Degree (or 15 Degrees) in each 5*th* or 10*th* Parallel of Latitude, hath to a Degree (or 15 Degrees) on the Equator. For example, in the firft Column of the Table towards the Left-Hand, are the Degrees of Latitude; over againft the 10th Degree, I find 59 Miles in the fecond Column, and 00 Minutes, or Fractions of a Mile, in the third Column, which fignifies that a Degree (or 15 Degrees) in the 10th Parallel of Latitude, contains but 59 Miles 00 Minutes of a Degree (or 15 Degrees of the Equator) which Length I take from the Scale I C or C K between my Compaffes, and fet off on each fide the Meridian, or Diameter N S, on the 10*th* Parallel

Again, in the Parallel of 20 Degrees, I find a Degree to contain 56 Miles 24 Minutes, or parts of a Mile, of a Degree in the Equator, and transfer that Length from the aforefaid Scale upon the 20th Parallel, the like is to be underftood of all the reft, and thofe Points being found and joined, will form the Meridians on the Gores   The fame Directions muft be followed in all other Proportions for the Breadth of the Gores, in chufing of which, obferve, that as it is manifeft from the Figure of the Globe, that a Paper fo large as $\frac{1}{12}$ of the Circumference of the Globe, cannot lie upon its Convexity, without crumbling, lapping over, or tearing, in the Application, therefore it will be better to ufe fome leffer Proportion, as L M, *a b*, or *c d* for note, the narrower they are, the more exactly they will fit the Globe. Note alfo, in drawing the Parallels from 10 to 30 Degrees of Latitude, right Lines will do well enough

A TABLE *fhewing in what Proportion the Degrees of Longitude decreafe in the Parallels of Latitude.*

Lat.	Mil	Min	Lat.	Mil	Min	Lat.	Mil	Min	Lat.	Mil	Min	Lat.	Mil	Min	Lat.	Mil	Min	Lat.	Mil	Min
0	60	0	13	58	28	25	54	24	37	47	56	49	39	20	61	29	4	73	17	32
1	59	56	14	58	12	26	54	0	38	47	16	50	38	32	62	28	8	74	16	32
2	59	54	15	58	0	27	53	28	39	46	36	51	37	44	63	27	12	75	15	32
3	59	52	16	57	40	28	53	0	40	46	0	52	37	0	64	26	16	76	14	32
4	59	50	17	57	20	29	52	28	41	45	16	53	36	8	65	25	20	77	13	32
5	59	46	18	57	4	30	51	56	42	44	36	54	35	26	66	24	24	78	12	32
6	59	40	19	56	44	31	51	24	43	43	52	55	34	24	67	23	28	79	11	28
7	59	37	20	56	24	32	50	52	44	43	8	56	33	32	68	22	32	80	10	24
8	59	24	21	56	0	33	50	20	45	42	24	57	32	40	69	21	32	81	9	20
9	59	10	22	55	36	34	49	44	46	41	40	58	31	48	70	20	32	82	8	20
10	59	0	23	55	12	35	49	8	47	41	0	59	31	0	71	19	32	83	7	20
11	58	52	24	54	48	36	48	32	48	40	8	60	30	0	72	18	32	84	6	12
12	58	40																85	5	12
																		86	4	12
																		87	3	12
																		88	2	4
																		89	1	4
																		90	0	0

The exact Geometrical Way of drawing the Parallels and Meridians on the Gores.

Becaufe in the Method before laid down, the true Centers of the Parallels are not exact-*Plate 18.* ly in thofe Points found as there directed, nor the Points in them the Points by which the *Fig. 1.* Meridians muft pafs · therefore I think it proper here to exhibit the Geometrical Manner of drawing them truly.

Suppofe S B to be the Semidiameter of the Globe, with which defcribe the Quadrant B I, and continue out the Semidiameter S I, both ways   Make S A equal to $\frac{1}{4}$ of the Circumference, the Point A of which, will be the Pole of the Gore   Then divide the Quadrant B I into 90 equal Parts or Degrees, to every of which draw the Tangents *i* 80, *k* 70, *l* 60, *m* 50, &c until they meet the Radius S I continued. Again, having divided the Line A S (equal to $\frac{1}{4}$ of the Circumference of the Globe) into 90 equal Parts, (I have only divided it into 9) and numbred them as *per* Figure, take the Length of the Tangent *i* 80 between your Compaffes, and fetting one Foot in the Point 80 of the Line A S, the other will fall upon the Point *a* in the faid Line continued out beyond A, which will be the Center of the 80*th* Parallel paffing thro the Point 80 in the Line A S.

Moreover,

Moreover, to find the Center of the 70th Parallel, take the Tangent *k* 70 between your Compasses, and setting one Foot in the Point 70 of the Line A S, the other will fall on the Point *b* in the Line A S continued, which will be the Center of the 70th Parallel, passing thro the Point 80 in the Line A S

In like manner, to find the Center of the 60th Parallel, take the Tangent *l* 60 between your Compasses, and set it off from the Point 60 in the Line A S, and you will have the Center *c* for the 60th Parallel, passing thro the Point 60 Proceed thus for finding the Centers *d*, *e*, *f*, *g*, &c. of the Parallels 50, 40, 30, 20, &c about each of which Centers respective Arcs being drawn, the Parallels will be had.

The Reason of this Operation for finding the Centers of the Parallels, is this, If a Sphere or Globe hath revolved upon a Plane, in such manner that every Point of the Periphery of some lesser Circle of it, has touched the said Plane, and the Point which in the beginning of the Motion was contiguous to the Plane, became to be contiguous to it again, then the Points on the Plane, that were contiguous to the Points of the Periphery of the aforesaid lesser Circle, will be in the Circumference of a Circle, whose Center will be the Vertex of a right Cone, lying on the aforesaid Plane, the Base of which will be the said Circle; and consequently the Vertex will be determined in the Plane, by continuing a right Line raised on the Circle's Center perpendicularly till it cuts the aforesaid Plane.

How to draw the Meridians.

Having drawn the Sines 10 *p*, 20 *q*, 30 *r*, 40 *s*, &c divide the Radius B S into 360 equal Parts, or make a Diagonal Scale of that Length, whereby 360 may be taken off Then having assumed S C for half the Breadth of the Gore, suppose $\frac{1}{24}$ of the Circumference of the Equator, take S *x* (the Sine Complement of 80 deg) between your Compasses, and applying this Extent on the Radius B S, or the Diagonal Scale, see how many of those Parts that the Diameter is divided into, that Extent takes up Then take $\frac{1}{24}$ of those Parts, and with the Quotient as so many Degrees make the Arc 10 L off, which will give the Point L in the Parallel of 10 Degrees, thro which the Meridian must pass.

Again, take S *w* between your Compasses, and see how many of the Parts that the Radius B S is divided into, it contains, then take $\frac{1}{24}$ of those Parts, and with the Quotient, as so many Degrees, make the Arc 20 M off, which will give another Point M, thro which the same Meridian must pass in the 20th Parallel.

In like manner, to find the Point N in the Parallel of 30 Degrees, thro which the Meridian must pass, take S *u* (the Sine Complement of 60 Degrees) in your Compasses, and see how many of the Parts that the Radius B S is divided into, then taking $\frac{1}{24}$ of those Parts, with the Quotient as so many Degrees, make the Arc 30 N off.

Proceeding in this manner, you may find other Points in the other Parallels, thro which the Meridian must pass Which Points being afterwards joined, the quarter of the Meridian A N C will be drawn, and therefore one quarter of the Gore, and consequently the other three Quarters of the Gore will be easily limited

Method of ordering the Circumpolar Papers.

The Circumpolar Papers were formerly not cut out by themselves, till Artists found it hard to make the Poles, or Points of the Gores, fall nicely in the North and South Poles, whence, to help that Inconveniency, they made Circular Papers serve to cover the Superficies of the Globe between the Polar Circles, the Parallels on which Papers are all Concentric Circles, and the Meridians Right Lines yet finding still so big Papers not to fit the Globe's Convexity, but wrinkle about the edges, they have extended them from the Poles only to the Parallels of 70 Degrees. But neither will it do yet, because the Longitude decreases disproportionally, the further off the Poles. If the Diameter of a Polar Paper extends to 10 Degrees from the Pole only, that Paper will lie flat upon the Globe's Convexity, without any sensible stretching or contracting : But if it extend to or beyond the 70th Parallel, you must take another Course

Fig. 2. Suppose A P B to be half of a Gore, 12 of which will cover a Globe About the Point P with an extent to the 70th Parallel, describe a Circle, which from the Points G or F, divide into 12 equal Parts ; or which is the same, continue every other Meridian in the Parallel 80 to the Parallel 70, and by the aforementioned Table set off on each Side these 12 Meridians, the true Longitude of each 10 Degrees in the Parallel of 80, or, which will save that trouble, transfer the Distance from C to G, or from G to D upon the Parallel of 70 Deg. in the Polar Paper, for that is the extent of 10 Degrees in that Parallel; and, as is manifest from the Figure, there will lie between each twelfth part of the Circumference F G, a narrow slip of Paper which must be cut out, and then the Paper being laid upon the Globe, the Parts will naturally close whereas, for want of this care taken, we commonly see the Polar Papers wrap over and wrinkle, besides, the Points of the Meridians on the Polar Papers seldom meet those of the Meridians of the Gores, except now and then by chance.

From this one rough Draught you may transfer the rest of the Gores that are to make up the Surface of the Globe, by which the trouble of projecting a New Scheme for every

Gore

Plate XVII

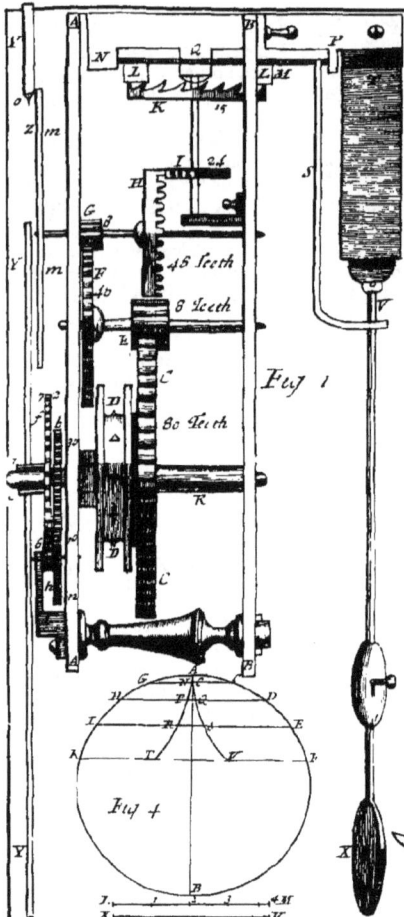

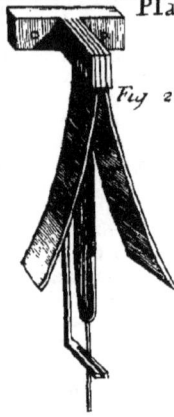

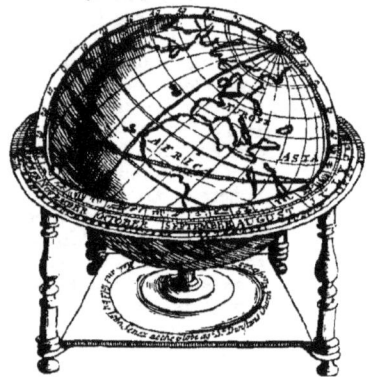

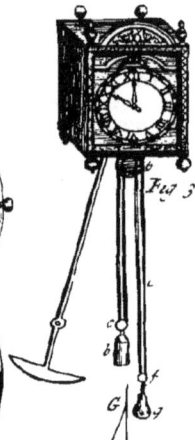

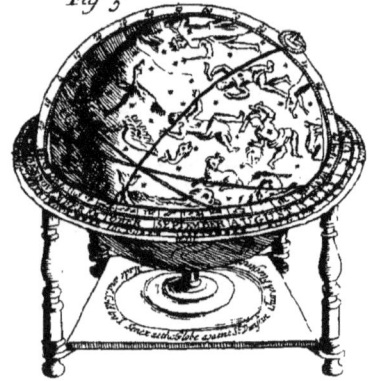

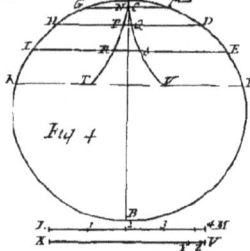

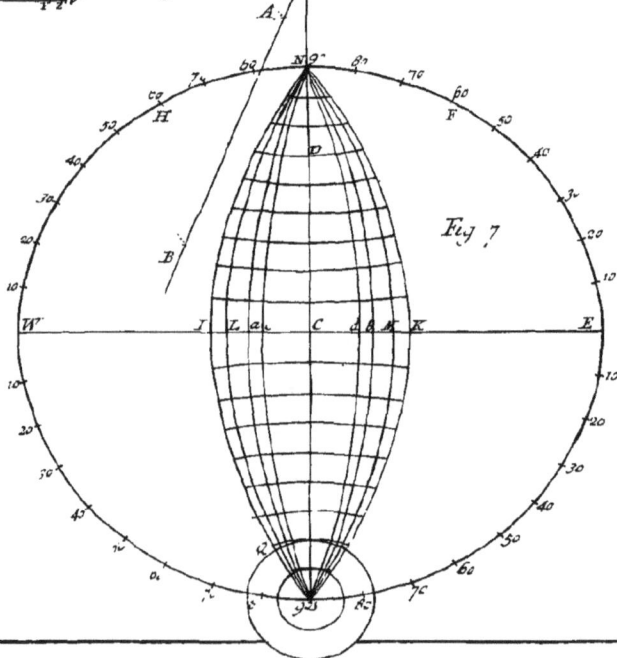

Gore will be avoided. Obferve to do it with great care, for a fmall Error will, when the Gores are all joined, appear very fenfible. Then becaufe the Gores in all make 12, you may divide your Projections upon three Sheets of large Paper, allowing four Gores to each Sheet

Draw an Eaft and Weft Diameter thro every Sheet, in each of which fet off the Diftance Fig 2. from I to K, of *Fig* 7 *Plate* 17. with your Compaffes four times, without fhifting the Points In the middle of each erect Perpendiculars, and transfer 70 Degrees thereon (allowing the Polar Papers to include 20 Degrees from the Poles) Northwards and Southwards from the Center, which is the Interfection of the Equator with the ftreight Meridians or Perpendiculars, for Northern and Southern Latitude

From the aforefaid Semi-gore, take the Diftance between the Point of each 10th Parallel in the Perpendiculars, and in the Meridians A C, B D, and in the fair Draught defcribe Arcs to the Right and Left, upon the Points in the Perpendiculars.

Then placing one foot of your Compaffes in the Point A or B, extend the other to the Point of the Meridians and Parallels Interfection, and as you go along, transfer the Diftances upon the Copies from the correfpondent Points of the Equator into the Arcs, and the Places where they cut will be the Points thro which the Meridians and Parallels muft be drawn And that Meridian, among all the Papers which is pitched upon for the firft, let be divided equally from the Equator to G, and then in the Polar Papers to the Poles, into Degrees or Minutes, numbering each 10th or 5th Degree, with the Degrees of Latitude, minding to draw three Lines to diftinguifh it from other Meridians. The fame muft be obferved in defcribing the Ecliptick or Equator, on which laft every 5th or 10th Degree, till you come to 180 Degrees, muft be figured Eaftward and Weftward from the firft Meridian.

When all the Papers are finifhed fo far as relates to the Meridians and Parallels, you muft next draw the Ecliptick, and becaufe that Circle interfects the Meridians in fuch and fuch Parallels of Declination, and the Meridians cut the Equator in the Degrees of Right Afcenfion; therefore by help of a Table of the Declination of thofe Points of the Ecliptick that cut the Meridian, and the Right Afcenfion of the fame Points, find the Declination over-againft the Right Afcenfion, which fhews thro what parts of the Meridians the Ecliptick Arcs muft pafs, and draw Right Lines thro the Points of Interfection, which Lines will form the Ecliptick on the Globe

A TABLE of *Right Afcenfion* and *Declination* of every 15 *Degrees* of the *Signs*.

	Deg.	Deg.	Min.		Deg	Min.
Aries	15	13	48		5	56
Taurus	0	27	54		11	30
Taurus	15	42	31		16	23
Gemini	0	57	48		20	12
Gemini	15	73	43		22	39
Cancer	0	90	00	Add 180 Degrees for the fix other Signs	23	30
Cancer	15	106	17		22	39
Leo	0	122	12		20	12
Leo	15	137	29		16	23
Virgo	0	152	6		11	30
Virgo	15	166	12		5	56

Seek the Right Afcenfion as Longitude, and the Declination as Latitude, and where they interfect is the refpective Point of the Ecliptick

Proceed next to infert the Stars on the Gores for the *Celeftial Globe*, and *Places* on thofe for the Terreftrial Globe, by help of moft approved Aftronomical and Geographical Tables and Maps, according to their refpective Longitude and Latitude, which may eafily be effected by finding the Meridian and Parallel of the Star or Place, and the Point where they interfect each other, will be the exact Situation thereof

The Rhumb Lines (which always make the fame Angles with the Parallels they are drawn thro) may be infcribed by *Wright*'s Card, or Loxodromick Tables, found in fome Books of Navigation, as thofe in *Newhoufe*. Trade Winds are beft defcribed from Dr *Halley* in the *Philofophical Tranfactions* the Conftellations may be drawn by a Celeftial Globe.

Your Projectures of the Heaven and Earth being finifhed, you may either apply them to a particular Pair of Globes, or have them engraved in Copper-Plates.

C H A P. II.

Of Astronomical and Geographical Definitions, and the Uses of the Globes.

BEfore I lay down the Uses of the Globe, it will be proper to exhibit the following Definitions, necessary to be known in order to understand their Uses

Definition I The *Latitude of any Place*, is an Arc of the Meridian of that Place, intercepted between the Zenith and the Equator, and this is the same as an Arc of the Meridian intercepted between the Pole and the Horizon, and therefore the Latitude of any Place is often expressed by the Pole's Height, or Elevation of the Pole. the Reason of which is, that from the Equator to the Pole, there always being the Distance of 90 Degrees, and from the Zenith to the Horizon the same Number, and each of these 90 containing within it the Distance between the Zenith and the Pole, that Distance therefore being taken away from both, must leave the Distance from the Zenith to the Equator equal to the Distance between the Pole and the Horizon, or the Elevation of the Pole above the Horizon

Definition II. Latitude of a Star or Planet, is an Arc of a great Circle reckoned on the Quadrant of Altitude, laid through the Star and Pole of the Ecliptick, from the Ecliptick towards its Pole

Definition III. Longitude of a Place is an Arc of the Equator intercepted between the Meridian ; or it is more properly the Difference, either East or West, between the Meridians of any two Places, accounted on the Equator

Definition IV Longitude of a Star, is an Arc of the Ecliptick, accounted from the beginning of *Aries* to the Place where the Star's Circle of Longitude crosseth the Ecliptick, so that it is much the same as the Star's Place in the Ecliptick, accounted from the beginning of *Aries*

Definition V Amplitude of the Sun or of a Star, is an Arc of the Horizon intercepted between the true East or West Points of it, and that Point upon which the Sun or Star rises or sets

Definition VI Right Ascension of the Sun, or of a Star, is that part of the Equinoctial reckoned from the beginning of *Aries*, which rifeth or setteth with the Sun or Star in a Right Sphere but in an Oblique Sphere it is that part of a Degree of the Equinoctial, which comes to the Meridian with it, (as before) reckoned from the beginning of *Aries*

Definition VII A right or direct Sphere, is when the Poles are in the Horizon, and the Equator in the Zenith : the Consequence of being under such a Position of the Heavens as this (which is the case of those who live directly under the Line) is, that the Inhabitants have no Latitude nor Elevation of the Pole, they can nearly see both the Poles of the World   All the Stars in the Heaven do once in twenty-four Hours rise, culminate, and set with them, the Sun always rises and descends at Right Angles with the Horizon, which is the Reason they have always equal Days and Nights, because the Horizon doth exactly bisect the Circle of the Sun's Diurnal Revolution

Definition VIII. A Parallel Sphere, is where the Poles are in the Zenith and Nadir, and the Equinoctial in the Horizon, which is the Case of such Persons, if any such there be, who live directly under the North or South Poles

And the Consequences of such a Position are, that the Parallels of the Sun's Declination will also be Parallels of his Altitude, or Almacanters to them   The Inhabitants can see only such Stars as are on their side the Equinoctial, and they must have six Months Day, and six Months continual Night every Year, and the Sun can never be higher with them than 23 Degrees, 30 Minutes, (which is not so high as it is with us on *February* the 10*th*)

Definition IX An oblique Sphere, is where the Pole is elevated to any Number of Degrees less than 90 and consequently the Axis of the Globe can never be at Right Angles to, nor in the Horizon ; and the Equator and Parallels of Declination, will all cut the Horizon obliquely, from whence it takes its Name

Oblique Ascension of the Sun or Stars, is that Part or Degree of the Equinoctial reckoned from the beginning of *Aries*, which rises and sets with them in an oblique Sphere

Ascensional Difference, is the Difference between the right and oblique Ascension, when the lesser is substracted from the greater

On the Terrestrial Globe.

Definition X A Space upon the Surface of the Earth, reckoned between two Parallels to the Equator, wherein the Increase of the longest Day is a quarter of an Hour, is by some Writers called a Parallel.

Definition

Definition XI And the Space contained between two fuch Parallels, is called a Climate : Thefe Climates begin at the Equator, and when we go North or South, till the Day becomes half an Hour longer than it was before, they fay we are come into the firft Climate, when the Days are an Hour longer than they are under the Equator, we are come to the Second Climate, &c thefe Climates are counted in Number 24, reckoned each ways from the Poles.

The Inhabitants of the Earth are divided into three forts, as to the falling of their Shadows.

Definition XII *Amphifcii,* who are thofe which inhabit the Torrid Zone, or live between the Equator and Tropicks, and confequently have the Sun twice a Year in their Zenith ; at which time they are *Afcii,* i e have no Shadows, the Sun being vertical to them thefe have their Shadows caft to the Southward, when the Sun is in the Northern Signs, and to the Northward when the Sun is in the Southern Signs reckoned in refpect of them

Definition XIII *Heterofcii,* who are thofe whofe Shadows fall but one way, as is the Cafe of all fuch as live between the Tropicks and Polar Circles, for their Shadows at Noon are always to the Northward in North Latitude, and to the Southward in South Latitude

Definition XIV *Perifcii,* are fuch Perfons that inhabit thofe Places of the Earth that lie between the Polar Circles and the Poles, and therefore have their Shadows falling all manner of ways, becaufe the Sun at fome time of the Year goes clear round about them The Inhabitants of the Earth, in refpect of one another, are alfo divided into three Sorts

Perioeci, who are fuch as inhabiting the fame Parallel (not a great Circle) are yet directly oppofite to one another, the one being Eaft or Weft from the other exactly 180 Degrees, which is their Difference of Longitude Now thefe have the fame Latitude and Length of Days and Nights, but exactly at contrary Times, for when the Sun rifeth to one, it fets to the other

Antoeci, who are Inhabitants of fuch Places, as being under a Semi-circle of the fame Meridian, do lie at equal Diftance from the Equator, one towards the North, and the other towards the South Now thefe have the fame Degree of Latitude, but towards contrary Parts, the one North and the other South, and therefore muft have the Seafons of the Year directly at contrary Times one to the other

Antipodes, who are fuch as dwell under the fame Meridian, but in two oppofite and equidiftant Parallels, and in the two oppofite Points of thofe two Parallels, fo that they go Feet againft Feet, and are diftant from each other an intire Diameter of the Earth, or 180 Degrees of a great Circle. Thefe have the fame Degree of Latitude, but the one South, the other North, and accounted from the Equator a quite contrary way, and therefore thefe will have all things, as Day and Night, Summer and Winter, directly contrary to one another

USE I *To find the Latitude of any Place*

Bring the Place to the Brafs Meridian, and the Degrees of that Circle, intercepted between the Place and the Equinoctial, are the Latitude of that Place either North or South

Then to fit the Globe fo that the wooden Horizon fhall reprefent the Horizon of that Place, elevate the Pole as many Degrees above the wooden Horizon, as are contain'd in the Latitude of that Place, and it is done ; for then will that Place be in the Zenith

If after this you rectify the Globe to any particular time, you may by the Index know the time of Sun-rifing and Setting with the Inhabitants of that Place, and confequently the prefent Length of their Day and Night, &c

USE II *To find the Longitude of a Place*

Bring the Places feverally to the Brafs Meridian, and then the Number of Degrees of the Equinoctial, which are between the Meridians of each Place, are their Difference of Longitude either Eaft or Weft

But if you reckon it from any Place where a firft Meridian is fuppofed to be placed, you muft bring the firft Meridian to the Brazen one on the Globe, and then turn the Globe about till the other Place come thither alfo. reckon the Number of Degrees of the Equinoctial intercepted between the firft Meridian, and the proper one of the Place, and that is the Longitude of that Place, either Eaft or Weft

USE III *To find what Places of the Earth the Sun is Vertical to, at any time affigned.*

Bring the Sun's Place found in the Ecliptick on the Terreftrial Globe to the brazen Meridian, and note what Degree of the Meridian it cuts, then by turning the Globe round about, you will fee what Places of the Earth are in that Parallel of Declination (for they will all come fucceffively to that Degree of the brazen Meridian), and thofe are the Places and Parts of the Earth to which the Sun will be Vertical that Day, whofe Inhabitants will then be *Afcii,* that is, their erect Bodies at Noon will caft no Shadow

Of

Of the Celeftial Globe.

USE IV *To find the Sun's place in the Ecliptick in any given Day of the Month, by means of the Circle of Signs on the wooden Horizon*

Seek the Day of the Month upon the Horizon, obferving the Difference between the *Julian* and *Gregorian* Calendars, and then againft the faid Day you will find, in the Circle of Signs, the Sign and Degree the Sun is in the faid Day This being done, find the fame Sign and Degree upon the Ecliptick on the Superficies of the Globe, and the Sun's place will be had   *Note*, If the Sun's place be required more exactly, you muft confult an Ephemeris for the given Year, or elfe calculate it from Aftronomical Tables

USE V. *The Sun's Place for any Day being given, to find his Declination*

Bring the Sun's Place for that Day to the Meridian, and then the Degrees of the Meridian, reckoned from the Equinoctial either North or South to the faid Place, fhew the Sun's Declination for that Day at Noon, either North or South, according to the time of the Year, *viz* from *March* the 10th to *September* the 12th, North, and from thence to *March* again, South

USE VI *To find the Sun's Amplitude either Rifing or Setting.*

Having rectified the Globe to the Latitude of the Place, that is, moved the brazen Meridian till the Degree of Latitude thereon be cut by the Plane of the wooden Horizon, bring the Sun's Place to the faid Horizon either on the Eaft or Weft fide, and the Degrees of the Horizon, reckoned from the Eaft Point, either North or South, give the Amplitude fought, and at the fame time you have in the Circle of Rhumbs the Point that the Sun rifes or fets upon.

USE VII *To find the Sun's Right Afcenfion*

Bring the Sun's Place to the brazen Meridian, and the Degrees intercepted between the beginning of *Aries*, and that Degree of the Equinoctial which comes to the Meridian with the Sun, is the Right Afcenfion, which if you would have in time, you muft reckon every 15 Degrees for one Hour, and every Degree four Minutes

Note, The Reafon of bringing the Sun's place to the Meridian in this Ufe, is to fave the trouble of putting the Globe into the Pofition of a Right Sphere for properly Right Afcenfion is that Degree of the Equinoctial, which rifes with the Sun in a Right Sphere But fince the Equator is always at Right Angles to the Meridian, if you bring the Sun's place thither, it muft in the Equinoctial cut his Right Afcenfion

USE VIII *To find the Sun's Oblique Afcenfion*

Having rectified the Globe to the Latitude, bring the Sun's Place to the Eaft-fide the Horizon, and the Number of Degrees intercepted between that Degree of the Equinoctial, which is now come to the Horizon and the beginning of *Aries*, is the Oblique Afcenfion Now the leffer of thefe two Afcenfions being taken from the greater, the Remainder is the afcenfional Difference, which therefore is the Difference in Degrees between the Right or Oblique Afcenfion, or the Space between the Sun's Rifing or Setting, and the Hour of fix Wherefore the afcenfional Difference being converted into Time, will give the time of the Sun's Rifing and Setting before or after fix.

USE IX *To find the time of the Sun's Rifing or Setting in any given Latitude*

Having firft brought his Place to the Meridian, and the Hour-Index to twelve at Noon, bring his Place afterwards to the Horizon, either on the Eaft or Weft-fide thereof, then the Hour-Index will either fhew the time of his Rifing and Setting accordingly Now the time of the Sun's Setting being doubled, gives the Length of the Day, and the time of his Rifing doubled, gives the Length of the Night

USE X *To find the Sun's Meridian Altitude, or Depreffion at Midnight, in any given Latitude*

Bring his Place to the Meridian above the Horizon, for his Noon Altitude, which will fhew the Degrees thereof, reckoning from the Horizon, and to find his midnight Depreffion below the North Point of the Horizon, the Point in the Ecliptick oppofite to the Sun's prefent Place, muft be brought to the South part of the Meridian above the Horizon, and the Degrees there intercepted between that Point and the Horizon, are his midnight Depreffion.

USE XI *To find the Sun's Altitude at any time of the Day given*

Rectify the Globe, that is, bring the Sun's Place to the Meridian, and fet the Hour-Index to twelve, and raife the Pole to the Latitude of the Place above the Horizon This being done, fit the Quadrant of Altitude, that is, fcrew the Quadrant of Altitude to

the

the Zenith, or in our Latitude fcrew it fo that the divided Edge cut 51 deg 32 min on the Meridian reckoned from the Equinoctial. Then turn the Globe about till the Index fhews the given time, and ftay the Globe there ; after which, bring the Quadrant of Altitude to cut the Sun's Place in the Ecliptick, and then that Place or Degree of the Ecliptick will fhew the Sun's Altitude on the Quadrant of Altitude.

USE XII *To find the Sun's Altitude, and at what Hour he is due Eaft or Weft.*

Rectify the Globe, and fit the Quadrant of Altitude Then bring the Quadrant to cut the true Eaft Point, and turn the Globe about till the Sun's Place in the Ecliptick cuts the divided Edge of the Quadrant of Altitude , for then that Place will fhew the Altitude, and the Index the Hour

USE XIII *The Sun's Azimuth, or when he is on any Point of the Compafs being given , to find his Altitude and the Hour of the Day*

Set the Quadrant of Altitude to the Azimuth given, and turn the Globe about till his Place in the Ecliptick touches the divided Edge of the Quadrant , fo fhall that Place give the Altitude on the Quadrant, and the Hour-Index the Time of the Day

USE XIV *To find the Declination, and Right Afcenfion of any Star.*

Bring the Star to the brazen Meridian, and then the Degrees intercepted between the Equinoctial and the Point of the Meridian cut by the Star, gives its Declinations And the Meridian cuts, and fhews its Right Afcenfion on the Equinoctial, reckoning from the beginning of *Aries*

USE XV *To find the Longitude and Latitude of any Star.*

Bring the Solftitial Colure to the brazen Meridian, and there fix the Globe , then will the Pole of the Ecliptick be juft under 23 deg 30 min reckoning from the Pole above the North Point of the Horizon, and upon the fame Meridian , there fcrew the Quadrant of Altitude, and then bring its graduated Edge to the Star affigned, and there ftay it fo will the Star cuts its proper Latitude on the Quadrant, reckoned from the Ecliptick , and the Quadrant will cut the Ecliptick in the Star's Longitude, or its Diftance from the firft Point of *Aries*

USE XVI *To find the time of any Star's rifing, fetting, or culminating, that is, being on the Meridian.*

Rectify the Globe, and Hour-Index, and bring the Star to the Eaft or Weft part of the Horizon, or to the brazen Meridian, and the Index will fhew accordingly the time of the Star's rifing, fetting or culminating, or of its being on the Meridian

USE XVII. *To know, at any time affigned, what Stars are rifing or fetting, which are on the Meridian, and how high they are above the Horizon, on what Azimuth or Point of the Compafs they are , by which means the real Stars in the Heaven may eafily be known by their proper Names, and rightly diftinguifhed from one another*

Rectify the Globe, and fit the Quadrant of Altitude, and fet the Globe, by means of the Compafs, due North and South , then turn the Globe and Hour-Index to the Hour of the Night affigned , fo will the Globe, thus fixed, reprefent the Face or Appearance of the Heavens for that time · whereby you may readily fee what Stars are in or near the Horizon, what are on or near the Meridian ; which are to the North, or which to the South, &c and the Quadrant of Altitude being laid over any particular Star, will fhew its Altitude and Azimuth, or on what Point of the Compafs it is, whereby any Star may eafily be known , efpecially if you have a Quadrant to take the Altitude of any real Star fuppofed to be known by the Globe,to fee whether it agrees with that Star which is its Reprefentative on the Globe or not.

USE XVIII *The Sun's Place given, as alfo a Star's Altitude, to find the Hour of the Night*

Rectify the Globe, and fit the Quadrant of Altitude , then move the Globe backwards or forwards, till the Quadrant cuts the Star in its given Altitude for then the Hour-Index will fhew the Hour of the Night And thus may the Hour of the Night be known by a Star's Azimuth, or its Azimuth by its Altitude.

USE XIX. *To find the Diftance between any two Stars*

If the Stars lie both under the fame Meridian, bring them to the brazen Meridian, and the Degrees of the faid Meridian comprehended between them, are their Diftance.

If they are both in the Equinoctial, or have both the fame Declination, that is, are both in the fame Parallel, then bring them one after another to the brazen Meridian, and the Degrees of the Equinoctial intercepted between them, when thus brought to the Meridian feverally, are their Diftance.

If the Stars are neither under the fame Meridian or Parallel, then either lay the Quadrant of Altitude from one to the other (if it will reach) and that will fhew the Diftance between them in Degrees; or elfe take the Diftance with Compaffes, and apply that to the Equinoctial, or to the Meridian

This Method of Proceeding will alfo fhew the Diftance of any two Places on the Terreftrial Globe in Degrees Wherefore to find how far any Place on the Globe is from another, you need only take the Diftance between them on the Globe with a Pair of Compaffes, and applying the Compaffes to the Equator at the beginning of *Aries*, or at the firft Meridian, you will there find the Degrees of their Diftance, which multiply'd by 70, and that will be their Diftance in Miles

---

CHAP. III.

Of SPHERES.

SECTION I.

Of the Ptolemaick Sphere.

Fig. 3.

THE third Figure of *Plate* 18, reprefents a Ptolemaick Armillary Sphere, made of Brafs, or Wood, confifting of the fame Circles that have been defcribed in Chapter I aforegoing, and having a round Ball fixed in the middle thereof, upon the Axis of the World, reprefenting the Earth. Upon the Surface of this Ball are drawn Meridians, Parallels, &c as likewife as many Kingdoms, Countries, Seas, &c with their Names, as can conveniently be depicted thereon. This Sphere revolves about the faid Axis, between the Meridian, and by this means not only fhews the Sun's diurnal and annual Courfe, &c about the Earth, according to the Ptolemaick Hypothefis, which fuppofes the Earth to be at reft, and the Sun to move about the fame ; but likewife by it any Problem relating to the Sun, may be folved, that can be done by the Globes And this any one that knows the Ufe of the Globes may likewife do.

SECTION II.

Of the common Copernican Sphere.

Fig. 4.

This Sphere ftands upon four brafs or wooden Feet, upon each of which are fixed the four ends of a brafs or wooden Crofs, upon which Crofs is faftened a large hollow brafs or wooden Circle, whofe Center is exactly over the Center of the Crofs. Upon the upper Plane of this Circle are the Calenders, and Circle of Signs defcribed, the fame as on the Horizon of the Globes. Clofe within the infide of this Circle is fitted a flat moveable Rundle, whofe Center is common with the Center of the Crofs The outmoft Limb of this Rundle is divided into 24 equal Parts, reprefenting the 24 Hours of Day and Night, numbered from the Index (of which more hereafter) towards the Right-hand with Numerical Letters from I to XII, and then beginning again with I, II, &c to XII again

There is a round Wheel fixed upon the Crofs, under the faid Rundle, whofe Convex Side is cut into a certain Number of Teeth Thro the Rundle, the Wheel on the Crofs, and the Crofs itfelf, is fitted a perpendicular Axis, about which the Rundle moves. This reprefents part of the Axis of the Ecliptick, and at the top thereof is placed a little Golden Ball, reprefenting the Sun

On the under fide of the moveable Rundle moves another Wheel, whofe Convex Side is cut into Teeth, and as the Rundle is turned about upon its Center, this Wheel is alfo turned about upon its Center, by the falling in of the Teeth on that Wheel fixed on the Crofs. Likewife near the outmoft Limb of the Rundle is fitted another Wheel, into which is fitted a Pedeftal, holding up a Sphere of feveral Parts, having a Terreftrial Globe inclofed therein, as fhall be fhewn hereafter The outmoft Limb of this Wheel is likewife cut into Teeth, fitted into the Teeth of the fixed Wheel , and fo as the Rundle moves round, this Wheel is carried about, and with it likewife the Earth, and all the Circles faftened upon the aforefaid Pedeftal

On one fide of this Rundle is faftened a little round Pin to turn about the Rundle by, and near this Pin, is an Index upon the Rundle, reaching to the outward Limb of the great hollow Circle, and fo at once may be applied to the Day of the Month in both Calenders, and alfo to the Degree of the Ecliptick the Sun is in that Day at Noon. *Note,* This Index is called the Index of the moveable Rundle On each fide of the Crofs is placed a Pillar, fupporting a broad Circle, reprefenting the Zodiack, with the Ecliptick in the middle

dle

dle thereof, as in the Ptolemaick Sphere   *Note,* This is called the Zodiack, in the Use of the Sphere.

Upon the aforesaid Pedestal are fastened two Circles cutting each other at Right Angles, representing the two Colures so placed, that the Points wherein they intersect each other stand directly upwards and downwards, and represent the Poles of the Ecliptick, the uppermost being the North, and the other the South   One of these Colures, *viz.* the Solstitial, hath a small Hour-Circle placed thereon, at the extremity of the Axis of the Earth   In the middle, between the two Poles of the Ecliptick, is a Circle broader than the Colures, cutting them at Right Angles, and this represents the Ecliptick, so called in the Use of the Sphere, and is divided into Degrees, figured with the Names and Characters of the. Signs, and having on the inward edge thereof several of the most notable fixed Stars, with the Names affixed to them, and each Star placed to the Degree and Minute of Longitude thereof, that it hath in Heaven.

Oblique to this Ecliptick $23\frac{1}{2}$ Degrees, on the inside, is fitted a thin Circle, representing the Equinoctial, and is divided into 360 Degrees, and having two parallel lesser Circles at $23\frac{1}{2}$ Degrees equally distant therefrom, representing the Tropicks.   On the inside of all these Circles, two thin Semi-circles (called Semi-circles of Latitude) are fitted in the Poles of the Ecliptick, so as one of them may move thro one half of the Ecliptick, *viz.* from *Cancer* thro *Aries* to *Capricorn*, and the other from *Cancer* thro *Libra* to *Capricorn*   the former of these may be called the vernal Semi-circle of Latitude, and the other the autumnal Semi-circle of Latitude   On the edge of these Semi-circles are depicted the same fixed Stars in their proper Longitude and Latitude, as are placed on the ecliptick Circle aforesaid, with their several Names affixed to them.

Thro the solstitial Colure at $23\frac{1}{2}$ Degrees from each Pole of the Ecliptick, goes a Wire, representing the Earth's Axis, having an Index placed on the end thereof, for pointing at the Hour, on the Hour-Circle placed on the solstitial Colure, as aforesaid   In the middle of this Axis is fixed a round Ball, representing the Earth, having Meridians, Parallels, &c and the Bounds of the Lands and Waters depicted thereon, as also the Names of as many Countries and Towns as can be placed with conveniency thereon   And in two opposite Points of the Equinoctial of this Ball, *viz.* 90 Degrees distant from the first Meridian, are fixed two small Pins, whereon a moveable Horizon is placed, in the East and West Points thereof, so that these Pins serve for an Axis to the Horizon · for on these Pins the Horizon may be elevated or depressed to any Degree the Pole is elevated above the Horizon   This Horizon slides on the North and South Points, within a brazen Meridian, hung upon the Axis of the Earth

Round this Meridian, on the outmost Side, is made a Groove, having a small brass Ring fitted therein, so as the upper side thereof is even with the upper side of the brazen Meridian   This small brass Ring is fastened to two opposite Points in the Horizon, *viz.* in the North and South, and serves as a Spring to keep it to the Degree of the Meridian you elevate the Horizon to   Upon two Pins on this small Ring, are likewise fastened two Semi-circles of Altitude, yet not so fastened, but that they may move as upon Centers, the one moving from North to South, thro the East-side of the Horizon, and the other the same way thro the West-side   This Motion is performed upon the two Pins aforesaid, as upon two Poles, which they represent, *viz.* the Poles of the Horizon, and therefore are so placed, that they may divide the upper and lower half of the Horizon into two equal Parts, and as the Horizon is moved, slide always into the Zenith and Nadir, and so become the Poles of the Horizon   These two Semi-circles of Altitude are divided into twice 90 Degrees, numbered at the Horizon upwards and downwards, and ending at 90 in the Zenith and Nadir

SECTION III.

The Use of the Copernican Sphere.

USE I   *The Day of the Month given, to rectify the Sphere for Use in any given Latitude, and to set it correspondent to the Situation of the Heavens*

Bring the Index of the moveable Rundle to the Day of the Month, and elevate the Horizon to the Latitude of the Place, then bring the Meridian to the Sun's Place in the Ecliptick, and the Index of the Hour-Circle to 12   Lastly, Bring the Center of the Earth, the Sun, or Golden Ball, in the Sphere, and the Sun in Heaven into a Right Line   Then will the Earth be rectified to its Place in Heaven, the Horizon to its Latitude on Earth, the Circles on the Sphere agreeable to those in Heaven, and the whole correspondent with the Heavens for that Day at Noon.

USE II   *The Day of the Month being given, to find the Sun's Declination*

Rectify the Earth's place (according to *Use* I) and then you will have the Sun's place in the Zodiack ; then bring the Meridian to the Sun's place in the Ecliptick on the Sphere, and the Number of Degrees comprehended between the Equinoctial and the Sun's place, are the Sun's Declination for that Day at Noon

USE

USE III *To find the Sun's Right or Oblique Aſcenſion for any Day at Noon*

Rectify the Earth's place to the Day of the Month, and bring the Meridian to the Sun's place in the Ecliptick, and the Number of Degrees on the Equinoctial contained between the vernal Colure, and the Sun's place, are the Right Aſcenſion ſought.

Now to find the Oblique Aſcenſion, turn the Earth till the Eaſt ſide of the Horizon ſtands againſt the Sun, and the Degree of the Equinoctial then at the Horizon, ſhews the Oblique Aſcenſion.

USE IV *To find the Sun's Meridian Altitude*

Bring the Index of the Rundle to the Day of the Month, and rectify the Horizon to the Latitude of the Place This being done, bring the Meridian to the Sun's place in the Ecliptick, and the Number of Degrees on the Meridian comprehended between the Horizon and the Sun's place, gives the Meridian Altitude ſought.

USE V *To find the Sun's Altitude at any time of the Day.*

Bring the Index of the moveable Rundle to the Day of the Month, and rectify the Horizon, and Hour-Index : then turn the Earth till the Hour-Index comes to the given Hour of the Day, and bring the vertical Circle to the Sun's place, and the Number of Degrees of the vertical Circle that tranſite the Sun's place, are his Altitude above the Horizon

USE VI. *The Sun's Altitude being given, to find the Hour of the Day*

Bring the Index of the Rundle to the Day of the Month, and rectify the Horizon and Hour-Index (as by *Uſe* I) then turn the Earth till you can fit the Horizon to the given Altitude upon the vertical Circle, directly againſt the Sun's place, then the Hour-Index will give the Hour of the Day, reſpect being had to the Morning or Afternoon

USE VII. *To find at what Hour the Sun comes to the Eaſt or Weſt Points of the Horizon*

Bring the Index of the moveable Rundle to the Day of the Month, and rectify the Horizon and Hour-Index (as by *Uſe* I) then bring the vertical Circle to the Eaſt Point of the Horizon, if it be the Sun's Eaſting you would enquire, or to the Weſt Point of the Horizon, if it be the Sun's Weſting This being done, turn the Earth till the vertical Circle comes to the Sun's place, then will the Index point to the Hour of the Day.

USE VIII *To find the time of the Sun's riſing or ſetting*

Bring the Index of the moveable Rundle to the Day of the Month, and rectify the Horizon, and Hour-Index Then turn the Earth Eaſtwards, till ſome part of the Eaſt-ſide of the Horizon ſtands directly againſt the Sun's place, then will the Hour-Index point to the time of the Sun's riſing. Again, Turn the Earth till ſome part of the Weſt-ſide of the Horizon ſtands directly againſt the Sun's place, then the Index of the Hour-Circle will ſhew the time of the Sun's ſetting.

USE IX. *The Hour of the Day given, to find the Sun's Azimuth*

Bring the Index of the moveable Rundle to the Day of the Month, and rectify the Horizon and Hour-Index Then turn the Earth till the Hour-Index points to the Hour of the Day given This being done, bring the vertical Circle to the Sun's place, and the Number of Degrees of the Horizon, that the vertical Circle cuts, counted from the Eaſt Point, either Northwards or Southwards, are the Degrees of the Sun's Azimuth before Noon Or the Number of Degrees of the Horizon that the vertical Circle cuts, counted from the Weſt-ſide of the Horizon, either Northwards or Southwards, give the Sun's Azimuth after Noon

USE X *To find in what Place of the Earth the Sun is in the Zenith, at any given time, as alſo in what ſeveral Places of the Earth the Sun ſhall ſtand in the Horizon at the ſame time*

Bring the Index of the moveable Rundle to the Day of the Month, and rectify the Hour-Index, then ſeek the Sun's Declination, and turn the Earth eaſtwards till the Index points to the given Hour, ſo ſhall the Number of Degrees of the Equinoctial that the Meridian paſſes thro while the Earth is thus turning, be the Number of Degrees of Longitude, eaſtwards from your Habitation, the Place ſhall have in the Parallel of the Sun's Declination

Now if you open a Pair of Calliper Compaſſes to 90 Degrees on the Equinoctial, and place one Foot in this Point of the Earth thus found, and turn the other Foot round about the Earth, all the Places that the Foot paſſes thro will at that time have the Sun in their Horizon.

Plate XVIII _fronting page 159_

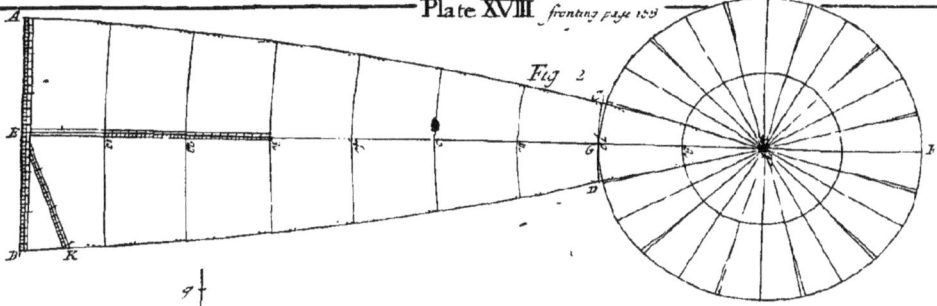

Fig 2

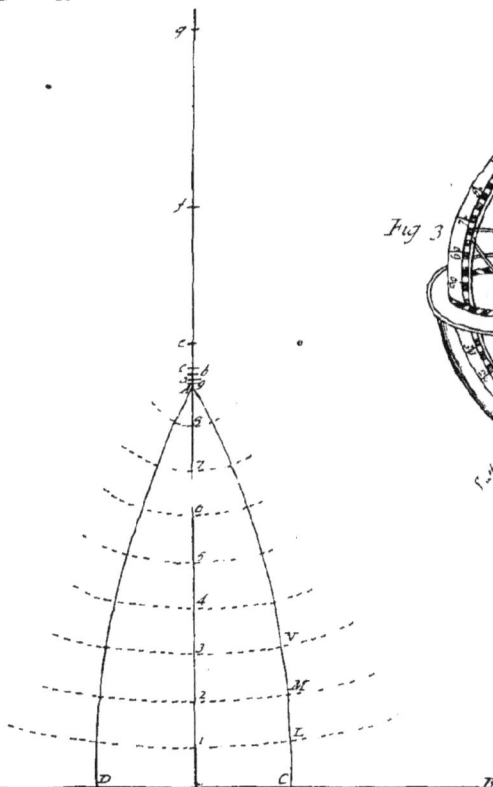

Fig 1

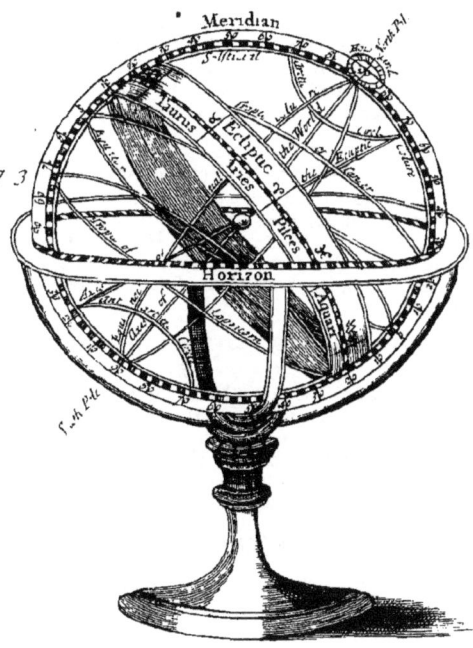

Fig 3

Meridian

Ecliptic

Horizon

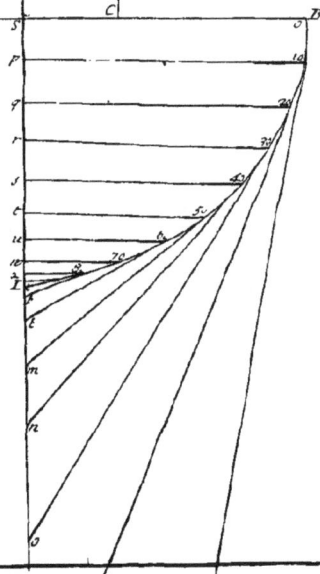

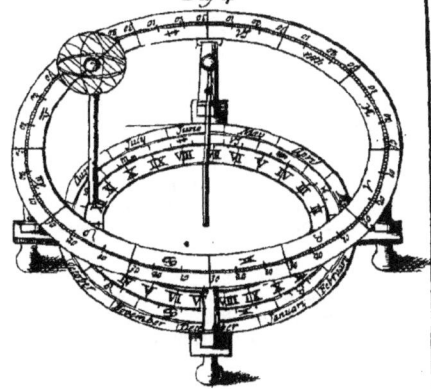

Fig 4

I. Senex sculpt

U S E XI *How to find the true Places of the Stars on the Sphere, as likewise their Longitude and Latitude*

Round the Plane of the Ecliptick, are placed feveral of the moft noted fixed Stars, according to their true Longitude, and along the two Semi-circles of Latitude, are the fame Stars placed according to their Latitude from the Ecliptick Whence if you would find the true place of any given Star in the Sphere, Firft feek the Star in the Ecliptick and likewife the fame Star on one of the Semi-circles of Latitude, and bring the edge of that Semi-circle to the Star in the Ecliptick, then will the Star on the Semi-circle of Latitude ftand in the fame Place and Situation on the Sphere, that it does in Heaven

U S E XII *To find the Declination, right and oblique Afcenfion of a Star*

Bring the proper Semi-circle of Latitude to the Star on the Ecliptick, and the Meridian to the Star on the Semi-circle of Latitude, and then the Number of Degrees on the Meridian, comprehended between the Equinoctial and the Star, are its Declination Likewife the Degree of the Equator, cut by the Meridian, is the Star's right Afcenfion But to find a Star's oblique Afcenfion, rectify the Horizon (as by *Ufe* I) and bring the proper Semi-circle of Latitude to the Star in the Ecliptick, and turn the Eaft-fide of the Horizon to the Star, then will the Degree of the Equator cut by the Horizon be the Star's oblique Afcenfion

U S E XIII *To find the Time of the Rifing and Setting of any Star in any given Latitude*

Bring the Index of the moveable Rundle to the Day of the Month, and rectify the Horizon and Hour-Index, then bring the proper Semi-circle of Latitude to the Star on the Ecliptick, and the Eaft-fide of the Horizon to the Star, this being done, the Hour-Index will fhew the Hour the Star rifes at, and if you bring the Weft-fide of the Horizon to the Star, the Index of the Hour-Circle will fhew the Time that the Star fets

U S E XIV *The Day of the Month, Hour of the Night, and Latitude of the Place being given, to know any remarkable Star obferved in the Heavens*

Bring the Index of the moveable Rundle to the Day of the Month, and rectify the Horizon and Hour-Index, then turn the Earth till the Index of the Hour-Circle comes to the Hour of the Night, and obferve the Altitude of the Star, and what Point of the Compafs it bears upon Afterwards bring the vertical Circle to the fame Point of the Compafs, and number the Star's Altitude on the vertical Circle, and try with the Semi-circle of Latitude what Star you can fit to that Altitude, for that is the Star in the Heavens

U S E XV *The Azimuth of any known Star being given, to find the Hour of the Night, and Almicanter of that Star*

Bring the Index of the moveable Rundle to the Day of the Month, and rectify the Horizon and Hour-Index, afterwards bring the Star to its place, and the vertical Circle to its known Degree of Azimuth This being done, turn the Earth till the vertical Circle comes to the Star, then the Index of the Hour-Circle will fhew the Hour of the Night, and the Degree of the vertical Circle cut by the Star will be its Almicanter.

S E C T I O N IV.

The Defcription and Ufe of the Copernican Sphere, called the Orrery.

The Outfide of this Inftrument, as appears by the figure thereof, is very beautiful, the Frame being of fine Ebony adorned with 12 Silver Pilafters, in the form of *Caryatides*, and with all the Signs of the Zodiack caft of the fame Metal, and placed between them the Handles are alfo of Silver finely wrought, with very nice Joints On the top of the Frame, which is exactly Circular, is a broad Silver Ring, on which the Figures of the twelve Signs are exactly graved, with two Circles accurately divided, one fhewing the Degrees of each Sign, and the other the Sun's Declination againft his place in the Ecliptick each Day at Noon *Plate 19 Fig 1*

The aforefaid Silver Plate, reprefents the Plane of the great Ecliptick of the Heavens, or that of the Earth's annual Orbit round the Sun, which, as it paffes thro the Center of the Sun, fo its Circumference is made by the Motion of the Earth's Center, and which, for the better advantage of view and fight, is in the Figure placed parallel to the Horizon.

S is a large gilded Ball, ftanding up in the middle, whofe Support A B makes with the Plane of the Ecliptick an Angle of about 82 Degrees This Support reprefents the Sun's Axis continued, about which he revolves in about 25 Days, and the Golden Ball reprefents the Sun itfelf placed pretty near the Center of the Earth's Orbit, fo that

C c c   when

when the Inſtrument is ſet a going, the Excentricity of the Earth, and the other Planets, may be in the ſame proportion as they are in the Heavens.

The two little Balls M and V, which ſtand upon two Wires at different Diſtances from the Sun, repreſent *Mercury* and *Venus* The reaſon why they are placed upon the ſaid two Wires, is only that their Centers may be ſometimes in, and always pretty near the Plane of the great Ecliptick, and this Poſition is contrived in order to ſhew what Appearances they do really exhibit in their ſeveral Revolutions round the Sun

The Globe E is of Ivory, and repreſents the Earth The Pin or Wire that ſupports it, repreſents the Earth's Axis continued, and makes an Angle of 66 ½ Degrees, with the Plane of the Ecliptick. And as the Earth in each of her annual Revolutions round the Sun, always keeps her own Axis parallel to itſelf, ſo when this Inſtrument is ſet a going, the little Ivory Earth will likewiſe do ſo too, in its Revolution round the Golden Sun S.

The little Ball *m* ſtanding upon a Wire, repreſents the Moon, and *a b* is a Silver Circle repreſenting her Orbit round about the Earth, the Plane whereof always paſſes thro the Center of the Earth, and there are ſeveral Figures graved upon it, ſhewing the Moon's Age, from one New Moon to the other

One half of the Moon's Globe is white, and the other black, that ſo her Phaſes may be repreſented for this Inſtrument is ſo contrived, that this little Moon will turn round its own Axis, at the ſame time as it moves in the Silver Orbit round the Earth E.

The whole Movement, which conſiſts of near 100 Wheels, is covered by a great Braſs Plate, having a hole in it, and there is a moveable Index on the Silver Ecliptick, on the former of which, are the common Solar Years denoted; and by taking the Inſtrument to pieces, it may be ſet to this preſent time, and the Planets, by means of an Ephemeris, may be ſet to any particular time alſo. So that if a Weight or Spring, as in a Clock, were applied to the Axis of the Movement, ſo as to make it move round once in juſt twenty-four Hours, the repreſentative Planets in the Inſtrument, viz. *Mercury*, *Venus*, the *Earth*, and the *Moon*, would all perform their Motions round the Sun, and one another, exactly in the ſame Order as their Originals do in the Heavens, and ſo the Aſpects, Ecliptes, &c of the Sun and Planets, would thereby be ſhewn for ever But becauſe this would be inſtructive only in that ſlow and tedious way, to ſuch as could have daily recourſe to it, therefore there is a Handle fitted to it, by which the Axis may be ſwiftly turned round, and ſo all the Appearances ſhewn in a very little time: for by turning the Handle backwards or forwards, what Ecliptes, Tranſits, &c have happened in any time paſt, or what will happen for any time to come, will be ſhewn, without doing any injury to the Inſtrument

One entire Turn of the Handle of this Inſtrument, anſwers to the diurnal Motion of the Earth about its Axis, and is meaſured by means of an Hour-Index, placed at the Foot of the Wire whereon the Earth is fixed, moving once round in the ſame time Alſo obſerve that the Contrivance of this Inſtrument is ſuch, that the Motion may be made to tend either way, forwards or backwards, and ſo the Handle may be turned about till the Earth be brought to any Degree or Point of the Ecliptick required

Again, As the Earth moves round, by turning the Handle, the Moon's Orbit riſes and falls about 5 Degrees above and below the great Ecliptick, that ſo her North or South Latitude may be exactly repreſented, and there are two little Studs placed in two oppoſite Points of the Moon's Orbit, repreſenting the Moon's Nodes

Now if the Handle, one Turn of which anſwers to one Natural Day, or twenty-four Hours, be turned twenty-five times about, then the Sun will have moved once round about its Axis Again, 365 ¼ of the Turns of the Handle will carry the Earth quite round the Sun, 88 will carry *Mercury* quite round, 244 will make *Venus* move once round the Sun, and about 27 ¼ Turns will carry the Moon round the Earth in her Orbit, which will likewiſe at the ſame time always turn the ſame Hemiſphere towards the Earth

And by thus revolving the Earth and Planets round the Sun, the Inſtrument may be brought to exhibit *Mercury*, and ſometimes *Venus*, as directly interpoſed between the Earth and the Sun, and then they will appear as Spots in the Sun's Diſk: and this Inſtrument ſhews alſo very clearly the Difference between the Geocentrick and Heliocentrick Aſpects, according as the Eye is placed in the Center of the Earth or Sun.

This Inſtrument likewiſe very plainly ſhews the Difference between the Moon's Periodick and Synodick Months, and the reaſon thereof, for if the Earth be ſet to the firſt Point of *Aries*, at which time ſuppoſe the firſt New Moon happens, and afterwards the Handle be turned 27 ¼ times about, we ſhall have the ſecond New Moon, and if at the Earth's place in the Ecliptick where this laſt New Moon happens, ſome Mark be made, and then the Handle be turned 27 ¼ times more, the Moon will be exactly brought again to interpoſe between the Earth and the Sun, that is, it will be New Moon with us. but the Line of the *Syzygy* will not be right againſt the aforeſaid Mark in the Ecliptick, but behind it, and it will require two Days time, or two Turns more of the Handle, before it gets thither The reaſon of this is plain, becauſe in this 27 ¼ Days, the Earth advances ſo far forwards in her annual Courſe, as is the Quantity of the Difference in time between the Moon's two Months.

If

If the Handle be turned about till the Conjunction or Opposition of the Sun and Moon happens in or near the Nodes, then there will be an Eclipse of the Sun or Moon. But in order yet further to shew the Solar Eclipses, and also the several Seasons of the Year, the Increase and Decrease of Day and Night, and the different Lengths of each in different parts of our Earth, there is a little Lamp contrived to put on upon the Body of the Sun, which casting, by means of a Convex Glass, (the Room wherein the Instrument is, being a little darkened) a strong Light upon the Earth, will shew at once all these things. First, how one half of our Globe is always illuminated by the Sun, while the other Hemisphere is in the dark, and consequently how Day and Night are formed by the Revolution of the Earth round her Axis. Also by turning round the Handle, you will see how the Shadow of the Moon's Body will cover some part of the Earth, and thereby shew, that to the Inhabitants of that part of the Earth there will be a Solar Eclipse.

When the Earth is brought to the first Degree of *Aries* or *Libra*, the reason of the Equality of Days and Nights all over the Earth, will be plainly shewn by this Instrument, for in these Positions, as the Earth turns about her Axis, just one half of the Equator, and all Parallels thereto, will be in the Light, and the other half in the Dark, and therefore the Days and Nights must be every where equal. for the Horizon of the Earth's Disk will be parallel to the Plane of the Solstitial Colure.

And when the Earth is brought to *Cancer*, the Horizon of the Disk, or that Plane which divides the Earth's enlightened Hemisphere from the darkened one, will not then be parallel to, but lie at Right Angles to the Plane of the Solstitial Colure. The Earth being now in *Cancer*, the Sun will appear to be in *Capricorn*, and consequently it will be our Winter Solstice. And as the Earth is turned either way about its Axis, the entire Northern frigid Zone, or all Parts of the Earth lying within the Artick Circle, are in the dark Hemisphere, and by making a Mark in any given Parallel, by the Earth's Diurnal Revolution, you will know how much longer the Nights are than the Days in that Parallel. And the contrary of this will happen, when the Earth is brought to *Capricorn*.

Therefore this Instrument delightfully and demonstratively shews, how thereby all the Phenomena of the different Seasons of the Year, and the Varieties and Vicissitudes of Night and Day, are solved and accounted for.

CHAP. IV.

Of an *Astronomical Quadrant, Micrometer, and* Gunter's *Quadrant.*

SECTION I.

THIS Figure represents an Astronomical Quadrant upon its Pedestal, with its Limb Fig 2. curiously divided Diagonally, and furnished with a fixed and moveable Telescope.

This Quadrant may be moved round Horizontally, by turning a perpetual Screw fitted into the Pedestal · For as this Screw is turned about by means of a Key, at the same time it causes the Axis A to turn, by the falling in of its Threads between the Teeth of a strong thick Circle on the said Axis.

Behind the Quadrant is fixed, at Right Angles to its Plane, a strong thick Portion of a Circle greater than a Semi-circle, having one Semi-circle of the outside thereof cut into Teeth. There is likewise another strong thick Portion of a Circle something greater than a Semi-circle behind the Quadrant, which is moveable upon two fixed Studs, at Right Angles to the former Portion, so that the Plane of this Portion may be parallel, inclined, or at Right Angles to the Plane of the Quadrant. On the side of this Portion, which is made flat next to the other fixed Portion, is a contrivance with a Screw and perpetual Screw, such that in turning the Screw the Threads of the perpetual Screw may be locked in between the Teeth of the fixed circular Portion, and by this means the Quadrant fixed to any Point, according to the direction of the Plane of the fixed Portion. And when the Quadrant is to be moved but a small matter in the aforesaid Direction, this may be done by turning the perpetual Screw with a Key.

The Outside of the abovementioned moveable circular Portion is cut into Teeth, and about the Center thereof the Axis A is moveable, according to the Direction of the Plane of the said Portion. In this Axis slides a little Piece carrying a perpetual Screw, whose Threads, by means of a Trigger, may be locked in between the Teeth of the moveable circular Portion. And so when the Axis is set in the Pedestal, the Quadrant may be fixed to any Point, according to the Direction of the Plane of the said moveable Portion.

Therefore

Therefore by these Contrivances the Quadrant may be readily fixed to any required Situation, for observing Celestial Phenomena, without moving the Pedestal

There is a Piece sliding on the Index, upon which the moveable Telescope is fastened, carrying a Screw and perpetual Screw, so that when the Telescope and Index are to be fixed upon any Point in the Limb of the Instrument, this may be done, by means of the Screw which locks the Threads of the perpetual Screw in between some of the Teeth cut round the Curve Surface of the Limb of the Instrument and when the Index and Telescope is to be moved a very minute Space backwards or forwards along the Limb, this is done by means of a Key turning a small Wheel fastened upon the aforenamed Piece, which is cut into a certain Number of Teeth, and whose Axis is at Right Angles to the Plane of the Quadrant, for this Wheel moves another (having the same Number of Teeth as that) which is at the end of the Cylinder whereon the perpetual Screw is and by this means the perpetual Screw is turned about, and so the Index and Telescope may be moved a very minute Space backwards or forwards along the Limb Note, The Number of Teeth the Curve Surface of the Limb is divided into, must be as great as possible, and the Threads of the perpetual Screw filling between them very fine, for the Exactness of the Instrument very much depends upon this

These Quadrants are commonly two Feet Radius, and all Brass, except the Pedestal and the perpetual Screws, the Telescopes have each two Glasses and Cross-hairs in their *Foci* ; and for the Manner of dividing their Limbs, &c See our Author's Quadrants

SECTION II.

Concerning a Micrometer.

Fig 3

This Micrometer is made of Brass A B C g is a rectangular Brass Frame, the Side A B being about 3 Inches long, and the Side B C, as likewise the opposite Side A g, are about 6 Inches, and each of these three Sides are $\frac{1}{4}$ of an Inch deep The two opposite Sides of this Frame are screwed to the circular Plate, which we shall speak of by and by

The Screw P having exactly 40 Threads in an Inch, being turned round, moves the Plate G D E F, along two Grooves made near the Tops of the two opposite Sides of the Frame, and the Screw Q having the same Number of Threads in an Inch as P, moves the Plate R N M Y along two Grooves made near the bottom of the said Frame, in the same direction as the former Plate moves, but with half the velocity as that moves with. These Screws are both at once turned, and so the said Plates moved along the same way, by means of a Handle turning the perpetual Screw S, whose Threads fall in between the Teeth of Pinions on the Screws P and Q Note, Two and a half Revolutions of the perpetual Screw S, moves the Screw P exactly once round

The Screw P turns the Hand *a*, fastened thereto over 100 equal Divisions made round the Limb of a circular Plate, to which the abovenamed two opposite Sides of the Frame are screwed at Right Angles The Teeth of the Pinion on the Screw P, whose Number are 5, takes into the Teeth of a Wheel, on the backside of the circular Plate, whose Number are 25 Again, On the Axis of this Wheel is a Pinion of two, which takes into the Teeth of another Wheel moving about the Center of the circular Plate, without side the same, having 50 Teeth This last Wheel moves the lesser Hand *b* once round the abovenamed circular Plate, in the $\frac{1}{100}$ part of the time the Hand *a* is moving round for because the Number of Teeth of the Pinion on the Screw P, are 5, and the Number of Teeth of the Wheel this Pinion moves round, are 20, therefore the Screw P moves four times round in the same time the said Wheel is moving once round Again, Since there is a Pinion of two takes into the Teeth of a Wheel, whose Number are 50, therefore this Wheel with 50 Teeth will move once round in the same time that the Wheel of 20 Teeth hath moved twenty-five times round ; and consequently the Screw P, or Hand *a*, must move a hundred times round in the same time as the Wheel of 50 Teeth, or the Hand *b*, hath moved once round

It follows from what hath been said, that if the circular Plate W, which is fastened at Right Angles to the other circular Plate, be divided into 200 equal Parts, the Index to which the Handle is fastened, will move five of these Parts in the same time that the Hand *a* has moved one of the hundred Divisions round the Limb of the other circular Plate and so by means of the Index *x*, and Plate W, every fifth Part of each of the Divisions round the other Plate may be known.

Moreover, Since each of the Screws P and Q have exactly 40 Threads in an Inch, therefore the upper Plate G D E F will move 1 Inch, when the Hand *a* hath moved forty times round, the four thousandth part of an Inch, when the said Hand hath moved over one of the Divisions round the Limb, and the twenty thousandth part of an Inch, when the Index *x* hath moved one part of the 200 round the Limb of the circular Plate W, and the under Plate R N M Y, half an Inch, the two thousandth part of an Inch, and the ten thousandth part of an Inch the same way, in the said respective times

Hence,

Hence, if the under Plate, having a large round Hole therein, be fixed to a Telescope, so that the Frame may be moveable together with the whole Instrument, except the said lower Plate, and the strait smooth Edge H I, of the fixed narrow Plate A B I H, as likewise the strait smooth Edge D E of the moveable Plate G D E F, be perceivable thro the round Hole in the under Plate, in the Focus of the Object-Glass, then when the Handle of the Micrometer is turned, the Edge H I of the narrow Plate A B I H, fixed to the Frame, and D E of the moveable Plate, will appear thro the Telescope equally to accede to, or recede from each other   And so these Edges will serve to take the apparent Diameters of the Sun, Moon, &c the manner of doing which is thus: Suppose in looking at the Moon thro the Telescope, you have turned the Handle till the two Edges D E and H I are opened, so as to just touch or clasp the Moon's Edges, and that there was twenty-one Revolutions of the Hand *a* to compleat that Opening   First say, As the focal Length of the Object-Glass, which suppose 10 Feet, is to Radius, so is 1 Inch to the Tangent of an Angle subtended by 1 Inch in the Focus of the Object-Glass, which will be found 28 min 30 sec   Again, Because there are exactly 40 Threads of the Screws in one Inch, say, If forty Revolutions of the Hand *a* give an Angle of 28 min 38 sec what Angle will twenty-one Revolutions give? The Answer will be 15 min 8 sec and such was the Moon's apparent Diameter, and so may the apparent Diameters of any distant Objects be taken

It is to be observed, that the Divisions upon the top of the Plate G D E F, are Diagonal Divisions of the Revolutions of the Screws, with Diagonal Divisions of Inches against them; and so as the said Plate slides along, these Diagonals are cut by Divisions made on the Edge of the narrow Plate K L, fixed to the opposite Sides of the Frame by means of two Screws These Diagonal Divisions may serve to count the Revolutions of the Screws, and to shew how many there are in an Inch, or the Parts of an Inch

SECTION III.
Of the Construction of Gunter's *Quadrant.*

This Quadrant, which is partly a Projection, that is, the Equator, Tropicks, Ecliptick, and Horizon, are Stereographically projected upon the Plane of the Equinoctial, the Eye being supposed to be placed in one of the Poles, may be thus made   Fig 4.

About the Center A describe the Arc C D, which may represent either of the Tropicks Again, Divide the Semidiameter A T so in E, that A E being Radius, A T may be the Tangent of 56 deg 46 min half the Sun's greatest Declination above the Radius or Tangent of 45 deg   To do which, say, As the Tangent of 56 deg 46 min is to 1000, so is Radius to 655   therefore if A T be made 1000 equal Parts, A E, the Radius of the Equator, will be 655 of those Parts   And if about the Center A, with the Distance A E, the Quadrant E F be described, this will serve for the Equinoctial

Now to find the Center of the Ecliptick, which will be somewhere in the left Side of the Quadrant A D (representing the Meridian) you must divide A D so in G, that if A F be the Radius, A G may be the Tangent of 23 deg 30 min the Sun's greatest Declination, therefore if A F be 1000, A G will be 434   And if about the Center G, with the Semidiameter G D, an Arc E D be described, this will be ¼ of the Ecliptick   And to divide it into Signs and Degrees, you must use this Canon, viz As Radius is to the Tangent of any Degree's distance from the nearest Equinoctial Point, so is the Cosine of the Sun's greatest Declination to the Tangent of that Degree's Right Ascension, which must be counted on the Limb from the Point B, by which means the Quadrant of the Ecliptick may be graduated

As, for Example, The Right Ascension of the first Point of ♉ being 27 deg 54 min lay a Ruler to the Center A, and 27 deg 54 min on the Limb, from B towards C, and where it cuts the Ecliptick, will be the first Point of ♉, and so for any other

The Line E T, between the Equator and the Tropick, which is called the Line of Declination, may be divided into 23 deg 30 min in laying off from the Center A, the Tangent of each Degree added to 45 deg   The Line A E being supposed the Radius of the Equinoctial   As suppose the Point for 10 Degrees of Declination be to be found, add 5 deg (half 10) to 45 deg and the Sum will be 50 deg   the Tangent of which will be (supposing the Radius 1000) 1192   therefore laying 1192 Parts from A, or 192 from E, and you will have a Point for 10 Degrees of Declination, and so for others

Most of the principal Stars between the Equator and Tropick of *Cancer*, may be put on the Quadrant by means of their Declination, and Right Ascension   As suppose the Wing of *Pegasus* be 13 deg 7 min and the Right Ascension 358 deg 34 min. from the first Point of *Aries*   Now if about the Center A, you draw an occult Parallel thro 13 deg. 7 min of Declination, and then lay a Ruler from the Center A thro 1 deg 26 min (the Complement of 358 deg 34 min to 360 deg) in the Limb B C, the Point where the Ruler cuts the Parallel, will be the Place for the Wing of *Pegasus*, to which you may set the Name, and the Time when he comes to the South.

D d d

There

There being Space fufficient between the Equator and the Center, you may there deſcribe the Quadrat, and divide each of the two Sides furtheſt from the Center into 100 Parts, ſo ſhall the Quadrant be generally prepared for any Latitude But before the particular Lines can be drawn, you muſt have four Tables fitted for the Latitude the Quadrant is to ſerve in.

Firſt, A Table of Meridian Altitudes for the Diviſion of the Circles of Days and Months, which may be thus made Conſider the Latitude of the Place, and the Sun's Declination for each Day of the Year, if the Latitude and Declination be both North, or both South, add the Declination to the Complement of the Latitude, if they be one North, and the other South, ſubſtract the Declination from the Complement of the Latitude, and you will have the Meridian Altitude for that Day As, in the Latitude of 51 deg 32 min. North, whoſe Complement is 38 deg 28 min the Declination on the 10th of *June* be 23 deg 30 min North, therefore add 23 deg 30 min to 38 deg 28 min and the Sun will be 61 deg 58 min the Meridian Altitude on the 10th of *June* Again, The Declination on the 10th of *December*, will be 23 deg 30 min South; wherefore take 23 deg 30 min from 38 deg 28 min and the Remainder will be 14 deg 58 min the Meridian Altitude on the 10th of *December* And in this manner may the Meridian Altitude for each Day in the Year be found, and put in a Table

Your Table being made, you may inſcribe the Months and Days of each Month on the Quadrant, in the Space left below the Tropick As, Laying a Ruler upon the Center A, and 16 deg 42 min the Sun's Meridian Altitude on the *1ſt* of *January*, in the Limb B C you may draw a Line for the end of *December* and beginning of *January*. Again, Laying a Ruler to the Center A, and 24 deg 34 min the Sun's Altitude at Noon the end of *January*, or firſt of *February*, on the Limb, and you may draw a Line for that Day And ſo of others

Now to draw the Horizon, you muſt find its Center, which will be in the Meridian Line A C, and if the Point H be taken ſuch, that if A H be the Tangent Complement of the Latitude, *viz.* of 38 deg 28 min. A F being ſuppoſed Radius; or if A F be ſuppoſed 1000, and A H 776 of thoſe Parts, then will H be the Center of the Horizon Therefore if about the Center H, with the Diſtance H E, an Arc be deſcribed cutting the Tropick T D, the ſaid Arc will repreſent the Horizon

The next thing done, muſt be to make a Table for the Diviſion of the Horizon, which may be done by this Canon, *viz.* As Radius is to the Sine of the Latitude, ſo is the Tangent of any Number of Degrees in the Horizon (which will be not more than 40 in our Latitude) to the Tangent of the Arc in the Limb which will divide the Horizon

As in our Latitude, 7 deg 52 min belong to 10 deg of the Degrees of the Horizon, therefore laying a Ruler to the Center A, and 7 deg 52 min in the Limb B C, the Point where the Ruler cuts the Horizon, will be 10 deg in the Horizon, and ſo of the reſt But the Lines of Diſtinction between every 5th Degree are beſt drawn from the Center H

The third Table for drawing the Hour-Lines, muſt be a Table of the Sun's Altitude above the Horizon at every Hour, eſpecially when he comes to the Equator, Tropicks, and other intermediate Declinations If the Sun be in the Equator, and ſo have no Declination, as Radius to the Co-ſine of the Latitude, ſo is the Co-ſine of any Hour from the Meridian to the Sine of the Sun's Altitude at that Hour

But if the Sun be not in the Equator, you muſt ſay, As the Co-ſine of the Hour from the Meridian is to Radius, ſo is the Tangent of the Latitude to the Tangent of a 4th Arc Then conſider the Sun's Declination, and the Hour propoſed, if the Latitude and Declination be both alike, and the Hour fall between Noon and Six, ſubſtract the Declination from the aforeſaid 4th Arc, and the Remainder will be a 5th Arc.

But if the Hour be either between Six and Midnight, or the Latitude and Declination unlike, add the Declination to the 4th Arc, and the Sum will be a 5th Arc Then as the Sine of the fourth Arc is to the Sine of the Latitude, ſo is the Co-ſine of the 5th Arc to the Sine of the Altitude ſought

Laſtly, You may find the Sun's Declination when he riſes or ſets, at any Hour, by this Canon, *viz.* As Radius is to the Sine of the Hour from Six, ſo is the Co-tangent of the Latitude to the Tangent of the Declination

As in our Latitude you will find, that when the Sun riſes at five in the Summer, or ſeven in the Winter, his Declination is 11 deg 36 min whence you will find the Sun's Meridian Altitude in the beginning of ♋ will be 61 deg 58 min. in ♊ 58 deg 40 min in ♉ 49 deg 58 min. in ♈ 38 deg. 30 min. &c but the beginning of ♋ and ♑ is repreſented by the Tropick T D, drawn thro 23 deg. of Declination, and the beginning of ♈ and ♎ by the Equator E F. Now if you draw an occult Parallel between the Equator and the Tropick, at 11 deg. 30 min. of Declination, it ſhall repreſent the beginning of ♉, ♍, ♏, and ♓ If you draw another occult Parallel thro 20 deg 12 min of Declination, it will repreſent the beginning of ♊, ♌, ♐ and ♒

Then lay a Ruler from the Center A thro 61 deg. 58 min of Altitude in the Limb B C, and note the Point where it croſſes the Tropick of ♋ Then move the Ruler to 58 deg. 40 min.

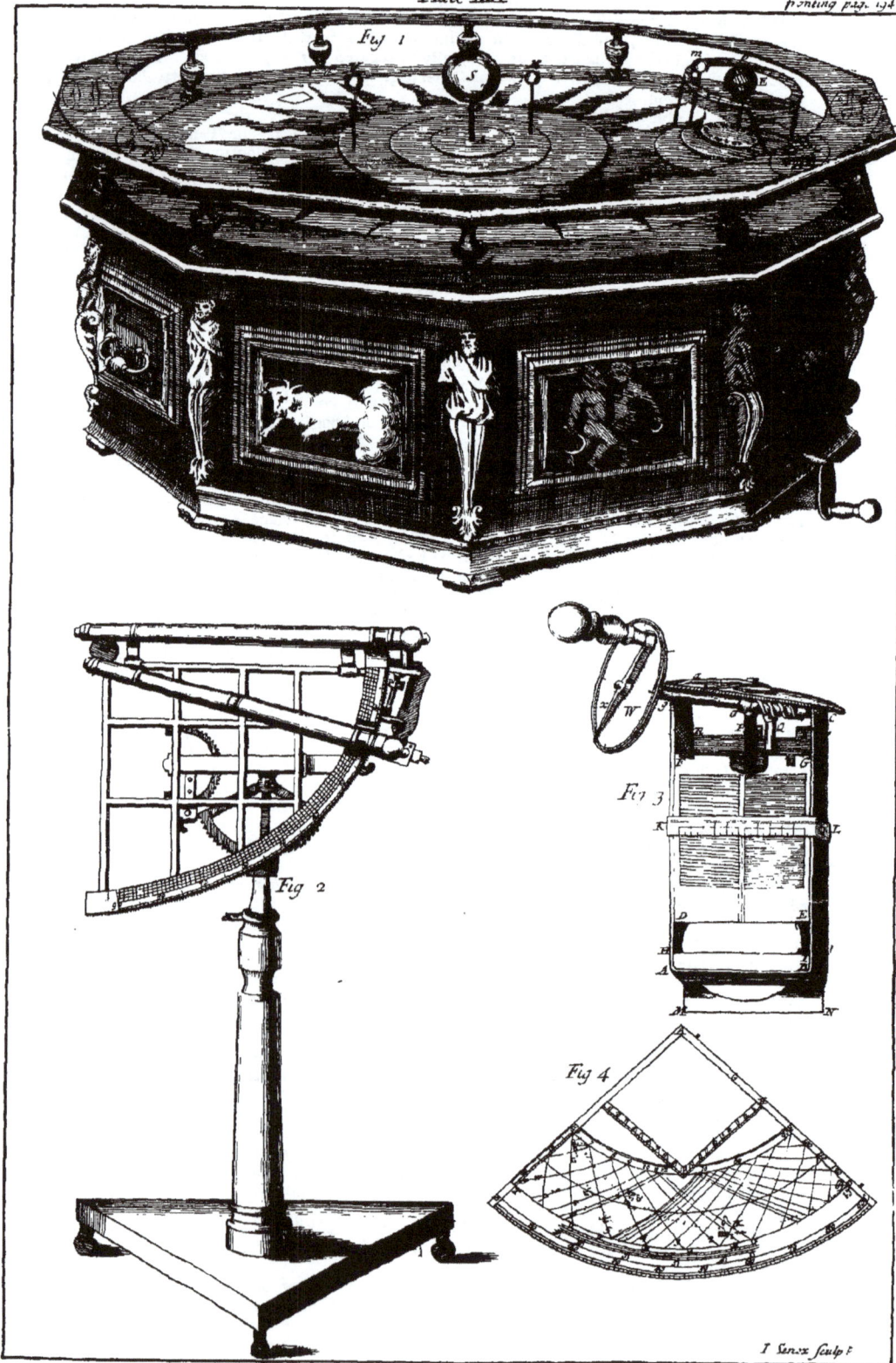

Plate XIX

Fig 1

S

Fig 2

Fig 3

Fig 4

I Senex sculp.

40 min and note where it croffes the Parallel of ♊, then to 19 deg 58 min and note where it croffes the Parallel of ♉, and again to 38 deg 28 min, noting where it croffes the Equator, and a Line drawn thro thefe Points will reprefent the Line of 12 in the Summer, while the Sun is in ♈, ♉, ♊, ♋, ♌, or ♍ In like manner, if you lay a Rule to A and 26 deg 58 min in the Limb, and note the Point where it croffes the Parallel of ♐, then move it to 18 deg 16 min and note where it croffes the Parallel of ♒ And again, to 14 deg 58 min noting where it croffes the Tropick of ♑, the Line drawn thro thefe Points fhall fhew the Hour of twelve in the Winter And in this manner may the reft of the Hour-Lines be drawn, only that of feven from the Meridian in Summer, and five in the Winter, will crofs the Line of Declination, at 11 deg 35 min and that of eight in the Summer, and four in the Winter, at 21 deg 38 min.

The fourth Table for drawing of the Azimuth Lines muft alfo be made for the Altitude of the Sun above the Horizon, at every Azimuth, efpecially when the Sun comes to the Equator, Tropicks, and fome other intermediate Declinations

If the Sun be in the Equator, and fo has no Declination, as Radius to the Co-fine of the Azimuth from the Meridian, fo is the Tangent of the Latitude to the Tangent of the Sun's Altitude at that Azimuth in the Equator

If the Sun be not in the Equator, as the Sine of the Latitude is to the Sine of the Declination, fo is the Co-fine of the Sun's Altitude at the Equator, at a given Azimuth, to the Sine of a 4*th* Arc

Now when the Latitude and Declination are both alike in all Azimuths, from the Prime Vertical to the Meridian, add this 4*th* Arc to the Arc of Altitude at the Equator But when the Azimuth is above 90 Degrees diftant from the Meridian, take the Altitude at the Equator from the 4*th* Arc When the Latitude and Declination are unlike, take the faid 4*th* Arc from the Arc of Altitude at the Equator, and then you will have the Sun's Altitude for a propofed Azimuth

Laftly, When the Sun rifes or fets upon any Azimuth, to find his Declination, fay, As Radius to the Co-fine of the Latitude, fo is the Co-fine of the Azimuth from the Meridian, to the Sine of the Declination

Now a Table being made according to the aforefaid Directions, if you would draw the Line of Eaft or Weft, which s 90 Degrees from the Meridian, lay a Ruler to the Center A, and 30 deg 38 min numbered in the Limb from C towards B, and note the Point where it croffes the Tropick of ♋, then move the Ruler to 26 deg 10 min and note where it croffes the Parallel of ♊, then to 14 deg 45 min and note where it croffes the Parallel of ♉; then to 0° and 0°, and you will find it crofs the Equator in the Point F, then a Line drawn thro thefe Points will be the Eaft and Weft Azimuth And fo may all the other Azimuths be drawn

Thefe Lines being thus drawn, if you fet two Sights upon the Line A C, and at the Center A hang a Thread and Plummet, with a Bead upon the Thread, the forefide of the Quadrant will be finifhed

SECTION IV.

The Ufe of Gunter's *Quadrant.*

USE I *The Sun's Place being given, to find his Right Afcenfion, and contrariwife*

Let the Thread be laid upon the Sun's Place in the Ecliptick, and the Degrees which it cuts in the Limb, will be the Right Afcenfion fought

For example, Suppofe the Sun's Place be the 4*th* Degree of ♊, the Thread laid on this Degree will cut 62 deg in the Limb, which is the Right Afcenfion required But if the Sun's Place be more than 90 deg from the beginning of *Aries*, the Right Afcenfion will be more than 90 deg And in this Cafe the Degrees cut by the Thread muft be taken from 180, to have the Right Afcenfion

Now if the Sun's Right Afcenfion be given, to find its Place, lay the Thread on the Right Afcenfion, and it will crofs the Sun's Place in the Ecliptick

USE II *The Sun's Place being given, to find his Declination, and contrariwife.*

Lay the Thread, and fet the Bead to the Sun's Place in the Ecliptick, then move the Thread to the Line of Declination, and there the Bead will fall upon the Degrees of the Line of Declination fought

For example, Let the Sun's Place be the 4*th* Degree of ♊, the Bead being firft fet to this Place, move the Thread to the Line of Declination, and there you will find the Sun's Declination 21 deg from the Equator

Now the Sun's Place being fought, in having the Declination given, you muft firft lay the Thread and Bead to the Declination, and then the Bead moved to the Ecliptick will give the Sun's Place fought.

USE

USE III *The Day of the Month being given, to find the Sun's Meridian Altitude, and contrariwise*

Lay the Thread to the Day of the Month, and the Degrees which it cuts in the Limb will be the Sun's Meridian Altitude

Suppose the Day given be *May* the 15*th*, the Thread laid upon this Day will cut 59 deg 30 min the Meridian Altitude sought

Again, If the Thread be set to the Meridian Altitude, it will fall upon the Day of the Month

As, suppose the Sun's Meridian Altitude be 59 deg 30 min the Thread set to this Altitude falls upon the 15*th* Day of *May*, and the 9*th* of *July*, and which of these two is the true Day, may be known by the Quarter of the Year, or by another Day's Observation for if the Sun's Altitude be greater, the Thread will fall upon the 16*th* of *May*, and the 8*th* of *July*, and if it prove lesser, then the Thread will fall on the 14*th* of *May*, and the 10*th* of *July*, whereby the Question is fully answered

USE IV *The Sun's Altitude being given, to find the Hour of the Day, and contrariwise*

Having put the Bead to the Sun's Place in the Ecliptick, observe the Sun's Altitude by the Quadrant, and then if the Thread be laid over the same in the Limb, the Bead will fall upon the Hour required For example, Suppose on the 10*th* of *April*, the Sun being then in the beginning of *Taurus*, I observe his Altitude by the Quadrant to be 36 deg place the Bead to the beginning of *Taurus* in the Ecliptick, and afterwards lay the Thread over 36 Degrees of the Limb, then the Bead will fall upon the Hour-Line of 9 and 3 and so the Hour is 9 in the Morning, or 3 in the Afternoon Again, If the Altitude be near 40 Degrees, the Bead will fall half way between the Hour-Line of 9 and 3, and the Hour-Line of 10 and 2 Wherefore it must be either half an Hour past 9 in the Morning, or half an Hour past two in the Afternoon, and which of these is the true Time of the Day, may be known by a second Observation For if the Sun rises higher, it is Morning, and if it becomes lower, it is Afternoon

Now to find the Sun's Altitude by having the Hour given, you must lay the Bead upon the Hour given (having first rectified or put it to the Sun's Place) and then the Degrees of the Limb cut by the Thread, will be the Sun's Altitude sought

Note, The Bead may be rectified otherwise, in bringing the Thread to the Day of the Month, and the Bead to the Hour-Line of 12

USE V *To find the Sun's Amplitude either rising or setting, when the Day of the Month or Sun's Place is given*

Let the Bead rectified for the time, be brought to the Horizon, and there it will shew the Amplitude sought If, for example, the Day given be the 4*th* of *May*, the Sun will then be in the 4*th* Degree of *Gemini* Now if the Bead be rectified and brought to the Horizon, it will there fall on 35 deg 8 min and this is the Sun's Amplitude of rising from the East, and of his setting from the West

USE VI *The Day of the Month or Sun's Place being given, to find the Ascensional Difference*

Rectify the Bead for the given time, and afterwards bring it to the Horizon, then the Degrees cut by the Thread in the Limb will be the ascensional Difference And if the ascensional Difference be converted into time, in allowing an Hour for 15 Degrees, and four Minutes of an Hour for one Degree, then we shall have the time of the Sun's rising before six in the Summer, and after six in the Winter, and consequently the Length of Day and Night may be known by this means.

USE VII *The Sun's Altitude being given, to find his Azimuth, and contrariwise*

Rectify the Bead for the time, and observe the Sun's Altitude Then bring the Thread to the Complement of that Altitude, and so the Bead will give the Azimuth sought upon or among the Azimuth Lines

And to find the Altitude by having the Azimuth given, having rectified the Bead to the Time, move the Thread till the Bead falls on the given Azimuth, then the Degrees of the Limb cut by the Thread, will be the Sun's Altitude at that time

USE VIII *The Altitude of any one of the five Stars on the Quadrant being given, to find the Hour of the Night.*

First, Put the Bead to the Star, which you intend to observe, and find how many Hours he is from the Meridian by *Use* IV then from the Right Ascension of the Star, substract the Sun's Right Ascension converted into Hours, and mark the Difference for this Difference added to the observed Hour of the Star from the Meridian, will shew how many Hours the Sun is gone from the Meridian, which is in effect the Hour of the Night

For

For example, The 15th of *May*, the Sun being in the 4th Degree of *Gemini*, I set the Bead to *Arcturus*, and observing his Altitude, find him to be in the West, about 52 deg high, and the Bead to fall upon the Hour-Line of two after Noon; then the Hour will be 11 Hours 50 min past Noon, or 10 Minutes short of Midnight. For 62 deg the Sun's Right Ascension, converted into Time, makes 4 Hours 8 min which if we take out of 13 Hours 58 min the Right Ascension of *Arcturus*, the Difference will be 9 Hours 50 min and this being added to two Hours, the observed Distance of *Arcturus* from the Meridian, shews the Hour of the Night to be 11 Hours 50 min.

Thus have I briefly shewn the Manner of solving several of the chief and most useful Astronomical Problems, by means of this Quadrant. As for the Manner of taking Altitudes in Degrees, as likewise the Use of the Quadrat, see our Author's Quadrant.

There are other Quadrants made by Mr *Sutton* long since, one of which (being in my Opinion the best) is a Stereographical Projection of ¼ of those Circles, or quarter of the Sphere between the Tropicks, upon the Plane of the Equinoctial, the Eye being in the North Pole.

The said quarter on the Quadrant, is that between the South part of the Meridian, and Hour of six, which will leave out all the outward part of the Almicanters between it and the Tropick of *Capricorn*, and instead thereof, there is taken in such a like part of the depressed Parallels to the Horizon, between the same Hour of six and Tropick of *Capricorn*, for the Parallels of Depression have the same Respect to the Tropick of *Capricorn*, as the Parallels of Altitude have to the Tropick of *Cancer*, and will produce the same Effect.

This Projection is fitted for the Latitude of *London* and those Lines therein that run from the Right-hand to the Left, are Parallels of Altitude, and those which cross them, are Azimuths. The lesser of the Circles that bounds the Projection, is one fourth of the Tropick of *Capricorn*, and the other one fourth of the Tropick of *Cancer*. There are also the two Eclipticks drawn from the same Point in the left Edge of the Quadrant, with the Characters or the Signs upon them, as likewise the two Horizons from the same Point. The Limb is divided both into Degrees and Time, and by having the Sun's Altitude given, we may find the Hour of the Day to a Minute by this Quadrant.

The Quadrantal Arcs next the Center contain the Calender of Months, and under them in another Arc is the Sun's Declination. So that a Thread laid from the Center over any Day of the Month, will fall upon the Sun's Declination that Day in this last Arc, and on the Limb upon the Sun's Right Ascension for that same Day. There are several of the most noted fixed Stars between the Tropicks, placed up and down in the Projection, and next below the Projection is the Quadrat and Line of Shadows, being only a Line of natural Tangents to the Arcs or the Limb, and by help thereof, the Heights of Towers, Steeples, &c. may be pretty exactly taken.

Now the Manner of using this Projection in finding the Time of the Sun's rising or setting, his Amplitude, Azimuth, the Hour of the Day, &c. is thus. Having laid the Thread to the Day of the Month, bring the Bead to the proper Ecliptick, (which is called rectifying of it) and afterwards move the Thread, and bring the Bead to the Horizon: then the Thread will cut the Limb in the time of the Sun's rising or setting before or after six. And at the same time the Bead will cut the Horizon in the Degrees of the Sun's Amplitude. Again, Suppose the Sun's Altitude on the 24th of *April* be observed 45 Degrees, what will the Hour and Azimuth then be? Having laid the Thread over the 24th of *April*, bring the Bead to the Summer Ecliptick, and then carry it to the Parallel of the Altitude 45 Degrees and then the Thread will cut the Limb at 55 deg 15 min. and so the Hour will be either 41 min past nine in the Morning, or 19 min past two in the Afternoon. And the Bead among the Azimuths shews the Sun's Distance from the South to be 50 deg. 41 min.

Note, If the Sun's Altitude be less than that which it hath at six a Clock, on any given Day, then the Operation must be performed among those Parallels above the upper Horizon, the Bead being rectified to the Winter Ecliptick.

There are a great many other Uses of this Quadrant, which I shall omit, and refer you to *Collins's* Sector upon a Quadrant, wherein its Description, and Use, together with those of two other Quadrants, are fully treated of.

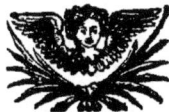

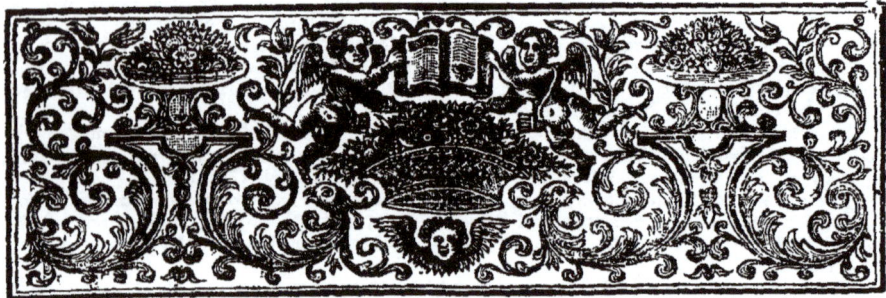

BOOK VII.

Of the Conſtruction and Uſes of Inſtruments
for Navigation.

CHAP. I.

Of the Conſtruction and Uſe of the Sea-Compaſs, and Azimuth
Compaſs.

SECTION I.

Plate 20.
Fig. 1.

THE firſt Figure ſhews the Compaſs Card, whoſe Limb repreſents the Horizon of the World. It is divided into four times 90 Degrees, and very often but into 32 equal Parts, for the 32 Points, whereof the four principal Points, which are called Cardinal ones, croſs each other at Right Angles, *viz.* the North, diſtinguiſhed by the *Flower-de-luce*, the South oppoſite thereto, and the Eaſt and Weſt. Now if each of theſe Quarters be biſected, we ſhall have the eight Rhumbs. Again, Biſecting each of theſe laſt Spaces, we ſhall have the eight Semi-Rhumbs. And laſtly, Biſecting each of theſe laſt Parts, we ſhall have the ſixteen Quarter-Rhumbs. The four Collateral Rhumbs take their Name from the four Principal Rhumbs, each aſſuming the two Names of thoſe that are nigheſt them : as, the Rhumb in the middle, between the North and the Eaſt, is called North-Eaſt, that between the South and the Eaſt, is called South-Eaſt; that between the South and the Weſt, is called South-Weſt; and that in the middle between the North and the Weſt, is called North-Weſt.

Alſo every of the eight Semi-Rhumbs aſſumes its Name from the two Rhumbs that be nigheſt it, as that between the North and North-Eaſt, is called North North-Eaſt; that between the Eaſt and North-Eaſt, is called Eaſt North-Eaſt, that between the Eaſt and South-Eaſt, is called Eaſt South-Eaſt, and ſo of others.

Finally, Each of the Quarter-Rhumbs has its Name compoſed of the Rhumbs or Semi-Rhumbs which are nigheſt to it, in adding the Word one-fourth after the Name of the Rhumb neareſt to it. For example; The Quarter-Rhumb neareſt to the North, and next to the North-Eaſt, is called North one-fourth North-Eaſt, that which is neareſt the North-Eaſt towards the North, is called North-Eaſt, one-fourth North, and ſo of others, as they appear abbreviated round the Card. Each Quarter-Rhumb contains 11 deg 15 min. the Semi-Rhumbs 22 deg 30 min and the whole Rhumbs 45 deg

The Inſide of this Card, which is ſuppoſed double, is likewiſe divided into 32 equal Parts, by a like Number of Radii, denoting the 32 Points, and the middle thereof, which is glewed upon a Paſteboard, hath a free Motion upon its Pivot, that ſo it may be uſed when the Declination or Variation of the Needle is found Note, The Outſide of this Card is placed upon the Limb of the Box.

The

The second Figure represents a piece of Steel in form of a Rhumbus, which serves for the Needle, and is fastened under the moveable Card with two little Pins, so that one of the ends of the longest Diameter of the said Rhumbs be precisely under the *Flower-de-luce.* This piece of Steel must be touched by a good Load-stone, so that one end may direct itself towards the North part of the World. The manner of doing which, we have already shewn in speaking of the Load-stone, and the Compass. *Note,* It is not so well to glew the said Needle under the Card, as some do, as otherwise to fasten it, because that causes a Rust very contrary to the magnetick Virtue.

The little Figure B, in the middle of the Rhumbus, which is called the Cap of the Needle, is made of Brass, and hollowed into a Conical Form. This Cap is applied to the Center of the Card, and is fastened thereto with Glew.

The third Figure represents the whole Compass, whereof A is a round wooden Box, about six or seven Inches Diameter, and four deep, (we sometimes make these Boxes square) *b b* and *c c* are two Brass Hoops, the greater of which being *b b*, is fastened to the Sides of the Box at the opposite Places B B. The other Hoop *c* C is fastened by two other Pivots at the Places C C, diametrically opposite to the Hoop *b b*, and these two Pivots go into Holes made towards the top of another kind of wooden Box, in which the Card is put. And by this means, this last Box, and the two Hoops, will have a very free Motion, so that when the great Box A is placed flat in a Ship, the lesser Box will be always horizontal, and *in equilibrio*, notwithstanding the Motion of the Ship. In the middle of the Bottom of this last Box, is placed a very strait and well pointed brass Pivot, on which is placed the Cap B of the Card, which Card having a very free Motion, the *Flower-de-luce* will turn towards the North, and all the other Points towards the other Correspondent Parts of the World. Finally, the Card is covered with a Glass, that so the Wind may have no power on it.

Use of the Sea-Compass

The Course that a Ship must take to sail to a proposed Place, being known by a Sea-Chart, and the Compass placed in the Pilot's Room, so as the two parallel Sides of the square Box be fixed according to the length of the Ship, that is, parallel to a Line drawn from the Poop to the Prow, make a Cross, or other Mark, upon the middle of that Side of the square Box perpendicular to the Ship's length, and the most distant from the Poop, that so the Stern of the Ship by this means may be directed accordingly.

Example. Departing from the Island *de Ouessant,* upon the Confines of *Brittany,* we desire to sail towards Cape *Finister* in *Galicia.* Now in order to do this, we must first seek (according to the manner hereafter directed) in a *Mercator's* Chart, the Direction or Course of the Ship leading to that Place, and this we find is between the South-West and the South South-West; that is, the Ship's Course must be South-West, one-fourth to the South. Therefore having a fair Wind, turn the Stern of the Ship, so that a Line tending from the South-West, one-fourth South, exactly answers to the Cross marked upon the middle of the Side of the square Box; and then we shall have our desire. And by this means, which is really admirable, we may direct a Ship's Course as well in the Night as in the Day, as well being shut up in a Room in the Ship, as in the open Air, and as well in cloudy Weather as fair, so that we may always know whether the Ship goes out of her proper Direction.

Of the Variation or Declination of the Needle

It is found by experience, that the touched Needle varies from the true North, that is, the *Flower-de-luce* does not exactly tend to the North part of the World, but varies therefrom, sometimes towards the East, sometimes towards the West, more or less, according to different Times, and at different Places.

About the Year 1665, the Needle at *Paris* did not decline or vary at all; whereas now its Variation is there above 12 Degrees North-westwardly. Therefore every time a favourable Opportunity offers, you must endeavour to observe carefully the Variation of the Needle, that so respect thereto may be had in the steering of Ships. If, for example, the Variation of the Needle in the Island *de Ouessant,* which was the supposed Place of departure in the abovementioned Example, was 10 Degrees, and if the Ship should exactly keep the Course of South-West, one-fourth to the South, instead of arriving at Cape *Finister,* it would come to another Country 10 Degrees more to the East.

Now to remedy this, you need only remove the Cross, upon the Side of the Box, shewing the Rhumb of Direction, more easterly by the Quantity of the Degrees of the Needle's Variation westwardly, and so as often as a new Declination, or Variation of the Needle be found, the place of the said Cross must be altered. *Note,* When the Box is quite round, a Mark must be made against the North and South on the Body of the said Box.

If likewise a Vessel departs from the *Sorlings,* in *England,* in order to sail to the Island of *Madera,* you will find by a Sea-Chart that her Course must be South South-West, but if at the same time the Variation of the Needle be six Degrees North Easterly, the Cross denoted upon the Edge of the Compass must be removed six Degrees towards the West, in order to direct the Ship according to her true Course found in the Chart.

But

But if a Sea Compafs be ufed, wherein the Pofition of the Needle may be altered, as that which hath a double Card, the *Flower-de-luce* of the Card muft be fixed, fo that its Point may fhew the true North, and then you will have it to alter every time there is a new Variation obferved   Now in this Cafe the Crofs upon the Edge of the Compafs muft not be altered

It is very neceffary, and principally in long Courfes, for Seamen to make Celeftial Obfervations often, in order to have the Variation of the Needle exactly, that the Direction of the Veffel may thereby be truly had, as likewife that they may know where they are, after having efcaped a great Storm, during which they were obliged to leave the true Courfe, and let the Veffel run according as the Wind or Currents drove her.

SECTION II.

Of the Azimuth Compafs.

Fig 4

This Compafs is fomething different from the common Sea-Compafs before fpoken of   For upon the round Box, wherein is the Card, is faftened a broad brafs Circle A B, one Semi-circle whereof is divided into 90 equal Parts or Degrees, numbered from the middle of the faid Divifions both ways, with 10, 20 *&c* to 45 Degrees, which Degrees are alfo divided into Minutes by Diagonal Lines and Circles: But thefe graduating Lines are drawn from the oppofite part of the Circle, *viz.* from the Point *b*, wherein the Index turns in time of Obfervation.

b c is that Index moveable about the Point *b*, having a Sight *b a* erected thereon, which moves with a Hinge, that fo it may be raifed or laid down, according to neceffity   From the upper part of this Sight, down to the middle of the Index, is faftened a fine Hypothenufal Lute-ftring, or Thread *d e*, to give a Shadow upon a Line that is in the middle of the faid Index

Note, The reafon of making the Index move on a Pin faftened in *b*, is, that the Degrees and Divifions may be larger, for now they are as large again as they would have been, if they had been divided from the Center, and the Index made to move thereon

The abovenamed broad brafs Circle A B, is croffed at Right Angles with two Threads, and from the ends of thefe Threads are drawn four fmall black Lines on the Infide of the round Box, alfo there are four Right Lines drawn at Right Angles to each other on the Card

This round Box, thus fitted with its Card, graduated Circle, and Index, *&c* is to be hung in the brafs Hoops B B, and thefe Hoops are faftened to the great fquare wooden Box C C

The Ufe of the Azimuth Compafs in finding the Sun's Magnetical Azimuth or Amplitude, and from thence the Variation of the Compafs

There are feveral ways of finding the Variation of the Needle, as by the rifing and fetting of the fame Star, or by the Obfervation of the two equal Altitudes of a Star above the Horizon, fince the faid Star, at each of thofe Times, will be equally diftant from the true Meridian of the World, or elfe by a Star's paffage over the Meridian

But thefe Methods are not much ufed at Sea   Firft, becaufe the Time wherein the Sun, or a Star, paffes over the Meridian, cannot be known precifely enough, for there is a great deal of Time taken in making Obfervations of the Sun's Altitudes, till he is found to have the greateft, that is, his Meridian Altitude.

Secondly, Becaufe the Sun's Declination may be confiderably altered, and alfo the Ship's Latitude between the Times of the two Obfervations of his equal Altitudes above the Horizon, Morning and Evening, or of his Rifing and Setting

Therefore the Variation of the Compafs may much better be found by one Obfervation of the Sun's magnetical Amplitude, or Azimuth.   But the Sun's Declination, and the Latitude of the Place the Ship is in, muft be known, that fo his true Amplitude may be had, his Altitude muft alfo be given, when the magnetick Azimuth is taken, that fo his true Azimuth may be had at that Time alfo

Now if the Obfervation be for an Amplitude at Sun-rifing, or an Azimuth before Noon, you muft put the Center of the Index *b c* upon the Weft Point of the Card within the Box, fo that the four Lines on the Edge of the Card, and the four Lines on the Infide of the Box, may agree or come together   But if the Obfervation be for the Sun's Amplitude, Setting, or an Azimuth in the Afternoon, then you muft turn the Center of the Index right-againft the Eaft Point of the Card, and make the Lines within the Box concur with thofe on the Card   Having thus fitted the Inftrument for Obfervation, turn the Index *b c* towards the Sun, till the Shadow of the Thread *d e* falls directly upon the flit of the Sight, and upon the Line that is along the middle of the Index, then will the inner Edge of the Index cut the Degree and Minute of the Sun's magnetical Azimuth, from the North or South

But note, that if the Compafs being thus placed, the Azimuth be lefs than 45 deg from the South, and the Index be turned towards the Sun, it will then pafs off the Divifions of

the

the Limb, and ſo they become uſeleſs as it now ſtands therefore you muſt turn the Inſtrument juſt a Quarter of the Compaſs, that is, place the Center of the Index on the North or South Point of the Card, according as the Sun is from you, and then the Edge thereof will cut the Degree of the Magnetick Azimuth, or Sun's Azimuth from the North, as before

The Sun's Magnetical Amplitude, (that is, the Diſtance from the Eaſt or Weſt Points of the Compaſs, to that Point in the Horizon whereat the Sun riſes or ſets) being obſerved by this Inſtrument, the Variation of the Compaſs may be thus found

Example Being out at Sea the 15th Day of *May*, in the Year 1715, in 45 Degrees of North Latitude, I find from Tables that the Sun's Declination is 19 deg North, and his Eaſt Amplitude 27 deg 25 min North. Now I obſerve by the Azimuth Compaſs, the Sun's Magnetical Amplitude at his riſing and ſetting, and find that he riſes between the 62d and 63d deg reckoning from the North towards the Eaſt part of the Compaſs, that is, between the 27th and 28th Degree from the Eaſt; and ſince in this Caſe the magnetical Amplitude is equal to the true Amplitude, I conclude that at this Place and Time, the Needle has no Variation

But if the Sun at his riſing ſhould have appeared between the 52d and 53d Degree from the North towards the Eaſt, his magnetical Amplitude would then be between 37 and 38 Degrees, that is, about 10 Degrees greater than the true Amplitude and therefore the Needle would vary about 10 Degrees North-Eaſterly If, on the contrary, the magnetical Eaſt Amplitude found by the Inſtrument ſhould be leſs than the true Amplitude, their Difference would ſhew that the Variation of the Needle is North-Eaſterly For if the magnetical Amplitude be greater than the true Amplitude, this proceeds from hence, that the Eaſt part of the Compaſs is drawn back from the Sun towards the South, and the *Flower-de-luce* of the Card approaches to the Eaſt, and ſo gives the Variation North-Eaſterly The reaſon for the contrary of this is equally evident

If the true Eaſt Amplitude be Southwardly, as likewiſe the magnetical Amplitude, and this laſt be the greater, then the Variation of the Needle will be North-Weſt, and if on the contrary, the magnetical Amplitude be leſs than the true Amplitude, the Variation of the Needle will be North-Eaſterly, as many Degrees as are contained in their Difference

What we have ſaid concerning North-Eaſt Amplitudes, muſt be underſtood of South-Weſt Amplitudes, and what we have ſaid of South-Eaſt Amplitudes, muſt be underſtood of North-Weſt Amplitudes

Finally, If Amplitudes are found of different Denominations, for example, when Amplitudes are Eaſt, if the true Amplitude be 6 deg North, and the magnetical Amplitude 5 deg South, then the Variation, which in this Caſe is North-Weſt, will be greater than the true Amplitude, it being equal to the Sum of the magnetical and true Amplitudes: and ſo adding them together, we ſhall have 11 Degrees of North-Weſt Variation Underſtand the ſame for Weſt Amplitudes

The Variation of the Compaſs may likewiſe be found by the Azimuth, but then the Sun's Declination, the Latitude of the Place, and his Altitude muſt be had, that ſo his true Azimuth may be found

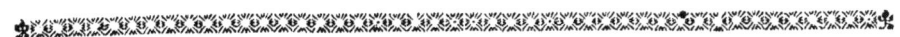

CHAP. II.

Of the Conſtruction and Uſe of Inſtruments for taking the Altitudes of the Sun or Stars at Sea.

Of the Sea-Aſtrolabe

THE moſt common Inſtrument for taking of Altitudes at Sea is the Aſtrolabe, which Fig. 5. conſiſts of a braſs Circle, about one Foot in Diameter, and ſix or ſeven Lines in thickneſs, that ſo it may be pretty weighty there is ſometimes likewiſe a Weight of ſix or ſeven Pounds hung to this Inſtrument at the Place B, that ſo when the Aſtrolabe is ſuſpended by its Ring A, which ought to be very moveable, the ſaid Inſtrument may turn any way, and keep a perpendicular Situation during the Motion of the Ship

The Limb of this Inſtrument is divided into four times 90 Degrees, and very often into halves, and fourths of Degrees

It is abſolutely neceſſary, that the Right Line C D, which repreſents the Horizon, be perfectly level, that ſo the beginning of the Diviſions of the Limb of the Inſtrument may be made therefrom. Now to examine whether this be ſo or no, you muſt obſerve ſome diſtant Object thro the Slits or little Holes of the Sights F and G, faſtened near the Ends of the Index, freely turning about the Center E, by means of a turned-headed Rivet I

F f f   ſay

say, you must observe the said distant Objects, in placing the Eye to one of the said Sights for example, to G then if the Astrolabe be turned about, and the same Object appears thro the other Sight F, without moving the Index, it is a sign the Fiducial Line of the Index is horizontal But if at the second time of Observation, the Index must be raised or lowered before the Object be espied thro the Sights, then the middle Point between the two Positions will shew the true horizontal Line passing thro the Center of the Instrument, which must be verified by several repeated Observations, before the Divisions of the Limb are begun to be made, in the manner as we have elsewhere explained.

Use of the Astrolabe.

The Use of this Instrument is for observing the Sun or Stars Altitude above the Horizon, or their Zenith Distance The manner of effecting which, is thus Holding the Astrolabe suspended by its Ring, and turning its Side towards the Sun, move the Index till the Sun's Rays pass thro the Sights F and G , then the Extremes of the Index will give the Altitude of the Sun in H, upon the divided Limb, from C to F, comprehended between the horizontal Radius E C and the Rays E F of the Sun, because the Instrument in this Situation represents a Vertical Circle. Now the Divisions of the Arcs B G or A F, shew the Sun's Zenith distance

The Construction of the Ring

Fig 6

This Figure represents a brass Ring or Circle, about 9 Inches in Diameter, which it is necessary should be pretty thick , that so being weighty, it may keep its perpendicular Situation better than when it is not so heavy, having the Divisions denoted in the Concave Surface thereof The little Hole C, made thro the Ring, is 45 Degrees distant from the Point of Suspension B, and is the Center of the Quadrant D E, divided into 90 Degrees, one of whose Radius's C E, is parallel to the Vertical Diameter B H of the Ring, and the other horizontal Radius C D, is perpendicular to the said Vertical Diameter

Now having found the said horizontal Radius C D very exactly, by suspending the Ring, &c Radius's must be drawn from the Center C to each Degree of the Quadrant D E, and upon the Points wherein the said Radius's cut the Concave Surface of the Ring, the correspondent Numbers of the Degrees of the Quadrant must be graved , and so the Concave Surface of the Ring, will be divided from F to G This Divisioning may be first made separately upon a Plane, and afterwards transferred upon the Concave Surface of the Ring

This Instrument is reckoned better than the Astrolabe, because the Divisions of the Degrees upon the Concave Surface are larger in proportion to its bigness, than those on the Astrolabe

The Use of the Ring

When this Instrument is to be used, you must suspend it by the Swivel B, and turn it towards the Sun A , so that its Rays may pass thro the Hole C This being done, the little Spot will fall between the horizontal Line C F, and vertical Line C G, upon the Degrees of the Sun's Altitude on the Inside of the Ring, reckoned from F to I

Of the Quadrant

Fig 7,

The Instrument of Figure 7, is a Quadrant about one Foot Radius, having its Limb divided into 90 Degrees, and very often each Degree into every 5th Minute by Diagonals There are two Sights fixed upon one of the Sides A E, and the Thread to which the Plummet is fastened, is fixed in the Center A I shall not here mention the Construction of this Instrument, because we have sufficiently spoken thereof in Chap V Book IV

Now to use this Instrument, you must turn it towards the Sun D, in such manner that its Rays may pass thro the Sights A and E, and then the Thread will fall upon the Degrees of the Sun's Altitude on the Limb, in the Point C, reckoned from B to C, and the Complement of his Altitude reckoned from E to C

Of the Fore-Staff, or Cross-Staff

Fig. 8.

This Instrument consists of a strait square graduated Staff A B, between two and three Foot in length, and four Crosses or Vanes F F, E E, D D, C C, which slide stiffly thereon The first and shortest of these Vanes F F, is called the Ten-cross or Vane, and belongs to that Side of the Staff whereon the Divisions begin at about 3 Degrees from the End A, (whereat the Eye is placed in time of Observation) to 10 Degrees Note, Sometimes the Thirty-cross E F is so made, as that the Breadth thereof serves instead of this Ten-cross

The next longer Vane E F, is called the Thirty-cross, and belongs to that Side of the Staff, whereon the Divisions begin at 10 Degrees, and end at 30 Degrees, and this is called the Thirty-side Half the length of the Thirty-vane will reach on this Thirty-side, from 30 deg to 23 deg 52 min and the whole length from 30 deg to 19 deg 47 min.

The

The next longer Vane D D, is called the Sixty-cross, and belongs to that Side of the Staff whereon the Divisions begin at 20 deg and end at 60 deg and is called the Sixty-side   The length of this Cross will reach on this Sixty-side, from 60 deg to 30 deg.

The longest Cross C C, is called the Ninety-cross, and belongs to that Side whereon the Divisions begin at 30 Degrees, and end at 90 Degrees, and is called the Ninety-side of the Staff · the Degrees on the several Sides of the Staff, are numbered with their Complements to 90 Degrees in small Figures

This Staff may be graduated Geometrically thus · Upon a Table, or on a large Paper Fig 9, pasted smoothly upon some Plane, draw the Line F G, the length of the Staff to be graduated, and on F and G raise the Perpendiculars F C and G D, upon which lay off the Length you intend for the half Length of one of the four Crosses, from F to C, and G to D, and draw the Line C D representing the Staff to be graduated   This being done, about the Center F, with the Semidiameter F G or C D, describe an eighth part of a Circle, which divide into 90 equal Parts   Then if Right Lines be drawn from the Point F, to each of the aforesaid Divisions, these Lines will divide the Line C D, as the Staff ought to be graduated

But if this Staff is to be graduated by the Table of natural Tangents, you must first observe, that the Graduations are only the natural Co-tangents of half Arcs, the half Cross being Radius; therefore divide the length of the half Cross into 1000 equal Parts, or 100000 if possible, according to the Radius of the Tables of natural Tangents   then take from this the Co-tangents, as you find them in the Table, and prick them from F successively, and your Staff will be graduated for that Vane. So do for the rest severally   If it be required to prick down the 80*th* Degree, the half of 80 is 40, and the natural Co-tangent of 40 deg is 119175, which take from the Scale or half Cross so divided, and prick it from F to P, and that will be the Point for 80 Degrees, &c   So again, To put on the 64*th* Degree, half of 64 is 32, and its Co-tangent is 160033, which take from the divided Cross (prolonged) prick it from F, and you will have the 64*th* Degree

Now that the Cross C D, when transferred to B, shall make the Angles C A D eighty Fig 10. Degrees, is demonstrable thus   Since C B the half Cross is Radius, and A B is by Construction the Tangent of 50 deg the Angle A C B is 50 Degrees, and since the Triangle A B C is Right Angled, the Angle B A C will be 40 Degrees   but the Angle D A C is double the Angle B A C; therefore the Angle D A C is 80 Degrees, and the Point B the true Point on the Staff for 80 Degrees   The same Demonstration holds, let the Cross be what it will.

If the Staff be to be graduated by any Diagonal Scale, measure half the Length of the Vane by the Scale, and say, As the Radius of the Tables 100000, is to the Measure of half the Cross, so is the natural Co-tangent of the half of any Number of Degrees desired to be pricked on the Staff, to the Space between the Center of the Staff F, and the Point for the Degrees sought

For example, Suppose half the Length of the Vane, measured on a Diagonal Scale, be 945, to find what Number must be taken off the Diagonal Scale for the 80*th* Degree The Co-tangent of 40 Degrees (half of 80) is 1191753, which being multiplied by 945, and divided by Radius, gives 11261   And this being taken from the Diagonal Scale, will give the Degrees desired

The Use of the Fore-Staff

The chief Use of this Instrument, is to take the Altitude of the Sun or Stars, or the Distance of two Stars, and the Ten, Thirty, Sixty and Ninety Crosses are to be used, according as the Altitude is greater or lesser, that is, if it be less than 10 Degrees, the Ten Cross must be used, if above 10, but less than 30 Degrees, the Thirty Cross must be used, and if the Altitude be judged to be above 30, but less than 60 Degrees, the Sixty Cross must be used   But when Altitudes are greater than 60 Degrees, this Instrument is not so convenient as others

To observe an Altitude

Place the flat End of the Staff to the outside of your Eye, as near the Eye as you can, Fig 11 and look at the upper End *b* of the Cross for the Center of the Sun or Star, and at the lower End *a* for the Horizon   But if you see the Sky instead of the Horizon, slide the Cross a little nearer to your Eye, and if you see the Sea instead of the Horizon, move the Cross a little further from your Eye, and so continue moving the Cross till you see exactly the Sun or Star's Center by the top of the Cross *b*, and the Horizon by the bottom thereof *a*   Then the Degrees and Minutes cut by the inner Edge *c* of the Cross, upon the Side of the Staff peculiar to the Cross you use, is the Altitude of the Sun or Star   But if it be the Meridian Altitude you are to find, you must continue your Observation as long as you find the Altitude increase, still moving the Cross nearer to your Eye, but when you perceive the Altitude is diminished, forbear any farther Observation, and do not alter your Cross, but as it stands, count the Degrees and Minutes on the Side proper to the Cross, and you will have the Meridian Altitude required, as also the Zenith Distance, by sub-
                                                                                                    stracting

ſtracting the ſaid Altitude from 90 Degrees, if it be not graduated on the Staff. To which Zenith Diſtance add the Minutes allowed for the Height of your Eye above the Surface of the Sea, according to the little Table in the Margin, or ſubſtract it from the Altitude, and then you will have the true Zenith Diſtance and Altitude.

Height of the Eye	Allowance.
Engliſh Feet	Min.
1	1
2	$1\frac{1}{4}$
3	2
4	2
5	$2\frac{1}{2}$
6	3
7	3
8	$3\frac{1}{4}$
9	$3\frac{1}{2}$
10	$3\frac{1}{4}$
12	4
16	4
20	5
24	$5\frac{1}{2}$
28	6
32	$6\frac{1}{2}$
36	7
40	7
44	$7\frac{1}{2}$
48	8

If it be hazy or ſomewhat thick Weather, the Fore-Staff may be uſed as above; but if the Sun ſhines out, the upper Limb of the Sun muſt be either obſerved, and afterwards his Semidiameter muſt be ſubſtracted from the Altitude found, or elſe a coloured Glaſs on the top of the Croſs muſt be uſed, to defend the Sight from the Splendour of the Sun

To obſerve the Diſtance of two Stars, or the Moon's Diſtance from a Star, place the Staff's flat end to the Eye, as before directed, and looking to both ends *a* and *b* of the Croſs, move it nearer or farther from the Eye, till you can ſee the two Stars, the one on one end, and the other on the other end of the Croſs Then ſee what Degrees and Minutes are cut by the Croſs on the ſide of the Staff proper to that Vane in uſe; and thoſe Degrees ſhew the obſerved Star's Diſtance

But that there may be no Miſtake in placing the Staff to the Eye, which is the greateſt Difficulty in the Uſe of this Inſtrument. Firſt, before Obſervation, put on the Sixty-croſs, and place it to 30 Degrees on its proper Side, and alſo the Ninety-croſs, ſliding to it 30 Degrees likewiſe on his Right Side · this being done, place the end of the Staff to the corner of your Eye, moving it ſomething higher or lower about the Eye, till you ſee the upper ends of the two Croſſes at once exactly in a Right Line, and alſo their lower ends, and that is the true Place of your Staff in Time of Obſervation

If the Sun's Altitude is to be obſerved backwards by this Inſtrument, you muſt have an horizontal Vane to fix upon the Center or Eye-end of the Croſs, as alſo a Shoe of Braſs for a Sight Vane, to fit on to the end of any of the Croſſes, then when you would obſerve, having put on the horizontal Vane, and fixed the Shoe to the end of a convenient Croſs, turn your back to the Sun, and looking thro the Sight in the braſs Shoe, lift the end of the Staff up or down, till the Shadow made by the upper end of the Croſs falls upon the ſlit in the Horizon-Vane, and at the ſame time you can ſee the Horizon through the Horizon-Vane Then the Degrees and Minutes cut by the Croſs on the proper Side, are the Altitude But if there be fixed a Lens, or ſmall double Convex-Glaſs, to the upper end of the Vane, to contract the Sun-beams, and caſt a ſmall bright Spot on the Horizon Vane, this will be found more convenient than the Shadow, which is commonly imperfect and double.

Of the Engliſh Quadrant, or Back-Staff

Fig 12.

This Inſtrument is commonly made of Pear-Tree, and conſiſts of three Vanes A, B, C, and two Arcs. The Vane at A is called the Horizon-Vane, that at B the Shade-Vane, becauſe it gives the Shadow upon the Horizon-Vane in Time of Obſervation, and that at C the Sight-Vane, becauſe in Time of Obſervation it is placed at the Eye The leſſer Arc D E is the Sixty Arc, and that marked F G is the Thirty Arc, both of which together make 90 Degrees, but they are of different Radius's The Sixty Arc D E is divided into 60 Degrees, commonly by every five, but ſometimes by ſingle Degrees. In Time of Obſervation, the Shadow-Vane is placed upon this Arc always to an even Degree

The Thirty Arc G F, is divided into 30 Degrees, and each Degree into Minutes by Diagonal Lines, and Concentrick Arcs. The Manner of doing which, I have already laid down elſewhere.

The Uſe of the Engliſh Quadrant

If the Sun's Altitude be to be taken by this Inſtrument, you muſt put the Horizon-Vane upon the upper End or Center A of the Quadrant, the Shade-Vane upon the Sixty Arc D E, to ſome Number of Degrees leſs than you judge the Co-altitudes will be by 10 or 15 Degrees, and the Sight-Vane upon the Thirty Arc F G This being done, lift up the Quadrant, with your Back towards the Sun, and look thro the ſmall Hole in the Sight-Vane C, and ſo raiſe or lower the Quadrant till the Shadow of the upper Edge of the Shade-Vane B falls upon the upper Edge of the ſlit in the Horizon-Vane A: if then at the ſame time the Horizon appears thro the ſaid ſlit, the Obſervation is finiſhed, but if the Sea appears inſtead of the Horizon, then remove the Sight-Vane lower towards F, but if the Sky appears inſtead of the Horizon, then ſlide the Sight-Vane a little higher and ſo continue removing the Sight-Vane, till the Horizon appears thro the ſlit of the Horizon-Vane,

Vane, and the Shadow of the Shade-Vane falls at the same time on the said Slit of the Horizon-Vane   This being done, see how many Degrees and Minutes are cut by the Edge of the Sight-Vane C, which answers to the Sight-Hole, and to them add the Degrees that are cut by the upper Edge of the Shade-Vane, and the Sum is the Zenith Distance or Complement of the Altitude   But to find the Sun's Meridian or greatest Altitude on any Day, you must continue the Observation as long as the Altitude be found to increase, which you will perceive, by having the Sea appear instead of the Horizon, removing the Sight-Vane lower, but when you perceive the Sky appear instead of the Horizon, the Altitude is diminished   therefore desist from farther Observation at that Time, and add the Degrees upon the Sixty Arc to the Degrees and Minutes upon the Thirty Arc, the Sum is the Zenith Distance, or Co-altitude of the Sun's upper Limb

And because it is the Zenith Distance or Co-altitude of the upper Limb of the Sun, that is given by the Quadrant, when observing by the upper Edge of the Shade-Vane, as it is customary to do, and not the Center, you must add 16 min the Sun's Semi-diameter, to that which is produced by your Observation, and the Sum is the true Zenith Distance of the Sun's Center   But if you observe by the lower part of the Shadow of the Shade-Vane, then the lower Limb of the Sun gives the Shadow, and therefore you must substract 16 min. from what the Instrument gives   but considering the Height of the Observator above the Surface of the Sea, which is commonly between 16 and 20 Feet, you may take five or six Minutes from the 16 Minutes, and make the allowance but 10 min or 12 min to be added instead of 16 min

Note also, The Refraction of the Sun or Stars causes them to appear higher than they are, therefore after having made your Observation, you must find the convenient Refraction, and substract it from your Altitude, or add it to the Zenith Distance, in order to have the true Altitude or Zenith Distance

If a Lens or double Convex-Glass be fixed in the Shade-Vane, which contracts the Rays of Light, and casts them in a small bright Spot on the Slit of the Horizon-Vane instead of a Shade, this will be an Improvement to the Instrument, if the Glass be well fixed, for then it may be used in hazy Weather, and that so thick an Haze, that an Observation can hardly be made with the Forestaff, also in clear Weather the Spot will be more defined than the Shadow, which at best is not terminated.

Of the Semi-circle for taking Altitudes at Sea

This Semi-circle is about one Foot in Diameter, and the Limb thereof is divided into 90 Fig. 13 Degrees only, each of which are quartered for 15 min   At A and B are two Sights fixed to the Extremes of the Diameter, and another at C, so adjusted as to slide on the Limb of the Semi-circle, that so the Sun's Rays may pass thro it when the Instrument is using

The Use of the Semi-circle

If an Altitude is to be taken forwards by this Instrument, the Eye must be placed at the Sight A, and then you must look thro the Sights A and B at the Horizon, and slide the Sight C on the Limb, till the Sun's Rays passing thro it, likewise come thro the Sight A to the Eye.   This being done, the Degrees of the Arc between B and C, shew the Sun's Altitude

But if the Sun's Altitude is to be taken backwards, which is the best way, because of its Splendour offending the Eye, you must place the Eye to B, and looking thro the Sights B and A, at the Horizon, you must slide the Sight C along the Limb, till the Sun's Rays coming thro it, fall upon the Sight A, and then the Arc B C will be the Sun's Altitude above the Horizon, as before

The Meridian Altitude or Zenith Distance of the Sun or Stars being found by Observation, to find the Latitude of the Place

Having observed with some one of the Instruments before spoken of, the Meridian Altitude or Zenith Distance of the Sun, or some Star, seek the Sun's Declination the Day of Observation   if it be North, substract the Sun's Declination found from the Sun's Altitude, and you will have the Height of the Equinoctial above the Horizon, and this Height taken from 90 Degrees, and you will have the Latitude of the Place   But if the Zenith Distance be added to the Declination of the Sun or Star, the Sum will be the Latitude of the Place

Again, If the Sun or Star have South Declination, you must add the observed Altitude to the Declination, and the Sum will be the Height of the Equinoctial above the Horizon, which taken from 90 Degrees, and the Latitude will be had   But if from the Zenith Distance be taken the Declination, the Remainder will be the Latitude of the Place

Lastly, If the Sun has no Declination, his Altitude taken from 90 Degrees, will be the Latitude, and so in this Case the Zenith Distance itself is the Latitude

Example The Sun being in the first Degree of *Cancer,* his Meridian Altitude at *Paris* is 64 deg. 30 min Zenith Distance 25 deg. 30 min. his Declination 23 deg. 30 min North Now if 23 deg. 30 min be taken from 64 deg. 30 min the Remainder is 41 deg for the Altitude of the Equinoctial, and so the Complement of 41 deg. to 90 deg is 49 deg the

Height

Height of the Pole or Latitude of *Paris*, but if the Zenith Diſtance 25 deg 30 min be added to the Sun's Declination 23 deg 30 min. the Sum will be 49 deg the Latitude of *Paris*, as before

Again, Suppoſe the 22*d* of *December* (New Stile) the Sun's Meridian Altitude at *Paris* is obſerved 17 deg 30 min and his Zenith Diſtance 72 deg. 30 min. his Declination is then 23 deg 30 min South, which added to 17 deg 30 min and the Sum is 41 deg whoſe Complement 49 deg is the Latitude of *Paris* Again, If from the Zenith Diſtance 72 deg. 30 min be taken the Declination, the Remainder will be 49 deg the Latitude of *Paris*, as before.

C H A P. III.

Of the Conſtruction and Uſes of the Sinecal Quadrant.

Plate 21
Fig 1

THIS Inſtrument is compoſed of ſeveral Quadrants, having the ſame Center A, and ſeveral parallel ſtrait Lines croſſing each other at Right Angles, both Quadrants and Right Lines being equally diſtant from each other Now one of theſe Quadrants, as B C, may be taken for a quarter or fourth part of any great Circle of the Sphere, and principally for a fourth Part of the Horizon and of the Meridian

If the Quadrant B C be taken for one-fourth part of the Horizon, either of the Sides, as A B, may repreſent the Meridian, that is, the Line of North and South And then the other Side A C, being at Right Angles with the Meridian, will repreſent the Line of Eaſt and Weſt All the other Lines parallel to A B are alſo Meridians, and all thoſe parallel to the Side A C, are Eaſt and Weſt Lines

The aforeſaid Quadrant is firſt divided into eight equal Parts by ſeven Radius's drawn from the Center A, which repreſent the eight Points of the Compaſs contained in one-fourth of the Horizon, each of which is 11 deg 15 min the Arc B C is likewiſe divided into 90 Degrees, and each Degree divided into 12 Minutes, by means of Diagonals, drawn from Degree to Degree, and ſix Concentrick Circles There is likewiſe a Thread, as A L, fixed to the Center A, which being put over any Degree of the Quadrant, ſerves to divide the Horizon as is neceſſary The Conſtruction of the reſt of this Inſtrument, is enough manifeſt from the Figure thereof

The Uſe of the Sinecal Quadrant.

There are formed Triangles upon this Inſtrument ſimilar to thoſe made by a Ship's Way with the Meridians and Parallels, and the Sides of theſe Triangles are meaſured by the equal Intervals between the Concentrick Quadrants, and the Lines N and S, E and O

Theſe Circles and Lines are diſtinguiſhed, by marking every fifth with broader Lines than the others, ſo that if every Interval be taken for one League, there will be five Leagues from one broad Line to the other, and if every Interval be taken for four Leagues, then there will be twenty Leagues, which make a Sea Degree, from one broad Line to the other

Let us ſuppoſe, for example, that a Ship has ſailed 150 Leagues North Eaſt, one-fourth North, which is the third Point, and makes an Angle of 33 deg 45 min with the North-part of the Meridian Now we have two things given, *viz* the Courſe, and Diſtance ſailed, by which a Triangle may be found on this Inſtrument ſimilar to that made by the Ship's Courſe, and her Latitude and Longitude; and ſo the other unknown Parts of the Triangle found And this is done thus

Let the Center A repreſent the Place of Departure, and count, by means of the Concentrick Arcs, along the Point that the Ship ſailed on, as A D, 150 Leagues from A to D; then the Point D will be the Place the Ship is arrived at, which note with a Pin This being done, let D E be parallel to the Side A C, and then there will be formed a Right-angled Triangle A E D, ſimilar to that made by the Ship's Courſe, difference of Latitude and Longitude, the Side A E of this Triangle gives 125 Leagues for the difference of Latitude Northwards, which make 6 deg 15 min reckoning 20 Leagues to a Degree, and one League for three Minutes And laſtly, the Side E D will give 83 leſſer Leagues towards the Eaſt, which being reduced in the manner hereafter ſhewn, will give the difference of Longitude, and ſo the whole Triangle will be known

Note, We call leſſer Leagues thoſe that anſwer to the Parallels of Latitude between the Equator and the Poles, which continually decreaſe the nearer they are to the Pole, and conſequently alſo the Degrees of Longitude; and therefore the nearer a Ship ſails to either of the Poles, the leſs way muſt ſhe make to alter her difference of Longitude any determinate Number of Degrees.

Since

Plate XX

Fig. 1

Fig. 2

Fig. 4

Fig. 5

Fig. 6

Fig. 3

Fig. 7

Fig. 9

Fig. 8

Fig. 11

Fig. 10

Fig. 12

Fig. 13

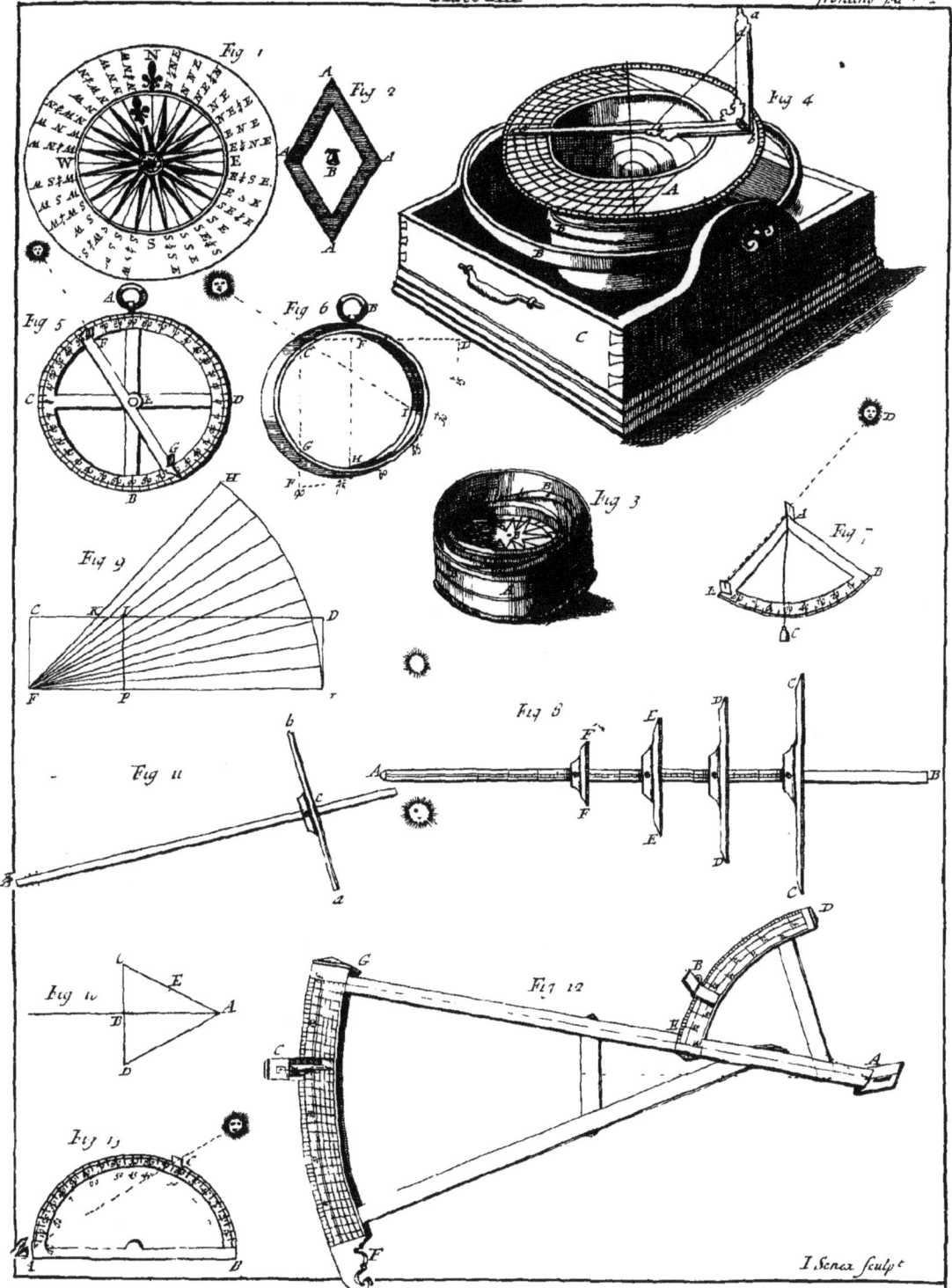

J. Senex sculpt

Since the Center A always reprefents the Place of departure, it is manifeft that when the Point D of arrival is found, be it in what manner foever, all the Parts of the Triangle A E D will afterwards be eafily determined

If the Sinecal Quadrant be taken for a fourth part of the Meridian, one Side thereof, as A B, may be taken for the common Radius of the Meridian, and the Equator, and the other fide A C, will then be half the Axis of the World The Degrees of the Circumference B C, will reprefent the Degrees of Latitude, and the Parallels to the Side A B perpendicular to A C, affumed from every Point of Latitude to the Axis A C, will be the Radius's of the Parallels of Latitude, as likewife the Sine-Complements of thofe Latitudes

If, for example, it be required to find how many Degrees of Longitude 83 leffer Leagues make in the Parallel of 48 deg you muft firft extend a Thread from the Center A, over the 48th deg of Latitude on the Circumference, and keeping it there, count the 83 Leagues propofed on the Side A B, beginning at the Center A Thefe will terminate at H, in allowing every fmall Interval four Leagues, and the Interval between the broad Lines twenty Leagues This being done, if the Parallel H G be traced out from the Point H to the Thread, the part A G of the Thread, fhews that 125 greater Leagues, or the equinoctial Leagues, make 6 deg 15 min in allowing 20 Leagues to a Degree, and three Minutes for one League, and therefore the 83 leffer Leagues A H, which make the difference of Longitude of the fuppofed Courfe, and which are equal to the Radius of the Parallel G I, make 6 deg 15 min of the faid Parallel

Let it be required, for a fecond example, to reduce 100 leffer Leagues into Degrees of Longitude on the Parallel of 60 Degrees Having firft extended the Thread from the Center A over the 60th Degree on the Circumference, count the 100 Leagues of Longitude on the Side A B, and the Parallel terminating thereon being directed to the Thread, the part of the Thread affumed from the Center, fhews that 200 Leagues under the Equator make 10 Degrees, that is, 100 Leagues in the Parallel of 60 Degrees make 10 Degrees of Longitude, fince every Degree of a great Circle is double to any Degree of the Parallel of 60 Degrees

On one Side of this Inftrument is put a Scale, called a Scale of *Crofs-Latitudes*, whofe Conftruction and Divifion is the fame as that of the Meridian Line of *Mercator's* Chart, of which we fhall fpeak by and by The Ufe of this Scale is to find a mean Parallel between that of Departure and that of Arrival

When a Ship has failed on an oblique Courfe, that is, neither exactly North, South, Eaft, or Weft, thefe Courfes, befides the North and South greater Leagues, give *leffer Leagues* eaftwardly and weftwardly, which muft be reduced to Degrees of Longitude But thefe Leagues were made neither upon the Parallel of Departure, nor upon that of Arrival, for they were made upon all the Parallels between thofe of Departure and Arrival, and are all unequal between themfelves, and confequently we are neceffitated to find a mean proportional Parallel between that of Departure and that of Arrival, which for this reafon is called a mean Parallel, and ferves to reduce Leagues made in failing a-crofs divers Parallels, into Degrees and Minutes of the Equator

Now there are feveral ways of finding fuch a mean Parallel, but I fhall only fpeak of that here, which is done by means of the Scale of *Crofs-Latitudes*, without Calculation, and is thus Let it be required, for example, to find a mean Parallel between that of 40 deg and that of 60 deg

Take, by means of a Pair of Compaffes, the middle between the 40th and 60th deg upon this Scale, and the faid middle Point will terminate againft the 51ft deg which confequently will be the mean Parallel fought

Note, Becaufe this Scale is in two Lines, you muft take the Diftance from 40 deg of Latitude to 45 deg which is on one Side, and lay it off upon fome feparate Right Line This being done, you muft take the Diftance from 45 deg to 60 deg which is on the other Side, and join thefe two Spaces together, then half of thefe two Lines being taken between your Compaffes, you muft fet one Foot upon the Number 60, and the other Point will fall upon 51 deg which will be the mean Parallel fought After which, it will be eafy to reduce the Leagues failed Eaftwardly into Degrees of Longitude, by the Sinecal Quadrant, confidered as a quarter of the Meridian, in the manner as we have laid down in the two Examples abovementioned

Of Mercator's Charts

This Figure reprefents a *Mercator's* Chart But before we give the Conftruction and Fig 2 Ufes thereof, it is neceffary to obferve that when a Ship fails upon any determinate Point of the Compafs, fhe always makes the fame Angle with all the Meridians fhe paffes over upon the Surface of the Terraqueous Globe

If a Ship fails North and South, fhe makes an infinitely acute Angle with the Meridian fhe defcribes, that is, fhe runs parallel to it, or rather fails upon it

If a Ship fails due Eaft and Weft, fhe cuts all the Meridians at Right Angles, for fhe either defcribes the Equator, or fome leffer Circle which is parallel thereto But if her Courfe be on any Point between the North and Eaft, North and Weft, South and Eaft, or South and Weft, then fhe will not defcribe a Circle, becaufe a Circle drawn oblique to the

Meridians,

Meridians, will cut all of them at unequal Angles, which the Ship muſt not do while ſhe ſails upon any determinate Point, unleſs North and South, or Eaſt and Weſt; therefore ſhe deſcribes a Curve, not circular, whoſe eſſential Property is to cut all the Meridians at the ſame Angle. And this is called a Loxodromick Curve, or only Loxodromy, and is a kind of Spiral, making an infinity of Revolutions towards a certain Point, which is the Pole, and every Turn thereof approaches nigher and nigher thereto. A Ship's Courſe then, except the two firſt abovenamed, is always a Loxodromick Curve, and is the Hypothenuſe of a Right-angled ſpherical Triangle, whoſe two other Sides are the Ship's Way in Longitude and Latitude. Now we have the Latitude commonly given by Obſervation, and the Loxodromick Angle by the Compaſs, therefore by Trigonometry we may find the Hypothenuſe, or the Way that the Ship has ſailed, &c.

But becauſe the Calculation of a Ship's Way by means of the Loxodromick Curve is troubleſome, therefore the Ancients ſought after ſome Method whereby a Ship's Way might be a ſtrait Line, which might nearly preſerve the Property of the Loxodromick Curve, which is, to cut all the Meridians under the ſame Angle. But they found this abſolutely impoſſible upon the account of the Meridians not being parallel between themſelves, as in reality they are not. And therefore they ſuppoſed the Meridians to be parallel ſtrait Lines, and ſo from this ſuppoſition it follows, that the Degrees of Longitude unequally diſtant from the Equator, are of the ſame bigneſs; whereas they really always diminiſh from the Equator, in a certain known Proportion, which is as Radius is to the Sine-Complement of the Latitude. But to retrieve this Error, they have ſuppoſed the Degrees of Latitude, which by the Nature of the Sphere are every where equal, to be augmented in the ſame Proportion as the Degrees of Longitude diminiſh. And ſo the Inequality which ought to be in the Degrees of Longitude of different Parallels, is thrown upon the Degrees of Latitude in the manner we are going to lay down.

Now Charts made in this manner are called *Mercator's* Charts, becauſe *Mercator* was the firſt that made them, and they are commonly eſteemed the beſt. for by the Experience of ſeveral Ages, it is found that Seamen ought to have very ſimple Charts, wherein the Meridians, Parallels, and Rhumb-Lines may be repreſented by ſtrait Lines, that ſo they may prick down their Courſes eaſily.

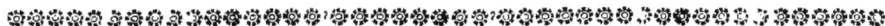

❀❀❀❀❀ ❀❀❀❀❀❀❀❀❀❀ ❀❀❀❀❀❀❀❀ ❀❀❀❀❀❀ ❀❀❀❀❀ ❀❀❀❀❀❀

CHAP. IV.
Of the Construction and Uses of Mercator's Charts.

Fig 2

IF the Degrees of Latitude are to be augmented as much as thoſe of Longitude are found enlarged by making them equal to the Degrees of the Equinoctial, the Secants muſt be uſed, which increaſe in the ſame Proportion as the Sine-Complements of the Latitudes, (which ought to repreſent the Degrees of Longitude) have been encreaſed, by making them equal to the Radius of the Equator, becauſe of the Parallelism of the Meridians: for the Sine-Complement of an Arc is to Radius, as Radius is to the Secant of that Arc.

As, aſſuming for one Degree of the Equator, and for the firſt Degree of Latitude, the whole Radius, or ſome aliquot part thereof, take for the 2d Degree of Latitude, the Secant of one Degree, or a ſimilar aliquot part of this Secant, and for the 3d Degree of Latitude, take the Secant of two Degrees, or the ſimilar aliquot part thereof, and ſo on.

When a Chart is to be made large, you muſt take, for 30 Minutes of Latitude, and 30 Minutes of the Equator, the Radius of a Circle or ſome aliquot part thereof, for one Degree of Latitude. This being done, you muſt add continually the Secant of 30 min for 1 ½ Degree of Latitude, the Secant of 1 Degree for 2 Degrees of Latitude, the Secant of 1 ½ Degree for 2 ½ Degrees of Latitude, or their ſimilar aliquot parts, and ſo proceed on. In doing of which, we uſe a Scale of equal parts, from which the Secants as they are found in Tables are taken off, by taking away ſome of the laſt Figures.

In theſe Charts the Scale is changed, according as the Latitude is; as, for example, if a Ship ſails between the 40*th* and 50*th* Parallel of Latitude, the Degrees of the Meridians between thoſe two Parallels will ſerve for a Scale to meaſure the Ship's Way, whence it follows, that there are fewer Leagues on the Parallels, the nearer they are to the Poles, becauſe they are meaſured by a Magnitude likewiſe continually increaſing from the Equator towards the Poles.

If, for example, a Chart of this kind be to be drawn from the 40*th* Degree of North Latitude to the 50*th*, and from the 6*th* Degree of Longitude to the 18*th*. Firſt draw the Line A B, repreſenting the 40*th* Parallel to the Equator, which divide into twelve equal Parts, for the 12 Degrees of Longitude, which the Chart is to contain. This being done, take a Sector or Scale, one hundred Parts whereof is equal to each of theſe Degrees of Longitude, and at the Points A and B raiſe two Perpendiculars to A B, which will repreſent two

parallel

parallel Meridians, and must be divided by the continual Addition of Secants As, for the Distance from 40 deg to 41 deg of Latitude, take 131½ equal Parts from your Scale, which is the Secant of 40 deg 30 min For the Distance from 41 deg to 42 deg take 133½ equal Parts from your Scale, which is the Secant of 41 deg 30 min For the Distance from 42 deg to 43 deg take 136, which is the Secant of 42 deg 30 min and so on to the last Degree of your Chart, which will be 154 equal Parts, viz. the Secant of 49 deg 30 min and will give the Distance from 49 deg of Latitude to 50 deg and by this means the Degrees of Latitude will be augmented in the same Proportion as the Degrees of Longitude on the Globe do really decrease

Having divided the Meridians, you may place the Card upon the Chart, for doing of which, chuse a convenient Place towards the middle thereof, as the Point R, about which, as a Center, describe a Circle so big that its Circumference may be divided into 32 equal Parts, for the 32 Points of the Compass Then having drawn a Line towards the Top of the Chart, parallel to the two divided Meridians, this will be the North Rhumb, and upon it a *Flower-de-luce* must be put, that thereby all the other Rhumbs or Points may be known, the principal of which ought to be distinguished from the others by broader Lines

After this, all the Towns, Ports, Islands, Coasts, Sands, Rocks, &c which form the Chart, must be laid down upon the same, according to their true Latitudes and Longitudes And if the Chart be large, there may several Cards be placed thereon, always with their North and South Lines parallel between themselves

The Use of Mercator's Charts

The chief Use of a Sea-Chart, is to find the Point of Departure therein, the Point arrived at, the Course, the Distance sailed, the Longitude and the Latitude, as we shall now explain by some Examples

Example I Suppose a Ship is to sail from the Island de Ouessant, in 48 deg 30 min of North Latitude, and 13 deg. 30 min of Longitude, to Cape *Finister* in *Galicia*, which is in 43 deg of Latitude, and 8 deg of Longitude Now the Point of the Compass the Ship must keep to, as also the Distance between the said two Places is required In order to do this, you must imagine a Line drawn from the Island de Ouessant to Cape *Finister*, and with a Pair of Compasses examine what Point on the Chart that Line is parallel to, and this Point, which is South-West, one-fourth South, is that which the Ship must sail on

But to find the Distance of the two Places, take between your Compasses the Extent of five Degrees on the Meridian against the beforenamed Course, that is, from the 43d deg to the 48th, and this will be a Scale of 100 Leagues This being done, set one Foot of your Compasses thus opened upon the Island de Ouessant, and the other Foot upon the occult Line tending to Cape *Finister*, making a little Mark thereon, and this Extent of the Compasses will give 100 Leagues of Distance Then take the Distance from the aforesaid Mark to Cape *Finister* between your Compasses, and placing one Foot upon the 43d deg of the Meridian, and the other Foot will fall upon 44 deg 45 min which amounts to 35 Leagues, and consequently the whole Distance between Cape *Finister* and the Island de Ouessant is 135 Leagues

Example II A Ship sailing from the Island de Ouessant South-West, one-fourth South, towards Cape *Finister*, and the Master-Pilot having examined the Force of the Wind, and the Number of Sails spread, and knowing by experience the swiftness of his Ship, has estimated her Way to have been 50 Leagues in 20 Hours Now to find the Point upon the Chart wherein the Ship is, he must take the Extent of 2½ Degrees, equivalent to 50 Leagues, between his Compasses, upon the Meridian, from the 46th deg to the 48½ deg This being done, if one Foot of the Compasses thus opened be set upon the Place of Departure, the other Foot will fall upon the Point T, the Place wherein the Ship is, on the Line of the Ship's Way But if the Longitude and Latitude of the Point T, or Place wherein the Ship is, be sought, he must place one Foot of the Compasses upon the Point T, and the other upon the nearest Parallel, and then conduct the Compasses thus opened perpendicularly along the Parallel to the Meridian and the Degree thereof whereat the Point of the Compasses comes to, will be the Latitude of the Point T And to find the Longitude of this Point, he must set one Foot of the Compasses therein, and the other upon the nearest Meridian Then if this Foot be slid along the Meridian (so that a Line joining the two Points be always parallel to itself) to the divided Parallel, he will have, upon that Parallel, the Longitude of the Point T

Because Meridians and Parallels are not drawn a-cross the Chart, to the end that the Rhumb-Lines may not be confused, therefore you may use a Ruler, which will produce the same Effect

Example III The Course being given, and the Latitude by Observation, to find the Distance sailed, and to prick down the Place of the Ship upon the Chart Suppose a Ship departed from the Island de Ouessant is arrived to a Place whose Latitude, by Observation, is found to be 46 Degrees, take, between your Compasses, the Distance from the 46th Degree of the Meridian to the 48½, which is the Latitude of the Place of Departure, over which 48½ Degree and the Island de Ouessant having laid a Ruler, slide one Foot of

the

the Compasses thus opened along the Side of this Ruler, till the other Foot interfects the Line of the Ship's Way, then the Point of Interfection S will be that whereat the Ship was at the Time of Obfervation   Now to find the Diftance failed, you muft extend the Compaffes from this Point S to the Place of Departure, and lay off this Extent upon the Meridian, which will reach from the 46*th* Degree to the 49*th*, and confequently the Diftance failed will be 60 Leagues, allowing 20 Leagues to a Degree

Example IV   The Latitude and Longitude of a Place being given, to find that Place in the Chart   Having placed one Foot of a Sea-Chart Compafs upon the known Degree of Latitude, and the other upon the nigheft Parallel, you muft place with your other Hand one Foot of another Pair of Compaffes upon the known Degree of Longitude on the Meridian, and the other Foot upon the neareft Meridian, and then flide both thefe Pair of Compaffes until their two Points meet each other · for then the Point of Concourfe will be that fought   This Operation is very much ufed by Seamen, for the Point where they are, being firft found by Calculation, or the Sinecal Quadrant, they can by this means prick down the Place of the Ship upon the Chart, and fo it will be eafy for them to find what Courfe the Ship muft fteer to continue on her Voyage.

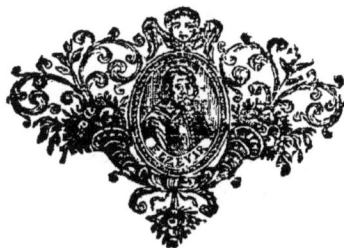

B O O K

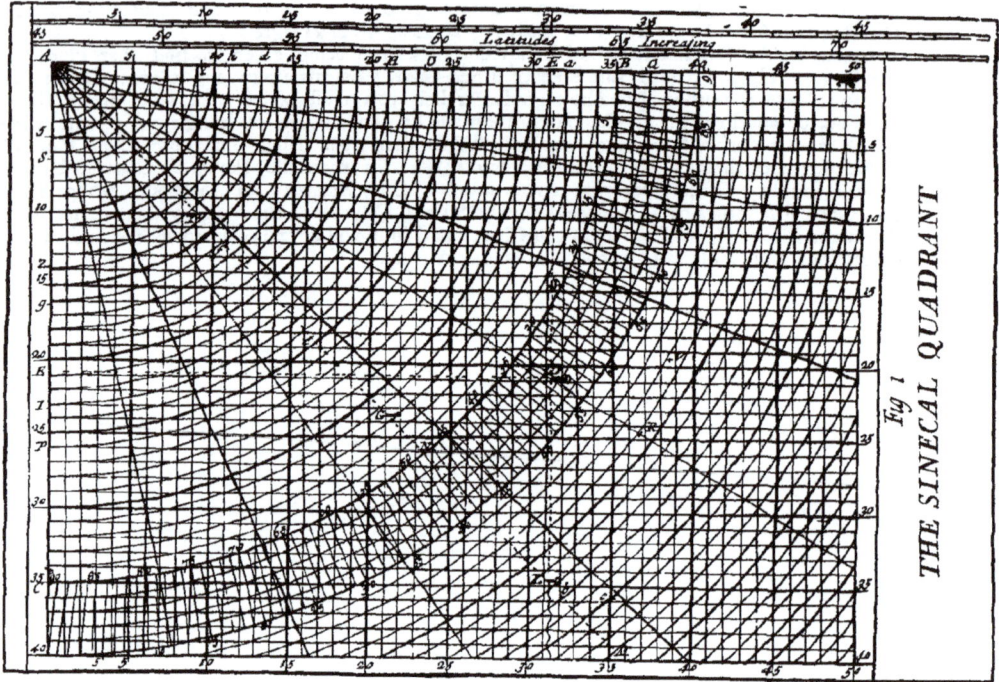

THE SINECAL QUADRANT

Fig 1

Latitudes Increasing

Plate XXI

fronting page 210

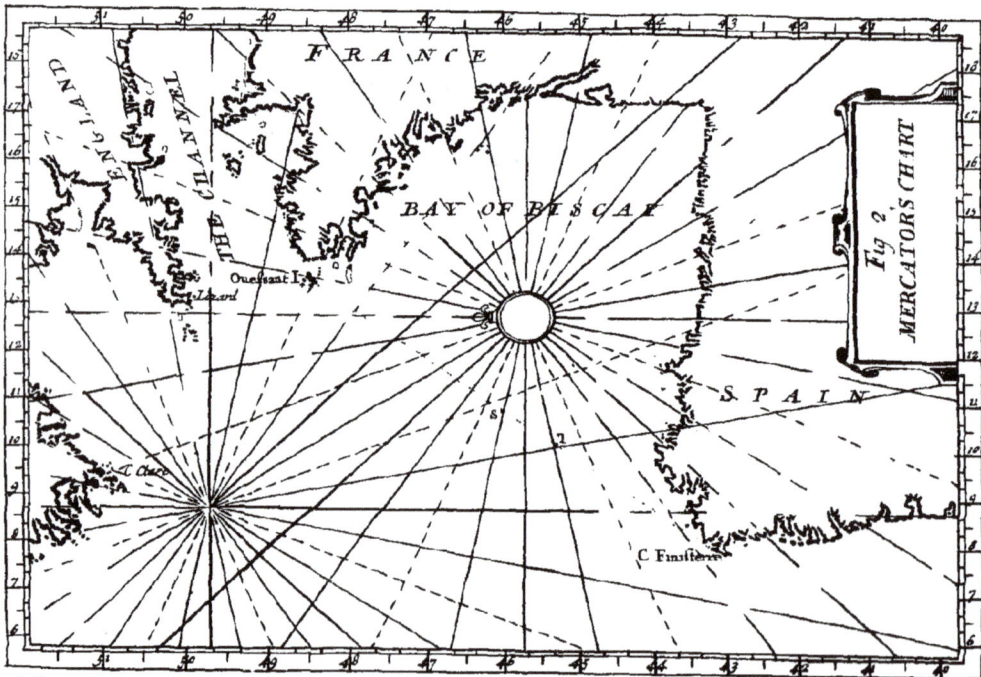

FRANCE

THE CHANNEL

ENGLAND

Oueşsant I.

BAY OF BISCAY

MERCATORS CHART

Fig 2

SPAIN

C. Clear

C. Finiſterre

I Senex ſculp.

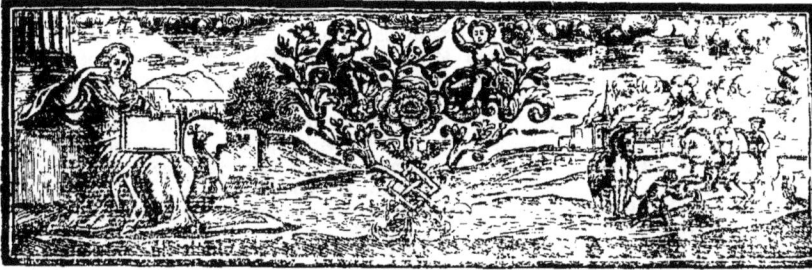

BOOK VIII.

Of the Construction and Uses of Sun-Dials.

Remarks and Definitions appertaining to Dialling.

UN-Dials take their Name from the principal Circles of the Sphere to which they are parallel as, a Horizontal-Dial is one parallel to the Horizon, an Equinoctial-Dial one parallel to the Equinoctial, a Vertical-Dial one that is parallel to a Vertical Circle, and so of others

There are two forts of Styles placed on the Surfaces of Dials, one is called a Right Style, which is a pointed Iron-Rod, that shews the Hour or Part on a Dial by the Shadow of its Extremity, and the other is called an oblique or inclined Style, or else the Axis, which shews the Time of Day upon a Dial by the Shadow of the whole Length thereof

The Extremity of the right Style of any Dial, represents the Center of the World and Equator, and the Plane of a Dial is suppofed to be as far distant from the Center of the Earth, as is the Length of the right Style For because the Sun's Distance from the Center of the Earth is fo great, and the Distance of any Point in the Earth's Superficies from the Center is fo fmall, compared with the Sun's Distance, therefore any Point on the Earth's Surface may without any fenfible Error be taken for its Center and fo the Extremity of the Style of any Dial may be taken for the Center of the Earth, and a Line parallel to the Axis of the World, which paffes thro the Extremity of the Style, may be confidered as the Axis of the World

The Hour-Lines, which are drawn upon Dial-Planes, are the Interfections of the faid Planes made by the Hour-Circles of the Sphere

The Center of a Dial, is the Interfection of its Surface with the Axis of the Dial paffing thro the Extremity of the Style parallel to the Axis of the World, and in this Center all the Hour-Lines meet each other

All Dial Planes may have Centers, except Eaft, Weft, and Polar ones, for on thefe the Hour-Lines are all parallel between themfelves

The Vertical Line of a Dial-Plane, is a Perpendicular drawn from the Extremity of the Style to the Foot thereof, but the Vertical Line of the Place wherein the Dial is, is a right Line perpendicular to the Horizon drawn thro the Extremity of the Style

Dials have likewife two Meridians, one of which is the fubftylar Line or proper Meridian of the Dial-Plane, becaufe its Circle paffes thro the Vertical Line of the Dial-Plane; and the other, which is the Meridian of the Place, hath its Meridian Circle paffing thro the Vertical Line of the Place

When a Dial declines neither to the Eaft or Weft, the fubftylar Line, or Meridian of the Plane, coincides with the Meridian of the Place or Hour-Line of 12, let the Surface of the Dial be Vertical, Horizontal, or even inclined upwards or downwards

The Horizontal Line of a Dial-Plane, is the common Section of the faid Plane, and a horizontal or level Line paffing thro the Extremity of the Stile, and the Equinoctial Line is the common Section of the Dial-Plane and Equinoctial Circle and this Line is always perpendicular to the fubftylar Line, and confequently if the Pofition of the fubftylar Line be known, and a Point of the Equinoctial Line be given, we may likewife have the Pofition of the Equinoctial Line and contrariwife, if the Equinoctial Line be given, we may have the

fubftylar

ſubſtylar Line, which is perpendicular thereto. *Note*, This ſubſtylar Line muſt paſs thro the Foot of the Style and the Center of the Dial.

The Hour-Line of ſix always paſſes thro the Interſection of the Horizontal and Equinoctial Lines in declining Dials, and ſo the ſaid Point of Interſection is one Point of the Hour-Line of ſix. *Note*, The Point wherein the Subſtyle and Meridian Lines meet, is the Center of the Dial.

When a Dial is to be drawn upon a Plane, you muſt firſt find the Poſition of the ſaid Plane, or of the Wall it is to be ſet up againſt, with regard to the Sun and the principal Circles of the Sphere. And this may be done, in obſerving ſeveral Times the ſame Day, at every 3 or 4 Hours interval, where the Shadow of the Extremity of a Style falls upon the Dial-Plane for by this means the Poſition of the Dial-Plane may be determined, and afterwards all the Hour-Lines, &c may be drawn thereon in the manner we ſhall hereafter ſhew. *Note*, The Exactneſs of a Dial very much depends upon theſe Points.

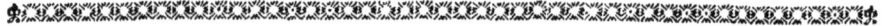

CHAP. I.

Of Regular and Irregular Dials, *drawn upon Planes and Bodies of different Figures.*

Plate 22
Fig 1

THIS Inſtrument repreſents a hollow Body, having 14 Planes, upon each of which a Dial may be drawn

The upper Plane A, is parallel to the Horizon, and ſo upon this a Horizontal-Dial is drawn, as well as upon the under Plane E, whereon the Sun ſhines but a very little   The Plane B is parallel to the Axis of the World, and makes an Angle of 49 Degrees with the Horizon of *Paris*, for the Latitude of which, all the Dials are ſuppoſed to be drawn. Now upon this Plane is drawn an upper Polar Dial, and upon the Plane F, which is oppoſite thereto, is drawn an under Polar Dial   The Plane C is parallel to the Prime Vertical, and ſince it faces the South, there is drawn thereon a South Vertical Dial   And upon the oppoſite Plane to this, which is towards G, and faces directly to the North, is drawn a Vertical North Dial, which cannot be repreſented in this Figure

The Plane H, which is parallel to the Equinoctial, and ſo makes an Angle with the Horizon of 41 deg *viz* the Complement of the Latitude of *Paris*, hath an upper Equinoctial Dial drawn upon it, and upon the oppoſite Plane D, is drawn an under Equinoctial Dial The Plane K is parallel to the Plane of the Meridian, and becauſe it directly faces the Weſt, a Meridional Weſt Dial is drawn thereon, and upon the oppoſite Plane to this is drawn a Meridional Eaſt Dial   The Plane I makes an Angle of 45 deg with the Meridian; and therefore there is drawn upon it a vertical Decliner, declining Southweſtwardly 45 deg and upon the oppoſite Plane to this is drawn a North-Eaſt Decliner of 45 deg   Finally, The Plane L declines North-Weſt 45 deg and its Oppoſite 45 deg South-Eaſt, and ſo upon theſe two Planes are drawn North-Weſt and South-Eaſt Decliners

The firſt Nine of the abovementioned Dials, are called Regular ones, and the Four others, which decline, are called Irregular Dials

The Axes of all theſe Dials are parallel to each other, and to the Axis of the World. We ſhall hereafter give the Conſtruction of all theſe Dials, as well as of thoſe on the following Inſtrument, of which we are going to ſpeak.

The Conſtruction of Dials drawn upon a Dodecahedron

Fig. 2.

This Figure is one of the five Regular Bodies, of which we have ſpoken in the firſt Book   This Body is called a Dodecahedron, and is terminated by 12 equal Pentagons, upon every of which may be drawn a Dial, except on the undermoſt

The Plane A being Horizontal, hath a Horizontal-Dial drawn thereon, whoſe Hour-Line of 12 biſects one of the Angles of the Pentagon   Upon the Plane B, which faces the South, is drawn a direct South-Dial, inclining towards the Zenith, or upwards 63 deg 26 min. The Center of this Dial is upwards, and the ſubſtylar Line is the Hour-Line of 12. The oppoſite Plane to this, is a North vertical one, inclining downwards or towards the Nadir 63 deg. 26 min. and ſo there is drawn thereon a North inclining Dial, whoſe Center is downwards

The Dial C, is a South-Eaſt inclining Recliner, whoſe Declination is 36 deg and Inclination to the Zenith 63 deg 26 min and its Center is downwards   The Dial D is a North-Eaſt Decliner of 72 deg. inclining towards the Nadir 63 deg. 26 min. the Center being upwards, and its oppoſite is a South-Weſt Decliner of 72 min inclining towards the Zenith 63 deg 26 min the Center being downwards.

The

The Dial E is a North-East Decliner of 36 deg and inclines towards the Zenith 63 deg 26 min the Center being downwards The opposite Dial to this, is a South-West Decliner of 36 deg and inclines towards the Nadir 63 deg 26 min its Center being upwards Finally, the Dial F is a South-East Decliner of 72 deg inclining towards the Zenith 63 deg 26 min the Center being downwards, and its opposite is a North-West Decliner of 72 deg inclining towards the Nadir 63 deg 26 min the Center thereof being upwards

All these Dials are furnished with their Axes, which are parallel between themselves, and to the Axis of the World

Now if one of these Bodies of Dials be set upon a Pedestal, in a Place well exposed to the Sun, and then be set right by means of a Compass or Meridian Line, drawn in the manner we shall hereafter shew, all the Dials that the Sun shines upon will shew the same Hour or Part at the same time by the Shadows of the Styles

But if a Dodecahedron of Dials be to be placed upon a Pedestal fixed in a Garden, it ought to be made of solid Matter, as Stone or good Wood, well painted to preserve it from Rain, &c therefore it will be here necessary to shew how to cut out a Dodecahedron

Take a Stone cut out into a perfect Cube, and divide each of the four Sides of its Faces Fig. 3. into two equal Parts by two Diameters A C, B D And at the Points A and C, make the Angles E A F, and H C G, each 116 deg 34 min that is, make Angles at the Points A and C, on each side the Diameter A C, of 58 deg 17 min each because all the Surfaces of the Dodecahedron make Angles of 116 deg 34 min with each other, therefore two Faces thereof being horizontally placed, all the others will incline 63 deg 26 min the Complement of 116 deg 34 min to 180 deg Now the Space between F and G, or E H, will be the Length of each side of the Pentagons, half of which, viz B F, must be taken and laid off both ways from the Point I to the Points Q and X And this must be done upon the Diameters crossing each other on all the other Faces of the Cube Afterwards the Stone must be cut away along the Diameters to the Extremities of the sides of the Pentagons for example, you must cut away the Stone down or all along the Diameter K M, in a Right Line to the Point Q in the first Surface of the Cube, as likewise all along the Diameter L N strait forwards to the Point S, and again all along the Diameter B D directly forward to the Point T And proceeding in this manner with the other Faces of the Cube, you may compleat your Dodecahedron But it will be very proper for a Person that has a mind to cut out one of these Bodies, to have a Pasteboard one before him, thereby to help his Imagination, that so he may know better what Angles and Sides to cut away

Cylinders may be cut likewise into Dodecahedrons, but let the Method above given suffice

We make also very curious Dials on the Faces of small brass Dodecahedrons

The Construction of an Horizontal Dial

The fourth Figure is an Horizontal Dial To make which, first draw the two Lines A B, Fig. 4. C D, cutting each other at Right Angles in the Point E, which will be the Center of the Dial, the Line A B the Meridian or Hour-Line of 12, and the Line C D the Hour-Line of 6 This being done, make the Angle B E F, 49 deg equal to the Elevation of the Pole at *Paris* (the Elevation of the Pole at *Paris* is but 48 deg 51 min but we neglect the nine Minutes, as being but of small Consequence in the Construction of Dials) and the Line E F will represent the Axis of the World In this the Point G must be chosen at pleasure, representing the Center of the Earth, and G H must be drawn at Right Angles to E F, cutting the Meridian or Hour-Line of 12 in the Point H This Line G H represents the Radius of the Equinoctial Now take H G between your Compasses, which lay off from H to B on the Meridian Line, and draw the Right Line L H K perpendicular to the Meridian, which will represent the common Section of the Equinoctial, and the Plane of the Dial then about the Point B, as a Center, describe the Quadrant M H, which divide into six equal Arcs, each of which will be 15 deg and draw the dotted Lines B 5, B 4, B 3, B 2, B 1 These will divide the Line L H into the Points 1, 2, 3, 4, 5, thro which Points, if Lines be drawn from the Center E of the Dial, you will have the Hour-Lines of 1, 2, 3, 4, and 5, on one side the Meridian, and because the Hour Lines equally distant on both sides from the Meridian make equal Angles with the Meridian, therefore if the Divisions 1, 2, 3, 4, 5, on one side the Meridian, be laid off from H towards K on the other side, and thro the Points where they terminate are drawn Lines from the Center F, these will be the Hour-Lines of 11, 10, 9, 8, 7 And if the Hour-Lines of 7 and 8 in the Morning are continued out beyond the Center, they will give the Hour-Lines of 7 and 8 in the Evening, and likewise the Hour-Lines of 4 and 5 in the Afternoon continued out in the same manner will give those of 4 and 5 in the Morning Note, Instead of drawing the Quadrant M H, we might, for greater facility, have only drawn an Arc greater than 60 deg for then if an Arc of 60 deg had been taken upon it from the Point H, by means of its Chord, which is equal to Radius, and the said Arc had been divided in four equal Arcs, each of 15 deg and another Arc of 15 deg had been added to that of 60 deg for the Hour of 5, we might have drawn the Lines B 1, B 2, B 3, &c as we have already done

Now

Now to draw the Half-hours, you must bisect each of the Arcs of 15 deg on the Quadrant M H, in order to have Arcs of 7 deg. 30 min and for the Quarters, each of these last Arcs must be again bisected, and thro each Point of Division occult Lines must be drawn from the Center B, cutting the Equinoctial Line K L Then if the Edge of a Ruler be laid thro these Points of Concourse and the Center E of the Dial, the Halfs and Quarters of Hours may be drawn

The Hour-Lines being drawn upon your Dial, you may give it what Figure you please, as a Parallelogram, regular Pentagon, &c

This Dial being fixed upon a very level Plane, that is, set parallel to the Horizon, exposed to the Sun, and its Hour-Line of 12 placed exactly North and South, as also the Style or Axis E H F being raised perpendicularly upon the Hour-Line of 12, so as F F be parallel to the Axis of the World · I say, if these things be so ordered, the Shadow of the Axis or Style will shew the Hour of the Day from Sun-rising to Sun-setting

The Construction of a Non-declining Vertical Dial

Fig 5

This Dial is parallel to the Prime Vertical, which cuts the Meridian at Right Angles, and passes thro the East and West Points of the Horizon. The Manner of drawing it is thus First draw the Lines E B and C D at Right Angles, the first of which shall be the Hour-Line of 12, and the other the Hour-Line of 6, then make the Angle B E F at the Point E, the Center of the Dial, equal to the Complement of the Elevation of the Pole, which at *Paris* is 41 deg and raise the Line I G perpendicularly on the Meridian, this will be the right Style, and the Point I is the Foot thereof, and G the Extremity, which, as above said, may be taken for the Center of the Earth and this Line both ways produced, will be the Horizontal-Line

From the Point G, in the Right Line E G F, which represents the Axis of the World, raise the Line G H at Right Angles thereto, cutting the Meridian in B. This Line G H shall represent the Radius of the Equinoctial, and the Line L H K, drawn thro the Point H, cutting the Meridian at Right Angles, represents the common Section of the Equinoctial and the Plane of the Dial Now make H B equal to H G, and about the Point B, as a Center, describe the Quadrant of a Circle M H, which divide into 6 equal Arcs, each of which will be 15 deg by dotted Lines, dividing the Line L K into unequal Parts, which shall be the Tangents of the said Arcs Finally, If thro those Points of Division and the Center E, you draw Lines, they will be the Hour-Lines on one side of the Meridian, and for drawing the Hour-Lines on the other side the Meridian, as also the Halves and Quarters of Hours, you must do as is shewn in the Horizontal-Dial

This Dial is set up against a Wall, or on a very upright Plane, directly facing the South, for which reason it is called a Meridional Vertical Dial: its Meridional or Hour-Line of 12 must be perfectly upright, and its Horizontal-Line level The Center thereof is upwards, and its Axis points towards the under Pole The opposite Dial to this, is a Vertical North one, having the Center downwards, and the Extremity of its Axis pointing to the upper Pole of the World The Construction of this latter Dial is the same as that of the other, the Hour-Lines and the Axis making the same Angles with the Meridian, as they do on that But the Sun shines but a small time upon this Dial, and this only in the Summer-time, viz in the Morning from his rising till he has passed the Prime Vertical, and in the Evening from the time he has again passed the Prime Vertical till his setting When the Sun describes the Summer Tropick, he rises at *Paris*, at 4 in the Morning, and comes to the Prime Vertical between 7 and 8 in the Morning, and in the Afternoon he repasses the Prime Vertical between 4 and 5, and sets at 8 Therefore we need only draw the Hour-Lines upon this Dial from 4 in the Morning to 8, and from 4 in the Afternoon to 8, at which time the Sun shines upon the Meridional Vertical Dial, but from about 8 in the Morning to about 4 in the Afternoon But when the Sun by his annual Motion is again come back to the Equinoctial, he will not shine at all upon the Vertical North Dial till after he has crossed the Equinoctial again ; and all this time he will shine upon the Meridional Vertical Dial from his rising to his setting

The Construction of a Polar Dial.

Fig. 6.

The *6th* Figure represents an upper Polar Dial, which is one that inclines upwards, but does not decline · for it is parallel to the Axis of the World, and the Hour-Circle of 6, which cuts the Meridian at Right Angles And for this reason the Hour of 6 in the Morning or Evening can never be shewn by this Dial, for the Shadow of the Style being then parallel to the Plane of the Dial, cannot be cast upon it This Dial likewise hath no Center, and the Hour-Lines are all parallel between themselves, and to the Axis of the World The Plane therefore being parallel to the Horizon of a right Sphere, passes thro the two Poles of the World, from whence comes the Name of a Polar Dial

The Manner of drawing this Dial is thus First draw the Line A B representing the Equinoctial, and I D at Right Angles thereto, for the Meridian or Hour-Line of 12 Then assume the Length of the Style at pleasure, according to the bigness of the Plane the Dial is to be drawn on, let this be C D, about the Extremity of which D describe a Quadrant, which

which divide into six equal Arcs, (or only describe an Arc of 60 Degrees, which divide into four Parts, of 15 Degrees each, for the four first Hours after Noon, and then add an Arc of 15 Degrees for the Hour of 5) This being done, draw dotted Lines from the Point D, thro the Divisions of the Circumference of the said Arc, to the Line A B, and then if Lines are drawn into the Points wherein the dotted Lines cut the Line A B, parallel to the Meridian, these Lines will be the Hour-Lines on one side the Meridian and if there be as many Parallels drawn on the other side of the Meridian, at the same Distances therefrom as the respective parallel Hour-Lines are on the other side, these will be the Hour-Lines on the other side of the Meridian The Style of this Dial must be equal in Length to C F, the Distance from the Hour-Line of 3 to the Hour-Line of 12, and may be made in figure of a Right-angled Parallelogram, as is that marked above the Letter K in the Figure of the Dial This Style is set upon the Hour-Line of 12, which for this reason is called the Sub-stylar Line

If a single Rod only be used for a Style, as that which is in the Point C of the Meridian, then the Hour will be shewn upon this Dial by the Shadow of the Extremity of the Style: whereas when a Parallelogram is used, we have the Hour shewn by the Shadow of one of its Sides, that is, by a right Line

An upper Polar Dial may shew the Hour from seven in the Morning to five in the Afternoon, and an under Polar one is useless, unless in the Summer, where the Hour is shewn thereby, from the Sun's rising to five in the Morning, and from seven in the Evening till his setting : and so for the Elevation of the Pole of *Paris*, the Hours of four and five in the Morning, and seven and eight in the Afternoon, are only set down upon this Dial, and these may be drawn as those on the upper Polar Dial, for the Distances of the Hour-Lines of four and five in the Afternoon from the Substyle, on the upper Polar Dial, are equal to the Distances of the Hour-Lines of four and five in the Morning from the Subftyle on the under Polar Dial Understand the same for the Hours of seven and eight in the Afternoon, and therefore there is no need of drawing the figure of this Dial. *Note*, The Distance of the Hour-Lines on these Dials depend upon the Breadth of the Style, or the Distance of the Point D from the Equinoctial Line

To set up this Dial at *Paris*, the Plane thereof must make an Angle of 49 deg with the Horizon, the upper one facing the Sky directly South, that so the Axis thereof may be parallel to that of the World, and the opposite Dial to this, *viz* the under Polar one faces downwards, the Morning Hours being towards the West, and the Afternoon ones towards the East, on both the upper and under ones

Now if the Horizontal Line is to be drawn upon this Dial, describe the Arc G H, about the Point F, the Extremity of the Style, equal to the Elevation of the Pole, *viz* 49 deg for the Latitude of *Paris*, and draw the Right Line F H, cutting the Meridian in the Point I, thro which draw the Horizontal Line L K, at Right Angles Now by means of this Line, we may know whether the Dial be well placed, and have its convenient Inclination, for if the Dial be inclined rightly, a Plane laid along the Horizontal Line, and supported by the Edge of the Style, will be level or parallel to the Horizon

A Polar Dial in a right Sphere is parallel to the Horizon, and in a parallel Sphere it is vertical or upright

The Construction of an Equinoctial Dial

An upper Equinoctial Dial shews the Hour but only six Months in the Year, *viz* from Fig 7 the Vernal Equinox to the Autumnal one, and the opposite Dial to this, which is an under Equinoctial one, shews the Hour during the other six Months of the Year, *viz* from the Autumnal Equinox to the Vernal one

The Plane of this Dial is parallel to the Equinoctial Circle, and is cut at Right Angles through the Center thereof by the Axis of the World.

The Construction of this Dial is thus · Draw two Right Lines A H, and E D, crossing each other at Right Angles, the first of which shall be the Hour-Line of 12, and the other the Hour-Line of 6, then about the Point A of Intersection describe a Circle, each quarter of which divide into six equal Parts, thro which, if strait Lines be drawn from the Center A, these Lines will be the Hour-Lines, because they each make equal Angles of 15 deg. and if each of these Angles be halved and quartered, the halves and quarters of Hours will be had

The Construction of an under Equinoctial Dial is the same as of an upper one, and in a parallel Sphere, *viz* where the Pole is in the Zenith, there is but one Equinoctial Dial, which will likewise be *there* an Horizontal one And in a right Sphere, *viz* where the two Poles are in the Horizon, these Dials are non-declining Vertical ones, and are set up against Walls, one of which faces the North Pole, and the other the South Pole, the Sun shining upon each six Months in the Year But in an oblique Sphere, as that which we inhabit, these Dials are inclined to the Horizon, and make an Angle therewith equal to the Complement of the Latitude, *viz* at *Paris*, an Angle of 41 deg

The Axis of an Equinoctial Dial is a strait Iron Rod going thro the Center of the Dial perpendicular to the Plane thereof, and parallel to the Axis of the World. The Length of
this

this Rod may be at pleasure, when it hath no other Use but shewing the Hour by the Shadow thereof, but when the Length of the Days, and the Sun's Place are to be shewn thereby, the said Rod must have a determinate Length, as we shall shew hereafter

The Construction of East and West Dials

Fig. 8

These Dials are parallel to the Plane of the Meridian, one of which directly faces the East, and the other the West. The 8th Figure is a West Dial, having the Hour-Lines parallel to each other, and to the Axis of the World, as in a Polar Dial, and their Construction is nearly the same as of the Hour-Lines on a Polar Dial.

This Dial is made thus. First draw the right Line A B, representing the Horizontal Line, and about the Point A, assume the Arc B C of a Radius at pleasure in this Line, equal to the Complement of the Latitude, or Height of the Equator above the Horizon, which at *Paris* is 41 deg. Then draw the Line C D, produced, as is necessary, from the Point C, and this Line shall represent the common Section of the Equinoctial and Plane of the Dial; after this, draw E D from the Point D, parallel to the Equinoctial Line, and this Line E D will be the Place of the Substyle, that is, the Line on which the Style must be placed, as likewise the Hour-Line of six. Now to draw the other Hour-Lines, assume the Point E at pleasure on the substylar Line, about which, as a Center, describe an Arc of 60 deg which divide into four equal Parts for 15 deg each, beginning from the substylar Line. After this, lay off as many Arcs of 15 deg as is necessary upon the said Arc both ways continued, and draw dotted Lines from the Center E thro all the Divisions of the Arc to the Equinoctial Line; then if right Lines be drawn thro the Points in the Equinoctial Line, made by the dotted Lines, parallel to the Hour-Line of 6, and perpendicular to the Equinoctial Line, these Lines will be the Hour-Lines. *Note,* This Dial shews the Time of Day after Noon to the setting of the Sun, and since the Sun sets (at *Paris*) at eight a-Clock in the Summer, we have pricked down the Hour-Lines from one to eight in this Dial, as appears per Figure.

The Construction of an East Dial is the same as of this, and there are pricked down the Hour-Lines upon it from the Sun's rising in Summer, viz. from four in the Morning to eleven. The reason that the Hour-Line of twelve cannot be drawn upon these Dials, is, because when the Sun is in the Meridian, his Rays are parallel to their Planes.

If a West Dial be drawn upon a Sheet of Paper, and then the said Paper is rendered Transparent by oiling, you will perceive thro the backside of the Paper an East Dial drawn entirely, only the Figures of the Hours must be altered, that is, you must put 11 in the place of 1, 10 in the place of 2, and so of others.

The Style of these Dials is a Brass or Iron Rod, in Length equal to F D, which is likewise equal to the Distance of the Hour of 3 from the Hour of 6. This Style is set upright in the Point D, and shews the Hour by the Shadow of its Extremity. These Dials, which may have likewise a Style in figure of a Parallelogram, as we have mentioned in speaking of Polar Dials, are set upright against Walls or Planes, perpendicular to the Horizon, and parallel to the Meridian, one of which directly faces the East, and the other the West, in such manner, that the Horizontal Line be perfectly level.

The Construction of Vertical Declining Dials

A Vertical Dial is one that is made upon a Vertical Plane, that is, a Plane perpendicular to the Horizon, as a very upright Wall.

Among the nine Regular Dials of which we have spoken, there are four of them Vertical ones, which do not decline at all, since they directly face the four Cardinal Parts of the World. It now remains that we here speak of Irregular Dials, some of which are vertical Decliners, others undeclining Decliners, and finally, others declining Incliners. Vertical Decliners are of four Kinds; for some decline South-eastwardly, the opposite ones to these, North-westwardly, others decline South-westwardly, and the opposite ones to these, North-eastwardly.

Now among the Irregular Dials, the vertical Decliners are most in use, because they are made upon or set up against Walls, (which commonly are built upright) or else upon Bodies whose Planes are upright, but before these Dials can be made, the Declinations of the Walls or Planes, on which they are to be made or set up against, must first be known or found exactly; and this may be done by some one of the Methods hereafter mentioned.

Fig. 9

Now suppose we know that a Plane (as that marked I of Figure 1) or upright Wall, declines 45 deg South-westwardly at *Paris*, or thereabouts, where the Pole is elevated 49 deg above the Horizon. It is required to draw a Dial for this Declination.

First, draw the Lines A B, C D, crossing each other at Right Angles in the Point E, the former of which shall be the Hour-Line of 12, and the other the Horizontal Line. About the Point E, as a Center, draw the Arc F N of 45 deg because the Plane's Declination is such, and since it is South-westwardly, the said Arc must be drawn on the Right-side of the Meridian, but if the Declination had been South-eastwardly, that Arc must have been

drawn

drawn on the Left-fide the Meridian   This being done, raife the Perpendicular F H from the Point F to the Horizontal Line, that fo we may have one Point of the Style therein, *viz* the Foot of the Style   Then take the Diftance E F between your Compaffes, and lay it off upon the Horizontal Line from E to O, and about the Point O, as a Center, defcribe the Arc E G equal to the Height of the Pole, *viz* in this Cafe 49 deg and draw the dotted Line O A to the Hour-Line of 12, then A will be the Center of the Dial thro which the Subftyle A H muft be drawn of an indeterminate Length   *Note*, This Subftyle is one of the principal Lines, by means of which a Dial of this kind is drawn, and upon which the whole exactnefs thereof almoft depends

Upon the Point H raife the right Line H I equal to H F, perpendicular to the Subftyle A H, and draw the right Line A I, prolonged, for the Axis of the Dial   Then let fall the Perpendicular K I to the Axis, cutting the fubftylar Line in K, and make K L equal to K I, and draw a right Line both ways thro the Point K, perpendicular to the Subftyle A K, this will reprefent the Equinoctial Line, and cuts the Horizontal Line in a Point thro which the Hour-Line of 6 muft pafs   Thus having already the Hour-Lines of 12 and 6, if the Operations hitherto performed have been done right, two dotted Lines L 6, and L N being drawn, will be at Right Angles to each other   Again, about the faid Point L, as a Center, defcribe the Quadrant of a Circle between the faid dotted Lines, whofe Circumference divide into 6 equal Arcs, of 15 Degrees each, and draw occult Lines thro the Points of Divifion to cut the Equinoctial Line, but to have the Morning Hour-Lines, and thofe after 6, prolong the Arc of the Quadrant both ways, and lay off as many Arcs of 15 Degrees upon it, as is neceffary, that fo occult Lines may be drawn from the Center L to cut the Equinoctial Line   Then if Lines are drawn from the Center A thro all the Points wherein the occult Lines cut the Equinoctial Line, thefe Lines thus drawn will be the Hour-Lines   *Note*, There muft be but 12 Hour Lines drawn upon any vertical declining Plane, for the Sun will fhine on any one of them but 12 Hours

Points in the Horizontal Line D C thro which the Hour-Lines muft pafs, may be found otherwife, by applying the Center of a Horizontal Dial to the Point F, in fuch manner, that the Meridian Line thereof coincides with the Line F E, and its Hour-Line of 6, with the Line F 6 for then the Points where the Hour-Lines of the Horizontal Dial cut the faid Line D C, will be the Points therein thro which the Hour-Lines muft be drawn from the Center A

The Hour-Lines of fix Hours fucceffively being given upon the Plane of any Dial whatfoever, the other Hour-Lines may be drawn after the following manner   Suppofe, in this Example, that the Hour-Lines from 6 to 12 are drawn, now if you have a mind to draw the Hour-Lines of 9, 10 and 11 in the Morning, which may be pricked down upon this Dial, draw a Parallel, as S V, from the Point V, taken at pleafure on the Hour-Line of 12, to the Hour-Line of 6, which fhall cut the Hour-Lines of 1, 2, and 3, in the Afternoon. This being done, the Diftance from V to the Hour-Line of 1 taken on this Parallel, and la'd off on the other fide, will give a Point in the faid Parallel thro which the Hour-Line of 11 muft be drawn ; likewife the Diftance V 2 will give a Point thereon, thro which the Hour-Line of 10 muft be drawn, and the Diftance V 3 will give a Point thro which the Hour-Line of 9 muft pafs   And fo if Lines are drawn from the Center of the Dial A thro the faid Points, they will be the Hour-Lines

In this manner likewife may be found the Points thro which the Hour-Lines of 7 and 8 in the Evening are drawn, in first drawing a Parallel to the Hour-Line of 12, cutting the Hour-Line of 6 in one Point, and meeting the Hour-Lines of 4 and 5 produced, for the Diftance from the Points where the Hour-Lines of 6 and 5 are cut by this Parallel, laid off on the other fide from the Point where the Hour-Line of 6 cuts the Parallel, will give a Point upon it thro which the Hour-Line of 7 muft be drawn   And the Diftance from the Points where the Parallel cuts the Hour-Lines of 6 and 8, laid off on the other fide on that Parallel, will give a Point therein thro which the Hour-Line of 8 muft pafs, and if Lines are drawn from the Center A thro thofe two Points found, they will be the Hour-Lines of 7 and 8 in the Evening   This is a very good way of drawing thofe Hour-Lines that are pretty diftant from the fubftylar Line, becaufe thereby we avoid cutting the Equinoctial very obliquely

The Conftruction of a South-Eaft vertical Decliner is the fame as of that which we have defcribed, excepting only that what was there made on the Right muft here be on the Left, and the Figures for the Morning Hours fet to thofe for the Afternoon. fo that if a South-Weft declining Dial be drawn upon a Sheet of Paper, and afterwards the Paper be oiled, that you may fee thro it, you will fee a South-Eaft Decliner thro the Paper, only the Figures fet to the Hour-Lines muft be altered, as, where the Figure of 1 ftands, you muft fet 11, where the Figure of 2, 10, where the Figure of 3, 9, and fo on   By this means the fubftylar Line, which falls between the Hour-Lines of 3 and 4 Afternoon, in Figure 9, will fall in this Dial between 8 and 9 in the Morning   And if the Plane's Declination had been lefs than 45 deg the Subftyle would have fallen yet nearer to the Meridian . but if, on the contrary, the Declination thereof had been greater, the Subftyle would have fallen more diftant from the Meridian, and pretty near the Hour-Line of 6   But when this

K k k   happens,

happens, the Hour-Lines fall ſo cloſe together near the Subſtyle, that we are obliged to make the Model of a Dial upon a very large Plane, that ſo the Hour-Lines may be very long, and the part of the Dial towards the Center taken away.

After the abovenamed manner, likewiſe may be drawn North-Eaſt and North-Weſt Dials; but theſe have their Centers downwards underneath the Horizontal Line, and properly are no other but South-Eaſt or South-Weſt Decliners inverted, as may be ſeen in Figure 10, which repreſents a North-Weſt Decliner of 45 deg drawn for the Plane L of Figure 1. and the ſubſtylar Line of this Dial muſt be between the Hours of 8 and 9 in the Evening, whence one Decliner only may ſerve for drawing four, if they have an equal Declination, tho to different Coaſts, two of, which will have their Centers upwards, and the other two their Centers downwards.

To draw the Subſtylar Line upon a Plane by means of the Shadow of the Extremity of an Iron-Rod, obſerved twice the ſame Day

Suppoſe the Subſtylar Line is to be found on the Decliner of Figure 9, firſt place obliquely upon the Dial-Plane, a Wire or Iron Rod, ſharp at the end, ſo that the Extremity thereof be perpendicularly over the Point H in the Plane This may be done by means of a Square.

Fig 9.

Now ſince this Figure is a South-Weſt vertical Decliner, therefore the Subſtylar Line thereon muſt be found among the Afternoon Hours, to the Right-hand of the Meridian; and conſequently, let us ſuppoſe the Shadow of the Extremity of the Iron-Rod at the firſt Obſervation to fall on the Point P, then about the Point H, the Foot of the Style, with the Diſtance H.P, deſcribe the circular Arc P R This being done, ſome Hours after the firſt Obſervation the ſame Day, obſerve when the Shadow of the Extremity of the Rod falls a ſecond time upon the aforeſaid Arc, which ſuppoſe in the Point Q then if the Arc P Q be biſected in the Point R, and a Right-line be drawn thro the Points R and H, this Line will be the Subſtyle, which being exactly drawn, and the Height of the Pole above the Horizon of the Place where the Dial is made for, being otherwiſe known, it will not then be difficult to compleat the Dial, for firſt, the Meridian or Hour-Line of 12 is always perpendicular to the Horizon, in vertical Planes, and the Point wherein the Meridian and Subſtylar Line produced meet each other, (as the Point A) will be the Center of the Dial The Horizontal Line is a level Line paſſing thro the Foot of the Style, as D H C

And to draw the Equinoctial Line, you muſt firſt form the Triangular Style A H I on the Subſtyle, whoſe Hypothenuſe A I is the Axis, and Side H I the right Style, then if I K be drawn from the Point I perpendicular to the Axis, meeting the Subſtylar Line in the Point K, and if thro K a Right Line M K N be drawn at Right Angles to the Stylar Line, this Line will be the Equinoctial, and the Point wherein it cuts the Horizontal Line will be always the Point thro which the Hour-Line of 6 muſt paſs Moreover, the Diſtance K L, laid off on the Stylar Line, will give the Point L the Center of the Equinoctial Circle. Now what remains to be done, may be compleated as before explained, and even the whole Dial may be drawn in one's Room, after the Poſitions and Concourſes of the principal Lines are laid off upon a Sheet of Paper, and the Angle which the Subſtylar Line makes with the Meridian or Horizontal Line be taken, for one is the Complement of the other

Now to prove whether the Equinoctial Line be drawn right, make the Angle B A O equal to the Complement of the Elevation of the Pole, viz. 41 deg for the Latitude of *Paris*, draw the Line A O to the Horizon, and make the Angle A O N a Right one, that ſo the Point N may be had in the Meridian or Hour-Line of 12, thro which the Equinoctial Line muſt paſs Thus having ſeveral Ways for finding the principal Points, one of them will ſerve to prove the other

When a Dial Plane declines South-eaſtwardly, the Subſtylar Line will be on the right Side of the Meridian In which Caſe it is proper to take notice, that in finding the Subſtylar Line, as above, to obſerve when the Shadow of the Extremity of the Rod falls upon the Plane, as ſoon as the Sun begins to ſhine thereon, as likewiſe to mind the Time very exactly when the Shadow of the Extremity of the Style comes again to touch the circular Arc; you may operate in this manner ſeveral Days ſucceſſively, in order to ſee whether the Poſition of the Subſtylar Line has been found exactly

When a Plane declines North-Eaſt or North-Weſt, the Shadows of the Extremity of the Iron Rod fall above the Foot of the Style, and ſo the Center of the Dial muſt be downwards Likewiſe the moſt proper Time for making theſe Operations is about 15 Days before or after the Solſtices, for when the Sun is near the Equinoctial, his Declination is too ſenſible, and the Operations leſs exact Neverthelefs the Equinoctial Line may be drawn upon a Plane, when the Sun is in the Equinoctial Points, and by that means a vertical declining Dial conſtructed, by the following Method.

To draw the Equinoctial Line upon a vertical Plane by means of the Shadow of the Extremity of an Iron-Rod.

The moſt ſimple and eaſy Method to draw the Equinoctial Line upon a Wall or Plane, is at the Time when the Sun is in the Equinoctial, (tho this may be done at any other

Time

Time by more complicated Methods) for when the Sun deſcribes the Equinoctial by his diurnal Motion, the Shadows of the Extremity of the Iron-Rod or Style, will all fall upon a Plane in a right Line, which is the common Section of the Equinoctial Circle of the Heavens and the Plane   Therefore if ſeveral Points, pricked down upon a Plane, made by the Shadow of the Extremity of the Rod, on the Day the Sun is in the Equator, be joined, the right Line joining them will be the Equinoctial Line, as the Line M N, in Figure 9   This being done, draw the right Line A H L thro the Foot of the Style at Right Angles to the Equinoctial Line, and this will be the Subſtylar, Line ⋅ Moreover, draw the level Line D H C thro the Foot H of the Style , this will be the Horizontal Line, and if H I be drawn equal to the Height of the right Style, and parallel to the Equinoctial Line and the Points K and L joined , and if A I be drawn at Right Angles to K I, then the Point A will be the Center of the Dial, and the upright Line A B the Meridian or Hour-Line of 12.   The common Section of the Equinoctial and Horizontal Lines, will likewiſe be the Point thro which the Hour-Line of 6 muſt paſs, and conſequently wherewith the Dial may be finiſhed   Note, The Angle H F E will be the Plane's Declination

To draw a Dial upon a Vertical Plane by means of the Shadow of the Extremity of an Iron-Rod or Style obſerved upon the Plane at Noon

A Style, as H I, (Vide Figure 9) being ſet up on a Wall or Dial Plane, whoſe Foot is H, and Extremity I , and if you know by any means when it is Noon, which may be known by a Meridian Line drawn upon a Horizontal Plane, as we ſhall mention hereafter, note where the Extremity of the Shadow of the Style H I falls upon the Plane at Noon, which ſuppoſe in the Point N, and thro this Point draw the Perpendicular A N B, which conſequently will be the Meridian of the Place or Hour-Line of 12 , then draw the level Line C H D, cutting the Meridian at Right Angles in the Point E , this will be the Horizontal Line   Again, Draw H F equal in Length to the right Style H I, and parallel to the Meridian , then take the Hypothenuſe E F between your Compaſſes, and lay it off upon the Horizontal Line from E to O, and make the Angle E O A equal to the Elevation of the Pole, viz. 49 deg and then the Point A will be the Center of the Dial

Likewiſe make the Angle E O N, underneath the Horizontal Line, equal to the Complement of the Elevation of the Pole, viz. 41 deg and the Point N on the Meridian Line will be that thro which the Equinoctial Line muſt paſs   Then if the right Line A H K be drawn thro the Center A, and the Foot of the Style H, this will be the Subſtylar Line , and if a Perpendicular be drawn thro the Point N to this Line, the ſaid Perpendicular will be the Equinoctial Line   Thus having found the principal Lines of the Dial, you may compleat it by the Methods before explained

This Method of drawing a Dial at any Time of the Year, by means of the Shadow of the Extremity of the Style H I obſerved at Noon, may ſerve, when it is not poſſible to find the Subſtylar Line by the Obſervations of the Shadows of the Extremity of an Iron-Rod or Style, which happens when Planes decline conſiderably Eaſtwards or Weſtwards

There are ſeveral other Methods of drawing Vertical Dials on Walls or Planes ⋅ but thoſe would take up too much time to mention in this ſmall Treatiſe, wherein we have only laid down the moſt ſimple and eaſy Methods of drawing Vertical Dials   And in order to draw Dials more exactly, we ſhall hereafter lay down Rules for calculating the Angles the Hour-Lines make at the Centers , and ſo the other Methods may be verified by theſe Rules

The Conſtruction of Non-declining inclining Dials

The Inclinations of theſe Dials are the Angles that their Planes make with the Horizon, and ſome of them face the Heavens, and others the Earth   There are likewiſe two Kinds of them with regard to the Pole , and two other Kinds with regard to the Equinoctial

If a Plane facing the South hath an Inclination towards the North, this Inclination may be leſs or greater than the Elevation of the Pole, for if the Inclination be equal to the Elevation of the Pole, this Dial-Plane will be an upper or under Polar one, whoſe Conſtruction we have already laid down

If the Inclination be leſs than the Elevation of the Pole, which at Paris is nearly 49 deg. and you would make a Dial upon a Plane facing the South, having 30 deg of Inclination towards the North, ſubſtract 30 deg from 49 deg and the Remainder 19 deg will be the Height of the Axis or Style above the Plane   Then if a Horizontal Dial be made upon this Plane for the Latitude of 19 deg. in the manner we have already laid down, we ſhall have an Incliner of 30 deg drawn, becauſe the ſaid Plane thus inclined is parallel to the Horizon of thoſe Places where the Pole is elevated 19 deg. and conſequently this muſt be a Horizontal Dial for thoſe Places.   The Center of this Dial is downwards, underneath the Equinoctial Line, and the Morning-Hour-Lines on the Left, and the Afternoon ones on the Right-hand of thoſe looking at them.

The under oppoſite Dial to this, which faces towards the North, is the ſame as the upper one facing towards the South, excepting only that the Center is upwards above the
                                                                            Equinoctial

Fig. 11, 12.

Equinoctial Line, and the Morning Hour-Lines on the Right, and the Afternoon ones on the Left-hand

If the Inclination of the Plane be greater than the Elevation of the Pole, suppose at *Paris*, and it be 63 deg substract the Elevation of the Pole 49 deg from 63 deg and the Remainder will be 14 deg and then make an Horizontal Dial for this Elevation of 14 deg. and you will have an Incliner of 63 deg the Center of the upper Plate facing towards the South, is upwards above the Equinoctial Line, the Morning Hour-Lines on the Left-hand, those of the Afternoon towards the Right, and in the opposite under Plane facing towards the North, the Center is downwards, the Morning Hours on the Right, and those of the Afternoon on the Left, as may be seen in Figure 11 and 12

If the Plane faces the North, and inclines Southwards, the Inclination thereof may be less or greater than that of the Equinoctial, for if it be equal, we need only make an upper or under Equinoctial Dial thereon, which is a Circle divided into 24 equal Parts, as is above directed in speaking of Regular Dials

If the Inclination be less than the Elevation of the Equinoctial, as, suppose a Plane at *Paris* inclines 30 deg. Southwardly, add the 30 deg of Inclination to 49 deg the Height of the Pole, and make an Horizontal Dial for the Elevation of 79 deg and your Dial will be drawn the Center of the upper Dial facing Northwardly, will be upwards, the Morning Hour-Lines on the Right-hand, the Afternoon ones on the Left, and on the opposite under Dial to this, the Center will be downwards, the Morning Hour-Lines on the Left, and the Afternoon ones on the Right-hand

Finally, If the Inclination, which suppose 60 deg be greater than the Height of the Equinoctial, add the Complement of the Inclination, which is 30 deg to the Elevation of the Equinoctial, which is 41 deg at *Paris*, and the Sum is 71 deg and make an Horizontal Dial for this Elevation of the Pole   The Center of the upper one of these Dials is downwards, the Morning Hour-Lines on the Right-hand, and the Center of the opposite under Dial is upwards, and the Morning Hour-Lines on the Left-hand

Note, The Meridian or Hour-Line of 12, is the Substylar Line of all Non-declining inclining Dials, passes thro their Centers at right Angles to the Hour-Lines of 6, and may be drawn by means of the Shadow of a Plumb-Line passing thro their Centers

There ought to have been eight Figures to represent all these different Dials, viz four for the upper ones, and four for the under ones, but since they are not difficult to be conceived or drawn, we have only represented two of them, with respect to the Dodecahedron on which we place them

The Construction of Declining inclining Dials

The Declination of a Dial is the Angle that the Plane thereof makes with the Prime Vertical, and its Inclination is the Angle made by the Plane thereof with the Horizon both of which we shall shew how to find hereafter

Now suppose, for example, that a Dial is to be drawn upon a Plane declining 36 deg South-eastwardly, and inclining 63 deg 26 min towards the Earth, as does the Plane C on the Dodecahedron of Figure 2

But before we shew how to draw this Dial, you must first observe that the Horizontal Line, which passes thro the Foot of the Style in Vertical Dials, must in no wise pass thro it in inclining Dials, for in upper Incliners facing the Heavens, this Line must be drawn above the Foot of the Style, and in under Incliners, facing the Earth, below the Foot of the Style. Secondly, The Meridian or Hour-Line of 12, in inclining Dials, does not cut the Horizontal Line at right Angles, as it does in Vertical Dials, but must be drawn thro two Points, one of which is found upon the Horizontal Line by means of the Angle of Declination, and the other upon a Vertical Line cutting the Horizontal one at right Angles

This last Point in upper Incliners is called the Zenith Point, because if the Sun was in the Zenith of the Place for which the Dial is made, the Extremity of the Shadow of the Style would fall upon that Point, which consequently will be underneath the Style of these Dials   And in under Incliners the said Point is called the Nadir Point, because if the Sun was in the Nadir, and the Earth transparent, the Extremity of the Shadow of the Style would touch that Point, which consequently will be above the Style, as in the proposed Dial

Thirdly, The Center of the proposed under Dial which declines South-eastwardly must be upwards, the Substylar Line to the Left-hand of the Vertical Line, and the Meridian among the Morning Hour-Lines, and so on the Right of the Vertical Line   The Centers of upper Dials declining South-westwardly must be likewise upwards, the Substylar Line on the Right-hand of the Vertical one, and the Meridian among the Afternoon Hour-Lines, and the opposite upper Dials to these, have their Centers downwards, and are no other but these Dials inverted   and therefore one of these four Dials is enough to be drawn

Fig 13. In order for this, let it be required to draw a Dial upon a Plane of the aforesaid Declination and Inclination   First, Draw the two Lines A B, C D, cutting each other at right Angles in the Point E ; then let C D be parallel to the Horizon, and upon it assume E F

at

at pleasure, for the Length of the right Style, whose Foot shall be E, and Extremity F, and about the Center F describe the Arc G H, equal to the Plane's Inclination, viz 63 deg 26 min and draw the right Line A F, likewise make the Angle G F I equal to the Complement of 63 deg 26 min viz 26 deg 34 min This being done, the Point A will be the Nadir, and one Point of the Meridian Line, and if a right Line M L N be drawn thro the Point L, parallel to C D, this will be the Horizontal Line, and if the Distance L F be taken between your Compasses, and laid off from L to O, the Point O will be the Center thro which Lines may be drawn dividing the Horizontal Line Again, About the Point O describe the Arc L P of 36 deg viz the Plane's Declination, and draw the Line O P cutting the Horizontal Line M L N in the Point 12, then if a right Line be drawn thro the Nadir A and this Point 12, the said Line A 12 will be the Meridian of the Dial or Hour-Line of 12 and moreover, if an Angle be made at the Point O on the Left-side of the Line A B, equal to the Complement of the Plane's Declination, which here is 54 deg you will have a Point on the Horizontal Line thro which the Hour-Line of 6, as likewise the Equinoctial Line, must pass

The next thing to be found is another Point, besides E the Foot of the Style, thro which the Substylar Line must pass, and in order for this, we need only find the Center of the Dial, after the following manner

Draw the Line M R from the Point M, (thro which the Hour-Line of 6 passes) at right Angles to the Meridian A 12, lay off the Distance O 12, from 12 to R, or else the Distance A F from A to R, draw the occult Line 12 R, and about the Point R describe the Arc N K, of 49 deg viz the Elevation of the Pole, then if R K be drawn cutting the Meridian in the Point K, this will be the Center of the Dial After this, the Substylar Line K E may be drawn, and if the Perpendicular M Q be drawn to this Line thro the Point M, the said M Q will be the Equinoctial Line Moreover, the Point in the Meridian Line thro which the Equinoctial Line must pass, may be found by making the Angle N R Q of 41 deg that is, the Complement of the Elevation of the Pole

The Positions of the principal Lines being thus found, it will not now be difficult to find the Points on the Horizontal or Equinoctial Lines thro which the Hour-Lines must be drawn, for if the Points are to be found upon the Horizontal Line, you must apply the Center of a Horizontal Dial to the Point O, in such manner, that the Hour-Line of 12 answers to the Line O 12, and the Hour-Line of 6 to the Line O 6 then the Points in the Horizontal Line M N, thro which the other Hour-Lines must be drawn, may be determined easily And if the Points thro which the Hour-Lines must pass on the Equinoctial Line be to be found, you must raise the Perpendicular E S on the Substyle equal to E F, and draw the Axis S K, and afterwards take the Distance T S between your Compasses, and lay off on the Substyle from T to V, then V will be the Center of the Equinoctial Circle, by means of which the Equinoctial Line may be divided, as we have directed in speaking of declining Dials, and the Hour-Lines drawn thro the Center of the Dial K Your Dial being thus made, you may draw a fair Draught thereof, wherein are only the principal Lines, and the Hour-Lines, as may be seen in the Pentagonal Figure marked 14

By means of this Dial three others of the same Declination and Inclination may be made The two under ones declining South-eastwardly and South-westwardly, have their Centers upwards, and the two upper ones, which decline North-eastwardly and North-westwardly, their Centers downwards, and are only the two former Dials inverted, as we have already mentioned

The Dial of Figure 15, represents that marked F in Figure 2, and is an upper Incliner of 63 deg 26 min declining South-eastwardly 72 deg and may be drawn by the abovesaid Method The Center of this Dial is upwards, and because it has a great Declination, the Hour-Lines will fall very close to one another near the Substylar Line, and therefore it ought to be drawn upon a large Plane, that so the Part thereof next to the Center may be taken away, and the Style and Hour-Lines terminated by two Parallels

There is another way of drawing Mechanically any sorts of Dials whatsoever, upon Polyhedrons or Bodies of different Faces or Superficies, without even knowing the Declinations or Inclinations of the Faces or Superficies, and that with as much exactness as by any other Methods whatsoever In order to do this, you must first make an Horizontal Dial upon one of the Planes or Faces that is to be set parallel to the Horizon, and set up the Style thereof upon the Hour-Line of 12, conformable to the Latitude of the Place After this, the Substylar Lines must be drawn upon all the Planes or Faces of the Polyhedron that the Sun can shine upon, that so Brass or Iron Styles, proportioned to the bignesses of the Planes or Faces, may be fixed upon them perpendicularly in such manner, that the Axes or upper Edges of the said Styles be parallel to the Axis of the Horizontal Dial This may be done in filing them away in right Lines by degrees, until their Axes, being compared with the Axis of a large Style similar to that of the Horizontal Dial placed level, (or held up so that its Base be parallel to the Horizon, by means of a Thread and Plummet hung to the Top of the Style) appear in a right Line with the Axis of the said Style.

Things being thus ordered, set your Polyhedron in the Sun, and turn it about, making the Shadow of the Axis of the Horizontal Dial fall upon each Hour-Line thereof successively,

and

and if at each of the respective Times right Lines be drawn along the Shadows of the Axes of the Styles of the other Faces of the Body upon the said Faces, these will be the same Hour-Lines upon each of the Faces of the Body, that the Shadow of the Style of the Horizontal Dial fell upon, on the Horizontal Dial. For example, Suppose the Shadow of the Axis of the Horizontal Dial falls upon the Hour-Line of 12, then at the same time draw Lines along the Shadows of the Styles upon the other Faces of the Body, and those Lines will be the Hour-Lines of 12 upon the said Faces   understand the same for others. This may be done likewise in the Night, by the Light of a Link moved about the Polyhedron.

There are great Stone Bodies cut into several Faces placed sometimes in *Gardens* having Dials drawn upon them, according to the abovesaid Method. And the Edges of the Stone which serve for Axes to some of these Dials, must be cut so as to be parallel to the Axis of the World.

The Arithmetical Construction of Dials by the Calculation of Angles

This Method is a great help for verifying any Operations in Dialling, wherein there is great Exactness required, and chiefly when we are obliged to make a small Model for drawing a large Dial   for an Error almost insensible in the Model, will become very considerable in the long Hour-Lines to be drawn upon a large Plane.

In the Construction of Regular Dials, as of the Horizontal one of Figure 4, the Divisions of the Equinoctial Line L K, are the Tangents of the Angles of the Quadrant M H, and the dotted Lines are their Secants; and therefore they may be pricked down by means of a Scale or Sector, in supposing the Radius H B 100   for then the Tangent H 1 of 15 deg. will be twenty-seven of the said Parts, H 2, the Tangent of 30 deg will be 58, H 3, the Tangent of 45 deg (equal to Radius) will be 100, H 4, the Tangent of 60 deg will be 173, and H 5, the Tangent of 75 deg will be 373 Parts   The Divisions on the other half of this Line for the Morning Hour-Lines are the same.

The Divisions for the halves and quarters of Hours may be found likewise upon the Equinoctial Line, by assuming the Tangents of the correspondent Arcs, which may be taken from printed Tables of natural Tangents, but from the Table of Secants we can deduce some Abbreviations   For example, the Line B 4, which is the Secant of 60 deg being double to Radius, if twice B H be laid off from B to 4, you will have the Point on the Equinoctial Line thro which the Hour-Line of 4 must be drawn   The said Secant laid off from 4 to L, will give likewise the Point in the Equinoctial Line thro which the Hour-Line of 5 must be drawn, &c

The Points thro which the half Hours must pass, may be found by means of the Secants of the odd Hours   For example, the Secant B 3, laid off at the Point 3 on the Equinoctial Line, will fall on one side upon the Point for half an Hour past 4, and on the other side, for half an Hour past 10, the Secant B 9, will give half an Hour past 7, and half an Hour past 1, B 11, will give half an Hour past 8, and half an Hour past 2, B 1, will give half an Hour past 3, and half an Hour past 9, B 7, will give half an Hour past 6, and half an Hour past 12, and lastly, B 5 will give half an Hour past 11, and half an Hour past 5.

The Division of the Equinoctial Line serves to make Horizontal and Vertical Dials exactly, but chiefly the undeclining Regular Dials, *viz.* the Polar East and West ones   for there need nothing be added to the facility of constructing Equinoctial Dials, because the Angles that the Hour-Lines make at the Center of the Dials are all equal between themselves.

The Angles that the Hour-Lines of a Horizontal Dial make with the Meridian in the Center of the Dial, may be found in the following manner by Trigonometry   As Radius is to the Sine of the Elevation of the Pole, so is the Tangent of the Distance of any Hour-Circle from the Meridian, to the Tangent of the Angle that the Hour-Line of that Hour makes with the Meridian or Hour-Line of 12, on the Horizontal Dial   For example, Suppose the Angle that the Hour-Lines of 1 and 11, make with the Meridian on a Horizontal Dial for the Latitude of 49 deg be required   form a Rule of Proportion whose first Term let be the Radius 100000, the second, the Sine of 49 deg which is 75471, and the third, the Tangent of 15 deg (*viz.* the Tangent of the Distance of the Hour-Circles of 11 and 1 from the Meridian) which is 26795   Now having found the fourth Term 20222, seek it in the Tables of Tangents, and you will find 11 deg 26 min stand against it   therefore the Angle that the Hour-Lines of 1 or 11 make with the Meridian, is 11 deg 26 min.

Thus may be found the Angles that all the Hour-Lines, and half Hour-Lines, &c make with the Meridian in the Center of a Horizontal Dial, *viz.* by as many Rules of Proportion, as there are Hour-Lines and half Hour-Lines, &c to be drawn, whose two first Terms are standing, to wit, the Radius, and the Sine of the Elevation of the Pole, and so you have but the third Term to seek in the Tables, that is, the Tangent of the Hour-Circle's distance from the Meridian, in order to find the 4*th* Term   You may take the Logarithms of those Terms if you have a mind to it, which will save the trouble of Multiplying and Dividing

The

The aforesaid Analogy may serve likewise for Vertical Dials, if the Sine Complement of the Elevation of the Pole, which is 41 deg about *Paris*, be made use of for the second Term, because any Vertical Dial at *Paris* may be considered as an Horizontal one for the Latitude of 41 deg

Moreover, the aforesaid Analogy holds for undeclining Inclining Dials, if the Sine of the Angle made by the Axis and Meridian Line at the Center of the Dial be used for the second Term of the Analogy. For example, Because the Dial B on the Dodecahedron of Figure 2, inclines 63 deg 26 min you must substract the Elevation of the Pole, which is 49 deg from 63 deg 26 min and then if you make an Horizontal Dial for the Latitude of 14 deg 26 min in taking 14 deg 26 min for the second Term of the Analogy, you may calculate the Angles that all the Hour-Lines make with the Meridian or Hour-Line of 12

A T A B L E *of the Angles that the Hour-Lines make with the Meridian at the Center of an Horizontal Dial*

Latitude	Hours										
	I and XI		II and X		III and IX		IV and VIII		V and VII		VI and VI
41 deg	9 d 58 m		20	45	33	16	48	39	67	47	90	00
49 deg.	11	26	23	33	37	3	52	35	70	27	90	00

To draw the principal Lines upon a Vertical Decliner by Trigonometrical Calculation

This manner of Calculation consists in the five following Rules

The Declination of a Plane being given, to find the Angle that the Substylar Line makes with the Meridian

Rule I As Radius is to the Sine of the Plane's Declination, so is the Tangent Complement of the Latitude, to the Tangent of the Angle made by the Substylar Line and Meridian in the Center of a Vertical Decliner And the Angle that the Substylar Line makes with the Horizon at the Foot of the right Style, is the Complement of this Angle Also the Angle that the Equinoctial Line makes with the Horizon at the Point wherein the Hour-Line of 6 cuts it, is equal to the Angle made by the Substylar Line and Meridian, and the Angle of the Equinoctial Line and Meridian is its Complement

Rule II To find the Angle which the Axis of the Dial makes with the Substylar Line, which may be called likewise the Height of the Pole above the Vertical Plane, say,

As Radius is to the Sine Complement of the Latitude, so is the Sine Complement of the Plane's Declination to the Sine of the Angle required Note, The Angle that the Axis makes with the right Style, is the Complement of this Angle, and the Angle that the Radius of the Equinoctial Circle makes with the right Style, is equal to the Angle that the Axis makes with the Substyle Also the Angle made by the Radius of the Equinoctial Circle and the Substyle, is the Complement thereof

Rule III To find the Arc of the Equinoctial or Angle between the Substylar Line and the Meridian in declining Dials, that is, the Difference between the Meridian of the Place, and the Meridian of the Plane, for the Substylar Line is the Meridian of the Plane, say,

As Radius is to the Sine of the Latitude, so is the Tangent Complement of the Plane's Declination to the Tangent of an Arc, whose Complement will be that required

Rule IV To find the Angle that the Hour-Line of 6 makes with the Horizontal Line, and the Meridian in the Center of the Dial, say,

As Radius is to the Sine of the Plane's Declination, so is the Tangent of the Latitude, to the Tangent of the Angle that the Hour-Line of 6 makes with the Horizon, the Complement of which, is that made by the Hour-Line of 6 and the Meridian

Rule V To find the Angles that the Hour-Lines make with the Substylar Line, and by this means, the Angles that they make with the Meridian in the Center of a Vertical Dial

This Proposition is founded upon this Gnomonick Principle, *viz.* that any Plane may be parallel to some Horizon, and consequently will be an Horizontal Dial for that Latitude, the Substylar Line being the Meridian, from which the proper Hour-Lines must be laid off on both sides

But before this can be done, the Angle that the Substyle makes with the Meridian must be found, by *Rule I* the Elevation of the Pole above the Plane, by *Rule II* the Arc of the Equinoctial between the Substyle and the Meridian, by *Rule III.* with the Difference or Degrees of the two first Distances from the Style, one being between the Substyle and the Meridian, and the other between the Substyle and the Hour-Line of 6 These being found, say,

As Radius is to the Sine of the Elevation of the Pole above the Plane, so is the Tangent of the Distance of any Hour-Circle from the Meridian of the Plane or Substylar Line to the Tangent of the Angle made by the Hour-Line of the proposed Hour-Circle and the Substylar Line in the Center of the Dial.

Note,

Note, If the Subftylar Line happens to fall upon any half or whole Hour, then the two firft Diftances of the Hour-Circles from the Subftylar Line will be each 7 deg 30 min. or 15 deg and in this Cafe, the Angles of the Hour-Lines of the Hour-Circles, equally diftant on both fides the Hour the Subftylar Line falls upon, will be equal on both fides the Subftylar Line

The Application of the precedent Rules to a Vertical Decliner of 45 deg South-weftwardly, in the Latitude of 49 deg (Vide Figure *9)*

` The Angle made by the Subftylar Line and the Meridian, will be found by the firft Rule 31 deg 35 min

The Angle of the Axis and Subftylar Line, by *Rule* II will be 27 deg 38 min and the Arc of the Equinoctial between the Meridian of the Place and the Meridian of the Plane, by *Rule* III will be found 52 deg 58 min and confequently the Subftylar Line falls between the Hour-Lines of 3 and 4 in the Afternoon , and the Angle made by the Hour-Line of 6 and the Meridian, is 50 deg 52 min

The Arc of the Equinoctial 52 deg 58 min being found, fubftract 45 deg which is the Arc of the Equinoctial anfwering to the Hour of 3, from it, and the Remainder 7 deg 58 min will be the Arc of the Diftance of the Hour of 3 from the Subftyle, and confequently 7 deg 2 min is the Diftance of the Hour of 4 from the Subftyle

Therefore to find the Angles that the Hour-Lines make with the Subftyle in the Center of the Dial, you muft begin with one of thefe Diftances, in faying, for example, As Radius 100000 is to the Sine of the Elevation of the Pole above the declining Plane, which in this Example is 27 deg 38 min whofe Sine is 46381, fo is the Tangent of 7 deg 2 min which is 12337, to a fourth Number, which fhall be found 5722, *viz* the Tangent of 3 deg 16 min and confequently the Angle that the Hour-Line of 4 makes with the Subftyle, is 3 deg 16 min and to find the Angle that the Hour-Line of 5 makes with the Subftylar Line, you muft firft add 15 deg to 7 deg 2 min and feek the Tangent of the Sum 22 deg 2 min and then proceed, as before, and you will find the Angle made by the Hour-Line of 5 with the Subftylar Line will be 10 deg 38 min the Angle of the Hour-Line of 6 with the fame, will be 19 deg 17 min the Angle of the Hour-Line of 7, 30 deg 44 min and the Angle of the Hour-Line of 8 in the Evening, 47 deg 35 min

But if the Angles that the faid Hour-Lines make with the Meridian or Hour-Line of 12 be required, you muft add 31 deg 35 min to each of the aforefaid Angles , and confequently the Angle that the Hour-Line of 4 makes with the Meridian, will be 34 deg 51 min the Hour-Line of 5, 42 deg 13 min the Hour-Line of 6, 50 deg 52 min the Hour-Line of 7, 62 deg 19 min and the Hour-Line of 8, 79 deg 10 min

Having calculated, in the abovefaid manner, the Angles made by the Hour-Lines on the other fide the Subftylar Line, with the faid Subftylar Line, you will find the Angle of the Hour-Line of 3, 3 deg 45 min that of the Hour-Line of 2, 11 deg 7 min that of the Hour-Line of 1, 19 deg 54 min that of the Hour-Line of 12, 31 deg 35 min that of the Hour-Line of 11, 48 deg 54 min that of the Hour-Line of 10, 75 deg 7 min. and that of the Hour-Line of 9, 106 deg 48 min

Now if 31 deg 35 min *viz* the Subftyle's Diftance from the Meridian, be taken from each of thefe laft Angles, then the Angle that the Hour-Line of 9 makes with the Meridian, will be 75 deg 13 min that of the Hour-Line of 10, 43 deg 32 min that of the Hour-Line of 11, 17 deg 19 min and fo of others

When the Declination of a Plane is very great, the Center of a Dial cannot then be pricked down conveniently thereon, fince the Hour-Lines will fall too near each other And in this Cafe they may be drawn between two Horizontal Lines, for the Angles that the Hour-Lines make with the faid Horizontal Lines, are the Complements of the Angles that the refpective Hour-Lines make with the Meridian

How to find the Declination of an upright or vertical Wall or Plane, by means of the Shadow of the Extremity of an Iron Rod or Style

Becaufe the Exactnefs of Vertical Dials chiefly depend on the knowledge of the Situations of the Walls on which they are to be made or fet up againft, with refpect to the Heavens, that is, their Declinations therefore it is very neceffary that their Declinations be found with all poffible exactnefs, which we fhall endeavour to do before we clofe this Chapter.

Preparations

You muft firft fix an Iron Rod or Wire in the Wall obliquely, having its Extremity fharp and pretty diftant from the Wall, as the Rod A I, whofe Extremity I is fharp. *Vide* Fig 9

Secondly, The Foot H of the Style muft be pricked down upon the Dial Plane This Point is that wherein the Perpendicular H I drawn from the Extremity of the Rod or Style meets the Plane of the Dial You muft likewife draw the Vertical Line H F paffing thro that Point, which reprefents the perpendicular Vertical to the Plane of the Dial, and alfo the Horizontal Line D C cutting the faid Vertical Line at right Angles, in the Foot of the Style

Style H   This being done, measure exactly the Length of the right Style H I or H F, its equal, that is, measure the Distance from the Foot of the Style to its Extremity, with some Scale divided into small Parts   Then having observed where the Extremity of the Shadow of the Iron Rod falls upon the Wall at different Times in the same Day, as at the Points 2, 3, 4, you must measure the Distance of each Extremity of the Shadow from the Horizontal Line with the Scale : as, for example, the Distance from the Point 2 to the Point Z in the Horizontal Line, as likewise the Distance from the same Point to the Vertical Line passing thro the Foot of the Style, as from the Point 2 to the Point X; and then you must set down the Numbers found orderly in a Memorial, that so they may be made use of in the following Analogies

But to prick down upon the Wall nicely the Shadow of the Extremity of the Rod or Style, you must use the following Method, which I had from M *de la Hire*   Fasten a little Tin-Plate, having a round hole therein, near the Extremity of the Rod, in such manner, that the Extremity of the Iron Rod be exactly in the Center of the said round hole, and the Plate exposed directly to the Sun, then you will see a little Oval of Light upon the Wall in the Shadow of the Plate   and if you draw quickly with a Pencil, a light Tract upon the Wall about the said Oval of Light, which is moving continually, the Center of the said Oval may be taken for the true Shadow of the Extremity of the Rod

Having thus marked the Points 2, 3, 4, whereat the Extremity of the Shadow falls, you must find the Amplitude, and the Sun's Altitude answering to each of them, and set them down in the Memorial

Note, The Amplitude that we mean here, is the Angle that the height of the Style or Rod makes with the Line drawn from each of the observed Extremities of the Shadow to the Horizontal Line (for each of these Lines represents upon the Wall the vertical Circle the Sun is in at the Time of Observation)   This Angle is marked H F Z in the Figure, and is the Amplitude correspondent to the Point 2   Now to find this Angle, you must say, As the Height of the Rod or Style is to the Distance from the Extremity of the Shadow to the vertical Line   so is Radius to the Tangent of the Amplitude   And by making this Analogy for each Extremity of the Shadow of the Rod observed at different Times, the correspondent Amplitudes will be had, and must be set down in one Column in the Memorial

Then to find the Sun's Altitude above the Horizon, you must take the Complement of the Amplitude, and the Distance of each observed Extremity of the Shadow from the Horizontal Line   This being done, say, As the Height of the Style is to the Sine Complement of the Amplitude, so is the Distance of the Extremity of the Shadow from the Horizontal Line, to the Tangent of the Sun's Altitude above the Horizon, which being found for the Times of each Observation of the Shadow of the Iron Rod, set them down orderly in one Column

Note, If the Extremity of the Shadow observed falls upon the vertical Line passing thro the Foot of the Style, there will then be no Amplitude, and in this Case you will have the Sun's Altitude by one Rule only, in saying, As the Height of the Style is to the Distance of the Extremity of the Shadow from the Foot of the Style, so is Radius to the Tangent of the Sun's Altitude.

After this, you must find the Distance of each observed Vertical or Azimuth Line from the Meridian, and in order to do this, the Sun's Declination must be had for the Times wherein the Extremities of the Shadow were taken   if it be at the time of the Solstices, the same Declination will serve for all the Extremities of the Shadow observed in one Day, but if the Sun be in the Equinoctial, you must have his Declination for each time of the Observation of the Extremity of the Shadow, in taking the Parts proportional

Now the Sun's Declination being had, you must take the Complement thereof, as likewise the Complement of his Altitude, and the Complement of the Latitude, and add them all three together, and take half the Sum, and from this half Sum take the Complement of the Sun's Altitude, and the Remainder will be a first Difference   and moreover, if the Complement of the Latitude be taken from the said half Sum, you will have a second Difference   This being done, say, As the Sine Complement of the Latitude is to the Sine of the first Difference, so is the Sine of the second Difference to a fourth Sine   and as the Sine Complement of the Sun's Altitude is to Radius, so is that fourth Sine found to another Sine, which being multiplied by Radius, and the Square Root of the Product, will be half the Distance of the Extremity of the Shadow observed, or of its vertical Line from the Meridian or Hour-Line of 12

This Distance being found in Degrees and Minutes, we may have the Declination of any Wall, which here is the Angle H F E, by some one of the five following Cases

First, If the Extremity of the Shadow of the Style is between the vertical Line passing thro the Foot of the Style, and the Hour-Line of 12, as is the Point 2 in this Example, which was observed some time in the Afternoon, then you must add the Amplitude to the Distance of the vertical Line from the Meridian

Secondly, If the Extremity of the Shadow falls beyond the vertical Line passing thro the Foot of the Style, as here the Point 3 does, you must substract the Amplitude from the Distance of the vertical Line from the Meridian, to have the Declination of the Wall.

Thirdly, If the observed Extremity of the Shadow be found exactly upon the vertical Line passing thro the Foot of the Style, then there will be no Amplitude, and its Distance from the Meridian will be the Wall's Declination.

Fourthly, If the Extremity of the Shadow is on this side of the Meridian, as here the Point 4 is, which was observed before Noon, the Amplitude will be greater than the Declination, to have which, you must substract from the Amplitude the Distance of the Vertical Line from the Meridian.

Fifthly, If the Extremity of the Shadow was observed precisely at Noon, the Wall's Declination would then be equal to the Amplitude, and since the Sun's Declination, and the Latitude is known, it will be easy to know whether the Altitude observed any Day be the greatest for that Day, that is, whether it be the Sun's Meridian Altitude. *Note*, What we have said is easily applicable to all Declinations, whether Eastwards or Westwards, if the Line of Midnight be used instead of that of Noon, when Walls decline North-East or North-West.

An Example will make all this manifest: in order to which, let us suppose, that, in a Place where the North-Pole is elevated, or, which is all one, where the Latitude of the Place is 48 deg. 50 min. we have observed the Extremity of the Shadow of an Iron-Rod upon a very upright Wall about the time of the Summer Solstice, whose Distance from the vertical Line passing thro the Foot of the Style is 100 equal Parts of some Scale, and the Height of the Style 300 of the same Parts.

The Operation by Logarithms

The Logarithm of 100	20000000
The Logarithm of Radius	100000000
The Sum	120000000
The Logarithm of 300	24771212
The Remainder	95228788

This Number remaining is the Logarithm Tangent of 18 deg. 26 min. for the Amplitude of the observed Extremity of the Shadow, and the Complement thereof is 71 deg. 34 min.

Then to find the Sun's Altitude, suppose the Distance from the Extremity of the Shadow observed to the Horizontal Line be 600 of the aforesaid equal Parts.

The Logarithm Sine of 71 deg. 34 min.	99771253
The Logarithm of 600	27781512
The Sum	127552765
The Logarithm of 300	24771212
The Remainder	102781553

This remaining Number is the Logarithm Tangent of 62 deg. 13 min. the Sun's Altitude.

	Deg.	Min.
Then suppose the Complement of the Latitude is	41	10
The Complement of the Declination of the Sun	66	45
The Complement of the Height of the Sun	27	45
The Sum	135	42
Half of the Sum	67	51
The Complement of the Latitude	41	10
The first Difference	26	41
Again, taking from	67	51
The Complement of the Sun's Altitude	27	47
We shall have the second Difference	40	4

The first Analogy.

The Logarithm Sine of the first Difference 26 deg. 41 min.	96523035
The Logarithm Sine of the second Difference 40 deg. 4 min.	98086690
The Sum	194609725
The Logarithm Sine of 41 deg. 10 min. substract	91883919
The fourth Sine remaining	96425800

The

The second Analogy

The Logarithm of Radius	——	——	——	10000000
The fourth Sine	——	——	——	96425806
The Sum	——	——	——	196425806
Subſtract the Logarithm Sine of 27 deg 47 min	——	——	——	96685064
The remaining Sine	——	——	——	99740742
The Sine of Radius	——	——	——	100000000
The Sum	——	——	——	199740742
The half of this Number for the Square Root	——	——	99887037 1

This laſt Number is the Logarithm Sine of 76 deg 4 min which being doubled, makes 152 deg 8 min but ſince this Angle is obtuſe, you muſt ſubſtract it from 180 deg and the remainder 27 deg. 52 min is the diſtance of the obſerved vertical Circle or Line from the Meridian · and becauſe the Extremity of the Shadow 2, for which the Calculation is ſuppoſed to be made, is between the vertical Line paſſing thro the Foot of the Style, and the Hour-Line of 12 ; you muſt add the aforeſaid 27 deg 52 min. to the calculated Amplitude 18 deg. 26 min to have the Declination 46 deg 18 min

The Declination of a Wall may be found by one Obſervation of the Extremity of the Shadow of a Style or Iron-Rod only , but it is better to make ſeveral Obſervations thereof in one Day, or in different Days, that ſo the Declination of the Wall may be calculated for each Obſervation, and the proportional Parts of the Differences ariſing may be taken if, for example, the Extremity of the Shadow of the Style hath been ſix times obſerved, you muſt take the one-ſixth part of the Differences produced by the Calculations, in order to have the true Declination of the Wall

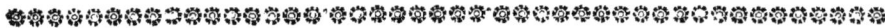

❀❀❀❀❀❀❀❀❀❀❀❀❀❀❀❀❀❀❀❀❀❀❀❀❀❀❀❀❀❀❀❀❀❀❀❀

C H A P. II.

Of the Conſtruction and Uſes of the Declinatory.

THIS Inſtrument is made of a very even Plate of Braſs or dry Wood, in figure of a Fig 16 Rectangle, about one Foot in length, and ſeven or eight Inches in breadth We draw the Diameter of a Semi-circle upon it parallel to one of the longeſt ſides of this Plate, viz parallel to A B, and we divide this Semi-circle into two Quadrants, containing 90 Degrees each, which we divide ſometimes into half Degrees, the Degrees being both ways numbered from the Point H, as may be ſeen in the Figure of the Inſtrument When this is done, we add an Index I to the ſaid Plate, which turns about the Center G, by means of a turn'd headed Rivet On the Fiducial Line of this Index we ſcrew a Compaſs, with the North-ſide towards the Center G, and likewiſe ſometimes a ſmall Horizontal Dial, whoſe Hour-Line of 12 turns to the Center G I ſhall ſay no more as to the Conſtruction of this Inſtrument, it being eaſy to underſtand, from what has been ſaid elſewhere in this Treatiſe

The Uſe of this Inſtrument in taking the Declinations of Planes

A Plane is ſaid to decline, when it does not face directly one of the Cardinal Parts of the World, which are North, South, Eaſt and Weſt , and the Declination thereof is meaſured by an Arc of the Horizon comprehended between the Prime Vertical, and the vertical Circle parallel to the ſaid Plane, if it be vertical, viz. perpendicular to the Horizon , for if a Plane be inclined, it can be parallel to no vertical Circle And in this Caſe, the Arc of the Horizon comprehended between the Prime Vertical, and that vertical Circle that is parallel to the Baſe of the inclined Plane, or elſe the Arc of the Horizon computed between the Meridian of the Place and the vertical Circle perpendicular to the Plane, is the Plane's Declination

There are no Planes, unleſs vertical or inclined ones, that can decline , for a Horizontal Plane cannot be ſaid to decline, becauſe the upper Surface thereof directly faces the Zenith, and its Plane turns towards all the four Cardinal Parts of the World indifferently

Now, in order to find the Declination of a Plane, whether vertical or inclined, you muſt draw firſt a level Line thereon, that is, a Line parallel to the Horizon, and lay the ſide A B of the Inſtrument along this Line · then you muſt turn the Index and Compaſs till the Needle fixes itſelf directly over the Line of the Declination or Variation thereof on the bottom of the Box This being done, the Degrees of the Semi-circle cut by the Fiducial Line of the

Index

Index gives the Plane's Declination towards that Coaſt ſhewn by the writing graved upon the Inſtrument If, for example, the Index be found fixed upon the 45th Degree, between H and B, and the end of the Needle reſpecting the North be directly over the Point S of its Line of Declination ; in this Caſe, the Plane declines 45 deg South-weſtwardly · but if in the ſame Situation of the Declinatory, the oppoſite end of the Needle, reſpecting the South, ſhould have fixed itſelf over the Point S of the ſaid Line of Declination, then the Plane would have declined 45 deg North-eaſtwardly

Again, If the Index be found between A and H, and the North-end of the Needle over the Point S of its Line of Declination, then the Declination of the Plane will be South-eaſtwardly , but if in this Situation of the Index, the South-end of the Needle fixes itſelf over the ſaid Point S, then the Plane will decline North-weſtwardly

If the Sun ſhines upon the Wall or Plane whoſe Declination is ſought, and the time of the Day be known exactly by ſome good Dial, as the Aſtronomick Ring Dial, we may find the Declination of the Wall or Plane by means of a ſmall Horizontal Dial faſtened on the Index, which muſt be turned till the Style of the Dial ſhews the exact Time of the Day, and then the Degrees of one of the Quadrants cut by the Fiducial Line of the Index, will be the Wall or Plaie's Declination and by this means may be avoided the Errors cauſed by the Compaſs, as well on account of the Variation of the Needle, as becauſe of Iron concealed near the Compaſs

When the Sun ſhines upon a Wall, we may find likewiſe the Subſtyle or proper Meridian by means of obſerving two Extremities of the Shadow of an Iron-Rod, in the manner ȝve have above mentioned, and afterwards the Declination, or elſe we may draw a Meridian Line upon an Horizontal Plane near the Wall, which being produced to the Wall, will be a means to find the Declination thereof, as alſo to find the Variation of the Needle Now the manner of drawing a Meridian Line is thus :

Fig M. Draw a Circle upon ſome level Plane, (ſuppoſe this to be repreſented by the Figure M) and in the Center thereof ſet up a ſharp Style very upright, or elſe fix a crooked Style in ſome Place, as A, in ſuch manner, that a Line drawn from its ſharp end to the Center of the ſaid Circle be perpendicular to the Plane of the Circle , which you may do by a Square But before you draw the Circle, it is neceſſary to know the Length of the Shadow of the Style, that ſo the Circumference of the Circle may be drawn thro the Extremity of the Shadow of the Style obſerved ſome time before Noon Now the Circle being drawn, ſuppoſe the Extremity of the Shadow touches the Circumference of the Circle in the Morning at the Point G, and about as many Hours after Noon as when in the Morning you obſerved the Extremity of the ſaid Shadow in G before Noon, you find the Extremity of the Shadow again to touch the Circumference of the Circle in F , then if the Arc F G be biſected in the Point C, and the Diameter B C be drawn, this Diameter will be a Meridian Line

If you have a mind to find a Meridian Line when the Sun is in the Equinoctial Line, there is no need of drawing a Circle, for all the Extremities of the Shadow of the Style will then be in a right Line, as E D, which is the common Section of the Equinoctial and the Horizontal Plane, and ſo any right Line, as B C, cutting E D at right Angles, will be a Meridian Line.

Thus having drawn a Meridian Line, if the Hour-Line of 12 of a Horizontal Dial be placed ſo as to coincide therewith, we may have the Time of the Day thereby · and therefore if at the ſame time the Index of the Declinatory be turned ſo, that the ſmall Horizontal Dial faſtened thereon ſhews the ſame Hour or Part, then the Degrees of the Circumference of the Inſtrument cut by the Index, will ſhew the Declination of the Wall or Plane Or elſe you may produce the aboveſaid Meridian Line till it cuts the declining Plane, for then it will make two unequal Angles with the Horizontal Line drawn upon the Plane, viz an acute and obtuſe Angle, which being meaſured with all the exactneſs poſſible, the Difference between either of theſe Angles and a right Angle, will be the Declination of the Plane For example, if the acute Angle be 50 deg and conſequently the obtuſe one 130 deg then the Difference between either of them and a right Angle, will be 40 deg. for the Declination of the Plane

If you have a mind to find the Variation of the Needle, apply one of the ſides of the ſquare Box of the Compaſs along the Meridian Line drawn on the Plane, and when the Needle is at reſt, obſerve how many Degrees the North Point thereof is diſtant from the *Flower-de-luce* of the Card , and theſe Degrees will be the Needle's Declination or Variation ; but this Variation will not laſt long, for it changes continually *Note*, When the Declinations of Planes be taken with a Compaſs, you muſt have regard to the Variation of the Needle, in letting it reſt over a Line ſhewing the Variation, which is drawn commonly on the bottom of the Compaſs-Box.

The Uſe of the Declinatory in taking the Inclinations of Planes.

This Inſtrument ſerves to take the Inclinations of Planes, as well as their Declinations, that is, the Angles the Planes make with the Horizon, and for this end there is a little Hole in the Center G, having a Plumb-Line faſtened therein

The

The 17*th* Figure ſhews the manner of taking the Declinations and Inclinations of Planes Fig 17. The Plane A, of this Figure, whereon the Declinatory is applied, is a vertical Meridional undeclining Plane   The Plane B declines South-weſtwardly 45 Degrees   The Plane C, is a direct Weſt one   The Plane D, declines 45 Degrees North-weſtwardly   And the other Declinations are taken in the ſame manner, in applying the Side A B of the Declinatory to them, ſo that the Plane of the Semi-circle may be parallel to the Horizon

Now to meaſure the Angle of a Plane's Inclination, you muſt apply ſome one of the other Sides of the Inſtrument to the Plane or Wall, and keeping the Plane of the Semi-circle perpendicular to the Horizon, ſee what Number of Degrees of the Circumference thereof the Plumb-Line plays upon, for theſe will be the quantity of the ſaid Angle of Inclination

If, for example, the Side C D be applied to the Plane E, and the Plumb-Line plays upon the Line G H, then the ſaid Plane will be parallel to the Horizon   But if the Side C A of the Inſtrument being applied on the Plane F, and the Plumb-Line plays, as *per* Figure, this Plane inclines 45 Degrees upwards   Again, If the Inſtrument being applied to the Plane G, and the Plumb-Line plays upon the Diameter, then this Plane is vertical   And laſtly, If the Side A C, being applied on the Plane H, and the Plumb-Line plays as *per* Figure, then the Inclination thereof will be 45 deg downwards

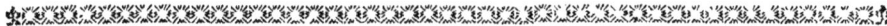

CHAP. III.

Of the Conſtruction and Uſes of Inſtruments, for drawing upon Dials the Arcs of the Signs, the Diurnal Arcs, the Babylonick *and* Italian *Hours, the Almacanters, and the Meridians of principal Cities.*

WE now proceed to deſcribe upon Dials certain Lines which the Shadow of the Extremity of the Style paſſes over, when the Sun enters into each of the 12 Signs of the Zodiack

Of the Trigon of Signs

The firſt Figure repreſents the Triangle or Trigon of Signs, made of Braſs or any other Plate 23 ſolid Matter, of a bigneſs at pleaſure   The Conſtruction of this is thus   Firſt draw the Fig 1. Line *a b*, repreſenting the Axis of the World, and *a c* perpendicular thereto, repreſenting the Radius of the Equinoctial, and about the Point *a* deſcribe the circular Arc *d c e* at pleaſure   This being done, reckon 23 ½ deg both ways from the Point *c* upon the ſaid Arc, for the Sun's greateſt Declination, and draw the two Lines, *a d*, *a e*, for the Summer and Winter Tropicks, likewiſe draw the Line *d e*, which will be biſected by the Radius of the Equinoctial in the Point *o*, about which, as a Center, draw a Circle, whoſe Circumference paſſes thro the Points *d* and *e* of the Tropicks, and divide the Circumference thereof in 12 equal Parts, beginning from the Point *d*   Then thro each Point of Diviſion equally diſtant from *d* and *e*, draw occult Lines parallel to the Radius of the Equinoctial Circle   Theſe Lines will interſect the Arc *d c* in Points thro which and the Center *a* Lines being drawn, theſe Lines will repreſent the beginnings of the Signs of the Zodiack, at 30 deg diſtance from each other

But to divide the Signs into every 10*th* or 5*th* Degree, you muſt divide the Circumference of the Circle into 36 or 72 equal Parts   After this, we denote the Characters of the Signs upon each Line, as appears *per* Figure   And when the Trigon is divided into every 10*th* or 5*th* Degree, we place the Letter of the Month to the firſt 10 Degrees of each Sign agreeing therewith

But the Trigon of Signs may be readier made by means of a Table of the Sun's Declination, for having drawn the two Lines *a b* and *a c* at right Angles, lay the Center of a Protractor on the Point *a*, with its Limb towards the Point *c*, and keeping it fixed thus, count 23 ½ deg on both ſides the Radius *a c*, for the Tropicks of ♋ and ♑, 20 deg 12 min. for the beginnings of the Signs ♌, ♊, ♐ and ♒, and 11 deg 30 min for ♉, ♍, ♏ and ♓ And in this manner we divide the Spaces for each Sign into every 10*th* or 5*th* deg by means of the following Table of the Sun's Declination   *Note,* The Equinoctial Points of ♈ and ♎ are placed at the end of the Radius of the Equinoctial *a c*

A TABLE of the Sun's Declination for every Degree of the Ecliptick.

Degrees of the Ecliptick	Signs ♈ ♎ D M.		Signs ♉ ♏ D M		Signs ♊ ♐ D M		Degrees of the Ecliptick
1	0	24	11	51	20	25	29
2	0	48	12	12	20	36	28
3	1	12	12	32	20	48	27
4	1	36	12	53	21	0	26
5	2	0	13	13	21	11	25
6	2	23	13	33	21	21	24
7	2	47	13	53	21	32	23
8	3	11	14	12	21	42	22
9	3	35	14	32	21	51	21
10	3	58	14	51	22	00	20
11	4	22	15	9	22	8	19
12	4	45	15	28	22	17	18
13	5	9	15	47	22	24	17
14	5	32	16	5	22	32	16
15	5	55	16	22	22	39	15
16	6	19	16	40	22	46	14
17	6	42	16	57	22	52	13
18	7	5	17	14	22	57	12
19	7	28	17	30	23	2	11
20	7	50	17	47	23	7	10
21	8	13	18	3	23	11	9
22	8	35	18	16	23	15	8
23	8	58	18	34	23	18	7
24	9	20	18	49	23	21	6
25	9	42	19	3	23	24	5
26	10	4	19	18	23	26	4
27	10	26	19	32	23	27	3
28	10	47	19	46	23	28	2
29	11	9	19	59	23	29	1
30	11	30	20	12	23	30	0
	♓ ♍		♒ ♌		♑ ♋		

By this Table we may know the Sun's Declination and Distance from the Equinoctial Points each Day at Noon, in every Degree of the Signs of the Zodiack, the greatest Declination being 23 deg 30 min tho at present it is but about 23 deg 29 min but a Minute difference is of no consequence in the Use of Dials. The Degrees of the first Column to the Left-hand, are for the Signs set down upon the top of the Table, and the Degrees in the last Column numbered upwards, are for the Signs set at the bottom of the Table.

Of the Trigon of Diurnal Arcs

The second Figure represents the Trigon of Diurnal and Nocturnal Arcs. These are drawn upon Sun-Dials by Curve Lines, like the Arcs of the Signs, and by means of them the Shadow of the Style shews how many Hours the Sun is above the Horizon, in any given Day, that is, the Length of the Day, and consequently the Length of the Night too, for this is the Complement of that to 24 Hours.

The Trigon of Signs is the same for all Latitudes, since the Sun's Declination is the same for all the Earth; but the Diurnal Arcs are different for every particular Latitude, and we draw as many of these Arcs upon a Dial, as there are Hours of Difference between the longest and shortest Days of the Year.

Fig. 2.   Now to construct the Trigon of Diurnal Arcs upon Brass or any other solid Matter, first draw the right Line R Z for the Radius of the Hour-Line of 12, or of the Equinoctial, and about the Point R, with any Opening of your Compasses taken at pleasure, describe the circular

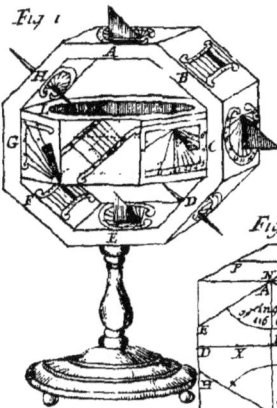

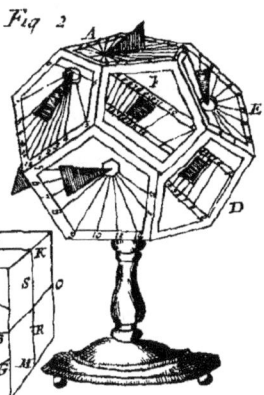

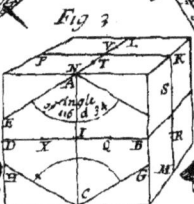

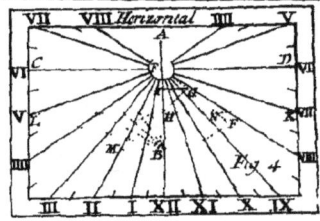

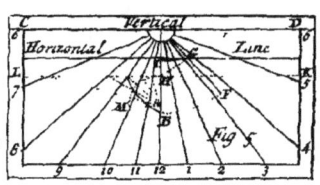

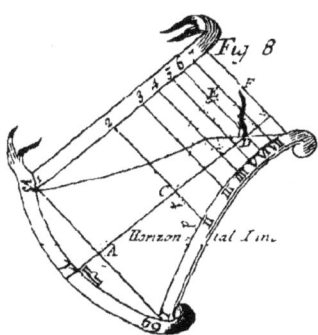

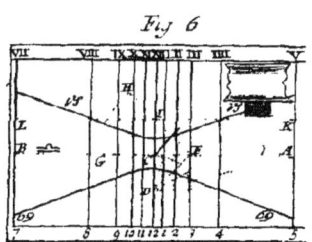

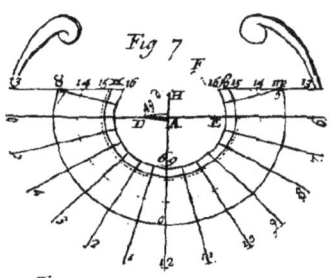

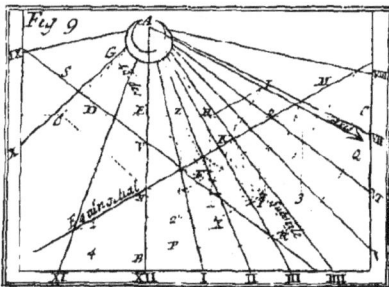

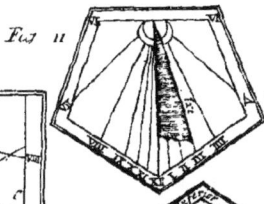

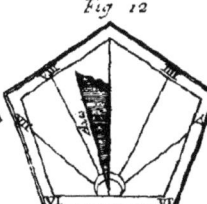

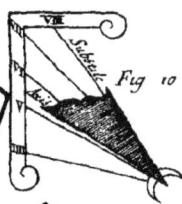

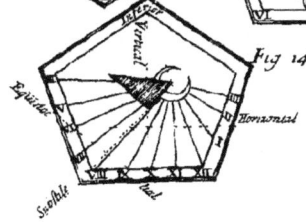

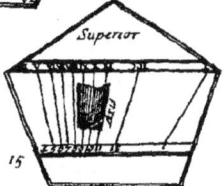

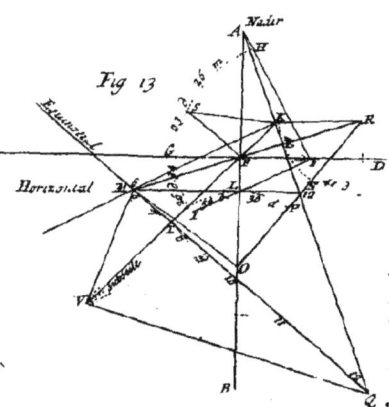

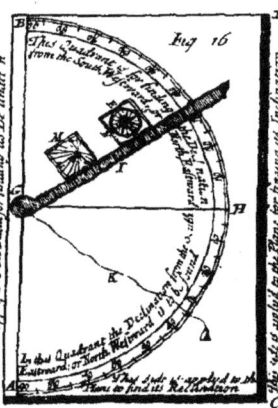

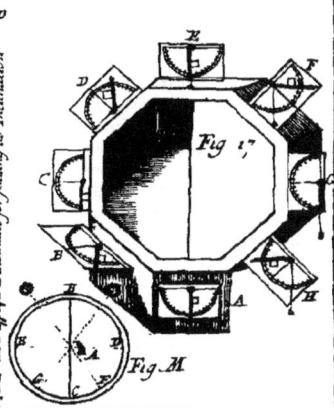

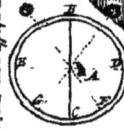

Plate XXII

fronting page 212

Circular Arc T S V, and lay off both ways thereon from the Point S, two Arcs, each equal to the Complement of the Latitude For example, if the Latitude be 49 deg make the Arcs S V, and S T, of 41 deg each. This being done, draw the right Line T X V, and about the Point X, as a Center, deſcribe the Circumference of a Circle T Z V Y, which divide into 48 equal Parts by dotted Lines, drawn parallel to the Radius of the Equinoctial R Z : then theſe Lines will cut the Diameter T X V in Points, thro which and the Point R, you may draw the Radius's of the Hours And ſince the longeſt Day at *Paris* is 16 Hours, and the ſhorteſt 8, you need but draw four Radius's on one Side the Line R Z, and a like Number on the other Side.

Moreover, the Angles that all the Radius's make at the Point R may be found Trigonometrically, by the following Analogy, *viz.* As Radius is to the Tangent Complement of the Latitude, ſo is the Tangent of the Difference between the Semidiurnal Arc at the time of the Equinox and the Arc propoſed, to the Tangent of the Sun's requiſite Declination. For example, Suppoſe it be required to draw upon the Trigon the diurnal Arc of 11 or 13 Hours, the Semidiurnal Arc is 5 ½ Hours, or 6 ½ Hours, and the Day of the Equinox the diurnal Arc is 12 Hours, and conſequently the Semidiurnal Arc is 6 Hours, and the Difference is half an Hour . therefore Radius muſt be put for the firſt Term of the Analogy, the Tangent of 41 deg (*viz.* the Complement of the Latitude of *Paris*) for the ſecond Term, and the Sine of 7 deg 30 min for the third Term Now the fourth Term being found, the Sun's Declination is 6 deg 28 min South, when the Day at *Paris* is 11 Hours long, and 6 deg 28 min North, when the Day is 13 Hours, and making three other Analogies, you will find that the Declination of the diurnal Arc of 10 Hours and 14 Hours, is 12 deg 41 min of 9 Hours and 15 Hours, 18 deg. 25 min. and of 8 Hours and 16 Hours, 23 deg 30 min

Of the Trigon with an Index

The third Figure repreſents the Trigon of Signs put upon a Rule or Index A, in order to draw the Arcs of the Signs upon great Dials The diurnal Arcs may be drawn likewiſe upon this Trigon, but the Arcs of the Signs and diurnal Arcs too muſt not be drawn upon one and the ſame Dial, for avoiding Confuſion In the Center of the Index there is a little hole thro which is put a Pin, that ſo the Inſtrument may turn about the Center of a Dial The Trigon ſlides along the Index, and may be fixed in any part thereof by means of the Screw B. The Arcs of the Signs with their Characters are round about the Circumference, and there is a fine Thread fixed in the Center thereof, in order to extend over the Radii quite to the Hour-Lines of a Dial, as we ſhall by and by explain Fig 3

The fourth Figure repreſents one half of a Horizontal Dial, having the Morning Hour-Lines to 12 a-clock thereon, and the Equinoctial Line C D This being enough of the Dial, for explaining the Manner of drawing the Arcs of the Signs thereon, by means of Figure 5, which repreſents a Trigon of Signs drawn upon a Plate, on which the Hour-Lines of an Horizontal Dial are adjuſted in the following manner Fig 4

Take the Length of the Axis V R of the Horizontal Dial between your Compaſſes, and lay it off on the Axis of the Trigon from O to C, after this, take the Diſtance from the Center V of the Dial to the Point C, wherein the Equinoctial Line cuts the Hour-Line of 12, and lay it off on the Trigon from C to *a*, and draw lightly the Line *c a* 12, cutting all the ſeven Lines of the Trigon This being done, take upon this Line the Diſtance from the Point *c* to the Interſection of the Summer Tropick, and lay it off from the Center V of the Dial on the Hour-Line of 12, and you will have one Point thro which the Summer Tropick muſt paſs, likewiſe take the Diſtance from the Point *c* to the Interſection of the Parallel of ♊, and lay it off on the Hour-Line of 12, from the Center of the Dial, and you will have a Point on the ſaid Hour-Line thro which the Parallel of ♊ muſt paſs, likewiſe aſſume all the other Diſtances on the Trigon, and lay them off ſucceſſively on the Hour-Line of 12 of the Dial, from the Center to the Point thro which the Winter Tropick paſſes, which muſt be the moſt diſtant from the Center of the Dial, and you will have the Points in the Hour-Line of 12 thro which each of the Parallels of the Signs muſt paſs And by proceeding in this manner with the other Hour-Lines, you will have Points in them thro which the Parallels of the Signs muſt paſs For example, Aſſume on the Hour-Line of 11 of the Dial, the Diſtance from the Center thereof to the Point wherein the Equinoctial Line cuts it, and lay this Diſtance off upon the Trigon from *c* towards *a*, and draw the right Ligne C 11, then take the Diſtances from the Point *c* to the Interſection of each of the Parallels of the Signs, and lay them off from the Center of the Dial, on the Hour-Line of 11, to the Points 2 2, &c and thoſe will be Points in the Hour-Line of 11, thro which the Parallels of the Signs muſt paſs. Underſtand the ſame for others

But becauſe the Hour-Line of 6 is parallel to the Equinoctial Line, make this likewiſe parallel to the Radius of the Equinoctial *o a* on the Trigon and to prick down the Line for the Hour of ſeven in the Evening, deſcribe an Arc about the Point C, as a Center, from the Line for the Hour of 6 to that for the Hour of 5, and lay off that Arc on the other ſide of the Line for the Hour of 6, and then you may draw the Hour-Line of 7, which will not meet the Summer Tropick Finally, The Line for the Hour of 8 muſt make the ſame Angle with the Line of the Hour of 6, as the Line for the Hour of 4 does; but

but it is uſeleſs to draw this Line for the Latitude of 49 deg becauſe this Line being parallel to the Tropick of ♋, cannot cut any one Radius of the Signs Now the Points thro
which the Arcs of the Signs muſt paſs, being found on the Hour-Lines of the Dial, you muſt
join all thoſe that appertain to the ſame Sign with an even hand, and you will have the Curved
Arcs of the Signs, whoſe Characters muſt be marked upon the Dial, as *per* Figure   *Note,*
We ſometimes ſet down the Names of the Months, and of ſome remarkable moveable Feaſts
upon the Dial   The Arcs of the Signs are drawn upon vertical Dials in this manner, but
here the Winter Tropick muſt be nigheſt to the Center of the Dial, and the Summer Tropick
furtheſt diſtant from it

It the Arcs of the Signs or diurnal Arcs are to be drawn upon a great Dial, the third Figure muſt be uſed in the following manner ·

Fig. 6

Faſten the Rule or Index to the Center of the Dial by a Pin, ſo that it may
be turned and fixed upon any Hour-Line, as may be ſeen in Figure 6 then having fixed the Center of the Trigon upon the Index, at a Diſtance from the Center
of the Index equal to the Diſtance from the Center of the Dial to the Extremity of the
Axis thereof, by means of the Screw R, take the Thread in one Hand, and with the other
raiſe or lower the Inſtrument upon the Plane of the Dial, ſo that the Thread extended
along the Radius of the Equinoctial of the Trigon, meets the Point wherein ſome Hour-
Line cuts the Equinoctial Line of the Dial, and in this Situation fix the Index   This being
done, extend the Thread along the Radius's of the Trigon, and prick down the Points upon
each Hour-Line of the Dial, thro which the Parallels of the Signs muſt paſs, both above and
below the Equinoctial Line, as we have done on the Hour-Line of 12 of the Dial repreſented in Figure 6   And if you do thus on all the Hour-Lines ſucceſſively one after the other,
and the Points marked thereon appertaining to the ſame Sign, be joined by an even Hand,
you will have the Parallels of the Signs upon the Surface of the Dial   But to make the
Points on the Hour-Line of 6, the Inſtrument muſt be turned ſo that the Fiducial Line of
the Index be upon the Hour-Line of 12, and the Radius of the Equinoctial Circle of the
Trigon parallel to the Hour-Line of 6   The Inſtrument being thus fixed, extend the
Thread along the Radius's of the Signs, until it cuts the Hour-Line of 6, and the Points
where it cuts the ſaid Hour-Line, will be thoſe thro which the Parallels of the Signs muſt
paſs in that Hour-Line

When the Arcs of the Signs are drawn on one ſide of the Dial, for example, on the
Morning Hour-Lines, you may lay off the ſame Diſtances from the Center on the Hour-Lines
of the other ſide the Meridian, as the Points denoted on the Hour-Line of 11 muſt be laid
off on the Hour-Line of 1, thoſe on the Hour-Line of 10 on the Hour-Line of 2; and ſo
draw the Arcs of the Signs on the other ſide of the Meridian   *Note,* The Arcs of the Signs
are drawn upon declining Dials in the ſame manner, it the Subſtylar Line be made uſe of inſtead of the Meridian, and the Diſtances from the Center be taken equal upon thoſe Hour-
Lines equally diſtant on both ſides of the Subſtyle from it

It the diurnal Arcs are to be pricked down upon a Dial inſtead of the Arcs of the Signs,
that is, the Length of the Days, we may likewiſe put thereon the Hour of the Sun's riſing
and ſetting, it the Length of the Day be divided into two equal Parts   For example, when
the Day is 15 Hours long, the Sun ſets half an Hour paſt 7 in the Afternoon, and riſes half
an Hour paſt 4 in the Morning, and ſo of others

It the Arcs of the Signs are to be drawn upon Equinoctial Dials, as on that of Figure 7,
Plate 22, take the length of the Axis of the Style A D, and lay it off upon the Axis of the
Trigon (of Figure 5 *Plate* 23) from O to P, and draw the Line P N parallel to the Radius of the Equinoctial, this ſhall cut the Summer Tropick and two other Parallels then
take the Diſtance from the Point P to the Interſection of the Tropick of ♋, and with that
Diſtance about the Center A of the Dial draw a Circle, which ſhall repreſent the Tropick of
♋   Take likewiſe the two other Diſtances on the Parallel of the Trigon, and draw two
other Circles about the Center of the Dial, the one for the Parallel of ♊ and ♌, and the
other for that of ♉ and ♍, which may be drawn upon an upper Equinoctial Dial   But if
this was an under Equinoctial Dial, then the above deſcribed Circles would repreſent the
Parallels of ♏, ♐, ♑, ♒ and ♓. but as for the Parallels of ♈ and ♎, they cannot be drawn
upon Equinoctial Dials, becauſe when the Sun is in the Plane of the Celeſtial Equator, his
Rays fall parallel to the Surfaces of Equinoctial Dials, and the Shadows of their Styles are
indefinitely protended.

The Horizontal Line is thus drawn · Firſt lay off the Style's length on the Hour-Line of
6, and about the Extremity D thereof, deſcribe the Arc E F (upwards for an upper Dial)
equal to the Latitude, *viz* 49 deg for *Paris*, and draw the Line D F, which ſhall cut the
Meridian in the Point H, thro which the Horizontal Line muſt be drawn parallel to the
Hour-Line of 6, as may be ſeen in Figure 7, *Plate* 22

The Uſe of this Line is to ſhew the riſing and ſetting of the Sun at his entrance into
the beginning of each Sign   For example, becauſe it cuts the Tropick of *Cancer* on the
Dial, in Points thro which the Hour-Line of 4 in the Morning, and 8 in the Evening paſſes,
therefore the Sun riſes the Day of the Solſtice at 4 in the Morning, and ſets at 8 in the
Evening at *Paris*.   Underſtand the ſame of others

To draw the Arcs of the Signs upon Polar Dials.

The Dial being drawn, (as appears in *Fig 6 Plate* 22) the dotted Radii of the Hours continued out till they meet the Equinoctial Line must be laid off successively upon the Radius of the Equinoctial of the Trigon of Signs (*Figure 5 Plate* 23) for drawing as many Perpendiculars thereon as there are dotted Radii, viz. one for the Hour of 12, and the five others for the Hours of 1, 2, 3, 4 and 5, which shall cut the Radii of the Signs of the Trigon This being done, take the Distances from the Radius or the Equinoctial of the Trigon upon the said Perpendiculars, to the Radius's of the other Signs, and lay them off upon the Hour-Lines of the Dial on both sides the Equinoctial Line A B For example ; Take the Distance 12 ♈, and lay it off on the Dial from the Point C upon the Hour-Line of 12, and you will have two Points in the said Line thro which the Tropicks must pass Likewise take the Space on the Trigon upon the Line 5 ♈ or ♋, and lay it off upon the Hour-Lines of 5 and 7 on both sides the Equinoctial Line of your Dial, and you will have Points in the Hour-Lines of 5 and 7, thro which the Tropicks must pass And in this manner may Points be found in the other Hour-Lines thro which the said Tropicks must pass , as also the Points in the Hour-Lines thro which the Parallels of the other Signs must be drawn, which being found must be joined   *Note*, We have only drawn the two Tropicks in the figure of this Dial for avoiding Confusion And the Parallels of the Northern Signs must be drawn underneath the Equinoctial Line, and the Southern Signs above it Also the diurnal Arcs are drawn in the same manner as the Arcs of the Signs are

How to draw the Arcs of the Signs upon East and West Dials

The Arcs of the Signs are drawn nearly in the same manner upon East and West Dials as upon Polar ones for example, let it be required to draw the Arcs of the Signs upon the West Dial of *Figure 8 Plate* 22 the dotted Radii of the Hours produced to the Equinoctial Line C D, must be laid off upon the Trigon of *Figure 1* (*Plate* 23) from the Point *a* upon the Radius of the Equinoctial, that so Perpendiculars may be drawn upon the Trigon cutting the Radius's of the Signs ; after this, you must take upon the said Perpendiculars the Distances from the Radius of the Equinoctial to the Intersection of the other Signs, and lay them off upon the Hour-Lines of the Dial, on both sides the Equinoctial Line For example, take the Space 6 ♈, or 6 ♋, and lay it off on both sides the Point D upon the Hour-Line of 6 on the Dial Proceed in this manner for finding Points in the other Hour-Lines thro which the Curve Parallels of the Signs must be drawn with an even Hand, so that the Northern ones be under the Equinoctial Line, and the Southern ones above it *Note*, The diurnal Arcs are drawn in the same manner , and we have only drawn the two Tropicks thereon for avoiding Confusion

The Construction of a Horizontal Dial, having the Italian *and* Babylonian *Hours , as also the Almacanters and Meridians described upon it*

Having already shewed the manner of pricking down the Astronomical Hours upon Sun-Dials, as also the Diurnal Arcs, and Arcs of the Signs, there may yet be several other Circles of the Sphere represented upon Dials, being pleasant and useful, which the Shadow of the Extremity of the Style passes over , as the *Italian* and *Babylonian* Hours, the Azimuths, the Almacanters, and the Meridians of principal Cities

The first Line of the *Italian* and *Babylonian* Hours is the Horizon, like as the first Line of the Astronomical Hours is the Meridian , for the *Italians* begin to reckon their Hours when the Center of the Sun touches the Horizon at his setting, and the *Babylonians* when he touches the Horizon at his rising

A general Method for drawing the Italian *and* Babylonian *Hours upon all kinds of Dials*

The Astronomical Hour-Lines, and the Equinoctial Line being drawn, as also a Diurnal Fig. 7. Arc or Parallel of the Sun's rising for any Hour, at pleasure, as, for the Hour of 4 at *Paris*, which Arc will be the same as the Summer Tropick, you may find two Points (as we shall shew here) in each of the aforesaid Lines, viz. one in the Equinoctial Line, and the other in the Diurnal Arc drawn, by means of which it will not be difficult to prick down the *Italian* and *Babylonian* Hour-Lines, because they being the common Sections of great Circles of the Sphere and a Dial-Plane, will be represented in right Lines thereon

Now suppose it be required to draw the first *Babylonian* Hour Line upon the Horizontal Dial of Figure 7, first consider that when the Sun is in the Equinoctial he rises at 6, and at 7 he has been up just an Hour, whence it follows, that the first *Babylonian* Hour-Line must pass thro the Point wherein the Astronomical Hour-Line of 7 cuts the Equinoctial Line, the second thro the Intersection of the Hour-Line of 8 , the third thro that of the Hour-Line of 9, and so of others

But when the Sun rises at 4 in the Morning, the Point in the Tropick of ♋, wherein the Hour-Line of 5 cuts it, is that thro which the first *Babylonian* Hour-Line must pass; the Intersection of the Hour-Line of 6 in the said Tropick, that thro which the second *Babylonian* Hour-Line must pass , the Intersection of the Hour-Line of 7 with the said Tropick, that Point thro which the third *Babylonian* Hour-Line must pass, and so of others Then if a

O o o   Ruler

Ruler be laid to the Point wherein the Hour-Line of 5 cuts the Tropick of *Cancer*, and on the Point in the Equinoctial Line cut by the Hour-Line of 7, and you draw a right Line thro them, this Line will reprefent the firft *Babylonian* Hour-Line. Proceeding in this manner for the other *Babylonian* Hour-Lines, you will find that the 8th *Babylonian* Hour-Line will pafs thro the Point the Tropick of *Cancer* is cut by the Aftronomical Hour-Line of 12, and the Point in the Equinoctial cut by the Hour-Line of 12, and the 5th *Babylonian* Hour-Line thro the Point in the faid Tropick cut by the Hour-Line of 7 in the Evening, and the Point in the Equinoctial Line cut by the Hour-Line of 5

One of the *Babylonian* Hour-Lines being drawn, it is afterwards eafy to draw all the others, becaufe they proceed orderly from one Aftronomical Hour-Line to the other, on the Parallel and the Equinoctial Line, as appears *per* Figure Finally, The Sun fets at the 16th *Babylonian* Hour, when the Day is 16 Hours long · he fets at the 12th when he is in the Equinoctial, and at the 8th when the Night is 16 Hours long, becaufe he always rifes at the 24th *Babylonian* Hour

You muft reafon nearly in the fame manner for pricking down the *Italian* Hour-Lines Here we always reckon the Sun to fet at the 24th Hour, and confequently, in Summer, when the Nights are but 8 Hours long, he rifes at the 8th *Italian* Hour; at the Time of the Equinox he rifes at the 12th *Italian* Hour, and in Winter, when the Nights are 16 Hours long, he rifes at the 16th *Italian* Hour and therefore the Hour-Line of the 23d *Italian* Hour muft pafs thro the Interfection of the Aftronomical Hour-Line of 7, and the Summer Tropick the Interfection of the Hour-Line of 5, and the Equinoctial Line, and the Interfection of the Hour-Line of 3, and the Winter Tropick But two of the faid Points are fufficient for drawing the faid *Italian* Hour-Line The 22d *Italian* Hour-Line paffes thro the Interfection of the Hour-Line of 6 in the Evening, and Summer Tropick, the Interfection of the Hour-Line of 4, and the Equinoctial Line, and the Interfection of the Hour-Line of 2, and the Winter Tropick. Proceeding on thus, you will find that the 18th *Italian* Hour-Line paffes thro the Points of the 12th Equinoctial Hour, that is, at the Time of the Equinox, it is Noon at the 18th *Italian* Hour, whereas at the Time of the Summer Solftice it is Noon at the 16th *Italian* Hour, and at the Winter Solftice it is Noon at the 20th *Italian* Hour, in all Places where the Pole is elevated 49 Degrees, as may be feen in the following Table

A TABLE *for drawing the* Babylonian *and* Italian *Hour-Lines upon* Dials.

Babylonian Hours	1	2	3	4	5	6	7	8.	9.	10	11	12	13	14	15	16
Paffing in the ♋ ♈ thro Parallel of ♑	5	6	7	8	9	10	11	12	1	2.	3	4	5	6	7	8
	7.	8	9	10	11	12	1	2	3	4	5	6	7	8	9	10
	9	10	11	12	1	2	3	4	5.	6	7	8	9	10	11	12
Italian Hours	23.	22	21	20	19	18	17	16	15	14	13	12	11	10	9	8
Paffing in the ♋ ♈ thro Parallel of ♑	7	6.	5.	4	3	2.	1	12.	11	10	9.	8.	7	6	5	4
	5.	4	3	2	1	12	11	10	9	8.	7	6.	5	4	3	2.
	3	2	1	12	11	10.	9	8.	7.	6	5	4	3	2.1.12		

The Ufe of the *Italian* Hour-Lines upon a Dial may be to find the Time of the Sun's fetting, in fubftracting the *Italian* Hour prefent from 24, and by the *Babylonian* Hours may be known the Time of the Sun's rifing

How to draw the Almacanters, and the Azimuths

Fig 7.
    The Almacanters or Circles of Altitude are reprefented upon the Horizontal Dial by concentrick Circles, and the Azimuths by right Lines terminating at the Foot of the Style B, which reprefents the Zenith, and is the common Center of all the Almacanters and therefore you need but divide the Meridian B XII into Degrees, the Extremity of the Style C being the Center, and the Tangents of thofe Degrees on the Meridian will be the Semidiameters of the Almacanters, which fhall terminate at the two Tropicks Now to find thefe Tangents, you may ufe a Quadrant like that of Figure 8 in this manner Lay off the Length of the Style C B from A to H, and draw the Line H I parallel to the Side A C of the Quadrant; then will this Line be divided into a Line of Tangents by Radii drawn from the Center A to the Degrees of the Limb. And thefe Tangents may be taken between your Compaffes, and laid off upon the Meridian Line B XII in fuch manner, that the 90th Degree anfwers to the Point B. But fince this Dial is made for the Latitude of 49 deg and fo confequently the Sun in his greateft Altitude there, is but 64 deg. 30 min you need only prick down this greateft Altitude, which will terminate at the Summer Tropick

This

'This being done, if one of the Circles of Altitude be divided into every 10th deg beginning from the Meridian B XII which is the 90th Azimuth, and thro these Points of Division right Lines are drawn to the Foot of the Style B these right Lines will represent the Azimuths or vertical Circles. We have not drawn them upon the Dial, for avoiding Confusion, but they may be eafily conceived

Now the Use of the Almacanters is to fhew the Sun's Altitude above the Horizon at any time, and of the Azimuths, to fhew what Azimuth or vertical Circle the Sun is in and this is known by obferving what Circle of Altitude or Azimuth Line, the Shadow of the Extremity of the Style of the Dial falls upon.

How to draw the Meridians or Circles of Terreftial Longitude upon the Horizontal Dial.

About the Point D, the Center of the Equinoctial Circle, defcribe the Circumference of Fig. 7. a Circle, and divide it into 360 equal Parts or Degrees, or only into 36 Parts, for every 10th Degree, then from the Hour-Line of 12, which reprefents the Meridian of the Place for which the Dial is made, viz *Paris*, count 20 deg Weftward for its Longitude, or Diftance from the firft Meridian paffing thro the Point G, on which having wrote the Number 360, prolong the Line G D to E, in the Equinoctial Line, and afterwards from the Center A draw the firft Meridian thro E, which paffes thro the Ifland *de Fer*, and fo of others But it will be eafier to draw the Meridians eaftwardly for every 5th or 10th Degree, and place thofe principal Cities upon them whofe Longitudes you know as, for example, *Rome* is 10 ½ deg more eaftwardly than *Paris*, *Vienna* 15 deg more eaftwardly than the faid City of *Paris*, and fo of other eminent Cities, whofe Differences of Meridians from that of *Paris*, are known by a good Globe, or Map, made according to the exact Obfervations of the Academy of Sciences

The Ufe of thefe Meridians on the Dial, is, to tell at any time when the Sun fhines thereon, what Hour then it is under any one of the faid Meridians, in adding to the time of Day at *Paris*, (for which the Dial is made) as many Hours as there are times 15 deg of Difference between the Meridians, and 4 min of an Hour for every Degree

For example, When it is Noon by this Dial at *Paris*, it will be One a-clock at *Vienna*, becaufe this City is more to the Eaft than *Paris* by 15 deg and confequently receives the Sun's Light fooner than *Paris* does And at *Rome* it will be 42 min paft 12, becaufe it is 10 ½ deg more eaftward than *Paris*, and fo of others Thefe Lines of Longitude reprefent the Meridians of the Places attributed to them, fo that when the Shadow of the Style falls upon any one of them, it will be Noon under that Meridian

---

C H A P. IV.

Of the Conftruction and Ufes of Inftruments for drawing Dials upon different Planes.

THE eighth Figure reprefents a Quadrant made of Brafs or any folid Matter, of a big- Fig. 8 nefs at pleafure, having the Limb divided into 90 Degrees The Ufe of this Quadrant may be to find the Lengths of Tangents, and by this means to divide a right Line into Degrees, as we did the Meridian of the Horizontal Dial (Fig 7) we may find likewife thereon the Divifions of the Equinoctial Line thro which the Hour-Lines muft pafs, in regular Dials, as alfo in declining Dials, if the Subftyle falls exactly upon a compleat Hour-Line, by laying off the Length of the Radius of the Equinoctial Circle, from the Center A to H or L, and drawing a right Line, as H I or L M, parallel to the Radius of the Quadrant A C For example, the Length L 1 or 11, anfwering to 15 deg of the Quadrant, fhall be the Tangent of the firft Hour-Line's diftance from the Meridian or Subftyle of the Dial, which being laid off upon the Equinoctial Line, whofe Radius is fuppofed equal to A L, will determine a Point therein thro which the faid Hour-Line muft be drawn L 12, anfwering to 30 deg of the Limb of the Quadrant, will be the Tangent of the fecond Hour-Line's diftance from the Meridian or Subftyle L 3, the Tangent of 45 deg will be that of the third Now if by this means you draw the Hour-Lines of three Hours fucceffively on each fide the Meridian or Subftyle, which in all make fix Hours fucceffively; thefe are fufficient for finding the Hour-Lines of the other Hours, according to the Method before explained in fpeaking of declining Dials, and which may be even applied to all regular Dials For example, If the Hour-Lines of fix Hours fucceffive be drawn upon an Horizontal Dial, as, from 9 in the Morning to 3 in the Afternoon, you may draw all the other Hour-Lines of the Dial by the aforefaid Method, as the Hour-Lines of 7 and 8 in the Morning, and 4 and 5 in the Afternoon, whofe Points in the Equinoctial Line are

some-

sometimes troublesome to be pricked down, and principally the Points of the Hour-Lines of 5 and 7, because of the Lengths of their Tangents

The Hour-Lines found by the abovesaid Method, which we shall not here repeat, will serve for finding of others , and these which are last found being produced beyond the Center, will give the opposite ones

The said Quadrant will serve moreover as a Portable Dial, since the Hour-Lines may be drawn upon it by means of a Table of the Sun's Altitude above the Horizon of the Place for which the Dial is to be made   See more of this in the next Chapter

The Construction of a moveable Horizontal Dial

Fig. 9.

This Instrument is composed of two very smooth and even Plates of Brass, or other solid Matter, adjusted upon each other, and joined together by means of a round Rivet in the Center A   The undermost Plate is square, the Length of the Side thereof being from 6 to 8 Inches, and is divided into twice 90 Degrees , by means of which, the Declinations of Planes may be taken   The upper Plate is round, being about 8 Lines shorter in Diameter than is the Length of the Side of the under Plate, and having a little Index joined to the Hour-Line of 12, shewing the Degree of a Plane's Declination

About the Center A is drawn an Horizontal Dial upon the upper Plate, for the Latitude of the Place it is to be used in, and the Axis B is so adjusted, that the Point thereof terminates in the Center A, wherein a small Hole is made for a Thread to come thro   There is also a Compass D fastened to this upper Plate, having a Line in the bottom of the Box, shewing the Variation of the Needle

The Use of the moveable Horizontal Dial

The Use of this Instrument is for drawing Dials upon any Planes, of whatsoever Situations , (as on declining inclining Planes, or both) in the following manner .

First draw a Horizontal or level Line upon the proposed Plane , place that side of the Square along this Line, whereon is wrote *the Side applied to the Wall*, and turn the Horizontal Dial till the Needle settles itself over the Line of Declination in the bottom of the Box ·
then extend the Thread along the Axis of the Dial till it meets the Plane, and the Point wherein it meets the said Plane will be the Center of the Dial   This being done, extend the Thread along each of the Hour-Lines of the Horizontal Dial that the Plane can receive, and mark the Points on the Horizontal Line upon the Plane, cut by the Thread   then if Lines be drawn from the Center found on the Plane thro each of those Points, those will be the respective Hour-Lines that the Thread was extended along on the Horizontal Dial, and must have the same Figures set to them   *Note,* If the Dial be vertical, not having any Declination, the Hour-Line of 12 will be perpendicular to the Horizontal Line of the Plane.

The Substylar Line is drawn thro the Center of the Plane, and the Angular Point of a Square, one Side whereof being laid along the Horizontal Line, and the other Side touching the Style of the Horizontal Dial.

Again, The Distance from the Side of the Square laid along the Plane to the Axis, is the Length of the right Style, which being laid along in the same Place at right Angles to the Substyle, you may draw the Axis from the Center to the Extremity thereof, which may be formed on the Plane by means of an Iron Rod, parallel to the Situation of the Thread extended along the Axis of the Horizontal Dial, and must be sustained by a Prop planted in the Plane perpendicular to the Substyle

If you have a mind to have a right Style only, some Point must be sought in the Substyle distant from the Center of the Dial, proportional to the bigness of the Dial, and an Iron-Rod must be set up perpendicularly therein   but the Point of this Rod must touch the Thread extended along the Axis   Finally, You may give what Figure you please to the Dial, and produce the Hour-Lines as is necessary, according to the bigness of the Plane. If a great Dial is to be drawn, you may place the Instrument at a Distance from the Plane it is to be drawn on ; but then you must take care that it be very level, and the Side thereof parallel to the Plane   And if North Dials are to be drawn, having first found the Declination of the Plane, for example, 45 deg North-westwardly, place the Index of the Dial over the Degree of the opposite Declination on the square Plate, *viz* over 45 deg South-eastwardly, then invert the whole Instrument, and extend the Thread along the Axis, that so the Center of the Dial may be found upon the Plane underneath the Horizontal Line, on which having pricked down the Points thro which the Hour-Lines must pass, you may draw them to the Center, and then proceed as before

The Construction of the Sciaterra

Fig. 10.

This Instrument is composed of an Equinoctial Circle A, made of Brass or any other solid Matter, adjusted upon a Quadrant B   The Point of the Hour of 12 of this Equinoctial Circle is fastened to one end of the Quadrant, and a little Steel Cylinder about two Lines in Diameter, serving for an Axis, and going thro the Center of the Equinoctial Circle, is so fixed to the other end C of the Quadrant, as to keep the said Equinoctial Circle fixed at right Angles to the Quadrant.

The

The Quadrant is divided into 90 deg. and is made to slide on the Top of the Piece L, according to different Elevations of the Pole The little Ball G is hung at the end of a Thread, whose other end is fastened to the Top of an upright Line on the Piece L, and so by means of this, and the Ball and Socket H, the Instrument may be set upright. The Piece I is of Steel, and the end thereof is forced into a Wall or Plane, to support the whole Instrument when it is to be used The Figure D is the Trigon of Signs put on the Axis, and turns about the same by means of a Ferril. This Trigon has a Thread F fastened to the Extremity thereof, and there is another Thread E fastened to the Center of the Dial. But note, we do not place the Trigon upon the Axis, unless when the Arcs of the Signs are to be drawn upon Dials

The Use of the Sciaterra.

You must first force the Steel Point I, into the Wall or Plane whereon a Dial is to be drawn, and place the Quadrant to the Degree of the Elevation of the Pole then you must take a Square Compass, and lay the Side thereof along the Plane of the Quadrant, and turn the Instrument until the Needle fixes itself directly over the Line of Declination, or if you have not a Compass when the Sun shines, and the Hour of the Day is known, turn the Instrument till the Shadow of the Axis falls upon the Hour of the Day upon the Equinoctial Circle

The Instrument being thus disposed, extend the Thread E from the Center along the Axis till it meets the Wall or Plane proposed, and there make a Point for the Center of the Dial: then extending the said Thread over each Hour of the Equinoctial, note the Points wherein it meets the Wall or Plane, and draw Lines from the Center (before found) thro them, and those will be the Hour-Lines After this, you may give the Dial what Figure you please, and set the same Figures upon the Hour-Lines as are upon the correspondent Hours of the Equinoctial Circle Note, The Style is set up in the manner we have mentioned in speaking of the moveable Horizontal Dial

If the Arcs of the Signs, or diurnal Arcs, are to be drawn upon the Dial, you must put the Ferril at the end of the Trigon upon the Axis, and fix it over each Hour of the Equinoctial one after another by means of the Screw . then extending the Thread F along the Lines appertaining to each Sign, mark as many Points on each Hour-Line on the Wall or Plane, and join them by curve Lines, which shall form the Arcs of the Signs, whereon must be set their respective Characters

The Arcs of the Signs may be otherwise drawn in the following manner : The Axis of the Dial being well fixed, chuse a Point in the same for the Extremity of the right Style, representing the Center of the Earth , and upon this Axis put the Ferril of the Trigon in such manner, that the Extremity of the right Style exactly answers to the Vertex of the Trigon, representing the Center of the Equinoctial and the World Then having fixed the Trigon by means of the Screw pressing against the Axis, turn it so that one of the Planes thereof (for the Signs ought to be drawn upon both sides) falls exactly upon the Hour-Lines one after another, and extend the Thread F along the Radius's of the Signs on the Trigon, and by means thereof mark Points upon each Hour-Line of the Wall or Plane and if these Points be joined, we shall have the Arcs of the Signs

Proceed thus for drawing North Dials, as likewise inclining and declining Dials, in observing to invert the Instrument when the Centers of the Dials are downwards.

The Construction of M Pardie's Sciaterra

This Instrument, which is made of Brass or other solid Matter, of a bigness at pleasure, Fig. 11. consists of four principal Pieces or Parts The first is a very even square Plate D, called the Horizontal Plane, because it is placed horizontal or level when using, having a round Hole E in the middle, wherein is placed a Pivot, upon which turns the second Piece, called the Meridional Plane, in such manner that the said Piece is always at right Angles to the Horizontal Plane On the narrow side C of this Piece is fastened a Plumb-Line, whose use is for placing the Instrument level The Top of this Piece is cut away into a concave Quadrant, both sides of which are divided into 90 deg beginning from the Perpendicular answering to the middle of the Pivot, and there is a pretty deep slit made down the middle of this Quadrant to receive a prominent Piece of a Semi-circle H, which is the third principal part, that so the said Semi-circle may be in the same Plane as the second Piece is, and likewise be raised or lowered according to different Elevations of the Pole The Diameter of this Semi-circle is called the Axis, and the Center thereof is simply called the Center of the Instrument, like as the Thread fastened thereto is called the central Thread The fourth Piece A is a very even Circle, both sides thereof being divided into 24 equal Parts, for the 24 Hours of the Day , and this is fixed at right Angles to the Semicircle H, and so moves along with it One of the sides thereof is called the upper-side, and the other the under-side. The Trigon of Signs is drawn (in the manner before explained) upon both sides of the Semi-circle, having the Point A, the Extremity of the Diameter of the Equinoctial Circle, for the Vertex thereof

The Use of this Instrument

Having first placed the Points of ♈ and ♎ of the Semi-circle upon the Degree of the Elevation of the Pole in the Place for which you would draw a Dial, set the Instrument upon a fixed Horizontal Plane, near to the Wall or Plane you are to draw a Dial on. Then turn the Meridional Plane till the Shadow of the Equinoctial Circle falls upon the Day of the Month or Degree of the Sign on the Axis the Sun is in. This being done, the Shadow of the said Axis or Diameter of the Semi-circle H, will shew the time of Day upon the Equinoctial Circle, and the whole Instrument will be well situated, the Meridional Plane answering to the Meridian of the Heavens, the Equinoctial Circle parallel to the Celestial Equinoctial Circle, and the Axis of the Dial parallel to the Axis of the World. This being done, extend the Thread F fastened to the Center, along the Axis to the Wall or Plane you are to draw a Dial on, and the Point wherein it meets the Wall will be the Center of the Dial. The said Thread thus extended will likewise give the Position of the Style or Axis of the Dial, for if an Iron Rod be placed in the said Point of Concourse, and in the same Situation as the Thread is, this will be the Style of the Dial; but if you have a mind to have a right Style only, you need but set up a Rod in the Wall or Plane, whose end touches the Thread extended along the Axis of the Instrument, and this Rod may have what Figure you please given to it, as a Serpent or Bird, provided the Extremity of the Bill thereof meets the said Thread.

Now to mark the Hour-Lines upon the Dial, extend the Thread from the Center over the Plane of the Equinoctial Circle along the Hour-Lines thereof one after another, until it meets the Wall: then if Lines be drawn from the Center of the Dial to the said Points of Concourse, these will be the Hour-Lines. But the Hour-Lines may be otherwise pricked down in the Night, by the light of a Link or Candle; for the central Thread being first extended along the Axis, and fastened to the Wall, afterwards move the Link till the Shadow of the Axis falls upon any given Hour upon the Equinoctial Circle, and then the Shadow of the said extended Thread upon the Wall will be the same Hour-Line, and by drawing a Line upon the Wall along the same with a Pencil, that will be the Hour-Line.

Proceed thus for drawing the other Hour-Lines. *Note,* This Method of drawing Dials is a very good one, particularly when a Surface is not flat and even, or when the Center of the Dial falls at a great Distance. You must observe likewise, that the Shadow of the Axis of the Instrument shews the Time of Day on the upper-side of the Equinoctial Circle from the 20th of *March* (N S) to the 22d of *September,* and on the under-side the other six Months, and the side of the Equinoctial Circle that the Sun shines upon, must always but just touch the Center of the Semi-circle

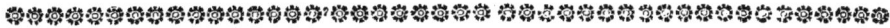

❀❀❀❀❀❀❀❀❀❀❀❀❀❀❀❀❀ ❀❀❀❀❀❀❀❀❀❀❀❀❀❀❀❀❀

CHAP. V.

Of the Construction and Uses of Portable Dials.

Of the Construction of a Globe

Fig. 12. THIS Figure represents a Globe, whereon are drawn the Meridians or Hour-Circles. There are divers sizes of them; the great ones are set up in Gardens, and are of Stone or Wood well painted, and the small ones are made of Brass, having Compasses belonging to them, and may be reckoned among the Number of Portable Dials

The manner of turning round Balls of any Matter is well known, but if a large Stone-Ball is to be made, that cannot be turned because of its Weight; first, you must roughly form it with a Chissel, and then take a wooden or brass Semi-circle of the same Diameter as you design your Ball. This being done, turn the Semi-circle about the Ball, and take away all the Superfluities with a Raspe, until the Semi-circle every where and way just touches the Superficies thereof, afterwards make it smooth with a Pumice-Stone or Sea-Dog Fish's Skin, &c.

The Globe being well rounded and made smooth, you must take the Diameter thereof with a Pair of Spheric Compasses, viz. such whose Points are crooked, which suppose the right Line A B; this Line is divided into two equal Parts in E by the vertical Line Z N, the upper Point whereof Z, represents the Zenith, and the lower one N, the Nadir. Now set one Point of the Spheric Compasses in E, and extend the other to A, and draw the Meridian Circle A Z B N; likewise setting one Foot of your Compasses in Z, with the last Opening describe the Circle A E B, representing the Horizon; and from the Point B to C count 49 deg the Elevation of the Pole on the Meridian, and setting one Foot of your Compasses in the Point C, representing the North Pole, extend the other to 41 deg on the Meridian below the Point B, and draw the Equinoctial Circle, likewise setting one Foot of your

your Compaffes, opened to the fame Diftance as before, upon the Point in the Meridian cut by the Equinoctial, you may draw the Hour-Circle of 6 paffing thro the Poles C and D By this means the Equinoctial fhall be divided into four equal Parts by the Meridian and Hour-Circle of 6, and if each of thefe four Parts be divided into fix equal Parts, for the 24 Hours of a Natural Day, and about the Points of Divifion as Centers, with the extent of a Quadrant of the Globe, Circles be defcribed, thefe will all pafs thro the Poles of the World C and D, and are the Hour-Circles. If you have a mind to have the half Hours or Quarters, each of the Divifions on the Equinoctial muft be divided into 2 or 4 equal Parts The Hour-Circles are numbered round the Equinoctial both above and below it, as appears *per* Figure

If the Parallels of the Signs are to be drawn upon the Globe, you muft count upon the Meridian both ways for the Equinoctial, the Declination for every Sign, according to the Table expreffed, as, for example, for the two Tropicks you muft count 23 deg 30 min from the Equinoctial, and about the Poles C and D, draw Circles on the Globe *Note,* The two Polar Circles muft be drawn at 23 deg 30 min from the Poles, or 66 deg 30 min from the Equinoctial

The Globe thus ordered muft be placed upon a Pedeftal proportionable to the bignefs thereof in a Hole made in the Nadir N, diftant from the Pole the Complement of its Elevation (*viz.* 41 deg) and fixed in a Garden, or elfewhere, well expofed to the Sun, fo as to be conformable to the Sphere of the World.

But if it be a fmall Portable Globe, we place a little Compafs upon the Pedeftal thereof, that fo the Globe may be fet North and South when the Hour of the Day is to be fhewn thereby, which is fhewn thereon without a Style, by the Shadow of the fame Globe · for the Shadow or Light thereon always occupies one half of the Globe's Convexity, when the Sun fhines upon it, and fo the Extremity of the Shadow or Light fhews the Hour in two oppofite Places If, moreover, the different Countries on the Earth's Superficies, as likewife the principal Cities, are laid down upon the Globe according to their true Latitudes and Longitudes, you may difcover any Moment the Sun fhines upon the fame, by the illuminated part thereof, what Places of the Earth the Sun fhines upon, and what Places are in darknefs The Extremity of the Shadow fhews likewife what Places the Sun is rifing or fetting at, and what Places have long Days, and what have fhort Nights you may likewife diftinguifh thereon the Places towards the Poles that have perpetual Night and Day. All this is eafy to be underftood by thofe who are acquainted with the Nature of the Sphere *Note,* This Dial is the moft natural of all others, becaufe it refembles the Earth itfelf, and the Sun fhines thereon as he does on the Earth

You may find the Hour of the Day otherwife, by means of a thin brafs Semi-circle divided into twice 90 deg adjufted to the Poles or Extremes of the Axis, by help of two little Ferrils This Semi-circle being turned about the Globe with your Hand, until it only makes a perpendicular Shadow upon the Globe, reprefents the Hour-Circle wherein the Sun is, and confequently fhews the Hour of the Day, and alfo what Places of the Earth it is Noon at that Time But in this Cafe the Number 12 muft be fet to the Meridian, and the Numbers 6 and 6 to the two Points wherein the Equinoctial cuts the Horizon · and this is the reafon why we commonly place two rows of Figures along the Equinoctial The Shadow of the two ends of the Axis, if they are continued out far enough beyond the Poles, and the Hours are figured round the Polar Circles, will likewife fhew the Hour *Note,* In order to make fmall Portable Globes univerfal, we adjuft Quadrants underneath them, that fo the Pedeftal may be flid according to the Elevation of the Pole This is eafy to be underftood

The Confiruction and Ufe of the Concave and Convex Semi-cylinder

Thefe Dials, which are made of different bignefles, the fmall ones of Brafs and the great ones of Stone or Wood, are very curious on account of their fhewing the Hour of the Day without a Style Their Exactnefs confifts very much in being very round and even both within fide and without.

The 13*th* Figure reprefents one of thefe Dials, fet upon and faftened on its Pedeftal, inclining to the Horizon under an Angle equal to the Elevation of the Pole, and directly facing the South and therefore the Hour-Lines and the Edges A B, *a b*, ferving as a Style, are all parallel between themfelves, and to the Axis of the World The whole Convex Cylinder is divided into 24 equal Parts, or twice 12 Hours, by parallel Lines, and the Concave Semi-cylinder is divided in 6 equal Parts by Right Lines, which are the Hour-Lines from 6 in the Morning to 6 in the Afternoon

Now when the Sun fhines upon this Dial, the Hour of the Day is fhewn on the Convex fide thereof, by the defect of Light, that is, by a right Line feparating the Light from the Shadow. But the Hour of the Day is fhewn in the Concave part of the Dial, by the Shadow of one of the Edges A B or *a b*, fo that when the Sun in the Morning is come to the Hour-Circle of 6, the Shadow of the eaft Edge *a b* will then fall upon the other Edge A B, which is the Hour-Line of 6 · and as the Sun rifes higher above the Horizon, the Shadow of the faid Edge *a b* will defcend and fhew the Hour among the Hour-Lines (*Note,*
The

Fig. 13.

The Figures on the Top are for the Morning Hours, and thofe on the Bottom for the Afternoon ones) When the Sun is come to the Meridian, he directly fhines into the Dial, and then the Edges will caft no Shadow . but when the Sun has paffed the Meridian, and defcends weftwards, the Shadow of the oppofite Edge A B will fhew the Hour from 12 to 6 in the Evening. If you have a mind to have the halves and quarters of Hours, you need but double or quadruple the Divifions

Small Dials of this kind have Compaffes belonging to them, that fo the Dials may be fet North and South

The Confruction and Ufe of the Vertical Cylinder.

This is a vertical Dial drawn upon the Superficies of a Cylinder by means of a Table of the Sun's Altitude above the Horizon at every Hour, when he enters into every 10th Degree of the Signs, according to the Latitude of the Place for which the Dial is to be drawn, and for this end the following Table is calculated for 49 Degrees of Latitude

A TABLE of the Sun's Altitudes for every Hour of the Day at his Entrance into every 10th Degree of the Signs, for the Latitude of 49 Degrees.

Hours. Signs.	XII		XI I		X II		IX. III		VIII IV		VII V		VI VI		V. VII.	
	D	M	D	M	D	M	D	M	D	M	D	M.	D	M	D	M
30 ♋	64	30	61	56	55	19	46	35	37	1	27	10	17	30	8	21
20 10	64	9	61	33	55	1	46	18	36	42	26	54	17	10	8	4
10 20	63	2	60	31	54	1	45	28	35	5	26	6	16	20	7	12
♊ ♌	61	12	58	49	52	34	44	7	34	39	24	50	15	6	5	50
20 10	58	48	56	30	50	29	42	14	32	53	23	6	13	20	3	57
10 20	55	52	53	42	47	57	39	55	30	41	20	57	11	11	1	40
♉ ♍	52	30	50	30	45	1	37	14	28	10	18	28	8	40		
20 10	58	51	46	48	41	44	34	13	25	19	15	43	5	44		
10 20	44	58	43	12	38	15	31	0	22	18	12	48	2	59		
♈ ♎	41	0	39	20	34	37	27	38	19	9	9	47				
20 10	37	2	35	26	30	58	24	15	15	58	6	42				
10 20	33	9	31	40	27	24	20	55	12	51	3	44				
♓ ♏	29	30	28	4	23	58	17	42	9	50	0	54				
20 10	26	8	24	46	20	51	14	45	7	6						
10 20	23	12	21	52	18	5	12	12	4	43						
♒ ♐	20	48	19	30	15	48	10	3	2	42						
20 10	18	48	17	44	14	6	8	27	1	13						
10 20	17	52	16	38	13	3	7	27	0	19						
♑ 30	17	30	15	15	12	42	7	8								

We now proceed to fhew the Confruction of the aforefaid Dial upon a Plane which afterwards may be made Cylindrical, or wrapped round a Cylinder, or this Dial may be made upon the Surface of a Cylinder itfelf, if the Lines be drawn thereon as upon a Plane

Fig. 14.

Defcribe the Right-angled Parallelogram A B C D upon a brafs Plate or Sheet of Paper, whofe breadth A B or C D let be nearly equal to the Circumference of the Cylinder it is to be wrapped round, and prolong the Line A B, upon which affume A E for the length of the Style, which fhall determine the length of the Cylinder Then about the Point E, as a Center, with the Radius E A, make a circular Arc equal to the Sun's Meridian Altitude at his entrance into *Cancer*, and draw the occult Line E D, determining the length or height of the Cylinder A D, but if this length was given, and the length of the Style required, you muft defcribe an Arc about the Point D, equal to the Complement of the Sun's greateft Meridian Altitude, which, if the greateft Altitude be 64 deg 30 min. will be 25 deg 30 min and draw the occult Line D E, which fhall determine the length of the Style E A, proportioned to the length of the Cylinder

This being done, divide the Arc A F into Degrees and Minutes, and draw occult Lines thro each of the Points of Divifion, from the Center E to the Line A D, that fo this Line may

may be made a Scale of Tangents But this Line may be otherwife divided, by fuppofing the Radius A E 100 or 1000 equal Parts, according to the length of the Cylinder, and taking the correfpondent Tangents from printed Tables, and laying them off from A.

Things being thus ordered, divide the Sides A B, D C into 6 equal Parts, and join the Points of Divifion by five parallel right Lines, which will reprefent the beginnings of the twelve Signs, then trifect each of thefe parallel Spaces for the 10th and 20th Degrees of each Sign Now by this means the beginnings of the Months may be fet upon your Dial, becaufe there will be no fenfible Error in fixing the Sun's entrance into every Sign the 20th Day of every Month, (N S) Then to prick down the Hour-Points upon all thefe Lines one after another, you muft ufe the foregoing Table· for example, to prick down the Hour-Point of 10 in the Morning, or 2 in the Afternoon, upon the Line A D reprefenting the Summer Tropick, you will find by the Table, that the Sun's Altitude at the time of the Summer Solftice at the Hours of 10 or 2, is 55 deg 19 min therefore you muft take the Tangent of 55 deg 19 min from your Scale of Altitudes A D, and lay off from the Side A B upon the faid Tropick, and then you will have a Point therein thro which the propofed Hour-Line muft pafs Again, To prick down the Hour-Point of the faid Hour of 2 upon another Parallel, fuppofe on that of the 1ft Degree of *Leo* or *Gemini*, you will find by the Table that the Sun's Altitude will then be 52 deg 34 min and the Tangent of thefe Degrees being taken from the Scale of Altitudes A D, and laid off upon the faid Parallel from A B, will give a Point therein thro which the Hour-Line of 2 muft pafs And if you proceed in this manner, and find Points in the other Parallels, and likewife on their Divifions of every 10th and 20th Degree, thefe Points joined will give the Curved Hour-Line of 10 in the Morning, or 2 in the Afternoon

And thus likewife may be found Points in the Parallels thro which the other Hour-Lines muft pafs, which being done, you muft join all thofe belonging to the fame Hour by an even Hand, and mark the Characters of the Signs, the firft Letters of the Months, as likewife the Hour-Figures, each in their refpective Places, as *per* Figure, and your Dial will be finifhed, which afterwards muft be wrapped about the Cylinder, or bent Cylindrically, fo that the Lines reprefenting the two Tropicks be parallel between themfelves.

The Style is faftened to a Chapiter ferving as an Ornament, and muft be moveable on the Line A B, that fo it may be placed at right Angles on the Degree of the Sign or Day of the Month This Dial being placed upright, or hung by a Ring, turn it to the Sun, fo that the Shadow of the Style may fall down right upon the Parallel of the Day you defire to know the Hour in, and then the Extremity thereof will fhew the Hour or Part

The Sun's Altitude may be fhewn likewife by this Inftrument thus· Put the Style upon the Scale of Altitudes, keeping the Cylinder fufpended or horizontally placed, and turn it about fo that the Style be towards the Sun, then the Shadow of the Extremity thereof fhall fhew the Sun's Altitude above the Horizon

The abovefaid Parallelogram may ferve likewife as a Dial, without being wrapped round a Cylinder, or turned up Cylindrically, if the Style be fo adjufted as to flide along the Line A B, that fo it may be fet over the Day of the Month, or Parallel of the Sign the Sun is in This is eafily done, in making a little Slit along the top of the Plate, and flatting the Foot of the Style, fo that it may flide in the faid Slit without varying its length Now if this Parallelogram be placed upright, and the Line A B level (which may be eafily done by means of a Plumb-Line faftened to one of the Sides) and you hold it thus in your hand, or fufpend it by a Ring, fo that it be directly expofed to the Sun, and the Shadow of the Style falls upon the Parallel of the Sign or Month, then the Extremity of the Shadow of the faid Style will fall upon the Hour

The Conftruction and Ufe of a Dial drawn on a Quadrant

This Figure reprefents a Portable Dial drawn on a Quadrant, whofe Conftruction we have Fig 8. thought fit to lay down here, fince it is made, as well as the Cylindrical Dial, by means of a Table of the Sun's Altitude calculated for the Latitude of the Place the Dial is made for

Firft, Divide the Limb B C of the Quadrant into Degrees, and about the Center A defcribe another Arc R S, reprefenting the Tropick of ♋ Likewife divide the Radius A B nearly into 3 equal Parts, and with the Diftance A D draw a circular Arc for the Tropick of ♑; divide the Space B D into 6 equal Parts, and defcribe the like Number of circular Arcs about the Center A, which fhall reprefent the Parallels of the other Signs, as they are denoted on the Side A C of the Quadrant The next thing to be done, is to draw the Hour-Lines. Let it be required (for example) to find a Point in the Tropick of ♋ thro which the Hour-Line of 12 muft pafs· By the above pofited Table, the Sun's Altitude (at *Paris*) at the faid time is 64 deg 29 min therefore take a Thread, or Ruler faftened to the Center A, and extend it to that Number of Degrees and Minutes on the Limb of the Quadrant, and where the Thread or Edge of the Ruler cuts the Tropick of ♋, will be one Point thro which the Hour-Line of 12 muft be drawn. Then feek the

Q q q   Sun's

Sun's Altitude when he enters into ♊, which being found 61 deg 12 min lay the Thread over 61 deg 12 min on the Limb, and where it cuts the Parallel of ♊, make a Mark; for a Point in the ſaid Parallel thro which the Hour-Line of 12 muſt paſs And if you proceed in this manner, Points may be found in the Parallels, or their Parts, (if the Quadrant be big enough) thro which the Hour-Line of 12 muſt paſs, as likewiſe all the other Hour-Lines, and if the Points be joined, the curve Hour-Lines will be had, and the Dial will be finiſhed, when there are two Sights fixed upon the Side A C.

The Uſe of this Quadrant.

Direct the Plane of the Inſtrument towards the Sun in ſuch manner, that his Rays may paſs thro the Holes of the Sights G G, and then the Plumb-Line freely playing, will ſhew the time of Day by interſecting the Parallel that the Sun is in But if you put a little Bead or Pin's Head upon the Plumb-Line, then you may extend the Thread from the Center, and ſlide the Bead thereon, and fix it over the Degree of the Sign or Day of the Month, and holding up the Quadrant, as before, the Bead will fall upon the Hour of the Day

The Conſtruction and Uſe of a Particular right-lined Dial

Fig. 15.

This Dial, which we call Particular, becauſe it ſerves but for one determinate Latitude, is made upon a very even Plate of Braſs, or other Metal, about the bigneſs of a playing Card The Conſtruction thereof is thus : Firſt, draw the two right Lines A B, C D, croſſing one another at right Angles in the Point E, about which, as a Center, with the Radius E C deſcribe the Circle C B D, and divide it into 24 equal Parts, beginning from the Point D, then thro each two Diviſions thereof equally diſtant from the Points C and D, draw parallel right Lines, which will be the Hour-Lines, whereof D R is that of 12, B E that of 6, and C M that of Midnight This being done, form the right-angled Parallelogram P M Q R, and draw the occult Line D R, making an Angle with C D equal to the Elevation of the Pole, *viz* 49 deg This Line ſhall repreſent the Radius of the Equinoctial, and by means thereof the Trigon of Signs muſt be formed, having D for its Vertex In order for this, produce the Hour-Line of the Sun's riſing in the longeſt Day of Summer, which here is the Hour-Line of 4, as likewiſe the Hour-Line of 6, until it meets the Radius of the Equinoctial Circle D R, then the Point in the Radius of the Equinoctial cut by the Hour-Line of 6, will be the Center of a Circle, whoſe Diameter ſhall be perpendicular to the ſaid Radius, and is terminated by the Interſection of the Hour-Line of 4 therewith This Circle being deſcribed, divide the Circumference thereof into 12 equal Parts, in order to form the Trigon of Signs, as is before explained in the third Chapter of this Book *Note*, The two Tropicks will be at the Extremities of the ſaid Diameter, each making an Angle of 23 deg 30 min with the Radius of the Equinoctial, the Vertex being the Point D Now the next thing to be done, muſt be to make a little ſlit along the Radius of the Equinoctial, that ſo a little Slider or Curſor may ſlide along it, having a little Hole drilled thro it for faſtening a Thread and Plummet with a Bead or Pin's Head on the Thread And after this, we place two Sights on the Extremities of the Line P Q.

The Uſe of this Dial.

Slide the Curſor, and fix the Hole in which the Thread is faſtened over the Degree of the Sign the Sun is in, or the Day of the Month, then flip the Bead or Pin's-head along the Thread, until it be upon the Hour-Line of 12. This being done, hold up your Inſtrument, lifting it higher or lower till the Sun ſhines thro the Holes of the Sights R and S, and the Thread freely plays upon the Plane thereof, then the Bead will fall upon the Hour of the Day.

The Conſtruction of a Univerſal right-lined Dial

Fig. 16.

This right-lined Dial, which ſerves for all Latitudes, is made of a bigneſs at pleaſure, upon a very even Plate of Braſs or other ſolid Matter The Conſtruction of it is thus : Draw the Lines A B, C D, cutting each other at right Angles in the Point E, about which, as a Center, deſcribe the Quadrant A F, which divide into 90 deg and with the Point E for the Vertex, make a Trigon of Signs according to the Method explained in *Chap* 2 Divide each Sign into 3 Parts, each being 10 deg and ſet the firſt Letters of the Months to the Places correſponding to them, by ſuppoſing (as we have already) that the Sun's entrance into every Sign is the 20*th* Day of the Month (N S.) for example, his entrance into ♈ the 20*th* of *March*, his entrance into ♉ the 20*th* of *April*, &c This may be without any ſenſible Error in ſo ſmall an Inſtrument Now draw dotted Lines from the Center E thro the Diviſions of the Quadrant A F, to the Line A G, which will divide it into Points, from which Parallels muſt be drawn to the Line A B, which ſhall be the different Latitudes or Elevations of the Pole, which muſt be only marked between the two Tropicks, as you ſee in the Figure, wherein they are drawn to every 5*th* deg. On both ſides the Point B lay off upon the Line B H, the Diviſions that the Radii of the Signs of

the

the Trigon make on the Line *a a*, reprefenting the Latitude of 45 deg that fo the Reprefentation of another Zodiack may be made upon the Line B H

Now the manner of drawing the Hour-Lines upon this Dial is thus Draw Lines thro every 15*th* deg of the Quadrant A F, parallel to E D, which is the Hour-Line of 6; and thefe Parallels will be the Hour-Lines from 6 in the Evening to 6 in the Morning, A L being the Hour-Line of Midnight And if the parallel Spaces be laid off on the other fide of the Hour-Line of 6, you will have the Hour-Lines from 6 in the Morning to 6 in the Evening And for drawing the half Hours, divide each 15*th* deg of the Quadrant A F into half, and draw Parallel Lines between the Hour-Lines

The Hour-Lines may be yet otherwife drawn, by means of a Circle, whofe Diameter is the Line A B, and whofe Circumference is divided into 24 equal Parts for the 24 Hours of the Day, or into 48, for the Half-Hours. For then if right Lines be drawn thro the oppofite Points of Divifion, parallel to E D, we fhall have the Hour-Lines, and thofe of the Half-Hours, as we have faid in the Conftruction of the former right-lined Dial

About the Point I, as a Center, draw an occult Quadrant, which divide into 90 deg and laying a Ruler to the Center I, and on each Divifion mark the fame Degrees upon the Sides G Q, and G S of the Inftrument   *Note*, By means of thefe Divifions we may find the Sun's Altitude above the Horizon, as we fhall fhew by and by R R are two Sights fixed on the Side G H And the Piece K is a fmall Arm or Index, made of 3 Blades of Brafs, fo joined to each other by headed Rivets, that they may have a Motion either to the right or left at the fharp end of this Arm is made a very little Hole, thro which goes a Thread with a Plummet at the end thereof, and a little Bead or Pin's Head thereon This little Arm is faftened to the Inftrument with a headed Rivet, that fo it may have a Motion at the place K

The Ufe of this Dial.

If the Hour of the Day be to be found by this Inftrument, you muft adjuft the end *a* of the Index on the Interfection of the Line of the Latitude of the Place, and the Degree of the Sign the Sun is in, or the Day of the Month, then extend the Thread, and flide the Bead to the fame Degree of the Sign in the little Zodiack, drawn on the Hour-Line of 12 B I This being done, hold the Inftrument up until the Sun fhines thro the Sights R R, and the Thread freely playing upon the Plane of the Inftrument, the Bead will fall upon the Hour of the Day

If the time of the Sun's rifing and fetting in all the Signs of the Zodiack for the Latitudes denoted upon the Inftrument be required, fix the end *a* of the Index on the Interfection of the Line of the Latitude of the Place, and the Degree of the Sign the Sun is in, then the Thread freely falling parallel to the Hour-Lines, will fhew the Hour of the rifing and fetting of the Sun For example, the end of the Index being fixed on the Interfection of the Sign of ♋, and the Line of the Latitude of 49 deg the Thread will fall along the Hour-Line of 4 in the Morning, or 8 in the Evening and this fhews, that about the 20*th* of *June*, (N S) the Sun rifes at *Paris*, at 4 in the Morning, and fets at 8 in the Evening, and fo of others

The Elevation of the Pole is found thus : Place the end of the Index on the Point I, and raife or lower the Inftrument until the Sun's Rays pafs thro the Holes of the Sights, then the Thread freely playing, will fhew the Sun's Altitude upon the Degrees on the fide Q S or Q G

All thefe kinds of Dials, that fhew the Hour of the Day by the Sun's Altitude, are convenient in this, that they fhew the Time of Day without a Compafs, but their common Imperfection is, that about Noon the Hour cannot be exactly determined by them, unlefs by feveral Obfervations to know whether the Sun increafes or decreafes in Altitude, and confequently whether it is before or after Noon

The Confiruction of a Horizontal Dial for feveral Latitudes

This Dial, which is made upon a very even and fmooth Plate of Brafs, or other folid *Plate* 24 Matter, hath a little Piece of Brafs in form of a Bird, the lower part of which is adjufted in two little knuckles, that fo it may be rendered moveable, and lie down upon the — *Fig* 1 Plane of the Dial This Bird is kept upright by means of a Spring that is underneath the Dial-Plate, which going thro a little fquare Hole in the Plate, keeps the Bird firm upon its Foot. There is a Style or Axis going into the Bird, which is double, the lower end of which goes into a little knuckle at the Center of the Dial, that fo the faid Style may be raifed or lowered, according to the Latitude There is on the Style a circular Arc, whereon the Degrees are fet down from 35 or 40 to 60   There is a Slit made along this divided Arc, paffing by the Eye of the Bird, that fo its Bill may be fet to the Degree of the Pole's Elevation, and fixed there. The Dial-Plate is hollowed in circular, that fo a Compafs may be added thereto, faftened underneath by two Screws. The Needle and the Glafs covering it, are placed in the fame manner as in other Compaffes, of which we have already fpoken.

The

The Surface of this Dial is divided into 4 or 5 Circumferences for the like Number of different Latitudes, according to some one of the Methods before laid down for drawing of Horizontal Dials, whereof that by the calculation of Angles is moſt in uſe for ſuch ſmall Dials as theſe. They may be drawn alſo by means of a Platform, upon which are ſeveral Dials divided by the Rules before given. But this is well known to the Inſtrument-maker.

The outmoſt Circumference, which is divided for 55 deg of Latitude, may well enough ſerve for thoſe Places contained between the 58 b and 53d deg of Latitude. The ſecond, which is divided for 50 deg of Latitude, may ſerve for Places contained between the 53d and the 47th deg of Latitude. The third, which is divided for 45 deg may ſerve for Places between the 47th and 42d deg. And the fourth, which is divided for 40 deg ſerves for Places contained between the 42d and 38th deg. of Latitude.

When a 5th Dial is drawn upon the Plate for the Latitude of 35 deg this ſerves for all Places contained between the 37th and the 32d deg of Latitude. Now by means of a good Map of the World, or Globe, you may ſee what Places theſe Dials will be in uſe, for that which is made for one Latitude, will ſerve for all Places round about the Earth, having the ſame North and South Latitude. We commonly grave underneath the Dial a Table of the principal Cities of the World with their Latitudes and Longitudes, that ſo the convenient Circumference on the Plate may be choſe, and the Axis of the Dial raiſed to the proper Elevation of the Pole.

The Uſe of this Dial

To find the Hour of the Day, raiſe or lower the Style, ſo that the end of the Bill of the little Bird may anſwer to the Degree of the Elevation of the Pole marked on the Style, as at *Paris* againſt the 49th Degree. The Style being thus raiſed, place the Dial parallel to the Horizon, that is, level, and turn it ſo to the Sun till the North Point of the Needle uſually marked with a little Ring, fixes itſelf over the Line of Declination, whereon is a *Flower-de-luce*, and *North* is writ. Then the Shadow of the Style will ſhew the Hour of the Day upon the Circumference divided for the Latitude of the Place. You muſt take care not to ſet the Dial near Iron, for this changes the Direction of the Needle.

The Conſtruction of a Ring Dial

Fig. 4.

Take a very round Ring of Braſs, or other ſolid Matter, about two Inches in Diameter, four or five Lines in breadth, and of a convenient thickneſs, and aſſume the Point A at pleaſure thereon (whereat there is a little Hole) about which, as a Center, deſcribe a Quadrant A D C, which divide into 90 Degrees. Then find the Sun's Altitudes in the foregoing Table at every Hour when he is in the Equinoctial for the Latitude of *Paris*, and laying a Ruler from the Center A thro thoſe Altitudes aſſumed on the Quadrant, you may draw Lines which will divide the concave Surface of the Ring into the Hour-Points. Now this Dial will be very good for the times of the Equinox, it being ſuſpended by the Ring B, ſo that the Line A D is upright.

But one of theſe Dials may be made for ſhewing the Hour of the Day at any other time of the Year, if the Hole A be made moveable. For doing of which, make the Arcs A E, A I, 23 deg. for the Signs ♉, ♍, ♏, and ♓, A F, A K, 40 deg 26 min for the Signs ♊, ♌, ♒, and ♐, and the Arcs A G, A L, 47 deg for the Signs ♋ and ♑. (The reaſon why we aſſume theſe Arcs double, is, becauſe Angles at the Circumference are but half thoſe at the Center.) Now by this means we ſhall have a kind of Zodiack upon the convex Surface of the Ring, whereon muſt be marked the Signs in their proper Places, or elſe the firſt Letters of the Months, that ſo the Hole A may be put to the Degree of the Sign, or the Day of the Month.

You muſt deſcribe likewiſe 7 Circles in the concave Surface of the Ring, whereof that in the middle will be for the Equinoctial, and the others for the other Parallels. This being done, about the Points A, E, F, G, I, K, L, as ſo many Centers, deſcribe Quadrants of 90 deg upon which Quadrants aſſume the Altitudes of the Sun every Hour when he is in every of the Signs, and produce the Radii drawn from the Centers to the Points of Aſſumption until they cut the Circumferences in the concave part of the Ring, and you will have Points thereon for the Hour-Lines which muſt be joined.

Note, Theſe Diviſions may be ſeparately drawn, and afterwards transferred on the Ring.

The Uſe of this Dial.

Place the moveable Hole at the Degree of the Sign wherein the Sun is, then holding the Ring ſuſpended, turn it towards the Sun, ſo that his Rays paſſing thro the Hole A, may fall upon the convenient Circumference of the Sign in the concave part of the Ring, and then you will have the Hour of the Day ſhewn.

To

Plate XXIII

Fig 1

Fig 2

Fig 3

Fig 4

Fig 5

Fig 6

Fig 7

Fig 8

Fig 9

Fig 10

Fig 11

Fig 12

Fig 13

Fig 14

Fig 15

Fig 16

Parallels of Declination

Meridian

This Side is applied to the Wall

Hours after Noon

Hours before Noon

D Horizontal Plane

The Diameter of the Cylinder

Length of the Style out of the Cylinder

Hours before Noon

I Senex sculp.t

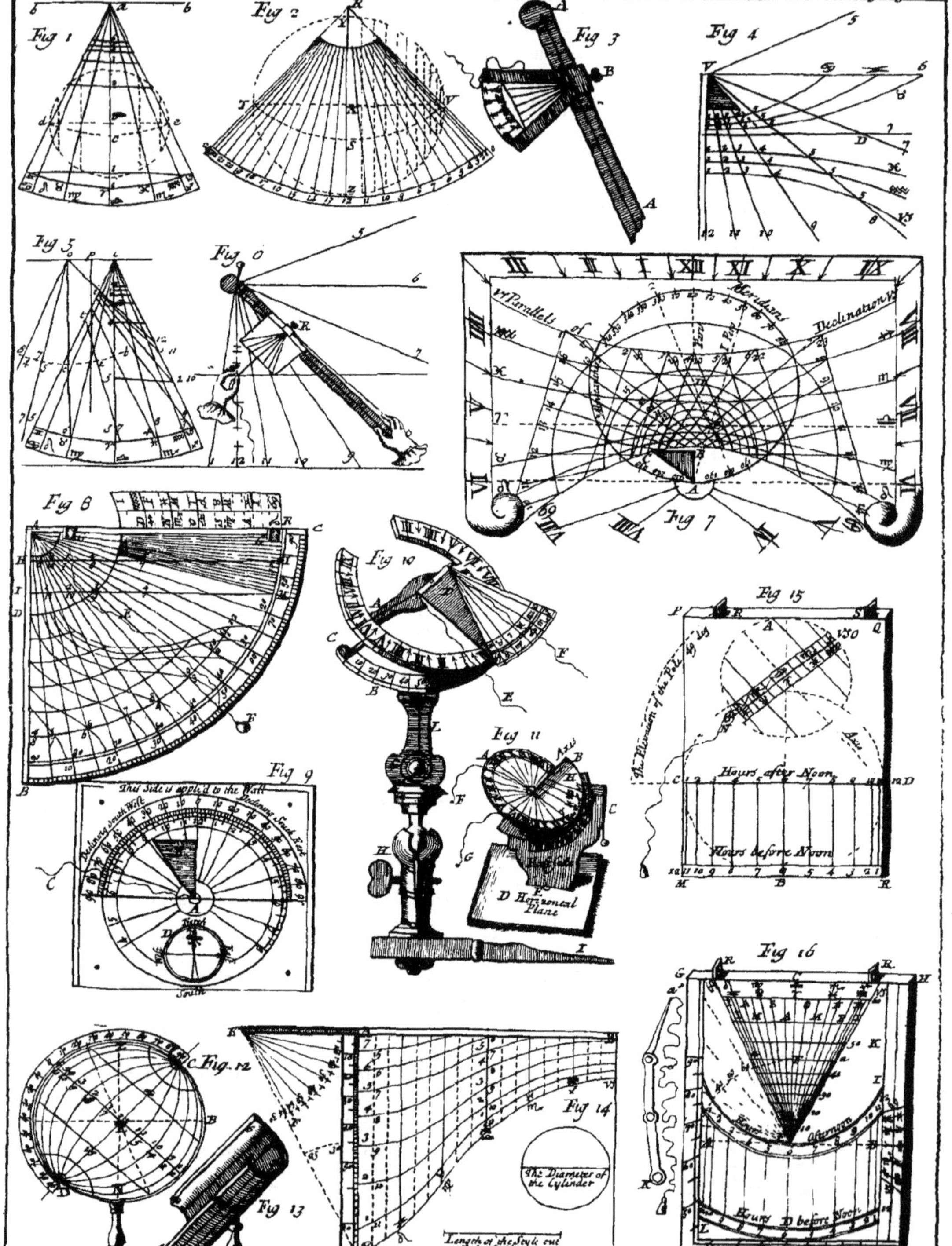

To describe the Hour-Lines upon another sort of Ring.

The fourth Figure represents this Ring compleat, and the Parallelogram A B C D, repre- Fig. 3 sents it laid open or stretched upon a Plane, that so the Hour-Lines may be pricked down thereon before it be turned up circularly

This Ring is made of a blade of Brass, or other solid Matter, being in length proportio- Fig. 4. nable to the Bigness you would have the Ring, and at least 4 or 5 Lines broad, with a proportionable thickness, and whose Extremes A C, B D, are cut at right Angles   About the Points C and D describe two Quadrants A L, M B, and divide each of them into 9 equal Parts, and from each opposite Division draw the Parallels of the Signs, whereof the Line C F D shall be for ♈ and ♎, A E B for the two Tropicks, and the others for the other Signs placed according to their order   Then bisect the Parallelogram A B C D by the Line E F, and draw the Line G H separately equal to E B, that so a Scale may be made thereof, which must be divided into 9 equal Parts, each of which must be subdivided into 10 equal Parts more by little dots, and so the said Scale will be divided into 90 equal Parts, answering to the 90 deg of a Quadrant. This being done, take the Degrees of the Sun's Altitude from the above posited Table of Altitudes, at every Hour when the Sun is in the Equinox, and the Solstices, for the Horizon of *Paris*. For example, When the Sun is in the 1st deg of ♋, his Meridian Altitude is 64 deg 29 min take 64 ⅔ equal Parts from the Scale G H between your Compasses, and lay them off upon the Brass Blade both ways from E to the Points I and K, as likewise from the Point F to the Points L and M, and join the Points I L and K M, by right Lines   then take from the Table the Sun's Altitude at the Hours of 1 and 11, when he is in the Summer Solstice, viz. 61 deg 54 min which here may be taken for 62 deg and opening your Compasses to the extent of 62 equal Parts of the Scale, lay them off upon A B from K towards L, and you will have a Point of the Hour-Lines of 11 and 1, likewise take 41 equal Parts or Degrees, for the Sun's Meridian Altitude when he is in the Equinoctial, and lay them off from M to O, and from L to N, and the Points N and O are those thro which the two Hour-Lines of 12 must be drawn Moreover, take 39 deg 20 min the Sun's Altitude when he is in the Equinox, at the Hours of 11 and 1, from the Scale, and lay them off from the said Points M and L upon the said Line C D, and you will have two Points in the Line C D, thro which the Hour-Lines of 11 and 1 must be drawn   And in this manner may Points be found in this Line, thro which the other Hour-Lines must pass

But now to find Points in the Line A B, or Tropick of *Capricorn*, on this side the Point E, thro which the Hour-Lines must be drawn, (for the Points of the same Line, on the other side of E, for the Tropick of *Cancer* may be found in the same manner as the Point for the Hour-Line of 11 and 1 was) you must take take 17 ½ Degrees, or equal Parts from the Scale, viz. the Sun's Meridian Altitude, when he is in the Tropick of *Capricorn*, and lay them off from I to P, and P will be the Point thro which the Hour-Line of 12 must pass; and so may the Points be found thro which the other Hour-Lines must be drawn.   Now if the Points found in the Lines A B, and C D, thro which the Hour-Lines pass, be joined by right Lines, these right Lines will be the Hour-Lines

But if you have a mind to be exacter, you may take the Degrees of the Sun's Altitudes at every Hour when he enters, and is in each 10th and 20th Degree of every Sign, and then find Points on the respective Parallels on the Dial thro which the Hour-Lines must be drawn, which will not be right Lines but Curves, and in this case the Dial will be exacter

Having drawn the Hour-Lines, you must Number them on both sides the Lines A B, C D, and also set down the Characters of the Signs, and the first Letters of the Months, each in their proper Place   When this is done, you must drill two little Holes in the Points R and S (viz. the middles of the Lines I L, K M) in a conical Figure, the greater Bases being outmost, that so the Sun's Rays may better come thro them, afterwards round or turn up the said Blade circularly, folder the Extremities A C, B D together, and place a Button, with a Ring in the middle of the Junction of the said Extremities, so that the whole Instrument be *in equilibrio*, which that it may, you must turn the outside thereof.

The Use of this Instrument

Hold the Ring suspended, and turn the Hole proper for the Time of Year towards the Sun, so that his Rays may fall upon the Parallel of the Sign he is in, the Day wherein you use the Instrument, and then the Hour of the Day will be shewn thereon by a bright Spot or Point of Light

Note, The Hole S is in use from the 20th of *March*, (N S) to the 22d of *September*, and the Hole R for the other six Months   We likewise write upon the convex Superficies of the Ring near the little Holes, the 20th of *March*, and the 22d of *September*, as appears in Figure 3 and, lastly, observe that these two last Dials are proper but for one Latitude.

The

The Conſtruction and Uſe of the univerſal Aſtronomical Ring-Dial

Fig 5.

This Inſtrument, whoſe Uſe is to find the Hour of the Day in any part of the Earth, by a bright Spot of the Sun's Light, is made of Braſs or other Metal, and conſiſts of two Rings or flat Circles turned both within ſide and without   The Diameter of theſe Rings, which ought to be broad and thick proportionable to their bigneſſes, are from two to ſix Inches   The outward Ring A repreſents the Meridian of any Place wherein one is, and there are two Diviſions of 90 Degrees thereon, which are diametrically oppoſite to each other, one whereof ſerves from our North Pole to the Equator, and the other from the Equator to the South Pole

The innermoſt Ring repreſents the Equator, and ought to turn very exactly within the outward one, by means of two Pivots or Pins put into Holes made diametrically oppoſite in the two Rings at the Points of the Hour of 12

There is a thin Riglet (called a Bridge) with a Curſor marked C, compoſed of two little Pieces that ſlide in an Aperture made along the middle of the ſaid Bridge, and which are kept together by two ſmall Screws   Thro the middle of this Curſor is a very little Hole drilled, that ſo the Sun may ſhine thro it   Now the middle of the ſaid Bridge may be conſidered as the Axis of the World, and the Extremities as the Poles of the World, and there are drawn on one ſide thereof the Signs of the Zodiack with their Characters, and on the other ſide the Days and Names of the Months, or only their firſt Letters, being placed according to the reſpect they have to the Signs   The Signs are divided into every 10th or 5th Degree, according to their Declination, by means of a Trigon already divided, the Vertex of which, or Extremity of the Radius of the Equinoctial, being within ſide the Equinoctial Circle, as at the Point F The two Pieces D D which are ſcrewed to the outermoſt Ring, ſerve to ſupport the Bridge or Axis which is moveable round, and are ſo ordered as that the innermoſt Ring may lie exactly within the outermoſt, and they both make as it were but one   The two Pieces E are alſo ſcrewed on the outermoſt Ring, and ſerve as Props to keep the Equinoctial Circle or inward Ring at right Angles to the Meridian or outermoſt Ring.

We ſhall not here repeat the manner of dividing the two Quadrants into Degrees, and the Equinoctial Circle into Hours, Halves and Quarters, having ſufficiently ſpoken of this elſewhere   We ſhall only add, that all the Diviſions of the Equinoctial Circle muſt be drawn upon the concave ſide thereof, which may be done by means of a piece of Steel turned up ſquare, according to the Curvature of the Circle

Near the outward Edges, on each of the two flat ſides of the Meridian, is made a Groove for the Piece G to ſlide therein, the middle of which is bent inwards, that ſo it may go into the ſaid Grooves   The two ſides of this Piece, which muſt be well hammered that they may have a good Spring, are made flat, in order to preſs againſt the convex Surface of the Meridian, that thereby the Piece G may be held faſt on any Degree of Diviſion of the Meridian   The Button thro which the Ring of Suſpenſion H goes, is riveted to the middle of the Piece G, ſo that it may turn round very freely, and by this means the Inſtrument be very perpendicularly ſuſpended by the Ring H   for this is one of the principal things in which the Exactneſs of the Inſtrument conſiſts

The Uſe of the Aſtronomical Ring-Dial

Place the ſhort Line *a* on the middle of the hanging Piece G over the Degree of the Latitude of the Place you are in upon the Meridian Circle, for example, over the 49th deg at *Paris*, and then put the Line croſſing the little Hole of the Curſor on the Bridge to the Degree of the Sign, or the Day of the Month you deſire to know the Hour of the Day in This being done, open the Inſtrument ſo that the two Rings or Circles be at right Angles to each other, and ſuſpend it by the Ring H, ſo that the Axis of the Dial repreſented by the middle of the Bridge be parallel to the Axis of the World

Turn the flat ſide of the Bridge towards the Sun, ſo that his Rays coming thro the little Hole in the middle of the Curſor, fall exactly on a Line drawn round the middle of the concave Surface of the Equinoctial Circle, or innermoſt Ring; and then the bright Spot or luminous Point ſhews the Hour of the Day in the ſaid concave Surface of the Ring

Note, The Hour of 12 cannot be ſhewn by this Dial, becauſe the outermoſt Circle or Ring being then in the Plane of the Meridian, it hinders the Sun's Rays from falling upon the innermoſt or Equinoctial Circle   You muſt obſerve likewiſe, that when the Sun is in the Equinoctial, you cannot then tell the Hour of the Day by this Dial, becauſe his Rays fall parallel to the Plane of the ſaid Equinoctial Circle   But this is but about one Hour every Day, and four Days in the Year

The Conſtruction and Uſe of a Ring-Dial with three Rings

Fig. 6.

This Inſtrument differs from the precedent one in nothing but only a third Ring or Circle, carrying the Sun's Declination.   The Ring A repreſents the Meridian of the Place you would uſe the Dial in, the Ring B repreſents the Equinoctial Circle, and the Ring D, which turns exactly within the ſaid Equinoctial Circle, produces the ſame effect, as the

Bridge

Bridge reprefenting the Axis of the World in the precedent Inftrument. The two Extremities of the Diameter of this laft Ring, or the two Points of the Circumference thereof, whereat it is faftened to the Meridian, anfwer to the two Poles of the World. On the oppofite Parts D D of the Circumference of this Circle, is denoted a double Trigon of Signs, whofe Center is the Vertex wherein all the Radius's reunite, the Arcs of each of which are fubdivided into every 10th or 5th Degree, to which may be likewife fubjoined the Days of the correfpondent Months.

The Index E is faftened to the Center of the innermoft Ring, having two Sights rivetted to the Extremities thereof, each having a fmall Hole drilled therein, for the Sun's Rays to pafs thro. Note, Dials compofed in this manner fhew the Hour of 12, becaufe the Index is without the Plane of the Meridian Circle. and when we make them large, as 9 or 10 Inches in Diameter, we divide the Equinoctial Circle into every 5th or every 2d Minute.

This Dial hath a Piece F like as the former Dial has, going into a Groove made on each fide the Meridian, to be flid to the Latitude of the Place. We fometimes fet thefe Dials upon Pedeftals, nearly like thofe of Spheres, which are flid to the Latitude, and in this Cafe they are placed upon an Horizontal Plain; we likewife add Compaffes to them, by which means the Variation of the Needle may be exactly known.

The Ufe of this Dial.

Place the little Line in the middle of the hanging Piece F to the Latitude of the Place wherein you have a mind to know the Hour of the Day, and the fiducial Line of the Index on the Day of the Month, or Degree of the Sign the Sun is in. Then open the Equinoctial Circle at right Angles to the Meridian, and holding the Inftrument fufpended, raife or lower the innermoft Circle, fo that the Sun's Rays may go thro the Holes of the two Sights; then the Line which is drawn along the middle of the Convexity of the faid Circle, will fhew the Hour or Part drawn in the middle of the Concavity of the Equinoctial Circle, even at all times of the Day.

This may likewife be done fomething more convenient, when the Inftrument is placed Horizontally upon its Pedeftal.

The Conftruction of a univerfal inclined Horizontal, and an Equinoctial Dial.

This Inftrument confifts of two Plates of Brafs, or other folid Matter, whereof the Fig. 7 under-one A is hollowed in about the middle, to receive a Compafs faftened underneath with Screws. The Plate B is moveable by means of a ftrong Joint at the Plate C. Upon this Plate is drawn a Horizontal Dial for fome Latitude greater than any one of thofe the Dial is to be ufed in, and having a Style thereon proportionable to that Latitude; for when the faid Plane B is raifed by means of the Quadrant, the Horizontal Plane muft always have a lefs Latitude than that the Dial is made for, or otherwife the Axis of the Style will have an Elevation too little.

Inftead of the Quadrant D we generally place but only an Arc from the Equator to 60 Degrees, which are numbered downwards, 60 being at the bottom, and for this Latitude of 60 deg we commonly draw the aforefaid Horizontal Dial. That Arc of 60 deg is faftened by two fmall Tenons, and may be laid down upon the Plate A, as likewife may the Style upon the Plate B, and both of thefe are kept upright by means of little Springs underneath the Plates. What remains of the Conftruction of this Dial, may be fupplied from the Figure thereof.

The Ufe of the inclined Horizontal Dial.

Raife the upper Plate B to the Degree of Latitude or Elevation of the Pole of the Place wherein you are, by means of the Graduations on the Quadrant D. Then if the Plane A be fet Horizontal, fo that the Needle of the Compafs fettles itfelf over its Line of Declination, the Shadow of the Axis will fhew the Hour of the Day. Note, We grave the Names of feveral principal Cities, as likewife their Latitudes and Longitudes, underneath the two Plates, in order to avoid the trouble of feeking them in Maps.

After the abovefaid manner, Equinoctial Dials are made Univerfal throughout the whole Earth; but here we muft have a whole Quadrant. The upper Plate is commonly in form of a hollowed Circle, which we divide into 24 equal Parts, for the Hours, each of which we fubdivide into 4 equal Parts, for the Quarters, all thefe being drawn in the Concavity of the Circle.

There is a Piece that goes thro the Circle, carrying the right Style, which is kept faft in the middle of the Circle by means of a little Spring faftened underneath the Circle, and by this means the right Style may be raifed above the faid Circle, and lowered underneath it. And when the Equinoctial Dial is drawn, we ufe the little Piece F for a Style, placed in the Center of the Circle. Note, The upper part of the Dial fhews the Hour of the Day from the 22d of *March*, (N. S) to the 22d of *September*, and the under part thereof the Hour of the Day, the other 6 Months of the Year.

The

The Uſe of the Equinoctial Dial.

You muſt place the Edge of the Equinoctial Circle to the Degree of the Elevation of the Pole, by means of the Quadrant, then if the Dial be ſet North and South by means of the Compaſs, the Shadow of the Style will ſhew the Hour of the Day at all times of the Year, even when the Sun is in the Equinoctial, becauſe the Circle is hollowed in

The Conſtruction of an Azimuth Dial

Fig. 8.

'This Dial, which is commonly made in the bottom of a Compaſs, is called an Azimuth Dial, becauſe it is made by means of the Azimuth's or Sun's Vertical Circles, upon a Plate of Braſs, or other ſolid Matter, parallel to the Horizon Firſt, draw the Line A B, repreſenting the Meridian, upon which deſcribe a Circle at pleaſure, half of which we ſhall only uſe here for drawing the Morning Hour-Lines, becauſe thoſe of the Afternoon are drawn after the ſame way. Divide this Circle into Degrees, beginning from the Point A, repreſenting the North Pole Then triſect the Semi-diameter A C, and take A D equal to two thirds thereof, which muſt be divided into 6 Parts, thro each Point of Diviſion, about the Center C muſt be drawn concentrick Arcs, repreſenting the Parallels of the Signs, the Arc H being the Summer Tropick, that neareſt to the Center C the Winter Tropick, and each of the others for two Signs equally diſtant from the Tropicks, as appears per Figure

The Parallels of the Signs may moreover be drawn, in deſcribing a Semi-circle upon the Line H D, which Semi-circle being divided into 6 equal Parts, you muſt let fall dotted Parallels upon the Line H D, theſe Parallels will divide the ſaid Line into unequal Parts, and if thro the Points of Diviſions Arcs be deſcribed about the Center C, theſe Arcs will be the Parallels of the Signs at unequal Diſtances from each other.

Now for drawing the Hour-Lines, the following Table of the Sun's Azimuths muſt be uſed, for example, to prick down a Point in the Tropick of *Cancer* thro which the Hour-Line of 11 in the Morning muſt be drawn, you will find the Sun's Azimuth will then be 30 deg 17 min and when he is in the firſt Degree of ♊, or laſt of ♌, his Azimuth at the ſame Hour is 27 deg 58 min and ſo of others Therefore if a Ruler be laid on the Center C, and on the 30th deg and 27 min of the outward divided Limb, the Edge of the Ruler will cut the Parallel of ♋, in a Point thro which the Hour-Line of 11 muſt paſs then keeping the Ruler to the Center, move it, and lay it over the 27th deg and 58th min of the outmoſt Limb, and you will have a Point in the Parallel of ♊ and ♌ thro which the Hour-Line of 11 muſt paſs, and in this manner may Points be found in the other Parallels thro which the Hour-Line of 11 muſt paſs, and alſo Points in all the Parallels thro which the other Morning Hour-Lines muſt paſs each of which Points belonging to the ſame Hours being joined, you will have the curved Hour-Lines on one ſide of the Meridian And to find the Points thro which the Afternoon Hour-Lines muſt paſs, take the Diſtances of each Point in the Parallels from the Meridian, and transfer them on the ſame Parallels continued out on the other ſide of the Meridian, becauſe the Sun's Azimuth at any two Hours equally diſtant on each ſide the Meridian, is the ſame

The Uſe of the Azimuth Dial

Turn the ſide B towards the Sun, ſo that the Shadow of the right Style planted in a Point without the Compaſs, and parallel to the Line of Noon, may fall along the Meridian Line ; then the Needle pointing exactly North and South, will ſhew the Hour of the Day in the Interſection thereof with the Parallel of the Sign the Sun is in, upon condition that the Needle has no Variation. But ſince the Needle varies now above 12 Degrees at *Paris*, you muſt place the Style in the Point E over the Line of Declination or Variation K I, and adjuſt the Shadow of the Style along the ſaid Line of Variation, and by this means the Error ariſing from the Needle's Variation will be avoided.

A T A B L E *of the Sun's Azimuth or Diſtance from the Meridian every Hour of the Day for the Latitude of* 49 *Degrees.*

Hours Signs	XI I D M.	X. II D M	IX. III D M	VIII IV D M	VII V D M	VI. VI D M	V VII D M	IV VIII D M
♋	30 17	53 40	70 30	83 57	95 20	105 56	111 28	127 26
♌ ♊	27 58	50 33	67 34	81 6	92 45	103 35	114 56	
♍ ♉	23 30	43 52	60 29	74 17	86 21	97 36		
♎ ♈	19 33	37 25	52 58	66 57	78 34			
♏ ♓	16 42	32 25	46 30	59 28	71 12			
♐ ♒	14 56	29 11	42 23	54 26				
♑	14 19	28 2	40 48					

The

The Construction and Use of the Analemmatick or Ecliptick Horizontal Dial

This is called an Analemmatick Dial, because it is made by means of the Analemma, which is the Projection or Representation of the principal Circles of the Sphere upon a Plane. The 9th Figure is the Analemma, and the 10th Figure represents the Dial compleat, which shews the Hour of the Day without a Compass.

Now to project the Analemma, upon a very even smooth Plate of Brass, draw the Lines Fig. 9. A B and C D, cutting each other at right Angles in the Point E, about which, as a Center, describe the Circle A C B D, representing the Meridian, its Diameter C D, the Horizon, and A B the Prime Vertical. Then assume the Arc D F equal to the Elevation of the Pole, which here is 49 deg and draw the Line E F representing the Axis of the World, likewise assume the Arc C G equal to the height of the Equinoctial 41 Degrees, and draw the Line G E for the Equinoctial. Assume the Arcs G H, G I, each of 23 deg. 30 min for the Sun's greatest Declination, and draw the Line H I cutting the Equinoctial in the Point Y, about which, as a Center, describe the Circle H L I K, or only half of it, which divide into 6 equal Parts, and thro each Point of Division draw Parallels to the Equinoctial, which continue out to the Horizon, then from the Sections made by the said Parallels on the Meridian, let fall the Parallels M, N, O and P to the Horizon, and from the Sections made by the said Parallels on the Axis, let fall the indefinite Perpendiculars S c, R b, Q a to the Horizon. This being done, take the Distance E M between your Compasses, with which setting one Foot in N, with the other make a small Arc upon the Line Q a, and with one Foot in O cut the Line R b with the other, then, continually keeping the Compasses opened to the extent E M, set one Foot in P, and cut the Line S c in the Point C.

Now to construct the little Zodiack, take the Distance ♊ C, and lay off from E towards A and B for the Tropicks of ♋ and ♑; again, lay off the Distance 46, from the Point E on one side, for the Parallel of ♊, and on the other side for the Parallel of ♒, and finally, take the Distance X a, for marking the Parallel of ♉ on one side, and that of ♓ on the other, and then the little Zodiack may be formed, as per Figure. Now to prick down the Hour-Points, you must describe the Circle M T Z V about the Center E, with the Distance E M, and divide the Circumference thereof into 24 equal Parts, as likewise the Circumference of the Meridian A C B D, and from each opposite Point of Division in the Meridian draw strait Lines parallel to A B, and in the Circle M T Z V, strait Lines parallel to C D, and thro the Intersections of these Lines that are nearest to the Meridian, draw lightly an Ellipsis from Point to Point, as you see in the Figure. These Points of Section will be the Hour-Points, those for the Morning being on the left, and those for the Afternoon on the right; and to have the half and quarter Hour-Points, the two Circles A C B D, M T Z V, must be divided into 96 equal Parts.

Things being thus prepared, transfer all the Hour-Points on another Brass Plate, and Fig. 10. form the Ellipsis B thereon, by lightly drawing Lines from Point to Point, and grave the proper Numbers upon it, as they are marked in the 10th Figure. Likewise transfer the Trigon of Signs upon the said Plate, taking each of the Distances between your Compasses, the one after the other, so that the Signs ♈ and ♎ be in the Line of the Hour of 6, and place the Characters of the Signs thereon, as also the first Letters of the Months, each one in their order. When this is done, you must adjust a Cursor C so as to slide along the middle of the Trigon. This Cursor carries the right Style D, which rises and falls by means of two small knuckles.

On the other part of this Plate, is drawn an Horizontal Dial according to the common Rules, for the same Latitude the Analemma is made for, and we place the Style or Axis E thereon upon the Hour-Line of 12, which rises, falls, and is kept upright by means of a small Spring underneath the Plate.

The Use of this Dial.

Set the Dial parallel to the Horizon, and put the Cursor with its right Style upon the Day of the Month, or Sign the Sun is in, then turn the Instrument until the same Hour be shewn upon the two Dials, which will be the Hour of the Day. If, for example, the Shadow of the Extremity of the right Style falls upon the 11th Hour on the Analemmatick Dial, and at the same time the Shadow of the Style of the Horizontal Dial falls likewise upon the 11th Hour, on the Horizontal Dial, then the true Hour of the Day will be that of 11. The Conveniency of this Dial consists in this, that the Hour of the Day may be found thereby without a Meridian Line, or Compass, but then it must be pretty large, to shew the Hour exactly.

The Construction of a universal Polar, East and West Dial.

This Instrument consists of a very strait and smooth circular Piece of Brass, or other Fig. 11. Metal, pretty thick, that so it may preserve its perpendicular Weight, as likewise that a Groove may be made round the Limb thereof, for a hanging-Piece to slide about the same, like that on the Astronomical Ring.

About

About the Center of the faid circular Piece defcribe the Circumference of a Circle, which divide into twice 90 Degrees. Then draw a right Line from the 90th Degree thro the Center, reprefenting the Equinoctial, near the top of which affume a Point at pleafure, thro which draw a right Line perpendicular to the Equinoctial Line, which fhall be the Hour-Line of 6. Then to have the other Hour-Lines, you muft lay off the anfwerable Tangents upon the Equinoctial Line both ways from the Point therein of the Hour-Line of 6, as the Tangent of 15 deg for the Hour-Points of 5 and 7, the Tangent of 30 deg for 4 and 8, the Tangent of 45 deg for 3 and 9, &c and if Lines be drawn thro thefe Points parallel to the Hour-Line of 6, thefe will be the Hour-Lines, and the Length of the right Style muft be equal to the Radius or Tangent of 45 deg. and muft be placed upright upon the Hour-Line of 6, at the Point wherein it cuts the Equinoctial Line

At the Points C C, on the Hour-Line of 9 in the Morning, and 3 in the Afternoon, are adjufted two fmall knuckles, in which is placed the Piece V, which may lie down upon the circular Piece, and likewife ftand at right Angles to it   Upon this Piece are pricked down the Hour-Lines of a Polar Dial, from 9 in the Morning to 12, and from 12 to 3 in the Afternoon   We fhall not here repeat the manner of drawing thefe Hour-Lines, for we have fufficiently fpoken of this already, as likewife how to draw the Arcs of the Signs; only obferve, that the Parallels of the Signs are divided into every 10th deg and the firft Letters of the Names of the Months are fet down in their proper Place

The Style B is adjufted to the circular Piece with a Joint, that fo it may be raifed or lie flat upon the faid Piece, but it muft be raifed fo that the Extremity thereof may be exactly over the Point in the Equinoctial Line cut by the Hour-Line of 6, and the Diftance of the faid Extremity from this Point equal to the Diftance from the Hour-Line of 9 to the Hour-Line of 6.

The Ufe of the faid Dial.

If you have a mind to find the Hour of the Day before Noon, place the little Line on the middle of the hanging Piece L upon the Latitude of the Place, on that Quadrant on the Right-hand of the Style B, raife the Style fo that the Extremity thereof be directly over the Interfection of the Equinoctial and the Hour-Line of 6, and its Diftance from that Point of Interfection equal to the Diftance from the Hour-Line of 9 to the Hour-Line of 6. Then holding the Dial fufpended by its Ring, expofe it to the Sun, fo that the Shadow of the Extremity of the Style falls upon the Day of the Month, and you will have the Hour of the Day upon the Eaft or Polar Dial. But if the Hour of the Day be required in the Afternoon, you muft put the hanging Piece on the Latitude of the Place upon the Quadrant on the left fide of the Style, and turn the Dial to the Sun fo that the Shadow of the Extremity of the Style falls on the Degree of the Sign or Day of the Month. Then you will have the Hour of the Day as before

Thus have I laid down the Conftruction and Ufes of Portable Dials, chiefly in ufe, which may be fet North and South, without a Compafs or Meridian Line   But before I clofe this Chapter, I fhall briefly defcribe fome other Portable Dials, which are curious enough, but are fomething difficult to make

The firft of thefe is a horizontal Dial of 2 or 3 Inches fquare, which we make of Brafs or any other folid Metal, for a given Latitude, and whofe Axis fhewing the Hour, is a Thread faftened at one end to the Center of the faid Dial, and the other end of which is hung to the top of a pretty thick Brafs Blade, placed at the Extremity of the Dial near the Hour-Line of 12   This Blade may lie down upon the Plane of the Dial, and is kept upright by means of a Spring underneath the Dial, and the Height of the Notch wherein the Thread lies above the Plane of the Dial, is equal to the Tangent of the Latitude

About a quarter of the Height of the faid Blade is adjufted thereon a Circle or Ring, proportioned to the bignefs of the Dial-Plate. This Ring is moveable by means of a Joint, and fo may lie down upon the Blade, and the Blade upon the horizontal Dial-Plane, and when the Inftrument is ufing, there is a Prop to keep this Ring at the Height of the Equinoctial, viz. 41 deg but when the Thread ferving for an Axis is extended, it muft exactly pafs thro the Center of this Ring

The Concavity of the Ring is divided into Hours, Halves and Quarters, as the Equinoctial Ring of the univerfal Ring-Dial is, and there is a Bead or Pin's Head put upon the Thread, that fo it may be moved to the Sign the Sun is in, and ferve as a Curfor to fhew the Hour of the Day in the middle of the Concavity of the Ring or Equinoctial.

Now to place the Bead to the Sign or proper Month, you muft have a feparate Brafs Riglet, having the Signs of the Zodiack, as alfo the Days of the Months drawn thereon in the manner they were drawn upon the Bridge of the univerfal Ring-Dial; and having placed the faid Riglet from the Center of the horizontal Dial along the Thread or Axis, flide the Bead to the Degree of the Sign the Sun is in, and then take away the Riglet, and fo will the Bead be placed for fhewing the Hour of the Day

On the backfide of the Blade is drawn an upright Line for a Plumb-Line to play on, that fo the Dial may be fet level   *Note*, This Dial may be rendered univerfal, if an Arc of a Circle divided into Degrees be adjufted behind the Blade by means of a Joint, fo as it

may

may lie upon the Blade, and the Point whereon the Plumb-Line is hung by the Center of the said Arc; for then the Dial may be set to the Latitude, by making the Plumb-Line fall upon the proper Degree on the circular Arc. It is proper also to observe, that the Hours from eight in the Evening to four in the Morning may be taken away from the Equinoctial Ring, that so this Dial may be of use at the time of the Equinox

The Use of the aforesaid Dial

Having placed the Bead to the Degree of the Sign the Sun is in, or Day of the Month, as before directed, expose the Dial to the Sun, and turn it to the right or left until the Shadow of the Bead falls upon the same Hour or Part, on the middle of the Concavity of the Equinoctial Ring, as the Shadow of the Thread or Axis does on the horizontal Dial; and then that will be the true time of the Day.

We make several other Portable Dials, as horizontal Astrolabes, being Projections of the Sphere upon the Plane of the Horizon; other Astrolabes vertically used by means of a Plumb-Line; horizontal Dials made by means of the Sun's Altitudes, which are likewise set North and South without a Compass, and whereon the Signs are drawn by right Lines issuing from the same Center, and the Hour-Lines, curve Lines, as likewise other Portable Dials, which are curious enough, whose Construction and Figures we reserve for another time

Horizontal Dials whereon are drawn the Signs, as that of *Fig 7. Plate 23.* may likewise be set North and South without a Compass, if the Dial be so placed in the Sun, that the Shadow of the Extremity of the right Style falls upon the Degree of the Sign the Sun is in, or Day of the Month. But here there is this Inconveniency, that the Distance of the Parallel of *Cancer* from the adjacent Parallels is so small, that the Space of 10 Days there cannot be distinguished So that when we have done all we can, it is scarce possible to make a Portable Dial that can be set North and South without a Compass or Meridian Line, without falling into one of these Inconveniencies, either of having the Hour-Lines near Noon too nigh each other, or not exactly shewing the Hour of the Day at the time of the Solstices, because of the small Difference that there is in the Sun's Elevations and Declination at those times.

CHAP. VI.

Of the Construction and Use of a Moon-Dial, and a Nocturnal or Star-Dial.

Of the Construction of a Horizontal Dial for shewing the Hour of the Night by the Moon

THIS is called a Moon-Dial, because by it you may tell in the Night by the Shadow *Fig 12.* of the Moon, what Hour-Circle the Sun is in It consists of two Pieces or Plates of Brass, or other solid Matter, of a bigness at pleasure. The under-Plate H, is in figure of a Parallelogram, and the upper one A is circular, turns about the shadowed Space L, and the Center B, and has a Horizontal Dial drawn upon it for the Latitude of the Place, according to the Rules before prescribed for drawing Horizontal Dials The under Plate hath a Circle thereon divided into 30 unequal Parts, for the Days of a Lunar Month. These Divisions are made thus, let D E be the Equinoctial Line by which the Horizontal Dial was drawn, and F the Center of the Equinoctial Circle, (or the Center by which the Equinoctial Line is divided) About this Center describe a dotted Circle, and divide it into 30 equal Parts, or half of it into 15, and having laid the edge of a Ruler on the Center F, lay it over each Point of the Divisions of the said Circle one after another, and prick down Points upon the Equinoctial Line, then lay the Ruler to the Center B, and on each Point of Division of the Equinoctial Line, and divide the Circle H, and when you have divided half of it, transfer the same Divisions on the other Semi-circle, and by this means the whole Circle will be divided into 30 unequal Parts for the 30 Days of a Lunar Month, about which Numbers must be graved, as they appear *per* Figure This being done, place the Axis B C answering to the Elevation of the Pole, and dispose it so that when it is set up it may not hinder the Hour-Plate from turning about the Center B

The Use of this Dial.

The Moon's Age must be found by an Ephemeris, or by the Epact, that so the Point of the Hour-Line of 12 on the Horizontal Dial may be applied to the Day of her Age in the Circle H of the under Plate

But before we go any further, you must observe, that the Moon by her proper Motion recedes Eastwards from the Sun every Day about 48 Minutes of an Hour, that is, if the Moon is in Conjunction with the Sun on any Day upon the Meridian, the next Day she

will

will croſs the Meridian about three quarters of an Hour and ſome Minutes later than the Sun . and this is the reaſon that the Lunar Days are longer than the Solar ones, a Lunar Day being that Space of Time elapſed between her Paſſage over the Meridian, and her next Paſſage over the ſame , and theſe Days are very unequal on account of the Irregularities of the Moon's Motion

Now when the Moon is come to be in Oppoſition to the Sun, ſhe will again be found in the ſame Hour-Circle as the Sun is, ſo that if, for example, the Sun ſhould be then in the Meridian of our Antipodes, the Moon would be in our Meridian, and conſequently would ſhew the ſame Hour on our Sun-Dials as the Sun would, if it was above the Horizon. But this Conformity would be of ſmall duration, becauſe of the Moon's retardation of about two Minutes every Hour. If moreover the Sun, at the time of the Oppoſition, be juſt ſetting above our Horizon, the Moon being diametrically oppoſite to it will be juſt riſing, &c and therefore to remedy the ſaid Retardation, we have divided the Circle H into 30 Parts

Now the Point of the Hour-Line of 12 on the Horizontal Dial being put to the Moon's Age, as above directed, and the under-Plate ſet North and South by means of a Compaſs or Meridian Line, the Shadow of the Style will ſhew the Hour of the Night, but to have the Hour more exact, you muſt know whether it is the firſt, ſecond or third Quarter of the Moon's Day that you ſeek the Hour in, that ſo the Point of the Hour-Line of 12 may be ſet againſt a proportionable part of one of the 30 Spaces or Lunar Days of the Circle H

The Table on the under-Plate H, is uſed for finding the Hour of the Night by the Shadow of the Moon upon an ordinary Dial To make this Table, draw 4 Parallel right Lines or Curves of any length, and divide the Space I I into twelve equal Parts for 12 Hours, and the two other Spaces K K into 15, for the 30 Lunar Days.

The Uſe of this Table

Firſt obſerve what Hour the Shadow of the Moon ſhews upon a Sun-Dial, then find the Moon's Age, and ſeek the Hour correſpondent thereto in the Table, and add the Hour ſhewn by the Sun-Dial thereto , then their Sum, if it be leſs than 12, or elſe its exceſs above 12, will be the true Hour of the Night For example , Suppoſe the Hour ſhewn upon the Sun-Dial by the Moon, be the *6th*, and her Age be 5 or 20 Days, againſt either of theſe Numbers in the Table you will find 4, which added to 6 makes 10, and ſo the Hour of the Night will be 10 Again, Suppoſe the Moon ſhews the Hour of 9 upon the Sun-Dial, when ſhe is 10 or 25 Days old, againſt 10 and 25 in the Table you will find 8, which added to 9, makes 17, from which 12 being taken, the Remainder 5 will be the true Hour ſought And ſo of others

To find the Moon's Age, you muſt firſt find the Golden Number, and this is done by adding 1 to the given Year, and dividing the Sum by 19, and the Remainder will be the Golden Number Then you muſt find the Epact, by means of the Golden Number, and this is done thus · Divide the Golden Number by 3, and each Unit remaining being called 10, will be the Epact, if the Sum be leſs than 30, but if above 30, 30 being taken from it, and the Remainder added to the Golden Number will be the Epact The Epact being found, the Moon's Age may be had after this manner · If the Moon's Age be ſought in *January*, add 0 to the Epact, in *February*, 2 ; in *March*, 1 , in *April*, 2 , in *May*, 3 , in *June*, 4 , in *July*, 5 , in *Auguſt*, 6 , in *September*, 8 , in *October*, 8 , in *November*, 10 , and in *December*, 10 · and the Sum, if it be leſs than 30, or the exceſs above 30, added to the Day of the given Month (rejecting 30 if need be) will be the Moon's Age that Day. For example, to find the Moon's Age the *14th* Day of *March*, in the Year 1716 (O S) the Golden Number is 7, and the Epact 17 , therefore adding 1 for *March* to 17, and the Sum will be 18 , and if to this 18 be added 14 for the Day of the Month, the Sum will be 32, from which 30 being taken, and the Remainder 2 will be the Moon's Age Note, This way of finding the Moon's Age is not ſo exact as we have it by the Ephemeris Likewiſe obſerve, that vertical Moon-Dials may be made in the manner as the horizontal ones are, but the Diviſions of 30 Parts upon Equinoctial Dials muſt be equal, and the moveable Circle divided into 24 equal Parts, &c

The Conſtruction of a Nocturnal or Star-Dial

The 13th Figure ſhews the Diſpoſition of the chief Stars compoſing the Conſtellation of *Urſa Major*, and *Urſa Minor*, about the Pole and the Pole-Star

The Nocturnal we are going to mention, is made by the Conſideration of the diurnal Motion, that the two Stars of *Urſa Major*, called his Guards, or the bright Star of *Urſa Minor*, make about the Pole, or the Pole Star, which at preſent is but about 2 deg diſtant from the Pole

Now to conſtruct this Inſtrument, you muſt firſt know the right Aſcenſion of the ſaid Stars, or in what Days of the Year they are found in the ſame Hour-Circle as the Sun is. This may be found, by Calculation, on a Globe, or a Celeſtial Planiſphere, by placing the Star in queſtion under the Meridian, and examining what Degree of the Ecliptick will be found at the ſame time under the Meridian. By this Method you will find that the

bright

bright Star or Guard of the Little Bear, was found twice in one Year with the Sun under the Meridian, *viz* in the Year 1715, once the *8th* of *May*, (N S.) above the Pole, and again the 8th of *November* below the Pole   Therefore in the faid two Days of the Year, the abovementioned Star will be in all the Hour-Circles at the fame time as the Sun is; and confequently will fhew the fame Hour   You will find alfo, that the two Guards of *Urfa Major* were found two other Days of the Year under the fame Meridian or Hour-Circle as the Sun, *viz.* the firft Day of *September* below the Pole, and the firft Day of *March* above it   And in thefe two Days the faid Stars will fhew the fame Hours as the Sun does; but becaufe the fixed Stars return to the Meridian every day about 1 deg. fooner than the Sun, or four Minutes of an Hour, which is two Hours *per* Month, it is this, which is to be obferved for having the Hour of the Sun, which is the Meafure of our Days.

Thefe things being premifed, it will not be difficult to make a Nocturnal or Star-Dial, in the following manner :

The Inftrument is compofed of two circular Plates applied on each other , the greater of which, having a Handle for holding up the Inftrument when ufing, is about two Inches and a half in Diameter, and is divided into twelve Parts for the twelve Months of the Year, and each Month divided into every *5th* Day , fo that the middle of the Handle exactly anfwers to the Day of the Year wherein that Star which is ufed has the fame right Afcenfion as the Sun has   If, for example, this Inftrument be made for the two Guards of *Urfa Major*, the firft Day of *September* muft be againft the middle of the Handle , and if it be made for the bright Star of *Urfa Minor*, the *8th* Day of *November* muft be againft the middle of the Handle   Therefore if you will have the Inftrument ferve for both thefe Stars, the Handle muft be made moveable about the faid circular Plate, that fo it may be fixed according to neceffity , and this is eafy to do by means of two little Screws

This being done, the upper leffer Circle muft be divided into 24 equal Parts, or twice 12 Hours, for the 24 Hours of the Day, and each Hour into Quarters, according to the Order appearing in the Figure   Thefe 24 Hours are diftinguifhed by a like Number of Teeth, whereof thofe whereat the Hours of 12 are marked are longer than the others, that fo the Hours may be counted in the Night without a Light

In the Center of the two circular Plates is adjufted a long Index A, moveable about the fame upon the upper Plate   Thefe three Pieces, *viz* the two Circles and the Index, are joined together by means of a headed Rivet, and pierced fo, that there is a round Hole thro the Center about two Inches diameter, for eafy feeing the Pole-Star thro it   *Note*, The Motions of the upper-Plate and Index ought to be pretty ftiff, that fo they may remain where they are placed when the Inftrument is ufing

The Ufe of this Inftrument

Turn the upper circular Plate till the longeft Tooth whereat is marked 12 be againft the Day of the Month on the under Plate , then bringing the Inftrument near your Eyes, hold it up by the Handle, fo that it leans neither to the Right or Left, with its Plane as near parallel to the Equinoctial as you can , and looking at the Pole-Star thro the Hole in the Center of the Inftrument, turn the Index about, till by the Edge coming from the Center, you can fee the bright Star or Guard of the Little Bear, if the Inftrument be adapted for that Star, and that Tooth of the upper Circle that is under the Edge of the Index, is at the Hour of the Night upon the Edge of the Hour-Circle, which may be known without a Light, by accounting the Teeth from the longeft, which is for the Hour of 12

You muft proceed in this manner for finding the Hour of the Night, when the Inftrument is made for the Guards of *Urfa Major*, which Stars are nearly in a right Line with the Pole-Star, are of the fame Magnitude, and are very ufeful for finding the Pole-Star.

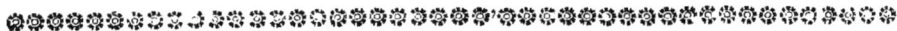

❀❀

C H A P. VII.

Of the Conftruction of a Water-Clock.

THIS Clock is compofed of a Metalline well foldered Cylinder, or round Box B, wherein is a certain quantity of prepared Water, and feveral little Cells, which communicate with each other by Holes near the Circumference, and which let no more Water run thro them than is neceffary for making the Cylinder defcend flowly by its proper Weight   This Cylinder is hung to the Points A A by two fine Cords of equal thicknefs, which are wound about the Iron Axle-tree D D, which Axle-tree goes thro the exact middle of

the

the Cylinder at right Angles to the Bases, and as it descends shews the Hour marked upon a vertical Plane on both sides of the Cylinder   The Divisions on this Plane are made thus . Having wound up the Cylinder to the top of the Plane from whence you would begin the Hour-Divisions, let it descend 12 Hours, reckoned by a Clock or good Sun-Dial, and note the Place where the Axle-tree is come to at the end of that time, and divide the Space the Axle-tree has moved thro in 12 equal Parts, each of which set Numbers to, for the Hours

We make likewise Clocks of this kind, that shew the Hour by a Hand turning about a Dial-Plate, as appears in the same Figure.   This is done by means of a Pulley four or five Inches in diameter, fastened behind the Dial-Plate on a Brass or Steel Rod, going thro the Center thereof ; one end of this Rod goes into a little Hole for supporting it, and at the other end is fixed the Hand shewing the Hour

The said Hand turns by means of a Cord put about the Pulley, one end of which supports the Axle-tree at the Place H, and at the other end is hung a small Weight F ; then as the Cylinder slowly descends, it causes the Pulley to turn about, and consequently the Hand, which by this means shews the Hour.

The Circumference of the Pulley must be equal to the Length the Axle-tree of the Cylinder moves thro during twelve Hours , and for this End you must take that Length exactly with a String, and then make the Circumference of the Pulley equal to the Length of the String, and so the Pulley and Hand will go once round in twelve Hours.   When the Cylinder descends a little too swift, and consequently the Hand moves too fast, then the Weight F must be made heavier ; and when it descends too slow, it must be made lighter.

The Construction of the Cylinder or Round Box

Fig 16

This Cylinder is sometimes made of beaten Silver, but commonly with Tin   The Diameter of each Base thereof is about 5 Inches, and the Height 2

The Inside of this Cylinder is divided into seven little Cells, (and sometimes into five) as the Figure shews   These little Cells are made by foldering seven Silver or Tin inclined Planes to each Base, and the concave Circumference of the Cylinder , each of which are about 2 Inches long, as B F, A L, E I, D H, C G   These Cells have such an Inclination when they turn about, that they receive the Water thro a little Hole in each Plane near the Circumference, and by this means let it run from one Cell to the other , so that as the Cylinder rolls, it descends, and shews the Hour upon a vertical Plane by the Extremity of the Axle-tree, which (as we have said) goes thro the square Hole M in the middle of the Cylinder   *Note*, In a Cylinder of the abovesaid bigness we usually pour seven or eight Ounces of distilled Water   But before the Water be poured in, you must take great care to well folder the inclined Planes to the Bases and Circumference   After this, the Water must be poured thro two Holes posited on one and the same Diameter, equally distant from the Center M, then these Holes must be well stopped with soldering, that so the Air may not get in, or the Water run out while the Cylinder is turning about.

You may perceive, by the Figure, that the inclined Planes within the Cylinder do not join each other, but end in G, H, I, L, F, that so when the Cylinder is winding up, the Water may run swiftly from one Cell to the other, and the Cylinder remain at any Height one pleases, because that at every Motion we give it when winding up, the Water running in a great Quantity thro the Openings, the Cylinder will presently assume its *Equilibrium*, which would not happen if the Cells were absolutely inclosed : for the little Holes in the inclined Planes, are not sufficient for letting the Water run thro them so swift as it ought, it going through them but by drops.

It is manifest, if this Cylinder was suspended by the Center of Gravity thereof, as would happen if the Surface of the Axle-tree should exactly pass thro the Center of the said Cylinder, it would remain at rest , and the Cause of its Motion is, that it is suspended without the Center of Gravity by the Cord's going about the Axle-tree, which ought not to be, with regard to the bigness of the Cylinder, and the quantity of Water in it, but about one Line, or one Line and a half, in thickness

From what has been said, it is evident that the Swiftness or Slowness of the Motion of the Cylinder depends upon the thickness of the Axle-tree, for the thicker the Axle-tree is, the slower will the Cylinder descend, and contrariwise, because it has more or less Excentricity, and consequently the Water will run more or less swift from one Cell to another , by which means the Force of its Motion will be more or less ballanced by the Weight of the Water contained in the opposite Cell

If you have a mind to see the Circulation of the Water in one of these Cylinders, you may have one made that shall have a Glass Base . but then it will be difficult to find a Matter that shall make the inclined Planes stick firm to this Glass Case, and this to the Circumference of the Cylinder

When the Cylinder is nearly descended to the bottom of the Cords, you must raise it up with your Hand, making it turn at the same time, so that the Cords may equally roll all along the Axle-tree, and that it be hung horizontally.

I

I have hinted before, that the Water poured into the Cylinder muſt be diſtilled, otherwiſe it muſt be often changed, becauſe it makes a Slime about the ſmall Holes thro which it runs, which hinders its running as it ſhould do

CHAP. VIII.

Of the Conſtruction of an Inſtrument, ſhewing on what Point of the Compaſs the Wind blows, without going out of one's Room.

YOU muſt affix to the Ceiling, Mantle-tree, or Wall of a Room, a Circle divided into 32 equal Parts, for the 32 Points of the Compaſs, ſo that the North and South Points thereof exactly anſwer to the Meridian Line, which may be eaſily done by a Compaſs Then there muſt be a Hand made moveable about the ſaid Circle, and this Hand muſt be turned about by an upright Axle-tree, which may be turned round by the leaſt Wind blowing againſt the Fane at the top thereof, above the Roof of the Houſe

But to explain this more fully, conſult *Fig* 17 The Wind turning the Fane A B, (which *Fig.* 17. ought to be of Iron) fixed to the top of the Axle-tree C D, turns this Axle-tree, which is placed upright, and ſuſtained towards the top by the horizontal Plane E F, which is a piece of Iron faſtened to ſome convenient Place for holding up the Axle-tree And at the bottom of the ſaid Axle-tree is placed a Steel ſquare G H, having a ſhallow ſmall Hole D made therein for the Point of the Axle-tree, which ought to be of tempered Steel for the Axle-tree to ſtand in, and move with the leaſt Wind The Pinion I K muſt have 8 equal Teeth for the 8 principal Winds The Teeth of this Pinion take into the Teeth of the Wheel M L, whoſe Number are 16 or 32, according to the Points denoted upon the Circle Y Z, and ſo this Wheel is turned about by the Fane, as alſo its Axis P Q, which being placed horizontally, goes thro the Wall T at right Angles to it, as alſo to the Circle of Winds Y Z, fixed to the Wall The Hand R ſhewing which way the Wind blows, is fixed to the end of this Axle-tree P Q, and turns along with it, and the Names of the Winds muſt be diſtinguiſhed by Capital Letters, as on Compaſs Cards

By the Diſpoſition of the whole Inſtrument it is eaſy to perceive, that when the Wind turns the Fane A B, this likewiſe turns the Axle-tree C D, which at the ſame time turns the Pinion I K, and the Pinion I K the Wheel L M, and this the Axis Q P, and Q P the Hand And ſo you may ſee which way the Wind blows, without going out of the Room

A ſhort Deſcription of the principal Tools uſed in making of Mathematical Inſtruments.

THE chief and moſt neceſſary Tool is a large Vice, ſerving to hold Work while it is filing, &c It is neceſſary that this Tool be well filed, that the Chops meet each other exactly, that they be cut like a File, be in good temperature, that the Screw be adjuſted as it ſhould be in its Box, and that the whole Tool be well fixed to a Bench There are alſo Hand-Vices of different bigneſſes, according to the Work to be filed

The Anvil, which ſerves for hammering Work upon, ought to be very ſmooth and of tempered Steel, and placed upon a great wooden Billot, ſo that it may not give way when it is working upon.

There are alſo Bench-Anvils for ſtrengthening and rivetting ſmall Work, ſome of theſe, which are called Bec's, and ſerve to make Ferrils upon, &c have one ſide Conical, and the other in figure of a ſquare Pyramid

Hand-Saws are made ſo as to have Branches drawing the Blades (which are of different bigneſſes) ſtraight by means of Screws and Nuts.

It is neceſſary to have good Files The rough ones made in *Germany* are the beſt; and the ſmooth and baſtard Files of *England* are very good. There are alſo ſmall rough and ſmooth Files, for filing Work Triangular, Square, Circular, Semi-circular, &c Raſps for

faſhioning

fashioning of Wood; several sorts of Hammers for straightening, smoothing, rivetting, &c of Work, Tapes and Plates for making Screws

Pincers and Knippers of several kinds Scissars of several sizes for cutting of Metals. Burnishing-Sticks for polishing Work. Steel-Drills of divers bignesses for making of Holes thro Work, having one end filed like a Cat's Tongue, and the other sharp These Drills are used different ways, for some of them are placed in a drilling Leath, which is composed of a small square Iron-Bar, and two little Poupets or Heads carrying a Pulley, wherein is placed the Drill in a square Hole going thro it, which is turned by means of a little Cat-gut Bow Note, This Tool is placed in a Vice when it is using Brass or Wood may be drilled also by putting it first into the Vice, and the Drill in a Pulley Then if the end of the Drill be put into a shallow Cavity made in a piece of Brass or Iron, placed against your Breast, and the Point thereof be put to the thing you would make a Hole thro, by turning the Drill swiftly about by means of the Bow, and at the same time pressing it with your Breast against the thing to be drilled, you will soon make a Hole thro it

The Leath is also of great use, the most simple of them is made of two Brass or Iron Poupets or Heads sliding along a square Iron-Bar, and a Support which also slides along the said Bar, upon which the Tools are laid when they are using At the top of the Poupets are two Screws of tempered Steel going thro them, which are fixed by means of Nuts When this Leath is to be used, it must be placed in a Vice, and the thing to be turned, between the two Points of the Screws, and if you have a mind to turn with your Hand, you must use a Cat-gut Bow

Great Leaths for turning with one's Foot are composed of two wooden Poupets, and two wooden side Beams, of a length and breadth proportional to the bigness of the Leath, which are sustained by two Pieces of Wood called the Feet of the Leath. These side Beams are placed level, about two or three Inches distant from each other, according to the bigness of the Poupets put between them, and the ends of them are adjusted upon the Feet, which are about four Foot high, and they are likewise joined underneath by two or three cross pieces of Wood, for rendering the Machine more stable and solid

The Poupets, which are two pieces of Wood of equal length and thickness, have one part of each cut so as to go in between the side Beams, and the other part, being the Head, is cut square, and solidly posited upon the side Beams, and that they may be very firm, there are Clefts of Wood drove with a Mallet into Mortice-holes at the bottom of the Poupets underneath the side Beams

In the Head of each Poupet is a tempered steel Point strongly inclosed in the Wood; so that when these two Points are brought to each other, they may exactly touch. There is likewise a wooden Bar going all along, which is sustained by the Arms of the Poupets, which may be lengthened and shortened at pleasure, and this serves as a Rest for the Tools, when they are using

Against the Ceiling, over the Leath, is fixed an Elastick wooden Rod, having at the end thereof a Cord fastened, which comes down to the Ground, and is fixed to the end of a piece of Wood, called the Treader

Now when you have a mind to work, the Cord must be put about the Piece to be turned, or about a Mandril adjusted to it, and pressing your Foot upon the Treader, you will turn the Work by means of the Rod which springs, then with proper Tools laid upon the Support, and against the Piece which is turning, you must first fashion it with coarse Tools, and finish it with fine ones

Because all Work cannot be turned between two Points, one of the Poupets must be taken away, and instead thereof must be placed a piece of Wood furnished with Iron, adjusted between the side Beams as the Poupets are, and instead of having a Steel Point has a very round Hole therein, in which goes the Colet of an Iron-Arbor, whose other end is sustained by the Steel-Point of the other Poupet.

The said Arbor is fifteen or eighteen Inches long, and is composed thus at the end, which is supported against the aforesaid piece of Wood, is a Screw of a very large Thread made round the Arbor, upon which are screwed on divers Brass Boxes, in which are held fast the pieces of Wood, which serve to place the several Works to be turned And at the other end of the said Arbor are made several Threads of Screws of different bigresses, that so Screws may be turned

Near the middle of the said Arbor, is placed a Mandril or wooden Pulley, about which goes a Cord There may be several other Pieces adjusted on this Arbor, for turning irregular Figures, as Ovals, Hearts, Roses, wreathed Pillars, &c All these Pieces are filed into the Figures that one would have them make, and have square Holes in the middle of them, which are adjusted to a Square near the end of the Arbor

When the Pieces are disposed on the Arbor, the pointed end thereof is placed in a little Hole in the Steel-Point of the Poupet, and the other end in the aforesaid wooden Piece (placed instead of a second Poupet) which is made so, that there are two Pieces which spring, and push the Figure backwards and forwards, and by this means move the Arbor backwards and forwards, more or less, according to the Figure, and this is the

Cause

Plate XXIV

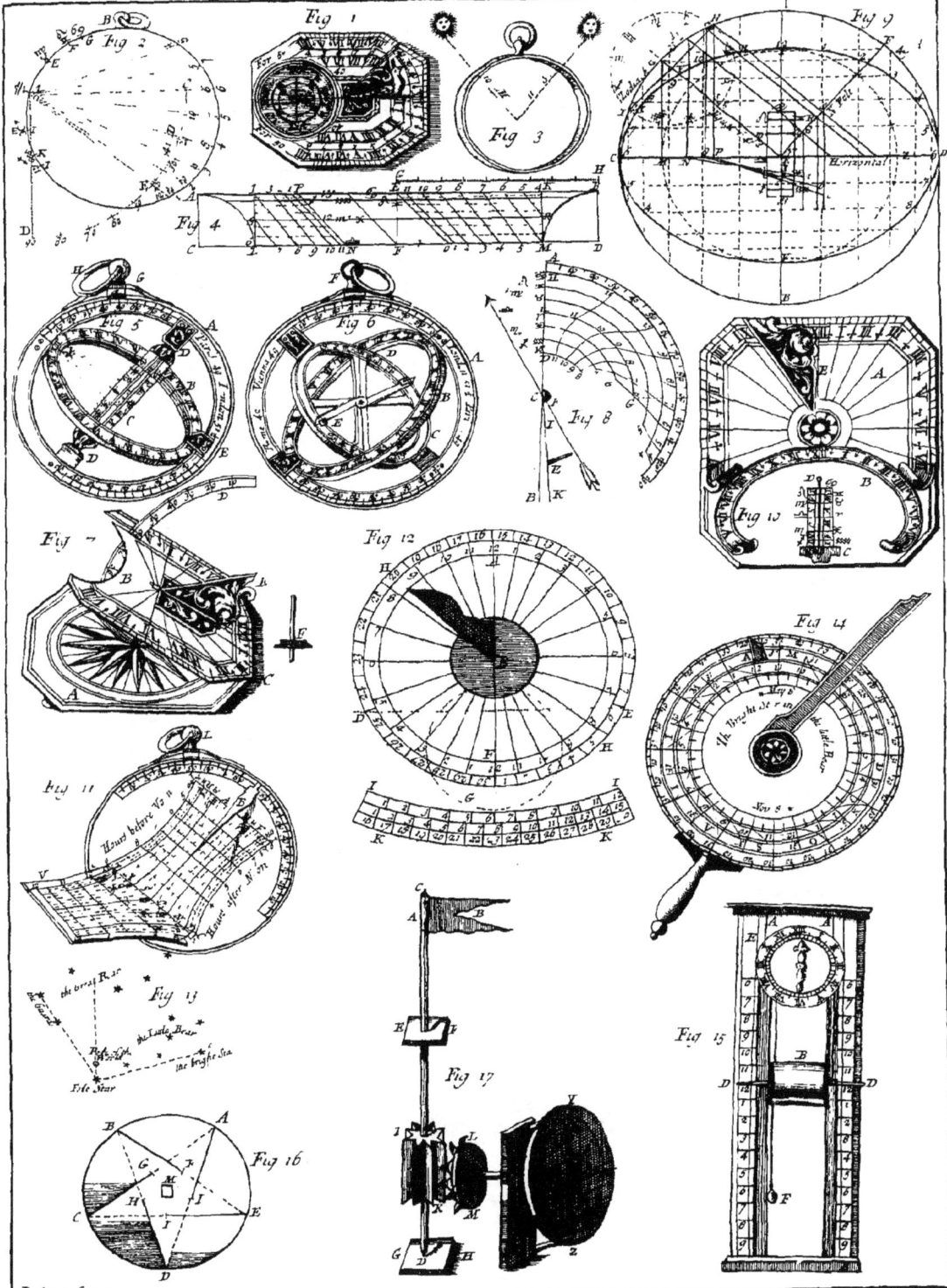

Cauſe that the Tool gives the proper Figure to the Work, which moves to it, or recedes from it, according to the Motion of the Arbor, for the Tool muſt always be held faſt upon the Support But ſince theſe kinds of Figures are ſeldom uſed for Mathematical Inſtruments, I ſhall ſay no more as to this way of turning

The principal Uſe of the ſaid Arbor, ſerves for turning of Rings, making of Grooves in Compaſſes, and other the like things And this may be done, in placing the Pieces to be turned upon the Wood belonging to the Boxes (of which we have already ſpoken) which are adjuſted on the Leath for receiving the ſaid Pieces *Note,* The Reſts or Supports of the Tools are likewiſe placed according as the Work requires, ſome before, and ſome ſideways.

Male and Female Screws are formed, by putting the proper Thread on the Arbor into a piece of Wood hollowed into a Screw of the ſame Thread, which is placed at the Poupet carrying the end of the Arbor. And the other end of the Arbor, where is a Colet of the ſame thickneſs, is put exactly into the Hole of the abovementioned piece of Wood, then if the Treader be put in motion by your Foot, the Work will move backwards and forwards, ſo as that you may form a Screw or a Nut, with toothed Tools made on purpoſe, according to the Threads marked upon the Arbor *Note,* For turning of Wood, Googes, Chiſſels, *&c.* are uſed But for Braſs and other Metals, ſmaller Tools of tempered Steel muſt be uſed, as Graving-Tools, *&c.*

Thus have I here, and in the Body of this Work, given a ſhort Account of the Tools commonly uſed in making of Mathematical Inſtruments. The others may be eaſily ſupplied according to Neceſſity But ſince they are uſually made by thoſe that uſe them, I ſhall here ſhew how to chuſe the beſt Metal for their Conſtruction.

The beſt Steel comes from *Germany* This ought to be without Flaws, Black-veins, or Iron-furrows You may know this by breaking of it, and ſeeing whether the Grain be very fine and equal

In forging of Tools, or any thing elſe of Steel, you muſt take care of over-heating them, and perform it as ſoon as poſſible, for the longer they are hot, the more will they be ſpoiled

When the Tools are forged and filed, and you have a mind to temper them, you muſt heat them red-hot till their Colour be ſomething redder than a Cherry, and then they muſt be tempered in Spring or Well-Water: the colder the Water is, the better And when they are cold, they muſt be taken out of the Water, and laid preſently upon a piece of hot Iron, ſo long, till the Colour they have contracted by tempering is loſt, and they become yellowiſh, and then they muſt be thrown again into the Water, without ſtaying till they become blue, becauſe they will loſe their Force

To temper Bundles of Files, or other Pieces of Iron, you muſt take Chimney-Soot, the oldeſt and groſſeſt being the beſt, and having finely powdered it, temper it with Piſs and Vinegar, putting a little melted Salt therein, until the whole be as a liquid Paſte The Soot being tempered, the Tools muſt be covered over with it, and this covered with Earth, and the whole Bundle thrown into a ſtrong Charcoal fire, and when it is become ſomething redder than a Cherry, it muſt be taken out and thrown into a Veſſel full of very cold Water, and then the Files will be ſufficiently hard.

We have already ſhewed the manner of ſoldering Braſs or Silver to each other, and we would have it here obſerved, that Iron may be ſoldered to Iron, by putting thin Braſs upon the Piece to be ſoldered, and the Powder of Borax, and then covering it all round with Charcoal, and heating it until we perceive the Braſs melts and runs

Note, Braſs cannot be hammered when it is hot, for it will break, but Copper is hammered cold or hot: but this is ſeldom uſed in making of Mathematical Inſtruments, becauſe Braſs is finer and more convenient. Braſs is made with red Copper and Calamin, which is a Stone giving a yellow Tincture to the Metal, and is found in the Country of *Liege,* and in *France*

Gold and Silver may be hammered cold or hot, and may be melted alſo nearly as Braſs is, and Mathematical Inſtruments are made with Gold and Silver in the ſame manner as with Braſs.

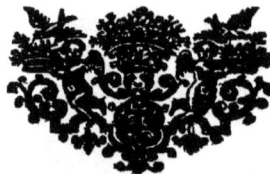

The

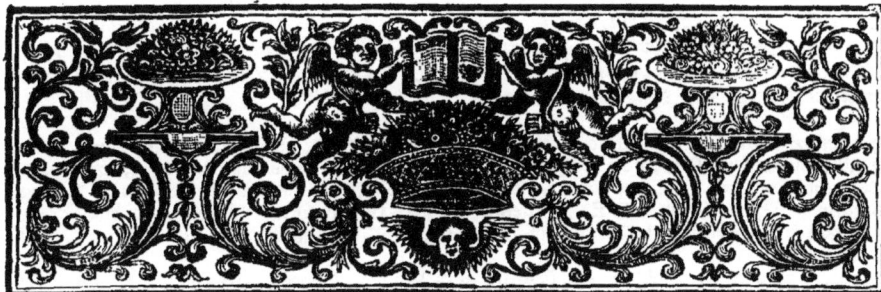

The Uſe of the Sector *in the Conſtruction of Solar Eclipſes.*

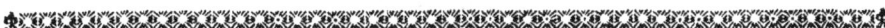

DEFINITION I.

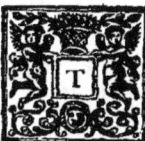

T HE Path of a *Vertex*, is that Circle of the Earth which any Place or *Vertex* on its Superficies deſcribes, in the Space of twenty-four Hours, by the Earth's diurnal Revolution. Whence the Paths of *Vertices* are Circles parallel to the Equator.

DEFINITION II

If a Plane be conceived to touch the Moon's Orbit in that Point, wherein a Line connecting the Centers of the Earth and Sun, interſects the ſaid Orbit, and ſtands at right Angles to the aforenamed Line : And if an infinite Number of right Lines be ſuppoſed to paſs from the Center of the Sun, thro this Plane to the Periphery of the Earth, to its Axis, as likewiſe to the Axis of the Ecliptick, and the Path of any *Vertex* ; the ſaid Lines will orthographically project the Earth's Diſk, its Axis, the Axis of the Ecliptick, and the Path of the *Vertex*, on the aforeſaid Plane : and this is the Projection we are to delineate. This being preſuppoſed, it will follow ;

1 That when the Sun is in ♋, ♌, ♍, ♎, ♏, ♐, the Northern half of the Earth's Axis projected on the aforeſaid Plane, viewed on that Side next to the Earth, lies to the Right-hand from the Axis of the Ecliptick · But if the Longitude of the Sun be in any of the ſix oppoſite Signs, it lies to the Left-hand from the Axis of the Ecliptick

2. When the Sun's apparent Place happens to be either in ♈, ♉, ♊, ♋, ♌, ♍, the North Pole lies in the *illuminate* or viſible part of the Diſk ; but otherways in the *obſcure*

3 When the Sun's Place in the Ecliptick is 90 Degrees diſtant from either Pole ; that is, when the Sun is in the Equator, *the Paths of the Vertices*, or all Circles of the Earth parallel to the Equator, will be projected in right Lines upon the ſaid Plane. but if the Sun's Place be leſſer than 90 Degrees, the ſaid Paths will be projected in Ellipſes upon the ſaid Plane, whoſe conjugate Diameters will be ſo much the leſſer, as the Place of the Sun is leſſer

4 *The tranſverſe Diameter of the Ellipſes* repreſenting any Path, is equal to double the right Sine of the Diſtance of the ſaid *Vertex* from the *Pole* ; that is, equal to twice the Co-Sine of the Latitude of the Place or *Vertex* but the *Conjugate*, to the Difference of the right Sines of the Sum, and Difference of the Diſtances of the Path and Sun from the Pole, that is, equal to the Sine of the Complement of the Sun's Declination added to the Co-Latitude of the Place, leſs the right Sine of the Difference of the Complement of the Sun's Declination, and the Co-Latitude of the Place.

5 The tranſverſe Diameter lies at right Angles to the Earth's Axis, and the conjugate coincides therewith

SECTION

SECTION I.

To reprefent in Plano, the Path of a Vertex in the Earth's Disk, whose Diftance from the North Pole is 38 deg. 32 min. the Sun's Place being in 10 deg. 40 min. 30 fec. of Gemini, femblable to that which will be projected on a Plane, touching the Earth's Orbit in that Point, by ftrait Lines produced from the Sun to the Earth.

HAving drawn the Semi-circle H E R, let it reprefent the Northern half of the Earth's *Plate 25.* illuminate Disk (becaufe the Sun is in *Gemini*) projected upon the faid Plane, the Sun its *Fig. 1.* Center, the Point therein oppofite to the Sun, H ⊙ R an Arc of the Ecliptick paffing through it. Upon ⊙ raife ⊙ E, perpendicular to the Ecliptick H R, and the Point E wherein it interfects the Limb of the Disk, will be the Pole of the Ecliptick, and ⊙ E its Axis

Again, Make ⊙ E equal to the Radius of a Line of Chords (by *Ufe* III *of the Line of Chords*) from which taking the Chord of 23 deg 30 min (the conftant Diftance of the two Poles) fet it off both ways from E to B and C, draw the Line B C, in which the Northern Pole of the World fhall be found

Make B A equal to A C, the half of this Line, the Radius of a Line of Sines and therein fet off the Sine of the Sun's Diftance from the folftitial Colure 19 deg 19 min. 30 fec from A to P, on the Left-hand of the Axis of the Ecliptick, (becaufe the Sun is in *Gemini*) and draw the Line ⊙ P, which will be the Axis of the Earth, and P the place of North-Pole in the illuminate Hemifphere of the Disk

Or the Angle E ⊙ I, which the Axis of the Earth and Ecliptick make with each other, may be more accurately determined by Calculation   For,

	deg.	min	fec	
As Radius —— to the Sine of the Sun's Diftance from the fol-	90	00	00	10,000000
ftitial Colure —— —— ——	19	19	30	9,5197331
So is the Tangent of the Sun's greateft Declination to the	23	30	00	9,637956
Tangent of the Inclination of the Axis —— ——	8	10	54	9,157687

Count the faid 8 deg 10 min 54 fec in the Limb of the Disk from E to I, on the Left-hand, and draw the Line ⊙ I, this fhall be the Axis, and the Point P wherein it interfects the Line B C, the place of the Pole in the illuminate Disk

The next thing required will be the Sun's Diftance from the Pole, or the Complement of his Declination, which will be found 67 deg 57 min 48 fec this, added to the Diftance of the Vertex from the Pole 38 deg 32 min. makes 106 deg. 29 min 48 fec and the fame 38 deg 32 min taken from 67 deg 51 min 48 fec gives 29 deg. 25 min 48 fec the Meridional Diftance of the Sun from the Vertex

Make ⊙ E the Radius of the Disk, to be the Radius of a Line of Sines, from which take the Sine of 73 deg 30 min 12 fec (the Complement of 106 deg. 29 min 48 fec to a Semi-circle) and fet it off in the Axis from ⊙ to 12, it there gives the Meridional Interfection of the Nocturnal Arc of the Path with the Axis

Take the Sine of 29 min 25 min 48 fec. from the fame Line of Sines, and fet it off the fame way from ⊙ to M, and it there gives the Interfection of the diurnal Arc of the Path with the Meridian   Whence M 12 will be the conjugate Diameter of the Path, it being the Difference of the Sines of 70 deg 30 min 12 fec and 29 deg 25 min 48 fec that is, the Difference of the Sines of the Sum, and Difference of the Diftances of the Path and Sun from the Pole, which will be the conjugate Diameter of any Path

Bifect 12 M in C, and through it draw 6 C 6 at right Angles to the Axis of the Globe; and then taking the Sine of 38 deg 32 min the Diftance of the Pole from the Vertex, fet it off from C both ways to 6 and 6, then the Line 6 6 will be the Tranverfe-diameter of the Path, and C 6 the Semi-diameter

Making C 6 equal to the Radius of a Line of Sines, if from the fame you take the right Sines of 15, 30, 45, 60, 75 Degrees, and fet them off feverally both ways from C in the Tranverfe-diameter, and from the Points fo found erect Perpendiculars, *a* 11, *a* 1, *a* 10, *a* 2, &c equal to the Co-fines of the faid Arcs, taken from a Line of Sines, whofe Radius fhall be C 12, equal to C M, you will have twenty-four Points given, through which the Ellipfis reprefenting the Path fhall pafs, which fhall alfo fhew the Place of the Vertex at every Hour of the Day In the fame manner may the Parts of an Hour be pricked down in the Path, in laying off the Sine of the Degrees and Minutes correfponding thereto from C towards 6, and then raifing Perpendiculars from the Points fo found in the Semi-tranfverfe, and fetting off from the faid Semi-tranfverfe each way upon the Perpendiculars, the

the Sines of the Complements of the Degrees and Minutes corresponding to the aforesaid Parts of an Hour As, for example, to denote half an Hour past 11 and 12, take the Sine of 7 deg. 30 min and lay it off on both sides from C to *b* and *b*; then take the Co-sine of 7 deg. 30 min. and having raised the Perpendiculars *b* +, lay off the said Sine-Complement from *b* to +, and you will have the Points in the Periphery of the Ellipsis, for half an Hour past 11, and half an Hour past 12; and in this manner may the Path be divided into Minutes, if the Ellipsis be large enough

Take this for another example; Suppose I would represent upon the Plane of the Earth's Disk, the Path of *Gibraltar*, whose Latitude is 35 deg 32 min North, and the Sun's Place is in 15 deg 45 min of *Leo*.

Fig. 2

Having, as before, drawn the Semi-circle H E R, for the Northern half of the Earth's illuminate Disk, and drawn ☉ E perpendicular to R H, as also drawn the Line C B, which is always equal to twice the Chord of the Sun's greatest Declination, 23 deg 30 min. you must next make A B equal to a Radius of a Line of Sines, and then lay off from A to P, on the Right-hand of the Axis of the Ecliptick, (because the Sun is in *Leo*) the Sine of the Sun's Distance from the solstitial Colure 45 deg. 45 min or, the Angle E ☉ I may be more nicely determined by Calculation, as was before directed, and then ☉ P I, will be the Axis of the World

Now the Sun's Distance from the Pole, or the Complement of his Declination is 73 deg 51 min which being added to the Complement of the Latitude 54 deg. 28 min the Sum will be 128 deg 19 min and this taken from 180 deg the Remainder will be 51 deg. 41 min also it 54 deg 28 min be taken from 73 deg 51 min the Difference will be 19 deg 23 min.

Then if you make the Semi-diameter of the Disk the Radius c a Line of Sines, and lay off from the Center ☉ to 12, the Sine of 51 deg 41 min the Point 12 in the Axis will be the Meridional Intersection of the Nocturnal Arc of the Path with the Axis, and if again you lay off the Sine of 19 deg 23 min from ☉ to M, you will have the Meridional Intersection of the Diurnal Arc of the Path with the Axis, whence M 12 will be the conjugate Diameter of the Elliptical Path

And if you bisect M 12 in C, and draw the Line b C 6 at right Angles to the Axis ☉ I, and then lay off the Sine Complement of the Latitude 54 deg 28 min from C to 6, on each side the Axis you will have the Transverse-diameter of the Path, which may be drawn and divided, as before directed, for that of *Fig* 1

Note, When the elevated Pole is in the obscure Hemisphere of the Earth, the diurnal Arc, or illuminated Part of the Path, is in that Part of the Ellipsis that lies nearest to the said Pole, but otherways in the more remote, and where the Ellipsis cuts the Limb of the Disk, are the Points on it from which the Sun appears to rise and set, &c. And because these Points are necessary to be found, when an Eclipse happens near Sun-rising or Sun-setting, they may be determined in the following manner

Fig 1.

Lay off the Sun's Declination 22 deg 2 min upon the Limb of the Disk from R to N, as also the Complement of the Latitude of 38 deg. 32 min from R to P, then draw the Line ☉ N, and from the Point P let fall upon the Diameter R H, the Perpendicular P Q, cutting the Line ☉ N in L This being done, take the Extent ☉ L, between your Compasses, and lay it off upon the Axis ☉ I from ☉ to K, then draw a Line both ways from the Point K, parallel to the transverse Axis C 6 of the Path, and the said Line will cut the Limb of the Disk in the Points *q p* of the Sun's rising and setting.

Or the Arc I *p* may be more accurately determined by Calculation, for in the Triangle ☉ Q L, right-angled at Q, are given the Angle Q L ☉, equal to the Sun's Distance from the Pole; and the Side Q ☉ equal to the Sine of the Latitude. To find the Side O L, which is equal to the Sine Complement of the Arc I *p*, the Canon is, As the Sine of the Sun's Distance from the Pole, is to Radius, so is the Sine of the Latitude to the Sine Complement of the Arc I *p*, or I *q*.

SECTION II.

HAving in the foregoing Section shewn how to draw the Path of any Vertex upon the Earth's Disk, as likewise to divide it, the next thing necessary to be given, in order to construct the Phases of a Solar Eclipse in any given Place on the Earth's Superficies, are,

I The apparent Time of the nearest Approach of the Moon to the Center of the Disk, or the Time of the Middle of the Eclipse

II The nearest Distance of the Moon's Center from the Center of the Disk in her Passage over it; which is equal to her Latitude at the time of the Conjunction.

III. The Semi-diameter of the Disk at the time of the Conjunction.

IV. The Moon's Semi-diameter at the same time.

V. The Sun's Semi-diameter.

VI. The Semi-diameter of the Penumbra.

VII. The

Plate XXV

Fig 1

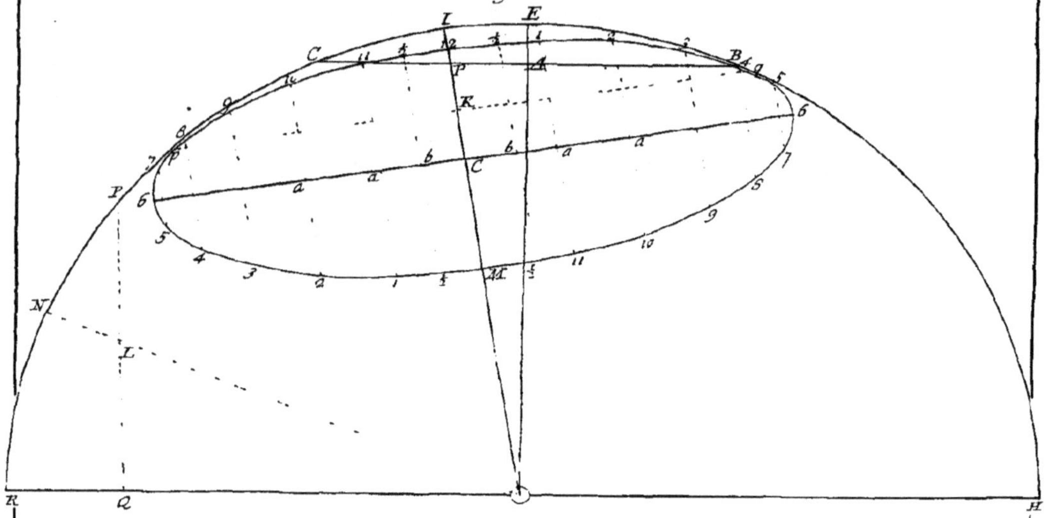

Fig 2

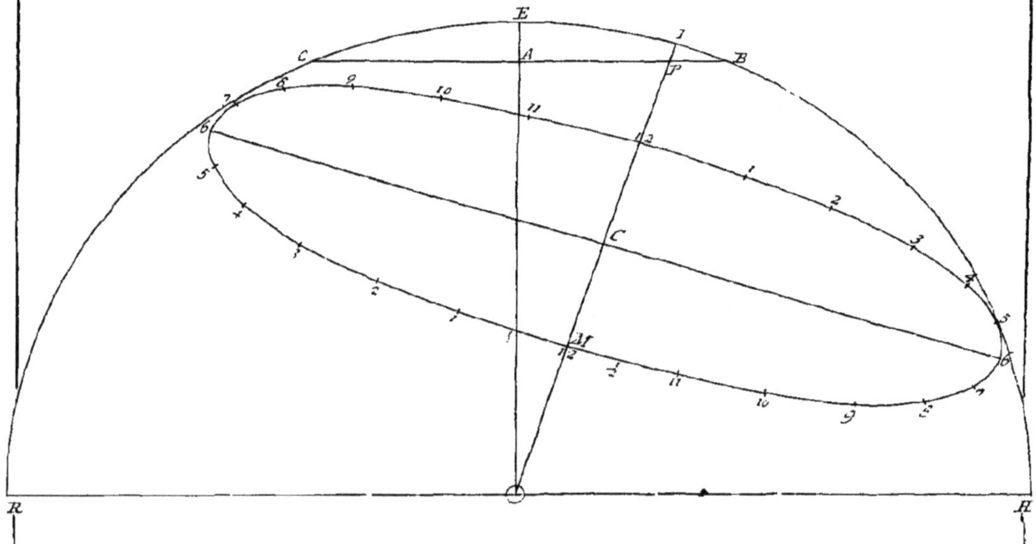

VII The Angle of the Moon's Way with the Ecliptick, which is equal to the Angle that the Perpendicular to the Moon's Way forms with the Axis of the Ecliptick, and if the Argument of Latitude be more than 9 Sines, or less than 3, the said Perpendicular lies to the Left-hand, if more, to the Right, from the Axis of the Ecliptick

VIII The hourly Motion of the Moon from the Sun at the time of the Conjunction.

Note, The Semi-diameter of the Disk is always equal to the Difference of the Sun and Moon's horizontal Parallaxes.

All these for the Solar Eclipse of *May* 11 1724. will be as follows ·

	Hours	min	sec.	
The apparent Time of the nearest Approach of the Moon to the Center of the Disk, will be	5	12	0	Afternoon
The nearest Distance of the Moon's Center from the Center of the Disk	0	32	14	
The Semi-diameter of the Disk	0	61	38	
The Moon's Semi-diameter	0	16	42	
The Sun's Semi-diameter	0	15	53	
The Semi-diameter of the Penumbra	0	32	35	
The Angle of the Moon's Way with the Ecliptick	0	5 deg	37 min	
The hourly Motion of the Moon from the Sun	0	35	18	

These being found from Astronomical Tables and Calculations, I shall shew how to draw the Line of the Moon's Way, or Path of the Penumbra, upon the Plane of the Earth's Disk, as it falls at the time of the Conjunction of *May* 11, 1724 and the manner of dividing the same, for *London, Genoa,* and *Rome*

Having drawn the Semi-circle H E R of the Earth's Disk, and the Paths of *London,* *Plate* 26. *Genoa,* and *Rome,* by the directions of the last Section, the Sun's Place being 61 deg Fig. 1. 38 min 45 sec and the Latitude of *London* 51 deg 31 min that of *Genoa* 44 deg 27 min and that of *Rome* 41 deg 51 min you must next draw the Perpendicular to the Moon's Way; which is done thus Take the Semi-diameter ⊙ H of the Disk between your Compasses, and open your Sector so, that the Distance from 60 to 60 of Chords be equal to that Extent; then taking 5 deg 37 min. parallel-wise from the Lines of Chords, (which is the Angle of the Moon's Way with the Ecliptick, or the Angle that a Perpendicular to her Way makes with the Axis E ⊙ of the same Ecliptick) lay them off upon the Limb of the Disk from F to F, on the Right-hand of the Axis of the Ecliptick, because the Argument of Latitude is more than three Sines, and the Line ⊙ F being drawn, will be the Perpendicular to the Moon's Way at the time of the general Conjunction, *May* 11, 1724.

Again Take the Semi-diameter of the Disk between your Compasses, and open the Sector so, that the Distance from $61\frac{38}{60}$, the Semi-diameter of the Disk, on each Line of Lines be equal to that Extent, then the Sector remaining thus opened, take between your Compasses the parallel Extent of $32\frac{14}{60}$, the nearest Approach of the Moon to the Center of the Disk, and lay it off from ⊙ to M, upon the Perpendicular to the Moon's Way, then, if upon the Point M, a Perpendicular, as M G, be drawn both ways, this will be the Line of the Moon's Way, or Path of the Penumbra

Now to divide the said Path into its proper Hours, which let be for *London* The middle of the General Eclipse, or the time when the Moon's Center will be at M, happens at 12 Minutes past 5 in the Afternoon say, As 1 Hour or 60 Minutes to 35 min 18 sec. the hourly Motion of the Moon from the Sun, so is 12 Minutes the time more than 5 in the Afternoon, to 7 min 3 sec the Motion from 5 a-clock to the midddle

Your Sector remaining open'd to the last Angle it was set to, take the Extent from $7\frac{1}{5}$ to $7\frac{1}{60}$ on each Line of Lines, and setting one Foot of your Compasses upon M, with the other make a Point on the Moon's Way to the Right-hand, and this shall be the Place of the Penumbra at 5 a-clock in the Afternoon at *London*, which therefore denote with the Number V

The hourly Motion of the Moon from the Sun is 35 min 18 sec therefore take the parallel Extent of $35\frac{18}{60}$, on the Line of Lines, between your Compasses, and setting one Foot upon V, with the other make Points on each side V, these shall shew the Place of the Moon's Center at the Hours of IV and VI, and if from these Points you farther set off the said Extent in the said Line, you may thereby find the Place of the Moon's Center for every Hour, whilst the Penumbra shall touch the Disk and if the Space between every Hour be divided into 60 equal Parts, you shall have the Place of the Moon's Center in the Line of her Way, to every single Minute of Time.

Or, you may take the Semi-diameter of the Disk between your Compasses, and make a Scale thereof, in dividing it, by means of the Sector, in the following manner: Open the Sector so, that the Distance between $61\frac{38}{60}$, the Semi-diameter of the Disk, and $61\frac{38}{60}$ on the Line of Lines, be equal to the Semi-diameter of the Disk. This Distance lay off from

X x x   A to

A to B: then your Sector remaining thus opened, take between your Compasses successively, the parallel Distances of each Division to $61\frac{3}{10}$, and lay them off from A towards B, every 5th of which Number, and your Scale will be divided into Minutes. And by the same Method you may divide each Minute into Parts, serving for Seconds, if your Scale be long enough. Now your Scale being divided, you may make use thereof, for drawing and dividing the Path of the Penumbra, without the Sector For $32\frac{4}{10}$ of these Parts of the Scale, give you the nearest Distance of the Moon's Center to the Center of the Disk. Also $7\frac{7}{10}$ Parts of the said Scale, will be the Distance of the Center of the Penumbra from the Point M, at five a-clock, and $35\frac{1}{10}$ of the Parts of the Scale, will be the Distance from Hour to Hour on the Path of the Penumbra

Now to fix Numbers upon the said Path of the Penumbra, representing the Hours when the Moon's Center will be at the said Hours, at *Rome* and *Genoa*, we must have the Difference of Longitude between *London* and the said two Places given, as also, whether they are to the East or West from *London*, the Difference of Longitude between *London* and *Rome*, is 12 deg 37 min and between *London* and *Genoa*, is 9 deg 37 min they being both to the East from *London* Each of these being reduced to Time, the former will be 50 Minutes, and the latter 38 Minutes, wherefore 5 a-clock for *Rome* on the Moon's Way, must be at 10 min. past 4, for *London*, and 6 a-clock at 10 Minutes past five, &c Understand the same for other Hours and Minutes I have noted the Hours for *Rome* under the Line of the Moon's Way, with *Roman* Characters. Again, 5 a-clock on the Moon's Way for *Genoa*, must be set at 22 Minutes past 5 for *London*, and 6 a-clock, at 22 Minutes past 6, &c. I have noted the Hours for *Genoa* with small Figures over the Line of the Moon's Way

Note, the 10 Minutes, and 22, are each of them the Complement of 50 Minutes, and 38 Minutes to 60 Minutes.

SECTION III

To determine the apparent Time of the Beginning or End of a Solar Eclipse, the Time when the Sun shall be eclipsed to any possible Number of Digits, the Inclination of the Cusps of the Eclipse, and the Time of the visible Conjunction of the Luminaries, in any given Latitude.

THE Paths of *London*, *Rome* and *Genoa*, as also the Path of the Penumbra being drawn and divided, as directed in the two last Sections for the great Eclipse of 1724, which will be a very proper Example for sufficiently explaining this Method, take between your Compasses the Semi-diameter of the Penumbra $32\frac{4}{10}$, from the Line of Lines on the Sector, it being first opened to the Semi-diameter of the Disk $61\frac{1}{10}$, or you may take it from your Scale, which being done, carry one Foot of your Compasses along the Line of the Moon's Way, from the Right-hand to the Left, wherein find such a Point, that if the said Foot be set, the other Foot shall cut the same Hour or Minute, in the Path of the Vertex of any given Place, then the Points in the Paths upon which either of the Feet of your Compasses stand, will shew the Time of the Beginning of the Eclipse at that Place

For example, If you carry the Semi-diameter of the Disk along the Line of the Moon's Way, you will find that one Foot of the Compasses being set at *a*, on the Moon's Way, which is 41 min past 5 in the Afternoon for *London*, the other Foot will fall on the Point *b* on the Path of *London*, which is likewise 41 min past 5 in the Afternoon, wherefore the Beginning of the Eclipse at *London* will be at 41 min past 5 in the Afternoon.

Again If you carry still on the Foot of your Compasses, they remaining yet opened to the Semi-diameter of the Disk, and find another Point on the Moon's Way, whereon if you fix one Point of your Compasses, the other shall cut the Path of the Vertex at the same Hour or Minute, which this stands upon in the Line of the Moon's Way, the Points whereon your Compasses stand in either Path, shall shew the Minute the Eclipse ends.

For example: One Foot of the Compasses being set to *g* in the Path of the Vertex, which is 29 min past 7 in the Afternoon, the other Foot will fall upon the Line of the Moon's Way, at the same Hour and Minute, viz 29 min past 7; therefore the Eclipse ends at *London* 29 min past 7 but take notice, that the Line of the Moon's Way should be continued further out beyond 7 a-clock, that so the Point of the Compasses may fall upon the proper Minute, to wit, 29.

Moreover: If one side of a Square be applied to the Ecliptick H R, and so moved backwards or forwards, until the other side of the said Square cuts the same Hour or Minute in the Path of the Vertex, and Line of the Moon's Way, this same Hour or Minute will be the Time of the visible Conjunction of the Luminaries at the given Place

For example, When the perpendicular side of the Square cuts the Path of the Moon's Way at *e*, which is 37 min past 6, the said side will likewise cut the Path of the Vertex for *London* at *c*, which is 37 min. past 6, therefore the Time of the visible Conjunction of the Luminaries at *London* will be 37 min. after 6.

Draw

Draw the Line *a b*, as alſo the Line ☉ *b*, this ſhall repreſent the vertical Circle, and the Angle ☉ *b a* will be the Angle that the vertical Circle makes with the Line connecting the Centers of the Sun and Moon, at the beginning of the Eclipſe at *London*

Draw the Line *g m*, to wit, join the Points in the Path of the Vertex, and the Path of the Moon's Way, which ſhews the end of the Eclipſe at *London*, and the Line ☉ *g*, then the Angle ☉ *g m*, will be that which the vertical Circle forms with the Line joining the Centers of the Luminaries.

Take the Semi-diameter of the Sun, *viz.* 15$\frac{54}{60}$ between your Compaſſes, either from your Sector, opened as before directed, to the Semi-diameter of the Diſk, or from your Scale, and with that upon the Center *c* (to wit, the Minute in the Path of *London*, whereat the Time of the viſible Conjunction happens) deſcribe a Circle, this Circle ſhall repreſent the Sun

Again, Take the Moon's Semi-diameter 6$\frac{44}{60}$ from your Sector, (remaining opened as before) or your Scale, and upon the Center *e* (to wit, the Minute in the Path of the Moon's Way, whereat the true Conjunction happens at *London*) deſcribe another Circle. This ſhall cut off from the former Circle ſo much as the Sun will be eclipſed, at the Time of the viſible Conjunction

From ☉ draw the Line ☉ *c v* This ſhall repreſent the vertical Circle, and *v* the vertical Point in the Sun's Limb, whereby the Poſition of the Cuſps of the Eclipſe, in reſpect of the Perpendicular paſſing thro the Sun's Center, are plainly and eaſily had

Produce *d c* till it interſect the Moon's Limb in *p*, then ſhall *p q* be the part of the Sun's Diameter eclipſed, at the time of the greateſt Obſcuration at *London* And if the Sun's Diameter be divided into 12 equal Parts, or Digits, you will find *p q* to be 11$\frac{55}{60}$ of thoſe Parts or Digits

Whence at *London*,

			H	M	Aftern
The Beginning of the Eclipſe, *May* 11 1724 at	—	—	05	41	
The viſible Conjunction of the Luminaries	—	—	06	37	
			Digits then 11$\frac{55}{60}$		
The End	—	—	—	07	29

After the ſame manner, the Beginning of the Eclipſe at *Genoa* will be 06 27
Viſible Conjunction, or middle of the Eclipſe — 07 20
The Sun will there ſet eclipſed, and the Eclipſe will be Total.

And the Beginning of the Eclipſe at *Rome* is — 06 42
The viſible Conjunction, or Middle, will there be when the Sun is ſet, and conſequently alſo the End.

I have, as you ſee in the Figure, alſo drawn a fourth Path for *Edinburgh*, whoſe Latitude is 55 deg 56 min and Longitude about 3 deg to the Weſt from *London* Wherefore for each Hour in the Moon's Way for *London*, you muſt account 12 min more for the ſame Hour at *Edinburgh*, that is, for example, 5 a-clock on the Line of the Moon's Way for *Edinburgh*, muſt ſtand at 12 min paſt 5 at *London* Underſtand the ſame for other Hours, &c

And by proceeding according to the Directions before given, you will find,

At *Edinburgh*,			H	M	Aftern.
The Beginning of the Eclipſe at	—	—	—	05	22
The Middle	—	—	{ 06	20	
			{ Dig then 11.		
The End	—	—	—	07	14

Note, The Path of the Moon's Way ought to be continued out further to the Left-hand, in order to determine the Time of the End of the Eclipſe at *Edinburgh*

If you have a mind to know at what Time any poſſible Number of Digits or Minutes ſhall be eclipſed at any Place in the Sun's antecedent or conſequent Limb, divide the Sun's Diameter into Digits or Minutes, and cut off the Parts required to be eclipſed from the Semi-diameter of the Penumbra; then take the remaining part of it between your Compaſſes, and carrying it along the Line of the Moon's Way, find the firſt Point in it, in which placing one Foot, the other will cut the ſame Hour in the Path of the Place that the fixed Foot ſtands upon; then the Hour and Minute in either Path upon which the Feet of your Compaſſes ſtand, will be the Time of that Obſcuration.

As, for example, Suppoſe it was required to find at what Time 6 Digits or $\frac{1}{2}$ of the Sun's Diameter ſhall be eclipſed in his antecedent Limb at *London*: Cut off $\frac{1}{2}$ of the Sun's Semi-diameter from the Semi-diameter of the Penumbra, and carrying the Remainder, as directed, you will find, that if one Point of your Compaſſes be ſet at 6 Hours 9 Minutes in the Afternoon, on the Path of the Moon's Way, the other Point will alſo fall upon the ſame Hour and Minute in the Path of *London*, and therefore the Time when the Sun's antecedent Limb

at

at *London* will be half eclipſed, will be at 9 Minutes paſt 6, and when its conſequent Limb will be half eclipſed, will be at 5 Minutes paſt 7

Fig 2.   Now to determine the Poſition of the Cuſps of the Eclipſe, for example, at *London*: Draw a Circle A D B E, repreſenting the Sun's Body, and the right Line A C B, repreſenting his vertical Diameter   This being done, lay off the Angle ⊙ *b a* upon the Sun's Limb from A to D, draw the Diameter E C D, and the Point D will be the firſt Point of the Sun's Limb obſcured by the Moon at the Beginning of the Eclipſe

Fig 3.   Again, To determine the Poſition and Appearance of the Eclipſe at the Time of the middle, or greateſt Obſcuration, take the Sun's Semi-diameter between your Compaſſes, and upon the Point C, deſcribe a Circle, then draw the vertical Diameter A C B, and make the Angle A C D equal to the Angle *v c p*, and draw the Diameter D C F   This being done, take the Moon's Semi-diameter between your Compaſſes, and having laid off from the Center C to E, the Diſtance *c e* in the firſt Figure, upon the Point E, as a Center, deſcribe an Arc cutting the Sun's Limb, and the Poſition and Appearance of the Eclipſe at the Time of the greateſt Obſcuration, or the middle, at *London*, will be as you ſee in the Figure

Laſtly, To determine the Poſition of the End of the Eclipſe, draw a Circle (as in the *4th* Figure) and croſs it with the vertical Diameter A C B, then make the Angle A C E equal to the Angle ⊙ *g m*, and draw the Diameter E D, then will the Point E on the Limb of the Sun, be that which is laſt obſcured, or whereat the Eclipſe ends

If you have a mind to find the Continuation of total Darkneſs at any Place where the Sun will be totally eclipſed, cut off the Semi-diameter of the Sun, from the Semi-diameter of the Penumbra, and taking the Remainder between your Compaſſes, carry it along the Line of the Moon's Way, and find the firſt Point in it, on which placing one Foot, the other will cut the ſame Hour in the Path of the Place, which Hour note down   Again; Carrying on further the ſame Extent of your Compaſſes, find two Points on the Paths of the Vertex and Moon's Way, which ſhall ſhew the ſame Hour and Minute on them both   This Time alſo note down, then ſubſtract the Time before found from this Time, and the Difference will be the Time of Continuance of total Darkneſs

F I N I S.

11 JU 62

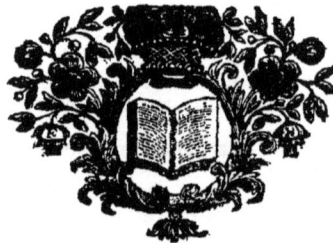

Plate XXVI

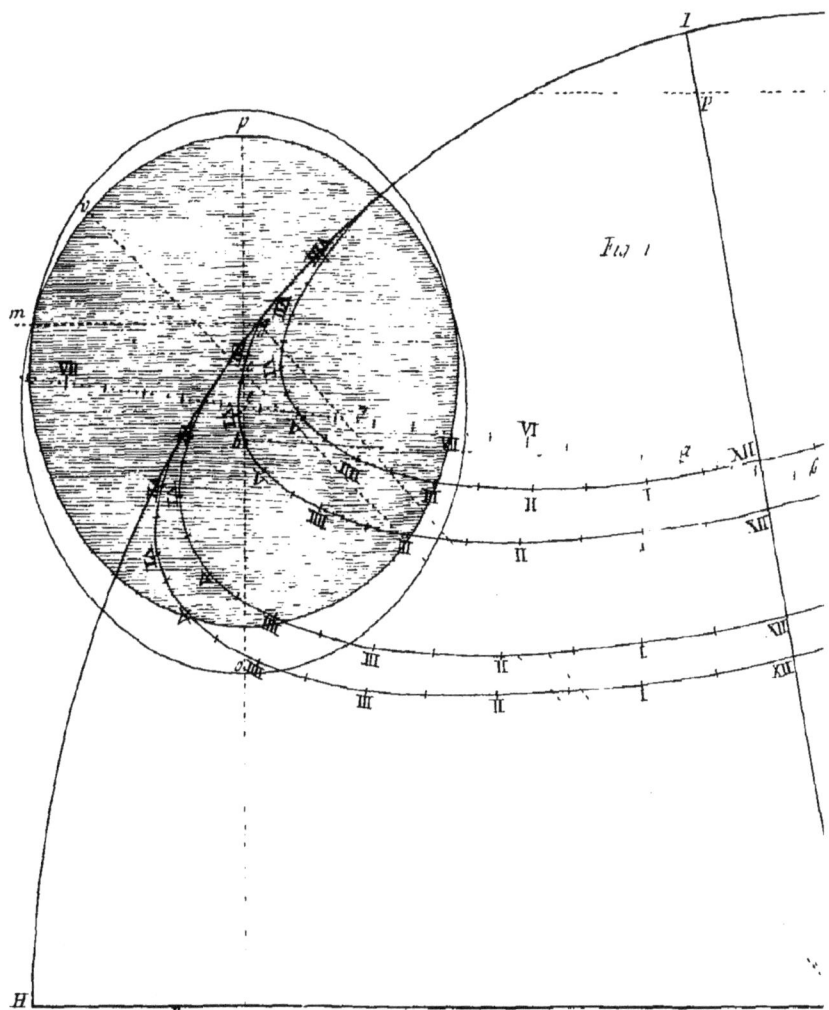

Fig 1

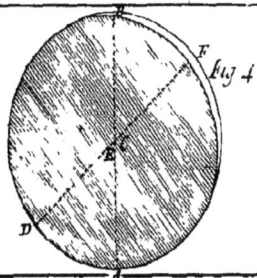

Fig 4

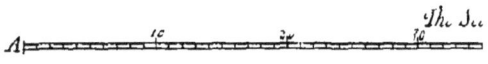

The Sc

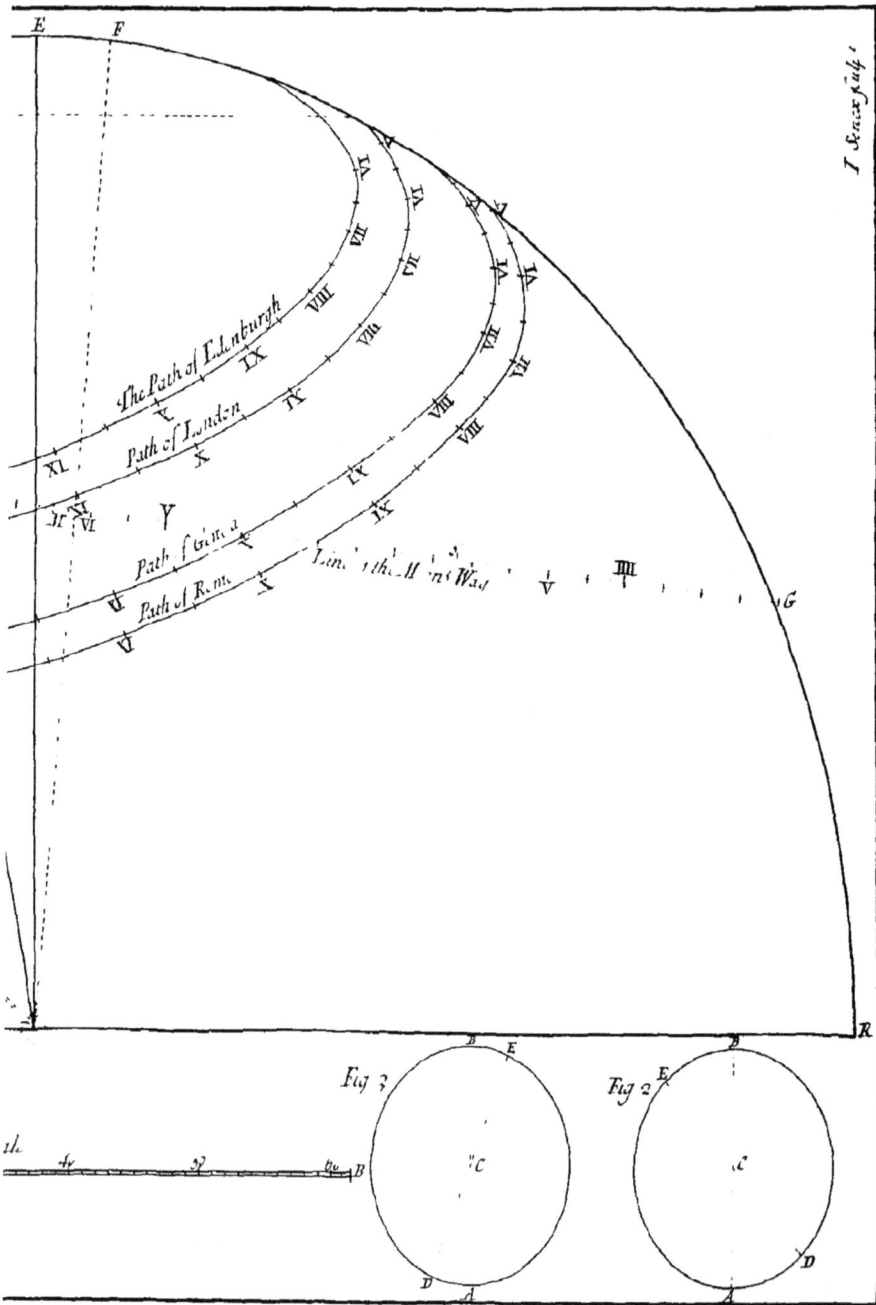

The Path of Edinburgh
Path of London
Path of Geneva
Path of Rome
Line of the Moon's Way

Fig 3.

Fig 2.

Lightning Source UK Ltd.
Milton Keynes UK
UKHW050743030323
417983UK00008B/423

9 781171 002567